MOSBY'S
MANUAL OF
UROLOGIC NURSING

MOSBY'S
M A N U A L   O F
UROLOGIC NURSING

Judith Lerner, RN, BS, CURN

Advisor for Patient Care Program Development,
Department of Urology,
Beth Israel Medical Center,
New York, New York

Zafar Khan, MD, FRCS

Associate Attending Urologist,
Physician in Charge—Urodynamics Laboratory,
Beth Israel Medical Center;
Assistant Professor of Urology,
Mount Sinai School of Medicine of CUNY,
New York, New York

with a foreword by
Elliot Leiter, MD, FACS
Director,
Department of Urology,
Beth Israel Medical Center;
Professor of Urology,
Mount Sinai School of Medicine of CUNY,
New York, New York

with **107** illustrations

The C. V. Mosby Company

ST. LOUIS • TORONTO • LONDON   1982

MOSBY

A TRADITION OF PUBLISHING EXCELLENCE

Editor: Pamela L. Swearingen
Assistant editor: Bess Arends
Manuscript editor: Marjorie L. Sanson
Book design: Nancy Steinmeyer
Cover design: Suzanne Oberholtzer
Production: Barbara Merritt, Linda R. Stalnaker

The C.V. Mosby Company
11830 Westline Industrial Drive, St. Louis, Missouri 63141

Library of Congress Cataloging in Publication Data

Lerner, Judith.
   Mosby's manual of urologic nursing.

   Bibliography: p.
   Includes index.
    1. Urological nursing—Handbooks, manuals, etc.
I. Khan, Zafar. II. Title. III. Title: Manual of
urologic nursing. [DNLM: 1. Urologic diseases—
Nursing. WY 164 L616m]
RC874.7.L47   610.73'69   81-18948
ISBN 0-8016-2947-0   AACR2

GW/VH/VH 9 8 7 6 5 4 3 2 1   05/D/635

To
Charlotte Jones
Head Nurse on Urology, 1966-1979

whose total commitment to quality patient care was an inspiration
to the doctors, to her patients, and,
most of all, to the nurses with whom she worked

Foreword

As medicine and surgery become ever more specialized and complex, the nursing care of patients requires a corresponding increase in expert knowledge and practice. Nowhere is this more evident than in the care of the urologic patient.

The last several years have seen the development of many new operative procedures, such as the implantation of penile prostheses and the application of microsurgical techniques to urologic conditions. Additionally, advances and changes in endoscopic procedures, catheter materials, catheter care, and a host of other critical areas demand that nurses develop and maintain the specialized knowledge and skills that make it possible to render informed, appropriate care.

This book by Ms. Lerner and Dr. Khan fills a gap that has long needed filling. Although information about urologic nursing is available in various publications, nowhere has it been presented in such detail and in such a convenient format. The authors have provided a thorough description of the actual and potential health-related problems that a urology patient encounters and an equally comprehensive approach to all aspects of the nursing management of these problems.

The book dovetails with the medical approach to patient management in that it provides medical and surgical information as the basis for many nursing interventions. It then defines the nursing methods to carry out the physician's orders and even specifies the nurse's contribution in assisting the physician to make necessary modifications in the orders. The brief descriptions of each surgical procedure, with emphasis on how it relates to nursing care (e.g., internal placement of drains, tubes, and conduits) are extremely enlightening for the nurse, especially since this aspect of urology is rarely included in nursing texts. Armed with a basic understanding of medical and surgical treatment, as well as detailed nursing knowledge, the nurse will be able to make decisions effectively and to act more independently. Furthermore, a thorough understanding of the normal expectations in the progress of the patient makes the nurse acutely aware of events for which the physician should be called.

The format is perhaps the most important element of this book. It is designed to facilitate rapid access to information so that questions can be answered as they arise in the clinical setting. It is arranged so that a brief answer to a nursing problem can be found at once. Next to it appears a detailed medical, surgical, or psychologic rationale for those who want a comprehensive understanding of urologic nursing.

I am proud to have had a small part in the preparation of this text; I am sure that it will become the standard by which all future urologic nursing manuals are measured.

Elliot Leiter, MD

Preface

The aim of this book is to provide information on urologic nursing in a rapidly accessible way that corresponds as closely as possible to actual clinical nursing practice. The nursing care plan format is used as the vehicle to convey this information because it provides a systematic approach to nursing actions required to resolve or prevent health-related problems the patient might experience in the course of treatment.

The book is designed for registered nurses who provide care for urology patients, as well as for students who are just being introduced to the field of urology. The fundamental aspects of caring for patients with urologic conditions are covered in the first 21 chapters. The following 30 chapters concentrate on the nursing management associated with a particular surgical procedure or medical diagnosis.

Certain liberties have been taken with the nursing care plan format to present as broad a picture of urologic nursing as possible. For example, a rationale section has been incorporated into the care plan to provide the factual or theoretical basis for the nursing actions. The concept of the nursing diagnosis, defined by the American Nurses' Association as a description of "actual or potential health problems which nurses are capable [of treating] and licensed to treat,"* has been modified slightly to identify more categories of nursing care and to cover as much information as possible. Certain nursing interventions begin with the phrase *be aware that,* which is more of an attitude than an action but is nonetheless an essential element in the systematic implementation of nursing care. Nursing interventions that require a physician's order have been listed in the care plan, followed by the phrase *as ordered.* Although they are not independent nursing actions, they are included to enable the nurse to visualize a more comprehensive system of patient care, and also to identify (and perhaps question) the management of a patient that is not taking place in the accustomed fashion.

Inherent in the use of a nursing care plan to convey a wide scope of information is the problem of individualized patient care. Protocols in medical and surgical management vary throughout the country and from hospital to hospital. In fact, numerous variations often exist within a particular institution. Therefore an attempt has been made to concentrate on the most common methods of patient management. In some cases specific details have been

---

*American Nurses' Association: The American Nurse **8**(11):9, Sept. 1, 1976.

purposely omitted. For example, precise definitions of time frames have been excluded. *Early postoperative period* includes nursing interventions applicable to the time in the patient's recovery when he has the maximum number of tubes, drains, dressings, etc. *Late postoperative period* contains nursing interventions associated with the removal of these mechanisms. *Convalescent period* applies to the last days of the patient's hospitalization and the first weeks at home, when patient teaching is the major focus of nursing care. The priority given to the nursing diagnoses within each time frame will vary according to the assessment of a particular patient's condition.

It would be impossible as well as unnecessary to mention every variation of nursing care for each urologic condition. The goal of this book is to enable nurses to provide comprehensive care by presenting standard nursing interventions for the common, expected problems the urology patient encounters, and to provide nurses with the basis of knowledge with which to formulate an individualized nursing care plan for each of their patients.

Judith Lerner
Zafar Khan

Acknowledgments

Dr. Khan and I would like to express our gratitude to the friends and colleagues who have helped to bring this book to fruition. In particular we wish to thank Dr. Elliot Leiter for his time and conscientious guidance throughout the past year and a half. We are also grateful to Dr. Maria A. Mieza, Attending Physician, Department of Radiology, Beth Israel Medical Center, and Dr. Sun H. Huh, Attending Physician, Radiation Therapy Department, Beth Israel Medical Center, for their help in compiling the x-ray films used as illustrations; Carol Schaeffer and Harry H. Lerner, for their creative assistance in the execution of the artwork; Elaine Doctorow, RN, Material Management Supervisor, Operating Room, Beth Israel Medical Center, for her efforts in locating illustrations from urologic supply companies; the staff at the Beth Israel library, whose cheerful assistance simplified the research considerably; the nurses on 6-Linsky, whose conscientious nursing practices inspired many of the nursing interventions; Professor Louise Jennings of Bellevue Hospital Nursing School, and Dean Gerald Freund of Hunter College of the City University of New York, who greatly facilitated my participation in nursing; and my husband, Dr. Richard Taylor, for his patience, critical evaluation, and knowledgeable suggestions.

Judith Lerner

AUTHORS' NOTE: The fashion in nursing publications today is to avoid consistent use of the pronoun "he" when referring to a patient. Because the great majority of urology patients are male, we have resisted this trend. The pronoun "she" is used only in relation to procedures that are limited to female patients.

Contents

Contents

Contents

WHERE TO FIND THE INFORMATION YOU ARE LOOKING FOR

The primary objective of this book is to make nursing information instantly available. We suggest that readers familiarize themselves with the basic layout of the chapters.*

NURSING DIAGNOSIS This is a statement of a patient's particular health-related problem, actual or potential, that is within the nurse's domain to treat.

Objectives of nursing intervention This is a general summary of the approach(es) used to resolve or prevent the problem.

Expected outcomes This is a list of measurable or observable indicators that the problem has either been obviated or adequately corrected by menas of nursing intervention.

Plan for implementation	Rationale
This column lists nursing activities aimed at resolution or prevention of the problem.	This column provides the medical, surgical, anatomic, psychologic, or theoretical framework on which the nursing interventions are based.

*Chapters 22 through 61 contain care plans with this format. The earlier chapters contain care plans that have been slightly modified to suit the particular topic being discussed.

UNIT I

ANATOMY AND PHYSIOLOGY
OF
THE GENITOURINARY SYSTEMS

Urology is the branch of medicine concerned with the urinary tract in the male and the female, and the reproductive organs of the male. The anatomy and physiology of the structures involved are covered in detail in most anatomy and physiology textbooks. The following discussion serves merely as a review and quick reference so that the nurse is familiar with the normal condition of the systems before having to deal with any pathologically affected organs.

It should be noted that nephrology, the branch of medicine concerned with specific pathologic conditions of the kidney, is a separate but overlapping field of study. Although renal function is a major aspect of both urology and nephrology, the nephrologist is primarily concerned with diseases of the kidney requiring medical management, such as nephritis and renal failure. The urologist treats renal conditions that are usually amenable to surgical correction.

CHAPTER 1

The urinary tract

The urinary tract consists of a pair of kidneys and ureters, a bladder, and a urethra. The entire system is extraperitoneal, that is, it lies behind and below the peritoneum.

The most superior organs are the kidneys, a pair of bean-shaped structures approximately 4½ inches long and 2½ inches wide (Fig. 1-1). The left one is often slightly larger than the right. They lie adjacent to the vertebral column at the level of the lower thoracic and upper lumbar vertebrae. Each is surrounded by perirenal fat and connective tissue (Gerota's fascia) with the adrenal gland lying on the upper pole of each kidney. Approximately half of

each kidney lies within the lower rib cage. The kidneys' lateral borders are convex, and the medial borders are concave. This indented portion of each kidney is the hilum, the area where blood vessels enter and leave the kidney. The ureter is also attached to the kidney at the hilum, posterior to the blood vessels. The renal arteries arise from the abdominal aorta and branch into smaller vessels within the kidney, bringing a third of the body's blood through the kidneys every minute. Each kidney consists of an outer layer, the cortex, and an inner portion, the medulla; they are often referred to as the renal parenchyma (Fig. 1-2, *A*).

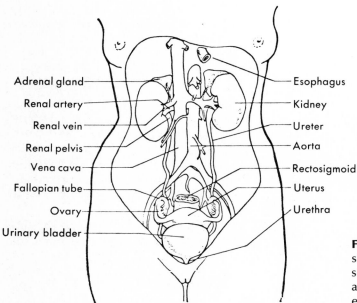

Adrenal gland — Esophagus
Renal artery — Kidney
Renal vein — Ureter
Renal pelvis — Aorta
Vena cava — Rectosigmoid
Fallopian tube — Uterus
Ovary — Urethra
Urinary bladder

Fig. 1-1. Female urinary tract. Right kidney usually is slightly lower than left. Ureters pass anterior to iliac vessels and posterior to uterine arteries. (From Winter, C., and Morel, A.: Nursing care of patients with urologic diseases, ed. 4, St. Louis, 1977, The C.V. Mosby Co.)

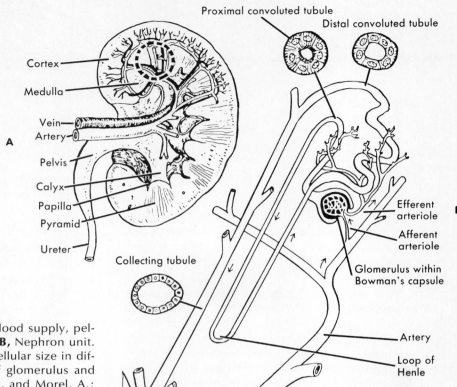

Fig. 1-2. Anatomy of kidney. **A,** Renal blood supply, pelvis, upper ureter, medulla, and cortex. **B,** Nephron unit. Note variations in luminal caliber and cellular size in different parts of tubule. Blood supply of glomerulus and tubule is also shown. (From Winter, C., and Morel, A.: Nursing care of patients with urologic diseases, ed. 4, St. Louis, 1977, The C.V. Mosby Co.)

The production of urine begins with the flow of blood from an afferent arteriole into the basic functional unit of the kidney, the nephron (Fig. 1-2, *B*). There are approximately 1 million of these microscopic structures in each kidney. A nephron consists of a glomerulus, a capsule (Bowman's capsule), and a tubule. The glomerulus is a capillary tuft through which a protein-free filtrate is removed from the blood. The capsule is an invaginated sac surrounding the glomerulus into which the filtrate flows. The tubule is an elongated, convoluted continuation of the capsule. The filtered blood leaves the nephron via the efferent arteriole, while the filtrate flows through the various portions of the tubule (the proximal convoluted tubule, the loop of Henle, the distal convoluted tubule, and the collecting tubule). Through a process of selective reabsorption and secretion at various points along the tubule, the filtrate is modified to form the final product, urine, which flows from the collecting tubules into the calyces and the renal pelvis. On gross observation it is these tubules which form the renal pyramids, whose bases are in the renal cortex and whose apexes form the papillae. Through the pores of the papillae, urine oozes into the minor calyces, which converge into two or three major calyces. These in turn unite to form the renal pelvis, the funnel-shaped portion of the kidney, which is contiguous with the ureter as it leaves the renal hilum. (It should be remembered that elimination of waste products is just one function of the kidney. Other functions include hormonal control of blood pressure; regulation of extracellular fluids, electrolytes, pH balance, and red blood cell production; and metabolism of vitamin D.)

Urine is propelled through the ureters, two hollow tubes approximately 12 inches long and ¼ inch wide, to the bladder via peristaltic action. At the ureterovesical junction the ureters run obliquely through the wall of the bladder for approximately ½ inch before opening into the lower portion of the bladder.

The bladder is a hollow muscular organ that normally lies within the pelvic cavity, but, when distended, it projects above the symphysis pubis. Its normal capacity is approximately 500 ml, but it is capable of considerable distention and may in some cases hold over 1000 ml of urine. Within the lower

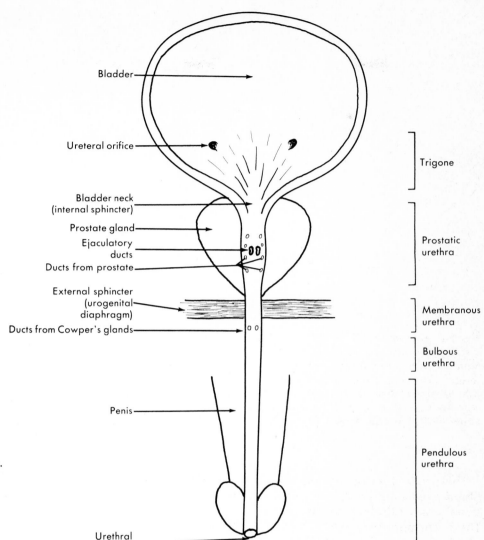

Fig. 1-3. Male bladder and urethra.

part of the bladder lies the trigone, a triangular area on the posterior wall delineated by the ureteral orifices and the bladder neck. Although there is no separate anatomic sphincter at the outlet of the bladder, the bladder neck is sometimes referred to as the internal sphincter, which has a major function in the process of micturition. Contraction of the bladder, and the subsequent expression of urine, is under voluntary and involuntary control. The nerves controlling the voiding reflex (i.e., the part of the mechanism that is independent of conscious control) originate in the sacral area of the spinal cord. The nerve supply to the bladder involves sympathetic and parasympathetic fibers.

On contraction of the bladder, urine flows through the bladder neck and into the urethra. The male urethra is approximately 8 inches long and is divided into four sections: prostatic, membranous, bulbous, and pendulous (Fig. 1-3). Numerous glands empty into the different portions. In the prostatic urethra these include the ejaculatory ducts from the seminal vesicles and ducts from the prostate gland. In the distal portions of the urethra Cowper's glands and Littre's glands produce secretions. In the female the urethra is approximately 2 inches long. Its meatus opens between the labia minora, anterior to the vaginal orifice (Fig. 1-4). Paraurethral glands and Skene's glands open into the female urethra.

5

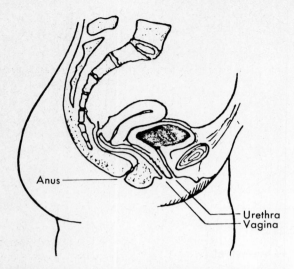

Fig. 1-4. Sagittal view of female pelvis showing relationship of urethra, vagina, and anus. (From Winter, C., and Morel, A.: Nursing care of patients with urologic diseases, ed. 4, St. Louis, 1977, The C.V. Mosby Co.)

The external urinary sphincter surrounds the membranous urethra in the male and the distal third of the urethra in the female. It is also known as the urogenital diaphragm and is a muscular structure under voluntary control. It normally functions in synchrony with the contraction of the bladder and relaxation of the bladder neck, as urine is expressed from the body.

CHAPTER 2

The male reproductive organs

The reproductive system of the male includes two testicles, two epididymides, two vasa deferentia, two seminal vesicles, a prostate gland, and a penis. The testicles are a pair of oval bodies measuring approximately 2 inches in length and 1 inch in width. Each is covered by a dense fibrous tissue (tunica albuginea) and is suspended from the spermatic cord within the scrotum. Muscle fibers in the scrotum and spermatic cord (the cremaster and dartos muscles) control small changes in the distance of the testicles from the body proper, responding to cold and other stimuli by contracting and pulling the testicles close to the perineum (cremasteric reflex).

Within the testicles testosterone and spermatozoa are produced. Testosterone is secreted by the Leydig cells into the bloodstream. Spermatogenesis takes place in the seminiferous tubules in the testicles, under the control of gonadotropic hormones and testosterone. It takes approximately 70 days for immature germ cells to become mature sperm. During the process, spermatozoa from each testicle are transferred into the corresponding epididymis, a cluster of long, narrow coiled tubules, tightly packed together along the posterior surface of each testicle (Fig. 2-1). Here the sperm undergo final maturation.

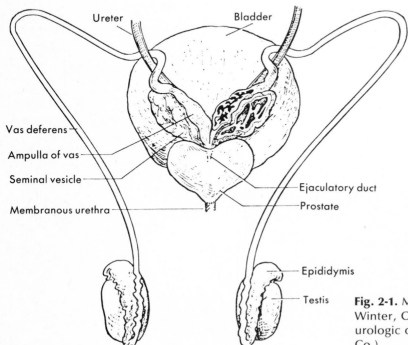

Ureter

Bladder

Vas deferens

Ampulla of vas

Seminal vesicle

Membranous urethra

Ejaculatory duct

Prostate

Epididymis

Testis

Fig. 2-1. Male reproductive system, posterior view. (From Winter, C., and Morel, A.: Nursing care of patients with urologic diseases, ed. 4, St. Louis, 1977, The C.V. Mosby Co.)

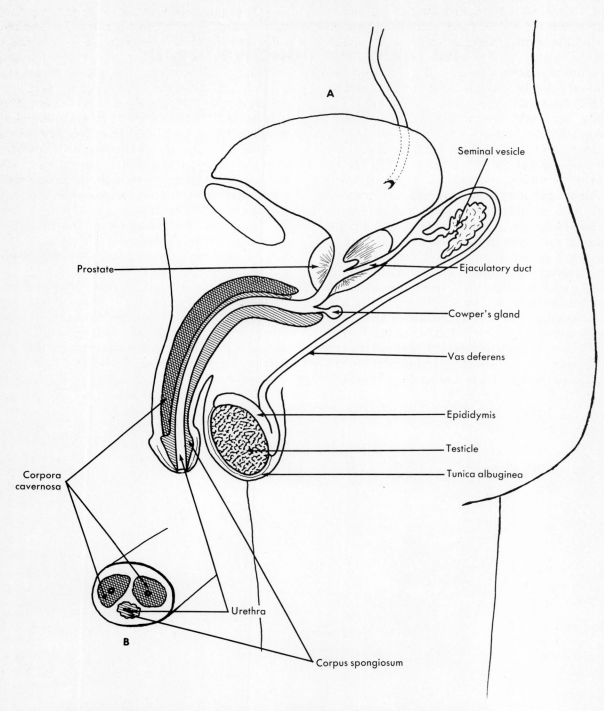

A

Seminal vesicle

Prostate

Ejaculatory duct

Cowper's gland

Vas deferens

Epididymis

Testicle

Tunica albuginea

Corpora cavernosa

B

Urethra

Corpus spongiosum

Fig. 2-2. Male genitourinary tract. **A,** Sagittal view. **B,** Cross section of penis showing erectile bodies.

Sperm from each testicle are then stored in the corresponding epididymis and vas deferens. The vas is a duct that conveys the sperm along the spermatic cord and into the pelvic cavity, where it joins the duct from the seminal vesicles to form the ejaculatory duct.

The seminal vesicles are a pair of structures whose secretions, along with the secretions from the prostate gland (located at the base of the bladder, surrounding the urethra), and the Cowper's glands (opening into the bulbous urethra), are combined with sperm and are released into the urethra as semen during emission. These secretions contribute to the transportation and the vitality of the sperm.

The distal portion of the urethra traverses the penis, an erectile structure composed of two lateral masses of erectile tissue (corpora cavernosa), and a ventral segment of erectile tissue (corpus spongiosum), bound together by fibrous tissue and covered with skin (Fig. 2-2). At the distal end is the cone-shaped glans penis, covered by a thin semimucous membrane and skinfold (prepuce or foreskin). Sexual arousal, as well as other stimuli, produces engorgement and distention of these tissues. The process of erection is thought to be controlled by parasympathetic nerve fibers. Emission (the release of seminal fluid into the urethra) and ejaculation (the rhythmic propulsion of semen out of the urethra at the time of orgasm) are thought to be controlled by the sympathetic nervous system.

References and bibliography

BIBLIOGRAPHY

Gardner, E., Gray, D.J., and O'Rahilly, R.: Anatomy—a regional study of human structure, ed. 4, Philadelphia, 1975, W.B. Saunders Co.

Lapides, J.: Fundamentals of urology, Philadelphia, 1976, W.B. Saunders Co.

Miller, M.A., and Leavell, L.C.: Kimber-Gray-Stockpole's anatomy and physiology, ed. 17, New York, 1977, MacMillan Publishing Co.

Smith, D.R.: General urology, ed. 9, Los Angeles, 1978, Lange Medical Publications.

Winter, C.C., and Morel, A.: Nursing care of patients with urologic diseases, ed. 4, St. Louis, 1977, The C.V. Mosby Co.

UNIT II

UROLOGIC DIAGNOSTIC PROCEDURES

Nurses frequently find diagnostic procedures to be the least familiar element in the management of a hospitalized patient because the majority of the procedures are administered in specialized departments. Although floor nurses usually are not directly responsible for the quality of the outcome of the tests, the preprocedure and postprocedure care of the patient is usually entirely within their domain. Understanding what happens to the patient while he is off the unit (and even understanding what happens to a specimen once it has been produced) enables nurses to provide the care that is most conducive to accurate test results, minimal side effects, and the absence of anxiety.

Certain guidelines apply to diagnostic procedures in general. The most fundamental is the scheduling of the procedures so that the effects of one do not distort the results of another. If a patient is to be scheduled for radiologic studies of the gastrointestinal tract as well as the urinary tract, the urinary tract x-ray examination should be performed first because residual barium in the gastrointestinal tract might interfere with visualization of the urinary tract. Furthermore, all blood and urine specimens for renal function tests should be collected prior to any x-ray examination requiring the use of contrast material, since its presence in the patient's blood and urine will cause temporary distortions of the test results.

If the patient is extremely anxious about a procedure despite nursing interventions to reduce the anxiety, the nurse should request that the physician order a sedative to be administered prior to the procedure, even if one is not usually required. This may also apply in cases where the patient is confused or for some other reason is unable to lie quietly for the length of time required to complete the test.

Any procedures requiring fasting and bowel preparations must be modified for children under 7 years of age. Food is usually withheld for only 4 to 6 hours, and cathartics are omitted. Sometimes an enema is given. If gas is found to be obscuring visualization of the urinary tract on the preliminary x-ray examination, a few ounces of formula or carbonated beverage may be given to push the gas aside.

A signed, informed consent document must be obtained from the patient (or, in the case of a minor, from a parent or legal guardian) prior to most, if not all, radiologic procedures, endoscopic manipulation, or surgery. In most cases this is done in the department where the procedure is to take place and **must** be done prior to the administration of any sedatives or analgesics.

The following unit consists of a small nursing care plan for each of the diagnostic procedures that might be performed on a urology patient by a physician.* The final chapter contains a list of the laboratory tests most commonly used in urology, a description of their function in diagnosing urologic conditions, and an enumeration of the nursing implications for each test.

---

*Biopsy of bladder tumor, prostatic nodule, and testicle (for infertility) appear in the unit on surgery for the particular organ.

CHAPTER 3

Radiologic studies

Plain film of the abdomen (kidneys, ureters, bladder [KUB]) (Fig. 3-1)

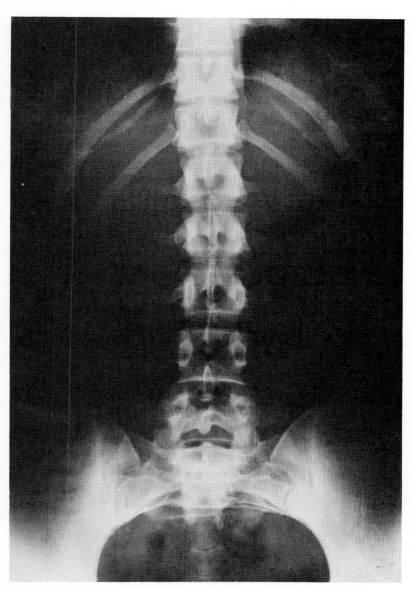

Fig. 3-1. Normal KUB x-ray film.

Purpose   After the initial history has been taken and a physical examination has been performed, a KUB film is frequently the next step in further evaluation. Although a diagnosis can rarely be made on the basis of this film alone, certain diagnoses can be excluded, and information can be obtained that will suggest the direction of further investigation. One of the most common indications for a KUB film is flank pain of acute onset. The x-ray film may show a radiopaque stone somewhere along the course of the ureters. Information about the size of the kidneys and the presence of masses may also be obtained, but ordinarily this evaluation requires contrast material and tomography. Abnormalities not related to the urinary tract that may be detected from a KUB examination may lead the physician to explore other avenues to determine the cause of the patient's complaints.

Relative contraindication   Pregnancy

NURSING DIAGNOSIS: Potential for adverse effects related to a plain film of the abdomen (KUB)

Objectives of nursing intervention
- Elimination of patient anxiety by means of psychologic preparation for the procedure
- Adequate cleansing of bowel (if ordered)

Expected outcomes
- Patient relaxed and cooperative throughout the procedure
- X-ray picture in optimal condition for diagnostic evaluation

Plan for implementation	Rationale
PHYSICAL PREPARATION	
None.	
or	
Provide a mild laxative as ordered on the evening before the procedure.	The physician may want the colon relatively empty of stool to obtain maximum visualization, especially if the patient is suspected of having urolithiasis.
PSYCHOLOGIC PREPARATION	
Explain to the patient what to expect during the procedure.	Prior knowledge of a procedure helps to decrease anxiety and enables the patient to participate more effectively in the procedure.
The patient will be placed in a supine position on the x-ray table and will be told to hold his breath when the picture is taken. The procedure takes a few seconds, and the patient will feel nothing. The exposure to radiation is minimal.	
POSTPROCEDURE CARE	
None required.	

Intravenous pyelogram (IVP) (Fig. 3-2) and nephrotomogram

Purpose   An intravenous pyelogram provides more detailed anatomic and physiologic visualization of the kidneys, ureters, and bladder than does the plain KUB film. Therefore it is a useful study whenever anatomic distortion is expected, for example, kidney and bladder tumors, urinary calculi, diverticula, vesical enlargement, and functional disturbances. Ability to excrete contrast medium gives a general reflection of renal function. The transport of the contrast medium through the ureters and the emptying of the bladder (postvoiding film) give valuable information about the entire function of the urinary tract.

Nephrotomography is usually performed with intravenous pyelography to provide more detailed information about structural abnormalities in the kidney. These x-ray films are of particular value because they focus on different planes of the kidney for precise visualization (as opposed to an IVP, which provides visualization of all depths at once).

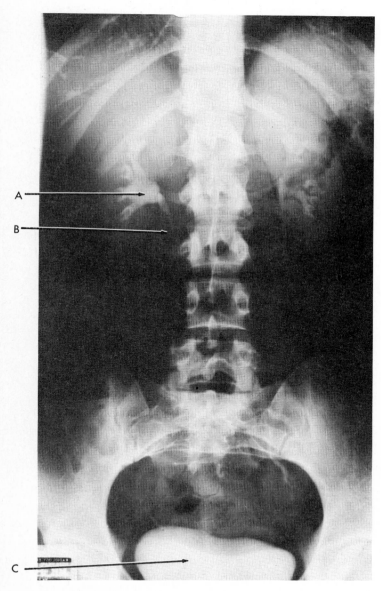

Fig. 3-2. Normal intravenous pyelogram. *A,* Renal pelvis; *B,* ureter; *C,* bladder.

| **Relative contraindications** | Pregnancy
Known or suspected hypersensitivity to compounds containing iodine
Renal failure
Uncontrolled diabetes mellitus
Multiple myeloma |

NURSING DIAGNOSIS: Potential for adverse effects related to intravenous pyelography

| **Objectives of nursing intervention** | Adequate cleansing of bowel
Elimination of patient anxiety by means of psychologic preparation for the procedure
Prevention or early detection and correction of complications |

| **Expected outcomes** | X-ray film shows clear view of the urinary tract
Patient relaxed and cooperative throughout the procedure
Urinary output normal in quantity and concentration within 3 hours after procedure |

Plan for implementation	**Rationale**
PHYSICAL PREPARATION	
1. Administer cathartic, as ordered. Castor oil is usually ordered to be administered in the evening prior to the x-ray examination.	The bowel must be relatively empty for adequate visualization of the urinary tract.
a. Explain the reason for the cathartic.	Many patients will refuse castor oil unless they receive a thorough explanation of why it is necessary.
b. Make the taste as palatable as possible by mixing it with soda, fruit juice, and/or crushed ice.	Most people find the taste of castor oil extremely unpleasant.
c. Place call-light within easy reach of the patient.	Castor oil usually produces a strong, and sometimes sudden, cathartic effect. Patients, particularly elderly ones,
d. Provide easy access to bathroom or bedpan.	may be incontinent if they cannot get to the bathroom or have a bedpan quickly.
2. Confirm with the physician any order for a cathartic if the patient has acute bowel inflammation, peptic ulcer, colitis, a colostomy, a ureterosigmoidostomy, or is very debilitated.	Catharsis is often contraindicated if these conditions are present because of the risk of gastric or intestinal irritation and perforation in the former conditions, and inability of the patient to withstand dehydration in the latter condition.
3. Prohibit oral intake after midnight prior to the procedure, as ordered.	The absence of solid food in the stomach reduces the risk of vomiting if the patient becomes nauseated from the contrast material. Also, mild dehydration results in better concentration of the contrast material and thus better visualization of the urinary tract on x-ray examination.
4. Reduce intravenous infusion rate if ordered.	
5. Confirm with the physician any order that would result in mild dehydration of the patient if any of the following conditions exist: a. The patient is elderly. b. The patient has severe diabetes mellitus c. The patient has multiple myeloma. d. The patient has any serious renal disease.	When any of these conditions are present, the patient may go into renal failure if dehydrated prior to IVP

Plan for implementation	**Rationale**

PSYCHOLOGIC PREPARATION

Explain to the patient what to expect during the procedure:	Prior knowledge of a procedure helps to decrease anxiety and enables the patient to participate more effectively in the procedure.
The patient will be given an intravenous injection of a contrast medium, and x-ray pictures will be taken in supine and oblique positions. There may be some discomfort during the injection, such as a warm flush, a salty taste in the mouth, nausea, and mild burning at the infusion site. In some cases a compression band will be placed around his waist to facilitate good visualization of the ureters.	
At the end of the procedure he will be asked to void, and one more picture will be taken. He should try to empty his bladder completely when he voids.	Usually a postvoiding film is taken to assess the presence of residual urine in the bladder.
The procedure takes approximately 30 minutes, but delayed pictures may be taken after a few hours. The exposure to radiation from one IVP series is not significant.	Initially a KUB is taken because a radiopaque stone may be obscured by contrast medium. After the dye is injected, pictures are taken at various intervals (e.g., 30 seconds, 1, 2, and 15 minutes), and right and left oblique films are taken, followed by a postvoiding film. Sometimes **nephrotomography** also is done for better visualization of the kidneys.

POSTPROCEDURE CARE

1. Be alert for indications of a hypersensitive reaction to the contrast medium. These include pruritus, sneezing, wheezing, dyspnea, and flushed skin.	Allergic reactions most commonly occur within a few minutes after administration of the contrast medium. It is unlikely that they will occur after the procedure is completed. They range from mild, transient rhinitis to severe anaphylaxis. Prompt recognition and treatment may be life saving.
2. If any of the above occur: a. Notify the physician. b. Have epinephrine, antihistamines, and corticosteroids on hand for rapid administration and a fully equipped emergency tray ("crash cart") readily available. c. Have oxygen readily available.	
3. Correct dehydration by encouraging oral fluids and increasing intravenous infusion rate as ordered.	Contrast medium is an osmotic diuretic. Therefore it produces moderate dehydration, which may be significant, especially if the patient was dehydrated prior to the procedure.
4. Expect the urine to be dark amber until the patient is well hydrated.	Concentrated urine will be present until dehydration is corrected.
5. Expect the specific gravity of the urine to be higher than normal for a few hours after the injection of the contrast medium.	During this period the urine contains contrast medium, which has a relatively high specific gravity.
6. Notify the physician if urine output is less than 30 ml per hour despite adequate intake.	The patient may be in renal failure, an uncommon but serious complication of intravenous pyelography.

Cystogram

Purpose The main function of a cystogram is to identify bladder disorders, such as tumors and diverticula. The presence of ureteral reflux of urine may also be visualized on this x-ray film.

Relative contraindications Pregnancy
Recent bladder surgery
Allergy to contrast medium is **not necessarily** a contraindication because it is not administered systemically

---

NURSING DIAGNOSIS: Potential for adverse effects related to cystography

Objective of nursing intervention Elimination of patient anxiety by means of psychologic preparation for the procedure

Expected outcomes Patient relaxed and cooperative throughout the procedure
X-ray pictures in optimal condition for diagnostic evaluation

Plan for implementation	Rationale
PHYSICAL PREPARATION	
None required.	
PSYCHOLOGIC PREPARATION	
Explain to the patient what to expect during the procedure.	Prior knowledge of a procedure helps to decrease anxiety and enables the patient to participate more effectively in the procedure.
A catheter will be inserted into the patient's urethra, and contrast medium (or air) will be instilled through the catheter into the bladder. X-ray films will be taken at various stages of filling in right and left oblique views, and an additional film will be taken after drainage of the medium. It should take approximately 10 minutes. The exposure to radiation is minimal.	
POSTPROCEDURE CARE	
None required.	

Voiding cystourethrogram (antegrade urethrogram)

Purpose   A voiding cystourethrogram provides all the information that a cystogram gives (see previous description) and identifies urethral disorders. Therefore urethral valves, strictures, and diverticula will also be visualized on this type of x-ray examination.

Relative contraindications   Pregnancy
Recent bladder or urethral surgery
Severe inflammatory condition of the urethra or bladder
Allergy to contrast medium is **not necessarily** a contraindication because it is not administered systemically

---

NURSING DIAGNOSIS: Potential for adverse effects related to voiding cystourethrography (antegrade urethrography)

Objective of nursing intervention   Elimination of patient anxiety by means of psychologic preparation for the procedure.

Expected outcomes   Patient relaxed and cooperative throughout the procedure
X-ray pictures in optimal condition for diagnostic evaluation

Plan for implementation	Rationale

PHYSICAL PREPARATION

None required.

PSYCHOLOGIC PREPARATION

Explain to the patient what to expect during the procedure.	Prior knowledge of a procedure helps to decrease anxiety and enables the patient to participate more effectively in the procedure.
A catheter will be inserted into the patient's urethra, and contrast medium will be instilled through the catheter into the bladder. X-ray films will be taken at various stages of filling in right and left oblique views. The catheter will then be removed and the patient will be asked to void. Pictures will be taken as the patient voids. The procedure takes approximately 15 minutes. The exposure to radiation is minimal.	

POSTPROCEDURE CARE

None required.

Retrograde urethrogram

Purpose   A retrograde urethrogram enables visualization of urethral strictures and diverticula and provides information about the presence of urethral injuries.

Relative contraindications   Pregnancy
Recent urethral surgery
Severe inflammatory condition of the urethra, bladder, or prostate
Allergy to contrast medium is **not necessarily** a contraindication because it is not administered systemically

---

NURSING DIAGNOSIS: Potential for adverse effects related to retrograde urethrography

Objective of nursing intervention   Elimination of patient anxiety by means of psychologic preparation for the procedure

Expected outcomes   Patient relaxed and cooperative throughout the procedure
X-ray pictures in optimal condition for diagnostic evaluation

Plan for implementation	Rationale
PHYSICAL PREPARATION	
None required.	
PSYCHOLOGIC PREPARATION	
Explain to the patient what to expect during the procedure.	Prior knowledge of a procedure helps to decrease anxiety and enables the patient to participate more effectively in the procedure.
The contrast medium is instilled into the urethra through a wide-mouth syringe. A special clamp is applied to hold the syringe and contrast material in place, and one or more x-ray pictures are taken. The clamp is then removed and the contrast medium spills out. The procedure takes approximately 15 minutes. The exposure to radiation is minimal.	
POSTPROCEDURE CARE	
None required.	

Renal angiogram

Purpose
The purpose of a renal angiogram is to visualize the vasculature of the kidneys. It provides the physician with information about the renal arteries and their branches and about the presence of renal masses, aneurysms, and congenital abnormalities of the kidneys.

Relative contraindications
Pregnancy
Known or suspected hypersensitivity to compounds containing iodine
Renal failure
Uncontrolled diabetes mellitus
Multiple myeloma

NURSING DIAGNOSIS: Potential for adverse effects related to renal angiography

Objectives of nursing intervention

Adequate cleansing of bowel

Elimination of patient anxiety by means of psychologic preparation for the procedure

Correction of dehydration after the procedure

Prevention or early detection and correction of complications

Expected outcomes

X-ray film shows clear view of the urinary tract

Patient relaxed and cooperative throughout the procedure

Absence of severe allergic reaction, hemorrhage, femoral artery occlusion, nausea, or abdominal discomfort

Urinary output normal in quantity and concentration within 3 hours after the procedure

Plan for implementation	Rationale
PHYSICAL PREPARATION	
1. Administer cathartic as ordered. Castor oil is usually ordered to be administered in the evening prior to the x-ray examination.	The bowel must be relatively empty for adequate visualization of the urinary tract.
a. Explain the reason for the cathartic.	Many patients will refuse castor oil unless they receive a thorough explanation of why it is necessary.
b. Make the taste as palatable as possible by mixing it with soda, fruit juice, and/or crushed ice.	Most people find the taste of castor oil extremely unpleasant.
c. Place call-light within easy reach of the patient.	Castor oil usually produces a strong and sometimes sudden cathartic effect. Patients, particularly elderly ones, may be incontinent if they cannot get to the bathroom or have a bedpan quickly.
d. Provide easy access to bathroom or bedpan.	
2. Confirm with the physician any order for a cathartic if the patient has acute bowel inflammation, peptic ulcer, colitis, a colostomy, ureterosigmoidostomy, or is very debilitated.	Catharsis is often contraindicated if these conditions are present because of the risk of gastric or intestinal irritation and perforation in the former conditions, and inability of the patient to withstand dehydration in the latter condition.

NOTE: A technique being introduced in the 1980s—digitalized intravenous angiography (DIVA)—will most likely replace renal angiography. A bolus of contrast material is injected into the central venous system via a central line, and a series of radiographs is made of the appropriate area. These images are displayed on and photographed from a television screen. The images are less sharp than those from standard angiography, but the procedure has the advantages of being faster and less expensive, and the problems of arterial emboli and bleeding from the puncture site are eliminated. The nursing care plan will be similar to that for an intravenous pyelogram unless unforeseen complications arise as the technique becomes more widespread.

Plan for implementation	**Rationale**
3. Prohibit oral intake after midnight prior to the procedure, as ordered.	The absence of solid food in the stomach reduces the risk of vomiting if the patient becomes nauseated from the contrast material. Also, mild dehydration results in better concentration of the contrast material and thus better visualization of the urinary tract on x-ray examination.
4. Reduce intravenous infusion rate if ordered.	
5. Confirm with the physician any order that would result in mild dehydration of the patient if any of the following conditions exist: a. The patient is elderly. b. The patient has severe diabetes mellitus. c. The patient has multiple myeloma. d. The patient has any serious renal disease.	When any of these conditions are present, the patient may go into renal failure if dehydrated prior to renal angiography.
6. Shave the pubic and groin area.	This reduces the number of bacteria near the cutdown site.
7. Be certain that a specimen of the patient's blood has been ordered for typing and cross-matching.	Hemorrhage occasionally occurs from this procedure. Blood should be available for the patient in case a transfusion is needed.
8. Determine location of pedal pulses; place an indelible mark over the area on each foot and make a note of the characteristics of the pulses in the patient's chart.	Pedal pulses are sometimes difficult to locate on certain individuals. Marking the exact location beforehand can expedite the nursing assessment after the procedure. Any changes in the pulse are easily identifiable if a baseline record is available.
9. Have the patient void immediately before the procedure.	The contrast material is an osmotic diuretic. Therefore the patient's bladder will fill relatively quickly during the procedure. Since this is a long procedure, starting with an empty bladder will avoid unnecessary discomfort.

Plan for implementation	**Rationale**

PSYCHOLOGIC PREPARATION

Explain to the patient what to expect during the procedure.

The patient will usually be given an injection of an analgesic (e.g., Demerol, 75 mg) prior to the procedure. A local anesthetic may also be administered to the area of the femoral artery. A needle will be inserted into the femoral artery, and a catheter will be inserted and advanced into the renal artery under fluoroscopic control. Contrast medium will be instilled into the renal artery, and x-ray pictures will be taken in rapid sequence as the medium passes through the renal vasculature. The patient may feel some discomfort while the catheter is being passed and may experience a hot flush, nausea, and a salty taste when the contrast medium is instilled. The catheter is then removed and a compression dressing is applied. The procedure takes approximately 2 hours.

Prior knowledge of a procedure helps to decrease anxiety and enables the patient to participate more effectively in the procedure.

POSTPROCEDURE CARE

1. Be alert for indications of a hypersensitive reaction to the contrast medium. These include pruritus, sneezing, wheezing, dyspnea, and flushed skin.

Allergic reactions most commonly occur within a few minutes after administration of the contrast medium. It is unlikely that they will occur after the procedure is completed. They range from mild, transient rhinitis to severe anaphylaxis. Prompt recognition and treatment may be life saving.

2. If any of the above occur:
   a. Notify the physician.
   b. Have epinephrine, antihistamines, and corticosteroids on hand for rapid administration, and a fully equipped emergency tray ("crash cart") readily available.
   c. Have oxygen readily available.

3. Be aware that hemorrhage is a potential complication and take the following precautions:
   a. Check the patient's pulse and blood pressure frequently (every 15 minutes for the first hour, every 30 minutes for the second hour, every hour for the next 4 hours, and then every 4 hours until the next day).
   b. Notify the physician if there is a drop in blood pressure of more than 20 mm Hg. (Slight fluctuation of the blood pressure is expected after this procedure due to irritation of the renal vasculature from the contrast medium).
   c. Check the dressing frequently (the same frequency as the blood pressure monitoring).

   d. Notify the physician if there is any bleeding or swelling at the puncture site. If either of the above is noted, apply pressure directly over the area.

Puncturing an artery can result in a hemorrhage. It the patient's clotting mechanisms are inadequate, a considerable amount of blood may be lost within a short time.

Initially a pressure dressing is placed over the puncture site. By the time the patient returns to the floor from the x-ray suite, it is usually replaced by an adhesive bandage. Although frank bleeding sometimes does occur, the development of a hematoma (bleeding into the surrounding tissue) is more common.

Plan for implementation	**Rationale**

4. Be aware that impairment of the circulation to the leg on the affected side is a potential complication, and take the following precautions:
  a. Monitor the temperature and color of the foot on the affected side by comparing with the uninvolved extremity.
  b. Monitor pedal pulse on the affected side and compare with baseline data.
  c. Notify the physician if the foot on the affected side becomes cold or pale or the pedal pulse is absent.
	Occlusion of the femoral artery or smaller arteries in the leg due to thrombosis and/or embolization of atheromatous plaques can severely impair circulation to the lower extremity. Prompt surgical intervention may be required.

5. Correct dehydration by encouraging oral fluids and by increasing intravenous infusion rates as ordered.	Contrast medium is an osmotic diuretic. Therefore it produces moderate dehydration, which may be significant, especially if the patient was dehydrated prior to the procedure.
6. Expect the urine to be dark amber until the patient is well hydrated.	Concentrated urine will be present until dehydration is corrected.
7. Expect the specific gravity to be higher than normal for a few hours after the injection of contrast medium.	During this period the urine contains contrast material, which has a relatively high specific gravity.
8. Ensure that the patient stays in bed for 8 to 12 hours after the procedure.	Bed rest is usually ordered because of the possibility of hemorrhage and unstable blood pressure.

9. If the patient complains of flank pain:
  a. Notify the physician at once.
  b. Obtain a urine specimen for a microscopic hematuria test.
  c. Be alert for anuria (if flank pain is bilateral).
	Flank pain and microscopic hematuria may indicate renal artery thrombosis, an unusual but potential complication of renal angiogram. If the condition is bilateral, anuria will occur. It requires surgical intervention.

10. Notify the physician if the patient complains of abdominal pain.	Although this may be a transient reaction to the contrast medium and therefore not serious, it may also indicate interference with the patient's visceral circulation.
11. Do not discontinue an intravenous line (even if the patient is tolerating food well) for at least 12 to 24 hours.	After 12 to 24 hours the risks of the above complications have diminished considerably. During this period, however, the intravenous line may be required if any emergency care must be given.
12. Monitor the urinary output for 2 to 3 days after the procedure.	This provides general information about the patient's renal function.
13. The morning after the procedure, obtain specimens for blood urea nitrogen, serum creatinine, and urine specific gravity tests.	These studies are usually ordered to ascertain that renal function has not been impaired by the procedure. There is a risk of acute tubular necrosis after renal angiography, particularly in elderly patients and those with diabetes.

Pedal lymphangiogram

Purpose   The purpose of a pedal lymphangiogram is to visualize the pelvic and paraaortic lymph nodes. It is used to determine metastatic invasion of these structures in patients with testicular, prostatic, or penile cancer. In many institutions this procedure is being replaced by computerized tomography (CT scan) of the area, since this newer procedure involves less risk for the patient and provides more reliable data (see p. 29).

Relative contraindications   Known or suspected hypersensitivity to compounds containing iodine
Inflammatory disease of the legs
Chronic edema of the legs
Pulmonary insufficiency

NURSING DIAGNOSIS: Potential for adverse effects related to pedal lymphangiography

Objectives of nursing intervention
- Adequate cleansing of bowel and cutdown sites
- Elimination of patient anxiety by means of psychologic preparation for the procedure
- Prevention or early detection and correction of complications

Expected outcomes
- X-ray film shows clear view of the abdominal lymphatic system
- Patient relaxed and cooperative throughout the procedure
- Absence of respiratory complications, infection, phlebitis, or lymphangitis

Plan for implementation	Rationale
PHYSICAL PREPARATION	
1. Administer cathartic as ordered in the evening prior to the procedure.	The bowel must be relatively empty for good visualization of the lymphatic system in the abdomen.
2. Wash the patient's feet.	Although a surgical prep will be done in the radiology department before the procedure, this reduces the amount of bacteria near the cutdown sites.
3. Shave any hair off the dorsal aspects of the feet.	

PSYCHOLOGIC PREPARATION

Explain to the patient what to expect during the procedure.

The patient will be given a subcutaneous injection into the interdigital skin on the dorsum of each foot. The injection contains approximately 1 ml of greenish dye that is taken up into the lymph vessels within 30 to 60 minutes and makes them visible. After administration of a local anesthetic, a small cutdown is performed to cannulate one lymph vessel in each foot, and contrast medium is then slowly infused (by gravity) into each vessel. There should be minimal discomfort during the procedure. Sutures are then applied to the cutdown sites and dressings are ap-

Prior knowledge of a procedure helps to decrease anxiety and enables the patient to participate more effectively in the procedure.

Plan for implementation	**Rationale**

plied. The first picture is taken a few hours after infusion of the contrast medium to visualize the lymph channels. By the next day the contrast medium is in the nodes, and another x-ray picture is taken. The procedure takes approximately 3 hours (plus a few minutes the following day). The exposure to radiation is not significant.

POSTPROCEDURE CARE

1. Be alert for indications of a hypersensitive reaction to the contrast medium. These include pruritus, sneezing, wheezing, dyspnea, and flushed skin.

Allergic reactions most commonly occur within a few minutes after administration of the contrast medium. It is unlikely that they will occur after the procedure is completed. They range from mild, transient rhinitis to severe anaphylaxis. Prompt recognition and treatment may be life saving.

2. If any of the above occur:
   a. Notify the physician.
   b. Have epinephrine, antihistamines, and corticosteroids on hand for rapid administration and a fully equipped emergency tray ("crash cart") readily available.
   c. Have oxygen readily available.

3. Be alert for symptoms of respiratory distress (cough, dyspnea, cyanosis) or shock.

Some of the contrast material may lodge in the lungs, resulting in pneumonitis or pulmonary emboli. Although this is a rare complication, it can be very serious, and prompt recognition and action are required.

4. If any of the above are present:
   a. Notify the physician at once.
   b. Have oxygen on hand for rapid administration if needed.

Plan for implementation	Rationale

5. Be alert for indications of infection.
  a. Monitor the patient's temperature every 4 hours.
  b. Report temperature elevation above 101°. (A low-grade fever may occur simply as a result of an inflammatory reaction to the contrast material without the presence of pathogenic organisms. In this case the fever is usually self-limiting, and the temperature is normal within 3 days.)
  c. Note the condition of the suture lines in the feet.
  d. Notify the physician if there is any evidence of inflammation (edema, erythema, exudate) around the suture lines.
	Although sterility is carefully observed during the cutdown procedure, there is always a risk of infection whenever the skin is broken and foreign material is instilled into the body.

6. Be alert for the following indications of lymphangitis and/or thrombophlebitis:
  a. A red, tender area on the lower extremity that is swollen and warm to the touch.
  b. Fever, accompanied by one or more of the aforementioned conditions.
	Inflammation of the lymph vessels occasionally is caused by irritation (or infection) from the contrast medium. Sometimes the superficial blood vessels are also involved.

7. If any of the preceding conditions are present:
  a. Notify the physician.
  b. Maintain orders for bed rest.
  c. Elevate the affected lower extremity.
  d. Do not massage the area.
 	
  e. Apply warm compresses as ordered.
	
	Elevation of the affected part decreases swelling.
	If infection is present, massage might spread it into the tissue spaces.
	Heat reduces inflammation.

8. Keep the dressings on the patient's feet clean and intact. If the sutures have not been removed by the fifth or sixth day, remind the physician of their presence.	It is easy to forget a few sutures because diagnostic studies and treatment of a potentially serious illness greatly outweigh their importance. Nonetheless, they must be removed or they will precipitate an inflammatory reaction that will require additional treatment.

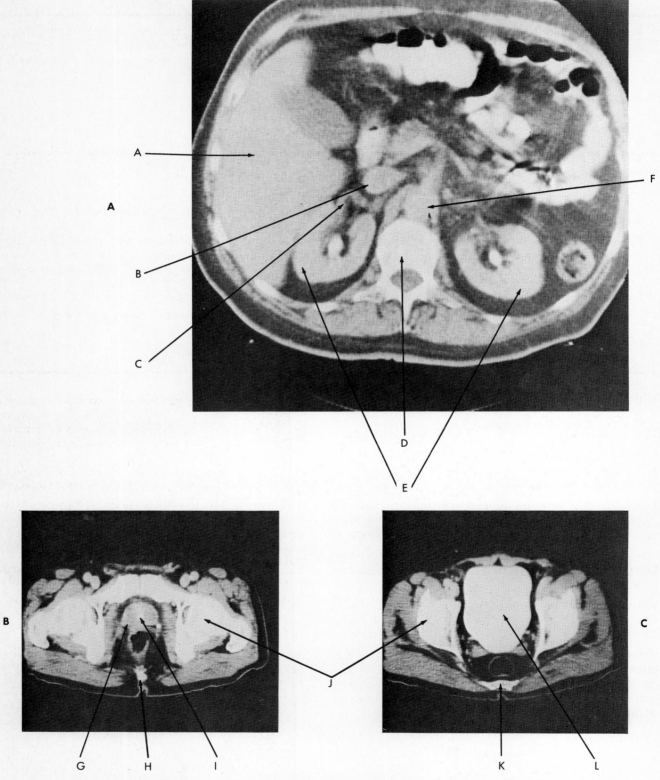

Fig. 3-3. Contrast-enhanced CT scans of kidney **(A)**, prostate **(B)**, and bladder area **(C)**. *A*, Liver; *B*, vena cava; *C*, renal artery; *D*, vertebra; *E*, kidneys; *F*, aorta, *G*, prostate; *H*, coccyx; *I*, urethra; *J*, head of femur; *K*, sacrum; *L*, bladder.

Computerized tomography (CT scan) (Fig. 3-3)

Purpose   Computerized tomography has a wide application in the diagnosis of urologic conditions, particularly in evaluation of renal tumors, testicular tumors, and prostatic cancer. Tissue densities can be measured accurately, and thus the nature and extent of the tumor can be determined.

Relative contraindication   Pregnancy

NURSING DIAGNOSIS: Potential for adverse effects related to computerized tomography (CT scan)

Objectives of nursing intervention
- Elimination of patient anxiety by means of psychologic preparation for the procedure
- Correction of dehydration after the procedure*

Expected outcomes
- Patient relaxed and cooperative throughout the procedure
- X-ray pictures in optimum condition for diagnostic evaluation
- Urinary output normal in quantity and concentration within 3 hours after the procedure.*

Plan for implementation	Rationale
PHYSICAL PREPARATION	
1. If ordered, prohibit oral intake prior to the procedure.	If the physician anticipates the use of contrast medium, he may prohibit oral intake for 3 or 4 hours prior to the procedure. Absence of solid food in the stomach reduces the risk of vomiting if the patient becomes nauseated from the contrast material.
2. If ordered, insert indwelling urethral catheter and rectal catheter immediately prior to the procedure.	Sometimes these tubes are inserted to distend the rectum and bladder so that they serve as landmarks. Usually this is only done if pelvic studies are required.
PSYCHOLOGIC PREPARATION	
Explain to the patient what to expect during the procedure.	Prior knowledge of a procedure helps to decrease anxiety and enables the patient to participate more effectively in the procedure.
The patient will be placed on a table that will move through the arch of an x-ray machine while pictures are taken.	
Sometimes contrast medium will be injected prior to the procedure as it is done before an intravenous pyelogram (p. 15). The patient will feel no discomfort (unless contrast medium is used). The procedure takes approximately 30 minutes.	The contrast medium sometimes helps to improve visualization of the urinary tract and to determine vascularity of soft tissues.

---

*Only applies if contrast medium was used during the procedure.

Plan for implementation	Rationale

POSTPROCEDURE CARE

1. Remove catheters from rectum and bladder.

2. Encourage fluids if contrast medium was used or if a catheter was inserted into the bladder. | Contrast medium is an osmotic diuretic that might cause dehydration. Increasing the flow of urine through the urinary tract also helps prevent any bacteria introduced during catheterization from multiplying and causing an infection in the urinary tract.

Loop-o-gram

Purpose A loop-o-gram is performed only on a patient who has an ileal or colon conduit. It enables the physician to visualize the length and width of the conduit and to determine the presence of ureteral reflux of urine.

Relative contraindication Pregnancy
Allergy to contrast medium is **not necessarily** a contraindication because it is not administered systemically

NURSING DIAGNOSIS: Potential for adverse effects related to a loop-o-gram

Objective of nursing intervention Elimination of patient anxiety by means of psychologic preparation for the procedure

Expected outcomes { Patient relaxed and cooperative throughout the procedure
X-ray picture in optimal condition for diagnostic evaluation

Plan for implementation	Rationale

PHYSICAL PREPARATION

None required.

PSYCHOLOGIC PREPARATION

Explain to the patient what to expect during the procedure. | Prior knowledge of a procedure helps to decrease anxiety and enables the patient to participate more effectively in the procedure.

A small catheter will be inserted into the stoma, and contrast medium will be slowly instilled. The filling is observed under fluoroscopy, and an x-ray picture is taken. The patient will not have any pain. The loop is then drained and the catheter is removed. The procedure takes approximately 10 minutes. The exposure to radiation is minimal.

POSTPROCEDURE CARE

None required.

Nephrostogram

Purpose
The purpose of a nephrostogram is to determine the patency of the ureter from a kidney into which a nephrostomy tube has been inserted. It is most commonly done after a nephrolithotomy or a pyeloplasty, prior to removal of nephrostomy drainage equipment.

Relative contraindications
Very recent renal or ureteral surgery (within 1 week)
Pregnancy
Allergy to contrast medium is **not necessarily** a contraindication because it is not administered systemically

---

NURSING DIAGNOSIS: Potential for adverse effects related to a nephrostogram

Objective of nursing intervention
Elimination of patient anxiety by means of psychologic preparation for the procedure

Expected outcomes
Patient relaxed and cooperative throughout the procedure
X-ray picture in optimal condition for diagnostic evaluation

Plan for implementation	Rationale
PHYSICAL PREPARATION	
None required.	
PSYCHOLOGIC PREPARATION	
Explain to the patient what to expect during the procedure.	Prior knowledge of a procedure helps to decrease anxiety and enables the patient to participate more effectively in the procedure.
A contrast medium will be instilled through the nephrostomy tube by gravity flow. The patient will feel no discomfort. X-ray pictures will be taken. The procedure takes approximately 15 minutes. The exposure to radiation is minimal.	
POSTPROCEDURE CARE	
Check the physician's orders regarding clamping of the nephrostomy tube.	If the x-ray film indicates patency, the tube is usually clamped for a trial period prior to its removal.

CHAPTER 4

Ultrasonic studies and combination ultrasonic and radiologic studies

Sonogram

Purpose   The main purpose of a sonogram is to differentiate between solid and cystic masses in the abdomen. The study uses ultrasound, whereby sound waves are bounced off tissue surfaces and an electronic image of echoes is reproduced on a screen. It is extremely useful in identifying renal tumors, renal cysts, and stones in the urinary tract.

Contraindications   None. However, a draining wound directly over the area to be studied may make the test more difficult to perform, since the procedure requires application of liberal amounts of oil to the surface of the skin and a transducer to be pressed against the skin.

NURSING DIAGNOSIS: Potential for adverse effects related to sonography

Objectives of nursing intervention
{ Elimination of patient anxiety by means of psychologic preparation for the procedure
Bladder adequately distended with urine (if pelvic studies are to be done)

Expected outcomes
{ Patient relaxed and cooperative throughout the procedure
Sonographic picture in optimal condition for diagnostic evaluation

Plan for implementation	Rationale

PHYSICAL PREPARATION

No physical preparation is required unless the sonogram is to be of the pelvic organs, in which case the patient should drink 1 L of fluid within 1 hour of the test and **not** empty his bladder.

A full bladder facilitates sonographic visualization of the pelvic organs.

PSYCHOLOGIC PREPARATION

Explain to the patient what to expect during the procedure.

An oil will be applied to the patient's abdomen and/or flank and a sound transducer will be moved over the area. The only discomfort will be a distended bladder (if pelvic sonogram is performed). The procedure takes approximately 10 minutes.

Prior knowledge of a procedure helps to decrease anxiety and enables the patient to participate more effectively in the procedure.

POSTPROCEDURE CARE

None required.

Renal cyst puncture, aspiration, and x-ray examination

Purpose   The purpose of this procedure is to aspirate the contents of a renal cyst so that it can be analyzed histologically and biochemically and to visualize the contours of the internal surface of the cyst radiographically.

Contraindications   None
Pregnancy is a contraindication to simultaneous radiographic studies

---

NURSING DIAGNOSIS: Potential for adverse effects related to puncture, aspiration, and x-ray examination of renal cyst

Objectives of nursing intervention
{ Elimination of patient anxiety by means of psychological preparation for the procedure
Absence or early detection and correction of complications

Expected outcomes
{ Patient relaxed and cooperative throughout the procedure
Absence of hemorrhage or infection

Plan for implementation	Rationale
PHYSICAL PREPARATION	
None required.	
PSYCHOLOGIC PREPARATION	
Explain to the patient what to expect during the procedure.	Prior knowledge of a procedure helps to decrease anxiety and enables the patient to participate more effectively in the procedure.
An oil will be applied to the area over the affected kidney and a sound transducer will be moved over the area. The position and size of the cyst will be determined, and the patient will be given a subcutaneous injection of local anesthetic into the area. Under sonographic control a special needle will be directed into the cyst, during which the patient might feel some discomfort. The contents of the cyst will be aspirated and sent for histologic and biochemical analysis. The patient will then be transferred to another room where contrast material will be instilled through the needle into the cyst, and subsequent x-ray pictures will be taken to visualize the internal contours of the cyst. The needle will then be removed and a dressing applied. The procedure takes approximately 30 minutes.	
POSTPROCEDURE CARE	

1. Be alert for indications of hemorrhage.
   a. Check the dressing every 4 hours.
   b. Monitor the blood pressure and pulse every 4 hours.
	Hemorrhage is a potential, but uncommon, complication after this procedure.

2. Check the patient's temperature every 4 hours and notify the physician of elevation above 101°.	Infection is also a potential, but rare, complication.

Antegrade pyelogram

Purpose This study is performed when there is an obstruction in the urinary tract and (1) retrograde studies are not possible because of the obstruction, and (2) intravenous pyelogram does not provide adequate visualization because of poor renal function. The process involves instillation of contrast medium into the renal pelvis or calyces, as opposed to retrograde pyelogram, which is performed cystoscopically through the lower end of the ureter (p. 49).

Relative contraindication Pregnancy

NURSING DIAGNOSIS: Potential for adverse effects related to antegrade pyelography

Objectives of nursing intervention
- Elimination of patient anxiety by means of psychologic preparation for the procedure
- Absence or early detection and correction of complications

Expected outcomes
- Patient relaxed and cooperative throughout the procedure
- X-ray pictures in optimum condition for diagnostic evaluation
- Absence of hemorrhage, extravasation of urine, or infection

Plan for implementation	Rationale
PHYSICAL PREPARATION	
None required.	
PSYCHOLOGIC PREPARATION	
Explain to the patient what to expect during the procedure.	Prior knowledge of a procedure helps to decrease anxiety and enables the patient to participate more effectively in the procedure.
An oil will be applied to the area over the affected kidney and a sound transducer will be moved over the area. The renal pelvis or a dilated calyx will be identified, and the patient will be given a subcutaneous injection of a local anesthetic into the area. Under sonographic control a special needle will be advanced into the renal pelvis (or calyx), during which the patient may feel some discomfort. The patient will then be transferred to another room where contrast medium will be instilled through the needle and x-ray pictures will be taken. If no obstruction (or only minimal obstruction) is seen on the x-ray film, the needle will be removed and a dressing applied.	

Plan for implementation	**Rationale**
Otherwise, a tube may be inserted for temporary drainage of urine. The procedure takes approximately 45 minutes. The exposure to radiation is minimal.	A nephrostomy tube attached to a collecting container may be inserted to allow drainage of the kidney and prevent further renal damage. This procedure, known as percutaneous nephrostomy (Fig. 4-1) is not to be confused with the surgical placement of a nephrostomy tube (see Chapter 26), which is an open procedure involving the various complications associated with general anesthesia and surgery. Care must be taken when changing the dressing not to dislodge the tube.

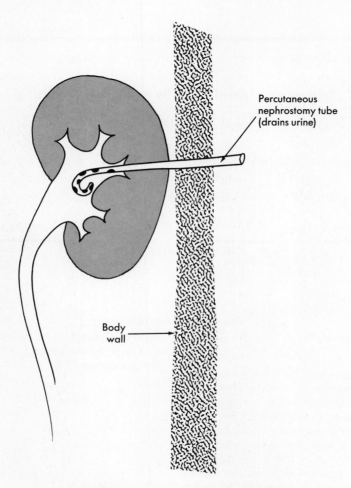

Percutaneous
nephrostomy tube
(drains urine)

Body
wall

Fig. 4-1. Percutaneous nephrostomy.

Plan for implementation	Rationale
	In some instances, percutaneous placement of a ureteral stent may, instead, be performed after antegrade pyelogram (Fig. 4-2). In this instance a self-retaining ureteral catheter is advanced into the ureter and extends into the bladder. This also allows the kidney to drain, but this type of mechanism is only employed in patients with a short life expectancy, since the catheter is left in place permanently. There is no external source of drainage and it does not require any specific nursing care.

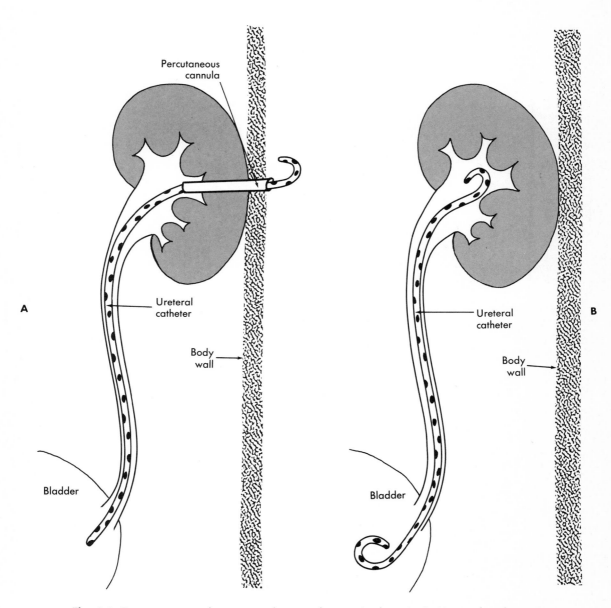

Fig. 4-2. Percutaneous placement of ureteral stent (catheter). **A,** Ureteral catheter inserted through percutaneous cannula. **B,** Ureteral catheter is advanced into bladder, and cannula is removed. Urine drains through the catheter into the bladder.

Plan for implementation	**Rationale**
POSTPROCEDURE CARE	

1. Notify the physician of any indications of hemorrhage. These include:
  a. Increasing pulse and respiratory rates, decreasing blood pressure, diaphoresis, pallor, and feelings of apprehension
  b. Bleeding from the puncture site
  c. Hematuria (even if it is only slightly pink)
	Hemorrhage is a potential complication after this procedure because the needle sometimes pierces a highly vascular portion of the kidney.

2. Notify the physician if the patient complains of flank pain or tenderness. This may be a symptom of extravasation of urine.	Extravasation is a potential complication because urine sometimes leaks into surrounding tissue through the puncture site in the renal pelvis or calyx.

3. Notify the physician of any symptoms of infection:
  a. Pain or tenderness in the area of the puncture site
  b. Temperature above 101°.
	Infection is a potential complication, although sterile procedure is observed for the placement of the needle and instillation of the contrast material.

4. Enforce orders for bed rest for 8 to 12 hours after the procedure.	Bed rest is usually ordered because of the possibility of hemorrhage.
5. Do not discontinue an intravenous line (even if the patient is tolerating food well) for at least 12 to 24 hours.	By the following day, the risk of hemorrhage has considerably decreased. During the first 12 to 24 hours, however, the intravenous line may be required if emergency care must be given.

CHAPTER 5

Radioisotope studies

Renal scan

Purpose The purpose of a renal scan is to assess the excretory function and the blood supply of the kidneys.

Relative contraindication Pregnancy

NURSING DIAGNOSIS: Potential for adverse effects related to a renal scan

Objective of nursing intervention Elimination of patient anxiety by means of psychologic preparation for the procedure

Expected outcome Patient relaxed and cooperative throughout the procedure

Plan for implementation	Rationale
PHYSICAL PREPARATION	
None required.	
PSYCHOLOGIC PREPARATION	
Explain to the patient what to expect during the procedure.	Prior knowledge of a procedure helps to decrease anxiety and enables the patient to participate more effectively in the procedure.
The patient will be given an intravenous injection of a radioactive isotope (various kinds are used) and will be placed in front of a machine that detects radioactivity. The radioactivity over both kidneys will be measured within a few seconds after the injection.	This reflects the blood flow to the kidneys.
Measurements of radioactivity are then repeated a few minutes later over the kidneys and bladder.	This reveals the excretory function of the kidneys.
Sometimes an injection of mannitol will be given at this point to facilitate excretion of the isotope, and additional measurements of radioactivity will be compared with the earlier ones. The entire procedure takes approximately 30 minutes.	This reveals abnormal delays in excretion caused by anatomic obstruction in the urinary tract.
POSTPROCEDURE CARE	
If mannitol was used in the procedure, encourage a high fluid intake for a few hours afterward.	Mannitol may have a mildly dehydrating effect.

Bone scan

Purpose	This study is done for urologic patients to determine the presence of metastatic infiltration of cancer into the bones.
Relative contraindication	Pregnancy

NURSING DIAGNOSIS: Potential for adverse effects related to a bone scan

Objective of nursing intervention	Elimination of patient anxiety by means of psychologic preparation for the procedure
Expected outcome	Patient relaxed and cooperative throughout the procedure

Plan for implementation	Rationale
PHYSICAL PREPARATION	
None required prior to injection of isotope.	
The physician may have the patient drink liberal amounts of water **after** the injection, **before** the scan is performed.	A high fluid intake facilitates excretion of the isotope from the kidneys, so there is less background activity.
PSYCHOLOGIC PREPARATION	
Explain to the patient what to expect during the procedure.	Prior knowledge of a procedure helps to decrease anxiety and enables the patient to participate more effectively in the procedure.
The patient will receive an injection of an appropriate radioactive isotope. Approximately 4 hours later, the patient will be placed in front of a machine that detects radioactivity.	It takes approximately this amount of time for the isotope to be taken up by the bones. Abnormal concentration of the isotope indicates disease, but this usually must be confirmed with a regular x-ray film of the skeleton.
POSTPROCEDURE CARE	
None required.	

CHAPTER 6

Urodynamic evaluation

Urodynamic evaluation: uroflowmeter, cystometrogram, electromyogram of external sphincter, urethral pressure profile, dynamic micturition study with videorecording (synchronous pressure flow measurement with videorecording), and pharmacologic urodynamic tests

Purpose
Urodynamic evaluation is a relatively new series of studies that provide information about the physiology of micturition. The tests are carried out after the patient has been examined and certain routine urologic investigations have been performed (e.g., urinalysis, urine culture, IVP, and cystoscopy). The indications for these studies are numerous, and patient selection depends on the physician's discretion. Patients with neurogenic bladder (defined by Lapides* as bladder dysfunction caused by "interference with the normal conduction of nerve impulses over one or more of the nerve tracts concerned with urination"), such as those with spinal cord injuries, multiple sclerosis, Parkinson's disease, and cerebral vascular accident, usually need full evaluation. Female patients with certain types of incontinence may undergo these studies to differentiate true stress incontinence from urgency incontinence, since the treatment is entirely different in each case. Male patients with symptoms of frequency and decreased urinary stream may require urodynamic evaluation to distinguish the most common cause of these symptoms (prostatic obstruction) from disorders such as neurogenic bladder or bladder neck dysfunction, which require totally different management. Children with diurnal incontinence (incontinence during the day and night) may need urodynamic tests to determine the cause of the problem, which may be a result of a previously undiagnosed neurogenic bladder, a functional disorder from faulty training, or other pathologic conditions.

Contraindications
Concomitant use of general anesthesia, strong analgesics or sedatives, cholinergic or adrenergic drugs
Severe urinary tract infection
Recent bladder surgery

---

*Lapides, J.: Fundamentals of urology, Philadelphia, 1976, W.B. Saunders Co., p. 210.

NURSING DIAGNOSIS: Potential for adverse effects related to urodynamic evaluation

Objective of nursing intervention	Elimination of patient anxiety by means of psychologic preparation for the procedure
Expected outcome	Patient relaxed and cooperative throughout the procedure

Plan for implementation	Rationale

PHYSICAL PREPARATION

1. Tell the patient he should not void before going to the urodynamic laboratory.

The patient will be asked to void as part of the initial evaluation.

2. Do not administer strong analgesics, sedatives, or cholinergic or adrenergic drugs within 6 to 8 hours of the tests.

These drugs affect the conduction of nerve impulses, thereby interfering with bladder function.

PSYCHOLOGIC PREPARATION

Explain to the patient what to expect during the procedure. (The following description is sequential and includes **all** urodynamic tests. In practice, the physician may eliminate some of the tests or change the order of the tests to suit the individual patient's needs. The nurse should keep the description as general as possible for this reason but still provide the patient with enough information for adequate psychologic preparation.)

Prior knowledge of a procedure helps to decrease anxiety and enables the patient to participate more effectively in the procedure. Although there is very little actual pain involved with these tests, the patient may feel considerable discomfort at times. This may be amplified by anxiety. Most patients cooperate better and experience less discomfort when they understand what is being done. The depth of explanation should depend on the patient's interest and ability to comprehend.

1. In the first part of the test the patient will be asked to void in a special bathroom. He should void in the same fashion as he usually does.

The patient will void into a funnel connected to a **uroflowmeter,** an electric device that calculates the rate at which the urine flows, the time taken to void, and the volume voided. This is recorded on a graph (Fig. 6-1). An abnormally slow rate may be an indication of outflow obstruction such as prostatic hyperplasia. An abnormally high rate may occur in patients with stress incontinence.

2. The patient will be placed on an examination table, and the physician will perform a modified neurologic assessment.

This is done to diagnose underlying neurologic disease.

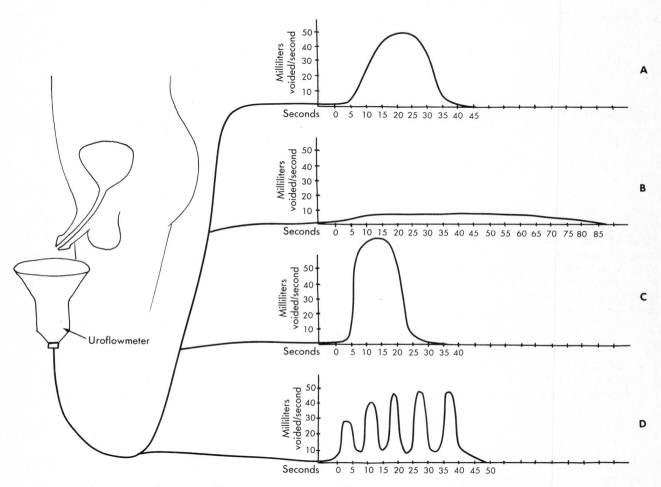

Fig. 6-1. Uroflowmeter flow curves. **A,** Normal flow pattern; normal rate and peak flow. **B,** Obstructed flow pattern; long voiding time and low peak. **C,** Superflow pattern; short voiding time and high peak. **D,** Abdominal flow pattern; voiding occurs only during periods of increased intraabdominal pressure (i.e., straining).

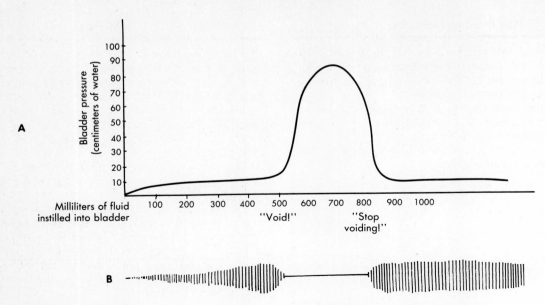

Fig. 6-2. Normal cystometrogram **(A)** and normal electromyogram **(B)** of external sphincter.

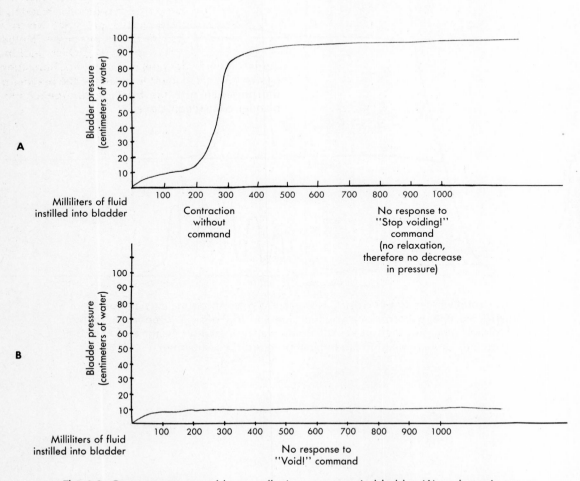

Fig. 6-3. Cystometrogram of hyperreflexive neurogenic bladder **(A)** and atonic neurogenic bladder **(B)**.

44

Plan for implementation	**Rationale**

3. A urethral catheter will be inserted, and the bladder will be filled with water (or sometimes carbon dioxide). Occasionally this procedure is done with a suprapubic tube instead of a urethral catheter.
 	
  a. The patient will be asked to notify the physician when be begins to feel a sense of fullness and then when his bladder actually feels full.
 	
  b. He will be asked to urinate and then asked to stop urinating at a certain point.
	After insertion of the catheter the volume of residual urine is noted. The catheter is connected to a transducer, and pressure changes are recorded on a graph, called a **cystometrogram.** This demonstrates changes in bladder pressure and how the patient perceives and responds to them. Normally, bladder pressure remains the same during the period that it is being filled until the volume reaches approximately 500 ml. When the patient is told to void, the pressure should increase abruptly because the bladder is contracting. The pressure should fall to the prevoiding level when the patient is told to stop voiding because the bladder should relax (Fig. 6-2, *A*). In a hyperreflexive neurogenic bladder, the pressure will increase before the volume reaches 500 ml (the bladder will contract spontaneously), and the pressure will remain high (no relaxation occurs) (Fig. 6-3, *A*). In an atonic neurogenic bladder, no bladder contraction occurs at all; thus the volume may be quite large (Fig. 8-3, *B*).

4. Sometimes the procedure may be performed with an additional catheter in the patient's rectum.	This is done to obtain a more precise evaluation of the bladder pressure. The catheter in the bladder enables measurement of the pressure within the bladder, but this also includes intraabdominal pressure, which may be quite high if the patient strains or coughs. Simultaneous measurement of rectal pressure (which indicates only intraabdominal pressure) and then the subtraction of this figure from the amount indicated in the bladder provides the physician with the **true** pressure generated by the bladder contraction alone.

Plan for implementation	**Rationale**

5. The patient may also have a needle electrode placed alongside the urethra (in a female patient) or inserted through the perineum into the external sphincter (in a male patient). The patient may feel some discomfort during the placement of the needle.

An **electromyogram** of the external sphincter may be obtained to determine sphincter activity during voiding. Normally this activity should completely disappear when the patient voids and should resume on the "stop voiding" command, indicating voluntary control of the sphincter (Fig. 6-2, *B*). A needle electrode provides the most satisfactory results, although a rectal plug or a surface electrode may also be used.

6. Sometimes an additional study is done by the slow withdrawal of the catheter through the urethra.

Urethral pressure profile indicates the prevailing pressure within the urethral lumen. It is done by connecting the catheter to a transducer and measuring the pressure while the catheter is withdrawn at a constant rate.

7. If the physician wants to visualize the functioning of the bladder, he may fill it with contrast medium (instead of water or carbon dioxide) and examine the patient with fluoroscopy.

This study is known as **dynamic micturition study with videorecording** or **synchronous pressure flow measurement with videorecording.** From the patient's point of view the preparations are similar to those for a cystometrogram. Instead of a catheter inserted in the bladder, two no. 8 feeding tubes are inserted via the urethra (or occasionally suprapubically). One is for measurement of intravesical pressure and the other is for filling the bladder with contrast material. The insertion of the EMG electrode is the same, and, if simultaneous urethral pressure profile is to be obtained, the technique is also the same. The difference with this procedure is that, under fluoroscopic control, the bladder filling and emptying are observed simultaneously with the recording of measurements of bladder pressure. The flow of contrast material through the lower tract may also be recorded on videotape, showing the location of any obstruction, and in cases of incontinence it would differentiate between neurogenic and anatomic disorders.

8. Sometimes the filling and emptying process will be repeated approximately 20 minutes after the physician gives the patient an injection of a medication.

Pharmacologic urodynamic tests consist of administration of bethanechol chloride (Urecholine), propantheline bromide (Pro-Banthine), or phentolamine (Regitine). One of these tests may be done if additional information is required. (See Appendix A for actions of these drugs.) A rise in bladder pressure after administration of bethanechol indicates the presence of denervation. Elimination of bladder contractions after administration of propantheline demonstrates the efficacy of this drug in controlling pathologic bladder contractions. A fall of urethral pressure after administering phentolamine indicates the usefulness of this drug in treating cases of abnormal urethral resistance. When this drug is tested, the urethral pressure profile test must be repeated.

POSTPROCEDURE CARE

None required.

CHAPTER 7

Cystoscopic procedures

Observation cystourethroscopy

Purpose
This procedure is performed to visualize the interior of the bladder and urethra. The indications for observation cystourethroscopy are numerous. They include pathologic bladder conditions such as tumors and stones and conditions of the urethra such as prostatic obstruction and urethral valves, polyps, tumors, strictures, and diverticula. The procedure is often done with local anesthesia in the cystoscopy suite. However, the physician may use general anesthesia if the patient is a child or if additional procedures are anticipated, such as retrograde pyelogram (p. 49) or biopsy.

Relative contraindication
Active urinary tract infection

NURSING DIAGNOSIS: Potential for adverse effects related to observation cystourethroscopy

Objectives of nursing intervention
- Elimination of patient anxiety by means of psychologic preparation for the procedure
- Prevention or early detection and correction of complications

Expected outcomes
- Patient relaxed and cooperative throughout the procedure
- Resumption of normal voiding pattern within 6 hours after the procedure
- Absence of severe voiding discomfort
- Absence of significant hematuria
- Temperature within normal range

Plan for implementation	Rationale
PHYSICAL PREPARATION	
None required.	

Plan for implementation	**Rationale**

PSYCHOLOGIC PREPARATION

Explain to the patient what to expect during the procedure.

Prior knowledge of a procedure helps to decrease anxiety and enables the patient to participate more effectively in the procedure.

The patient will be placed in a comfortable position on the examining table, on his back with his legs elevated on leg rests, with sterile drapes placed over his legs and body.

The patient must be positioned well on the table for safety and comfort. This includes padding the leg rests and having a pillow under his head. Sterility is extremely important whenever there is introduction of foreign elements into the urinary tract. Therefore sterile drapes and sterilization of all equipment are essential, and all personnel attending the patient should wear sterile gowns and caps.*

An intravenous injection of a mild sedative might be given, and a local anesthetic (lidocaine [2% Xylocaine HCl Jelly]) will be instilled into the urethra. After a few minutes to allow the anesthetic to take effect, a thin tube-like instrument (cystoscope) will be gently inserted into the urethra. While expanding the bladder with saline (via a tube running through the cystoscope) the physician will examine the bladder in a systematic fashion using different lenses.

Initially a urine specimen is collected for examination. The bladder is then distended with saline to enable visualization. Saline will be continuously flowing in and out of the bladder (via the cystoscope) throughout the procedure. The lenses used by the physician are a foroblique lens, which provides visualization at approximately 20 degrees, and a right-angle lens for 90-degree visualization.

The cystoscope will then be gradually withdrawn, and the lenses will be changed to examine the urethra.

For urethral visualization, foroblique and 0-degree lenses are used.

POSTPROCEDURE CARE

1. Explain to the patient that he may have some voiding discomfort (sensation of burning) for a few hours after the procedure, and it can be reduced by a liberal intake of fluids.

Irritation of the urethra is common after instrumentation. Dilution of the urine generally makes voiding less uncomfortable.

2. Monitor the volume and character of the urine for 24 hours after the procedure, and notify the physician if any of the following occur:
   a. The patient does not void for 6 hours after the procedure.†

Patients with considerable prostatic enlargement may go into urinary retention after the procedure because of urethral inflammation. If this is anticipated, some physicians insert an indwelling urethral catheter prophylactically.

   b. The patient is voiding small amounts with frequency and has suprapubic distention.†
   c. There is bright red blood in the urine.

This may indicate the patient is in retention with overflow.
Although light blood-tinged urine is not uncommon after cystoscopy, any frank bleeding is abnormal and requires medical attention.

3. Monitor the patient's temperature within 2 hours after the procedure and then every 4 hours for the next 24 hours.

Bacteremia can occur after any instrumentation of the urinary tract. This happens as a result of absorption of bacteria into the bloodstream through the urethra.

---

*Nursing care of the patient undergoing cystoscopy is covered in excellent detail in Morel, A., and Wise, G.J.: Urologic endoscopic procedures, ed. 2, St. Louis, 1979, The C.V. Mosby Co.
†Does not apply if the patient has an indwelling urethral catheter.

Plan for implementation	Rationale
4. Notify the physician if there is a temperature elevation above 101°.	Blood and urine specimens are often ordered to determine the type and sensitivity of the offending organism, and the patient is usually started on antibiotics.
5. Administer antimicrobial medication if ordered.	The physician may place certain patients on antimicrobial medication prophylactically, immediately after cystoscopy. Patients most prone to infection after urethral instrumentation are those who have residual urine or those with diabetes.

Retrograde pyelogram

Purpose A retrograde pyelogram is done to determine the exact location of a ureteral obstruction (i.e., a stone, tumor, or stricture) if it cannot be visualized on an intravenous pyelogram. (This occasionally happens because of poor renal function and failure to excrete the contrast medium adequately.) A CT scan is usually employed afterward to determine the density of the filling defect and thus distinguish between a stone and a tumor.

Relative contraindications Active urinary tract infection
Allergy to contrast medium is **not necessarily** a contraindication because it is not administered systemically

NURSING DIAGNOSIS: Potential for adverse effects related to retrograde pyelography

Objectives of nursing intervention

- Adequate cleansing of bowel
- Elimination of patient anxiety by means of psychologic preparation for the procedure
- Prevention or early detection and correction of complications

Expected outcomes

- Resumption of normal voiding pattern within 6 hours after procedure
- Absence of voiding discomfort
- Absence of hematuria
- Temperature within normal range

Plan for implementation	Rationale
PHYSICAL PREPARATION	
1. Administer cathartic as ordered.	The bowel must be relatively empty for adequate visualization of the urinary tract on x-ray examination.
2. Prohibit oral intake after midnight prior to the procedure.	General anesthesia is usually used for insertion of the ureteral catheter. An empty stomach reduces the risk of aspiration while the patient is anesthetized.

Plan for implementation	**Rationale**

PSYCHOLOGIC PREPARATION

Explain to the patient what will occur during the procedure.

After administration of anesthesia, the physician will insert a thin, tubelike instrument (cystoscope) into the patient's bladder, through the urethra, and instill a small amount of contrast medium into the obstructed ureter. X-ray pictures will be taken to visualize the ureter.

Prior knowledge of a procedure helps to decrease anxiety.

The affected ureter is catheterized (Fig. 7-1) to instill the contrast medium.

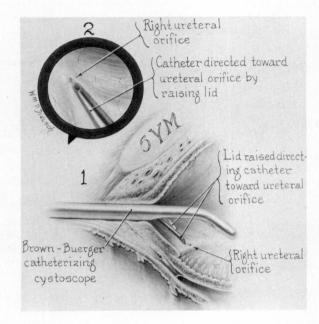

Fig. 7-1. Right ureteral catheterization. (Courtesy Mr. William P. Didusch and American Cystoscope Makers, Inc., Stamford, Conn.)

Occasionally an indwelling urethral catheter and ureteral catheter will be left in place for a few days to facilitate drainage of the obstructed ureter. The procedure takes approximately 60 minutes. The exposure to radiation is minimal.

If complete obstruction is found, sometimes an attempt is made to pass a ureteral catheter beyond the obstruction to drain the kidney. This will be left in place until definitive treatment has been decided on. It will be tied to an indwelling urethral catheter to help maintain its position in the ureter.

Plan for implementation	Rationale

POSTPROCEDURE CARE

1. If no catheters have been left in place:

   a. Explain to the patient that he may have some void-discomfort (sensation of burning) for a few hours after the procedure, and it can be reduced by a liberal intake of fluids.

   Irritation of the urethra is common after instrumentation. Dilution of the urine generally makes voiding less uncomfortable.

   b. Monitor the volume and character of the urine for 24 hours after the procedure, and notify the physician if any of the following occur:

   (1) The patient does not void for 6 hours after the procedure.

   Patients with considerable prostatic enlargement may go into urinary retention after the procedure because of urethral inflammation.

   (2) The patient is voiding small amounts with frequency and has suprapubic distention.

   This may indicate the patient is in retention with overflow.

   (3) There is bright red blood in the urine.

   Although light blood-tinged urine is not uncommon after retrograde pyelography, frank bleeding is abnormal and requires medical attention.

2. If the patient has a ureteral and indwelling urethral catheter in place, see Chapter 29, nursing diagnoses 4 and 5, for nursing care.

3. If a stone was found to be the source of obstruction, strain all urine.

   The stone may pass spontaneously. Chemical analysis will be required for the physician to determine a regimen for the prevention of future stones.

4. Administer prophylactic antibiotics as ordered.

   Antibiotics are usually given after retrograde pyelography because the risk of infection is relatively high.

CHAPTER 8

Diagnostic laboratory studies

Normal ranges for the most common tests are provided here. These values, however, may vary from one laboratory to another. The nurse is advised to follow the normal ranges specified by the particular laboratory.

Laboratory studies performed on blood

Test	Urologic application	Nursing considerations
Acid phosphatase (prostatic fraction) Normal range depends on method of assay	Elevation of this substance is often present in patients with carcinoma of the prostate that has extended beyond the prostatic capsule.	No special care required.
Alkaline phosphatase Normal range depends on method of assay	Elevation of this substance is present in the blood of patients with many conditions, including metastatic bone lesions.	No special care required.
Alpha-fetoprotein (AFP) (radioimmunoassay) 3000 ng/ml is minimum detectable level by gel-agar precipitation method	Elevation of AFP occurs in patients with testicular tumors. The test is used before and after orchiectomy. Continued elevation often indicates metastatic spread of the tumor. AFP is frequently referred to as a "tumor marker."	No special care required.
Activated partial thromboplastin time* Laboratory provides standard value (control) for each test	This test is usually routinely performed on all patients preoperatively to screen for coagulation disorders.	Anticoagulant (sodium citrate) is required in the specimen container. Immerse specimen in ice and send to the lab at once. Distorted values may occur from numerous medications. Heparin, antibiotics, sulfonamides, cathartics, and aspirin are among those which cause false positive (elevated) values. Antihistamines, barbiturates, chloral hydrate, corticosteroids, digitalis, certain diuretics, and vitamin K are among those which cause false negative (depressed) readings.
Creatinine Normal range: 1 to 1.5 mg/dl	Elevation of creatinine is often present in patients with impaired renal function. Glomerular filtration rate must be reduced by at least 50% for significant elevation to occur.	Any patient receiving aminoglycoside antibiotics should have serum creatinine levels evaluated three times per week because of the nephrotoxic effects of these drugs. Elevation of creatinine due to nephrotoxicity or hypersensitivity may also occur from numerous other medications, such as certain diuretics, phenobarbital, sulfonamides, tetracyclines, and cephalosporins.

*Partial thromboplastin time may be done instead.

Laboratory studies performed on blood—cont'd

Test	Urologic application	Nursing considerations
Cross-matching	This test is usually routinely performed preoperatively on all patients to determine blood compatibility in the event that a transfusion is required.	Follow hospital policy for precautions regarding transfusions. Take special care to provide all information requested by the lab, and write clearly on the lab slip. A transfusion with mismatched blood could have fatal consequences.
Fluorescent treponemal antibody absorption	This test is done to diagnose syphilis.	Send specimen to the lab at once. Hemolysis may interfere with accurate readings.
Human chorionic gonadotropin (HCG) (beta chain)	HCG (beta chain) is sometimes present in patients with testicular tumors. If it is present, the test is repeated after orchiectomy. Continued elevation often indicates metastatic spread of the tumor. In this context HCG is often referred to as a "tumor marker."	No special care required.
Hematocrit Normal ranges: Females, 38% to 45% Males, 40% to 50%	This test measures the percentage volume of red blood cells in whole blood. It is usually routinely performed on all patients preoperatively. It is also performed on patients who have undergone considerable blood loss to determine the need for a transfusion.	Do not withdraw blood from an extremity into which intravenous solution is infusing. Anticoagulant is required in the specimen container.
Hemoglobin Normal ranges: Females, 12 to 14.5 gm/dl Males, 14 to 16 gm/dl	This test measures the amount of hemoglobin in the blood. The indications are the same as for hematocrit.	Same as for hematocrit.
Hemoglobin electrophoresis	This test is done to determine the presence of sickle cell disease. Its relevance in urology concerns certain sequelae of the disease—hematuria and papillary necrosis.	Send specimen to lab at once. Anticoagulant is required in the specimen container.
Liver function tests Lactic dehydrogenase Cephalin-cholesterol flocculation (CCF) Serum aspartate aminotransferase (SGOT) Serum glutamic pyruvic transaminase	These tests relate indirectly to urology. In certain cases they provide information regarding renal tumors. Individuals with such tumors often develop disturbances in liver function.	Send specimens to lab at once. Withholding of food may be required prior to CCF test.
Platelet count Normal range (Brecher-Cronkite method): 150,000 to 400,000/mm^3	This test is usually routinely performed preoperatively on all patients to detect bleeding abnormalities caused by low platelet count. It may also be done on patients who have undergone blood loss to determine the need for a transfusion, and it is done at regular intervals for patients receiving chemotherapy or radiation therapy because these treatments suppress platelet production.	Anticoagulant is required in the specimen container.
Red blood cell count Normal ranges: Females, 4.0 to 5.0 million/mm^3 Males, 4.5 to 6.0 million/mm^3	This test is usually routinely performed on all patients preoperatively. Indications are the same as for platelet count.	Same as for platelet count.

Laboratory studies performed on blood—cont'd

Test	Urologic application	Nursing considerations
Sequential multiple analyzer (SMA) Normal ranges: Sodium: 136 to 145 mEq/L Potassium: 3.5 to 5.0 mEq/L Chloride: 98 to 106 mEq/L Bicarbonate: 21 to 28 mEq/L Calcium: 9 to 11 mg/dl Phosphorus: 3.0 to 4.5 mg/dl Glucose: 65 to 110 mg/dl	This series of tests provides information about the chemical composition of the plasma. SMA is actually an abreviation for the name of the instrument used to perform the test. It is capable of performing a variety of analyses at one time on a single sample of blood. This series of tests is usually routinely performed all patients preoperatively.	Send specimen to lab at once. If hemolysis occurs, serum potassium levels will be distorted. This test is usually done after 6 hours of fasting.
Testosterone Normal ranges: Females, 0.01 to 0.1 μg/dl Males, 0.3 to 1.0 μg/dl	Abnormal levels of testosterone are sometimes present in infertile patients.	No special care required.
Urea nitrogen Normal range: 10 to 20 mg/dl	Elevation of blood urea nitrogen (BUN) is often present in patients with impaired renal function. However, BUN levels are highly variable and cannot be used alone to evaluate renal function.	Various factors may cause abnormal BUN levels. Excessive intravenous fluids may cause lower readings; dehydration and rapid protein catabolism may cause elevations. Drugs that may raise BUN levels include aminoglycosides (in particular), various other antibiotics, sulfonamides, nitrofurantoin, and aspirin.
Uric acid Normal ranges: Females, 1.5 to 6.0 mg/ml Males, 2.5 to 8.0 mg/ml	This test may be ordered as part of the diagnostic study for patients with urinary calculi composed of uric acid to help determine the cause of the condition.	No special care required.
VDRL (Venereal Disease Research Laboratory)	This is a screening test for syphilis. In some hospitals it is routinely performed at admission.	No special care required.
White blood cell count Normal range: 4300 to 10,000/mm³	This test is usually routinely performed on all patients preoperatively. It may also be done if there is any evidence of infection (the count will be elevated) and will be performed at regular intervals if the patient is receiving chemotherapy or radiation therapy because these treatments suppress white blood cell production.	Anticoagulant is required in the specimen container.

Laboratory studies performed on urine

General guidelines

1. Timed specimens (i.e., those to be collected over a specified period, such as 12 or 24 hours) should be collected in the following way:
   a. Have the patient void; **discard** the urine; record the time. This is the starting time of the specimen collection and should be recorded as such on the laboratory slip.
   b. Collect **all** urine after this time for the specified time period.
   c. Have the patient void as close as possible to termination time (i.e., within 30 minutes), and include this urine in the specimen.
   d. Record the time of the last voiding. If the collection period was a few minutes longer or shorter than the required time, this is usually acceptable, but it must be stated as such on the laboratory slip (e.g., "12-hour urine specimen: started at 8 P.M. and ended at 7:45 A.M.").
2. Do not begin a 24-hour collection if the patient is scheduled to be off the floor for a considerable length of time (e.g., for x-ray examination) unless it can be ensured that any voided urine will be saved and included in the specimen. If any urine is discarded, the test is invalid.
3. Obtain 12-hour specimens overnight (e.g., 7 P.M. to 7 A.M.).
4. If the patient is menstruating, make a note of this on the laboratory slip so that blood in the urine is not assumed to be from the urinary tract; or reschedule the test.
5. Be aware that certain drugs may affect the color of the urine. Those most commonly used in urology include phenazopyridine (Pyridium), which turns the urine reddish orange; methylene blue, which turns the urine blue-green; and nitrofurantoin (Furadantin), which turns the urine brownish.
6. Be aware that cloudy urine does not necessarily indicate a urinary tract infection. Uninfected urine may become cloudy under the following conditions:
   a. Urine produced shortly after a meal may be cloudy due to the presence of phosphates or urates.
   b. Urine that stands at room temperature or is refrigerated for a period of time may develop a haze or cloudiness.

Test	Urologic application	Nursing considerations
Addis count	This is a test to evaluate the number of red and white blood cells and casts in the urine to follow the progress of patients with known renal disease (e.g., acute glomerulonephritis).	Collect the specimen over a 12-hour period (usually overnight) and preserve it in formalin. Send it to the lab as soon as it is completed. Fluid restrictions may be ordered for a 24-hour period prior to the test.
Calcium Normal range, without diet restrictions: 100 to 250 mg/24 hr	Patients with urinary calculi composed of calcium may require this test as part of the diagnostic study to determine the cause of their condition. A high urinary excretion of calcium may occur in hyperparathyroidism.	Indicate on the laboratory slip the type of diet the patient consumed during the 3 days prior to test. Collect the specimen over a period of 24 hours. Thiazide diuretics may interfere with test results, since they cause a decrease in calcium excretion.
Creatinine Normal ranges: Females, 0.6 to 1.5 gm/24 hr Males, 1.0 to 2.0 gm/24 hr	This test is usually performed as part of the creatinine clearance test for renal function. A blood sample is obtained during the period of urine collection, and the clearance rate (the volume of serum or plasma freed of creatinine during a specified period) is calculated.	Collect specimen over a 12- or 24-hour period. Encourage a liberal intake of fluids because a high urinary volume produces the most accurate results.

Laboratory studies performed on urine—cont'd

Test	Urologic application	Nursing considerations
Culture	This test is done to determine the presence of a urinary tract infection and to identify the infecting organism and appropriate antimicrobial treatment. Infections are associated with bacterial colony counts of 100,000 (10^5) or more per milliliter of urine. Pyuria (pus in the urine), combined with the above count, strongly suggests a urinary tract infection. The test is usually routinely performed on all patients.	Use sterile specimen container. Cleanse external portion of meatus thoroughly with soap and water or Betadine. Obtain a midstream specimen and send it to the lab within 30 minutes or refrigerate it. Specimens may also be obtained from a suprapubic tube or from an indwelling urethral catheter (see Chapter 11) but should never be taken from the collecting bag of a drainage system because this area may be contaminated.
Cystine	Patients suspected of having a genetic defect (cystinuria) that causes excretion of cystine in the urine will have this test. Cystine precipitates and forms urinary calculi. Normally there is no cystine in the urine.	Obtain a single voided specimen.
Cytology	This test is done on patients with known or suspected cancer anywhere in the urinary tract. Cells passed in the urine are examined for pathologic changes.	Obtain a single voided specimen, collected approximately 3 hours after previous voiding. Do not use a first voided specimen in the morning because the cells should not be exposed for many hours to cytotoxic properties in the urine. Place specimen in 70% alcohol (two parts alcohol to one part urine) and send to the lab at once.

Electrolytes
   Variable range for single
   voided specimens
	This test is done to assist in the evaluation of the patient's current electrolyte status.	Obtain a single voided specimen.

Electrophoresis	This test aids in determining the presence of cystinuria and aminoaciduria.	Obtain a single voided specimen.

17-Ketosteroids
   Normal ranges:
   Females, 4 to 14 mg/L/24 hr
   Males, 8 to 21 mg/L/24 hr
	These substances are metabolites of androgens. Their level may be elevated in patients with testicular cancer and abnormally low in patients with hypogonadism, nephrosis, or adrenal cortical insufficiency. The test is part of the study performed on patients with infertility.	Collect the specimen over a 24-hour period. Keep the specimen in a special container provided by the lab with the specific preservative. Refrigerate the specimen during the period of collection. The test may be invalidated if the patient is receiving corticosteroids and in some cases if he is under severe stress. Certain antibiotics, secobarbital, and numerous other medications may affect urinary levels of these substances.

Nitroprusside	This test aids in determining the presence of cystinuria.	Obtain a single voided specimen.
Oxalate Range depends on diet	Patients with urinary calculi composed of oxalate may require this test as part of the diagnostic study in determining the cause of the condition.	Collect the specimen over a 24-hour period.

pH
   Normal: 6.0
   Range: 4.5 to 7.5
	This test has a wide range of applications. It is most commonly done in urology as part of the evaluation of patients who have urolithiasis, since the acidity or alkalinity of urine predisposes the patient to certain types of stone formation.	This test may be affected by medications and dietary intake. Obtain a single voided specimen. Do not permit the specimen to stand at room temperature for more than 30 minutes prior to the test, or bacterial metabolism of urea will alkalinize the urine.

Laboratory studies performed on urine—cont'd

Test	Urologic application	Nursing considerations
Specific gravity Normal range: 1.010 to 1.025	This test provides information about the kidneys' ability to concentrate or dilute urine and indicates the patient's state of hydration.	Obtain a single voided specimen. Contrast medium used in certain x-ray examinations will cause elevation of specific gravity until the material is completely excreted. This usually occurs within 3 hours but may take as long as 24 hours.
Uric acid Range depends on diet	Patients with urinary calculi composed of uric acid may require this test as part of the diagnostic study in determining the cause of the condition.	Collect specimen over a 24-hour period with preservative in the container. Drugs that might interfere with the test include thiazide diuretics, aspirin, and x-ray contrast medium.
Urinalysis Normal findings: Blood: absent Glucose: absent Ketones: absent (may be present if the patient is fasting) Protein: absent Red blood cells: 1 to 3/HPF* White blood cells: 3 to 4/HPF* Oxalate or urate crystals: few	This test provides information regarding the balance of normal constituents of the urine and the presence of abnormal constituents such as red or white blood cells, casts, glucose, albumin, and acetone. It includes a microscopic and biochemical analysis as well as a gross examination of the urine. Usually it is routinely performed on all patients.	Obtain a single voided specimen. Send specimen to the lab at once. Refrigerate it if it cannot be sent within 1 hour. (If the specimen is permitted to stand at room temperature, the pH will rise from bacterial metabolism of urea, the glucose level will decrease from yeast or bacterial utilization, and blood cells and casts will disintegrate.)

*High-power field.

Miscellaneous laboratory studies

Test	Urologic application	Nursing considerations
Semen analysis Normal findings: Motility: > 70% progressive, forward Density: > 20 million/ml or 60 million/ejaculate Morphology: > 70% normal	This is part of the evaluation of a patient with infertility. It provides information concerning the concentration, motility, and morphology of sperm and the concentration of various other constituents in the fluid.	Obtain specimen after a period of at least 48 hours of sexual abstinence. Send specimen to the lab at once (a delay of more than 2 hours invalidates the test) and note time of collection on the lab slip. Avoid chilling the specimen.
Stone analysis	Composition of any calculi particles passed in the urine must be evaluated so that appropriate dietary instructions can be provided to prevent future stone formation.	Strain all urine from patients with urolithiasis who might pass the stone (i.e., patients with a stone less than 1 cm in diameter or patients with a stone of an undetermined size). Place specimen in a clean, empty test tube.
Wound exudate culture	A culture specimen should be obtained from any wound that drains purulent exudate to determine the infecting organism and the appropriate antimicrobial treatment.	Swab wound with sterile cotton-tipped applicator. Place specimen in a specially prepared bottle containing culture medium.
Tissue specimen	Any biopsy tissue, tissue appearing spontaneously in the urine (e.g., a sloughed papilla), or tissue removed from any other source must be examined microscopically.	Place all tissue particles in a preservative at once. Immersing them in a 10% volume of formalin is usually adequate, **except** for tissue from a testicular biopsy for infertility. In this case, Bouin's or Zenker's solution is used. Formalin will destroy the specimen.

References and bibliography

BIBLIOGRAPHY

Amelar, R.D., Dubin, L., and Walsh, P.C.: Male infertility, Philadelphia, 1977, W.B. Saunders Co.

Fischbach, F.T.: A manual of laboratory diagnostic tests, Philadelphia, 1980, J.B. Lippincott Co.

Hamburger, J., Crosnier, J., and Grünfeld, J.: Nephrology, New York, 1979, John Wiley & Sons.

Lapides, J.: Fundamentals of urology, Philadelphia, 1976, W.B. Saunders Co.

Morel, A., and Wise, G.J.: Urologic endoscopic procedures, ed. 2, St. Louis, 1979, The C.V. Mosby Co.

Resnick, M.I., editor: The Urologic Clinics of North America, vol. 6, no. 3, Philadelphia, 1979, W.B. Saunders Co.

Strand, M.M., and Elmer, L.A.: Clinical laboratory tests, ed. 2, St. Louis, 1980, The C.V. Mosby Co.

Thorn, G.W., et al.: Harrison's principles of internal medicine, ed. 8, New York, 1977, McGraw-Hill Book Co., Inc.

Tilkian, S.M., Conover, M.B., and Tilkian, A.G.: Clinical implications of laboratory tests, ed. 2, St. Louis, 1979, The C.V. Mosby Co.

Witten, D.M., Myers, G.H., and Utz, D.C.: Emmett's clinical urography, ed. 4, vols. 1-3, Philadelphia, 1977, W.B. Saunders Co.

UNIT III

MASTER CARE PLANS
FOR
THE UROLOGY PATIENT

The chapters in this unit were developed as an adjunct to many of the care plans in the book. Each chapter focuses on a specific aspect of nursing care required for almost all urology patients—hence the name **master care plan.** These care plans provide detailed instructions to elucidate related information presented in other chapters.

These master care plans should be used in conjunction with the care plans for a patient with a specific disorder. The details of the master care plan topics that apply solely to the particular disorder will appear only within the care plan relating to that disorder. For example, the fundamental aspects of care of a patient with a catheter will be identical, whether the patient has had a prostatectomy or fulguration of urethral warts. These nursing interventions are found in the master care plan. But there are also nursing interventions related to the catheter that are unique to each of these procedures. Such nursing interventions will appear within the chapter focusing on the particular procedure, preceded only by the list of nursing objectives and expected outcomes of the interventions discussed in the master care plan.

In this way the reader can avoid being encumbered by repetition of well-known information when studying a care plan for a specific disorder and concentrate on that aspect of the particular nursing problem which applies only to the disorder being discussed.

CHAPTER 9

Preoperative teaching

There is increasing evidence to indicate that comprehensive preoperative teaching considerably enhances the patient's well-being in the postoperative period. Redman[8] cites studies of the 1950s and 1960s which demonstrate that a reduction in postoperative pain and vomiting and a decrease in duration of hospitalization are associated with adequate preoperative information regarding what the patient can expect in the perioperative period and how he can take an active role in his recovery. More recent work by Boore[2], Felton et al.[3], Schmitt et al.[9], and Wong[13] indicates similar findings.

It appears that reduction of anxiety is the key factor in limiting these untoward postoperative events. The sources of anxiety are manifold and cannot all be alleviated by preoperative teaching. But some of the causes of anxiety, such as a sense of helplessness or fear of pain or the unknown, can be significantly reduced with thorough preoperative explanation.[4,10]

The subject of pain control deserves special mention. Pain is not only an extremely unpleasant experience for the patient but may also have deleterious effects on his convalescence (e.g., decreased respirations, limited activity). Thus every effort should be made to minimize the patient's fear and perception of pain. Telling the patient beforehand that there will be pain, but that medication will be available at the patient's request to control it, has been found to be the most successful approach toward reducing the anxiety related to the pain and thus decreasing the patient's perception of the pain itself.[9,12]

The following master care plan presents general guidelines for preoperative teaching of the urology patient. The preoperative teaching sections in subsequent care plans provide specific information pertinent only to the particular surgical procedure discussed.

PREOPERATIVE TEACHING
NURSING DIAGNOSIS: NEED FOR PREOPERATIVE TEACHING

Objectives of nursing intervention
1. If necessary, clarification of reason for hospitalization and type of surgery to be performed
2. Elimination of any negative or inaccurate notions regarding the forthcoming surgery
3. Explanation of preoperative tests and procedures
4. Psychologic preparation for general anesthesia (omit if the patient is to have spinal or local anesthesia)
5. Explanation of events expected in the early postoperative period
6. Explanation of body conditions expected in the early postoperative period
7. Identification of any known allergies

Expected outcomes
Verbal indication that explanations are understood
Verbal indication of optimistic expectations (within realistic limits) related to forthcoming surgery
Cooperation during preoperative tests and procedures
Verbal or behavioral indication of reduction of anxiety
Absence of postoperative complications
Absence of allergic reactions

NURSING OBJECTIVE 1. Clarification of reason for hospitalization and type of surgery to be performed

Plan for implementation	Rationale
1. Determine the extent of the patient's understanding of the forthcoming surgery by having him verbalize his perception of his condition and how he expects the surgery to help him.	The physician has discussed the forthcoming surgery with the patient prior to the patient's signing of the informed consent document. Signing of this form is a requirement in all hospitals prior to surgery and should be done before the nurse commences preoperative teaching. However, the patient may have numerous questions and uncertainties that he did not have an opportunity to discuss with his physician.
2. If deemed appropriate, provide a general description of the surgery and how it relates to the patient's condition.	This confirms or supplements what the physician has told the patient. Having such clarification will also enable the patient to provide information about himself to other health care providers if, at some time in the future, he is required to furnish his health history.

NURSING OBJECTIVE 2. Elimination of any negative or inaccurate notions regarding forthcoming surgery

Plan for implementation	Rationale
1. Determine if the patient has had any prior surgery and, if so, what is his perception of the experience.	This information provides the nurse with a frame of reference for presenting information in a manner that will minimize patient anxiety.
2. If the patient has had no prior surgery, take additional time in explaining all procedures.	The unknown is usually a source of considerable anxiety.
3. If the patient has had a negative experience with prior surgery, give as much reassurance as possible and correct any misconceptions the patient might have.	

NURSING OBJECTIVE 3. Explanation of preoperative tests and procedures

Plan for implementation	Rationale
1. Give a general description of the following diagnostic tests and procedures, and explain their purpose. (Depending on hospital policy and the patient's diagnosis, some of these tests and procedures may have been carried out prior to the patient's admission.) a. Routine preoperative blood and urine tests	See Unit two.

Plan for implementation	**Rationale**
b. Electrocardiogram and chest x-ray examination	These provide important guidelines for the anesthesiologist. Patients found to have cardiac irregularities or certain respiratory conditions may require spinal anesthesia rather than general anesthesia.
c. Additional urologic diagnostic procedures if the patient has obstructive uropathy or suspected tumor	See Unit two.

2. Give a general description of the following preoperative procedures:

a. An enema will be given in the evening prior to surgery.

An empty rectum reduces the risk of contamination of the surgical site during surgery. It also usually reduces postoperative discomfort by delaying the need to defecate for the next 24 to 48 hours.

b. The hair from the area surrounding the surgical site will be shaved prior to the surgery.

This reduces the bacterial count near the surgical site by eliminating the bacteria that adhere to the hair.

c. The consumption of food and fluids will be prohibited after midnight prior to surgery.

Preoperative fasting reduces the risk of aspiration of stomach contents during anesthesia and in the immediate period following the surgery.

d. The patient may be requested by his physician to refrain from smoking prior to surgery. The duration of abstinence ranges from 12 hours to 3 weeks, depending on the physician. Some do not request it at all.

The incidence of postoperative respiratory complications is considerably higher among smokers than nonsmokers.[1] However, medical data defining the optimum duration of abstinence prior to surgery are limited. Furthermore, the stress of being forbidden to smoke must be weighed against the possible (and unproven) benefits of short-term abstinence.

e. Antiembolic stockings or Ace bandages will be applied for the patient to wear during the surgery. They should be worn until the patient is ambulating well.

Many types of urologic surgery predispose the patient to deep vein thrombosis (see Chapter 13). Elastic stockings are often ordered as prophylaxis because they reduce venous stasis in the lower extremities.

f. An intravenous infusion of fluids will be started prior to surgery and will be continued until the patient is able to eat. Once the diet is well tolerated, the infusion is usually removed, and any medication given by this route will then be administered orally or intramuscularly.

This prevents dehydration and provides a route for the administration of anesthetics and certain postoperative medications.

g. An injection containing a sedative, an analgesic, and/or a drying agent will be given approximately 1 hour before the surgery begins, while the patient is still in his room. The purpose is to relax the patient, reduce oral and bronchial secretions, and enhance the effects of anesthesia. The patient should be aware that:

(1) The medication will probably make him drowsy, but it is not the anesthetic.

Occasionally, patients who have never had surgery before think that the preoperative medication is all they will receive with regard to anesthesia, and they become apprehensive because they are still awake when they are taken to the operating room.

(2) The medication may make the patient's mouth dry, but he should not drink.

Some patients need to be reminded that their stomachs must be empty prior to surgery.

(3) The patient must stay in bed after the medication is given and should call the nurse if he needs anything.

Most hospitals have this rule for the patient's safety. He may become unsteady on his feet after certain preoperative medications and could fall and injure himself.

NURSING OBJECTIVE 4. Psychologic preparation for general anesthesia (omit if the patient is to have spinal or local anesthesia)

Plan for implementation	Rationale
1. Allow the patient to communicate his feelings about general anesthesia.	The fear of general anesthesia is one of the most common causes of preoperative anxiety. Although complete alleviation of anxiety may not be possible, it can be considerably reduced by allowing the patient to verbalize his feelings and by providing reassuring information. Patients often harbor the following concerns: a. Fear of revealing personal information while unconscious. b. Fear of waking up in the middle of the operation. c. Fear of going to sleep and **not** waking up. d. Fear of postoperative nausea and vomiting.
2. Provide reassurance and the following information if the patient expresses apprehension: a. It is unusual for patients to talk while under anesthesia. When they do, it is usually unintelligible. b. Throughout the period that the patient is unconscious and in the immediate postoperative period, the patient will be under close surveillance and will not be left alone until he has fully regained consciousness. The anesthesiologist will control the amount of anesthesia throughout the surgery to ensure that the patient does not regain consciousness during the operation and will bring the patient quickly up to consciousness soon after the operation is completed. c. Postoperative nausea and vomiting do not always occur, and, if they do, they can usually be controlled with medication.	
3. Notify the physician if the patient exhibits excessive anxiety about the surgery.	The physician or anesthesiologist is often able to alleviate the anxiety by additional discussion and reassurance.

NURSING OBJECTIVE 5. Explanation of events expected in the early postoperative period

Plan for implementation	Rationale
Explain the events the patient can expect during the early postoperative period. In general:	
1. He will regain consciousness in the recovery room where nurses will be checking his pulse and blood pressure frequently. He will stay in the recovery room until he is fully conscious.	The patient is less likely to become alarmed by the unaccustomed attention if he knows in advance that this is routine procedure.
2. He will be encouraged to cough and breathe deeply. (Demonstrate abdominal breathing and obtain a satisfactory return demonstration from the patient.)	This helps to prevent atelectasis and to mobilize secretions. Some patients have difficulty with abdominal breathing, and the time for them to practice effective coughing is **before** the surgery.
3. Until the patient is permitted out of bed, he will be encouraged to turn from side to side, sit up, and flex and relax his leg muscles.	Any activity that enhances circulation and reduces stasis of blood helps to prevent deep vein thrombosis.
4. The patient will be encouraged to get out of bed as soon as possible (as ordered by his physician). Within the limits of his particular condition he will be expected to walk increasing distances each postoperative day (as tolerated). He should consider this part of his therapy.	Early mobilization reduces the incidence of deep vein thrombosis (see Chapter 13). In addition, it is heartening for the patient to see his activity level increasing and know he is taking an active role in his recovery. However, patients should be told beforehand that they will be expected to be out of bed soon after surgery because, in most cases, they will not feel like it when the time comes. This is particularly true of elderly people, who constitute a large portion of urology patients. They sometimes think that if they stay in bed and "rest" they will "get stronger." They often need to be convinced that just the opposite is true, and that bed rest results in disuse atrophy of the muscles and a decreased tolerance to activity once it is resumed.

NURSING OBJECTIVE 6. Explanation of body conditions expected in the early postoperative period

Plan for implementation	Rationale

1. Describe conditions relating directly to the surgical site, such as dressings, drains, and catheters. (See the preoperative teaching section of the care plan for each specific surgical procedure for this information.)

2. Describe changes in body functions. These include:
   a. Urination
      (1) In most cases after urologic surgery the patient will have an indwelling urethral catheter.

   This promotes complete drainage of the bladder and facilitates accurate measurement of urinary output.

      (2) A patient who does not have a catheter will be given a urinal or bedpan while bed rest is required.
      (3) Blood-tinged urine is expected after most kinds of urologic surgery.

   Prior knowledge of unusual coloration of urine will prevent unnecessary anxiety.

   b. Defecation
      (1) It is unlikely that the patient will have a bowel movement during the first 48 hours after surgery because of the preoperative enema and fasting.

   It is particularly important to mention this to elderly patients, who often become anxious if they do not move their bowels daily.

      (2) A bedpan will be provided, if it should be needed, while bed rest is required.

   Patients who have never been hospitalized before are sometimes very anxious about this aspect of their care.

      (3) If the patient has not had a bowel movement for 72 hours after surgery, he should notify the nurse.

   Analgesics, immobility, stress, and other factors may cause constipation, which is usually treated with a laxative on the third or fourth day after surgery.

3. Provide the following information regarding postoperative pain:

   The patient should feel that any pain will be effectively and safely handled. He should also understand that he will be expected to play a role in the control of his pain.

   a. Some pain at the surgical site is expected but can be controlled with medication.

   Unanticipated pain is usually a greater source of anxiety than is awareness of forthcoming pain, especially if the patient knows medication will be available to relieve it.

   b. Pain medication is usually ordered to be given every 3 or 4 hours **as needed,** and the patient is expected to tell the nurse when he has pain.

   Some patients assume pain medication is given routinely and wait for it in silence, despite the presence of pain. Others do not want to appear cowardly or bothersome, so they do not ask for medication. Knowing what is expected of them helps patients handle the pain more effectively. The awareness that they will have a degree of control over their pain also helps reduce the anxiety arising from the sense of powerlessness often experienced by hospitalized patients.

   c. The patient should request pain medication before the pain becomes very intense.

   Pain is harder to control once it has become severe.[6]

   d. If the patient voices concern about becoming addicted to pain medication, explain that control of pain is the most important consideration, and analgesics used for this purpose, and for this duration of time, will not result in addiction.

   Although present data are not definitive, it is estimated that less than 1% of patients receiving meperidine hydrochloride (Demerol) every 4 hours for 10 days will become addicted.* Equivalent doses of analgesia are rarely required for more than 3 or 4 days after most types of surgery[12] except for extensive procedures.

---

*Addiction is defined as "a behavioral pattern of compulsive drug use characterized by overwhelming involvement with the use of the drug, the securing of its supply, and a tendency to relapse after withdrawal."[5]

Plan for implementation	Rationale
e. If the patient has only mild pain, he should specify this to the nurse, and a nonnarcotic analgesic will be given.	Narcotics have numerous side effects (see Appendix A) and should not be given indiscriminately. Furthermore, although addiction is unlikely, some degree of dependence* will occur after continued narcotic administration for a few days.[7,11] This means that some patients might experience mild withdrawal symptoms when the narcotic medications are discontinued, such as restlessness, sleeplessness, or rhinorrhea.

*Physical dependence is defined as "a need for the continued administration of the narcotic in the sense that continued administration is necessary to prevent the development of physiologic disturbances known as the abstinence or withdrawal syndrome."[7]

NURSING OBJECTIVE 7. Identification of any known allergies

Plan for implementation	Rationale

1. Determine the existence of any allergies the patient might have.
  a. Ask the patient if he is aware of being allergic to anything.
  b. Specifically mention the following possible allergens:
    (1) Antibiotics	

(1) Antibiotics	Allergic reactions to certain antibiotics, particularly to penicillin and related drugs, may be very severe. Because there is a considerable choice of antibiotics from which to choose, a different drug can easily be substituted if the patient requires antibiotic therapy.
(2) Iodine compounds	A skin reaction to the surgical prep (usually povidone-iodine is used) can be prevented by using a different antiseptic agent.
(3) Adhesive tape	Although tape reactions are usually not serious, they can be very uncomfortable for the patient. Paper tape is usually well tolerated.
2. Record the presence of any known allergies on the patient's chart and medication sheet.	
3. If the patient is allergic to tape or iodine, place a conspicuous note on the **front** of his chart when he goes to the operating room.	This alerts the operating room staff to the need for changes in their usual regimen.

CHAPTER 10

Discharge preparations

Discharge preparations are essential components of nursing care that are too frequently neglected in deference to the more immediate needs of the patient. The requirement that discharge preparations be implemented as soon as possible after admission has helped to integrate discharge planning into the early period of hospitalization so that there is adequate time for referrals and thorough patient teaching.[1]

Although most urology patients resume their previous life-styles within a few weeks after discharge, there is often a considerable amount of patient education required when the patient leaves the hospital. Deciding in advance when and how the discharge instructions will be presented allows for individualized teaching plans that take into account the patient's particular needs, problems, capabilities, and limitations and promotes effective teaching sessions. In contrast, teaching that is done in the hours directly preceding the patient's discharge is rarely effective because the patient is either anxious about leaving the supportive environment of the hospital or is excited about going home. Either state of mind may reduce the ability to learn. Ideally, the information the patient must have on discharge should be taught over a period of a few days so that the patient has time to integrate it and ask questions. Furthermore, the data should be written so that misunderstanding can be virtually eliminated.

The following two-part care plan presents general guidelines for discharge preparations for the urology patient. The discharge planning and discharge teaching sections in the subsequent care plans provide specific information that is pertinent only to the particular condition or surgical procedure discussed in the chapter.

DISCHARGE PREPARATIONS
Discharge Planning
NURSING DIAGNOSIS: NEED FOR DISCHARGE PLANNING

Objectives of nursing intervention
1. Early commencement of discharge planning
2. Accurate estimate of time required for all discharge teaching

Expected outcome
Smooth transition of care after discharge

Discharge Teaching
NURSING DIAGNOSIS: NEED FOR DISCHARGE TEACHING

Objectives of nursing intervention
1. Explanation of basic information about medications to be taken at home
2. Explanation of information regarding follow-up care
3. Explanation of residual effects of the condition and/or treatment
4. Explanation of instructions concerning postdischarge activities
5. Explanation of symptoms that constitute a reason to contact the physician
6. Review of admitting diagnosis and mode of treatment

Expected outcomes
Accurate return verbalization and/or demonstration of all material learned
Smooth transition of care after discharge
Absence or early detection of complications arising after discharge
Ability to provide future health care practitioners with important data about health history

Discharge planning

NURSING OBJECTIVE 1. Early commencement of discharge planning

Plan for implementation	**Rationale**

1. Obtain the following information regarding the patient's current health status before hospitalization. This includes:
  a. Health care needs
  b. Degree of self-sufficiency
  c. Presence of household member and/or "significant other" who is able to provide assistance
	Information about the patient's current level of functioning is essential to the formulation of an appropriate discharge plan. It provides a point of reference for establishing realistic goals.

2. If deemed necessary, begin the referral process by contacting appropriate community health services or other organizations. Most patients hospitalized for urologic conditions, however, will be able to resume their former level of functioning after a relatively short convalescent period. Therefore professional care, other than the follow-up care by the physician, is usually not required. (See individual care plans for exceptions.)	

NURSING OBJECTIVE 2. Accurate estimate of time required for all discharge teaching

Plan for implementation	**Rationale**
1. Provide the patient with a general overview of what he will be required to know on discharge.	Teaching that is done shortly before discharge is more effective if the patient is already somewhat familiar with the information. This also gives the nurse an opportunity to assess the patient's pace of learning and to estimate the amount of time required to complete all the required teaching.
2. Determine the patient's present level of knowledge.	
3. Estimate the patient's rate of learning. Take into consideration the high level of anxiety of most patients on admission, especially if surgery is to be performed. This anxiety may reduce an otherwise normal learning rate.	

Discharge teaching

NURSING OBJECTIVE 1. Explanation of basic information about medications to be taken at home

Plan for implementation	Rationale
Provide the patient with instructions about the medication he is to take after discharge.	Patients convalescing after treatment for a urologic condition are frequently given a prescription for a mild analgesic and an antibiotic. Those being treated for urolithiasis may also be given medication to inhibit future stone formation.
1. Write out basic action, administration schedule, and dosage of each medication. (See Appendix A for specific drugs frequently used in urology.)	
2. Discuss important side effects.	
3. If the patient is given an antibiotic, emphasize the importance of taking the medication for the entire length of time prescribed.	Termination of antibiotic administration before the prescribed treatment time may result in the development of drug-resistant strains of the microorganism and persistent infection.

NURSING OBJECTIVE 2. Explanation of information regarding follow-up care

Plan for implementation	Rationale
1. Provide the patient with written information concerning the time, date, and location of the follow-up appointment with the physician in the office or urology clinic. It is usually scheduled for 2 to 4 weeks after discharge.	
2. Describe the purpose of the appointment. (See individual care plans for specific details.)	Some patients will disregard follow-up care (especially if they are feeling well) unless they are aware of its importance.
3. If the patient does not have a private physician, give him the name and phone number of one specific person he can contact (e.g., the resident physician in charge of his care or the enterostomal therapist) in the event that he has any questions or problems.	

Plan for implementation	Rationale
4. Inform the patient if arrangements have been made with the Visiting Nurse Service, and assure him that the nurse caring for him will have all pertinent information.	The transition from hospital to home care is often a source of considerable anxiety for the patient who depends on skilled nursing care. This anxiety is often reduced if the patient knows there is good communication between the nurse to whom he became accustomed in the hospital and the visiting nurse.
5. When applicable, provide the patient with information concerning services available within the community, such as local chapters of the American Cancer Society or United Ostomy Association. (See p. 147 for more information on these particular organizations.)	

NURSING OBJECTIVE 3. Explanation of residual effects of the condition and/or treatment

Plan for implementation	Rationale
Explain to the patient what to expect for a few weeks after discharge and that it is normal and no cause for alarm. This will vary according to the patient's diagnosis and treatment (see individual care plans for specific residual effects). In general, after urologic surgery the patient may experience:	Because of the anxiety many patients experience once they are "on their own" after discharge, symptoms of which they had only been vaguely aware during hospitalization often become threatening after they leave the hospital. They need reassurance that these symptoms are part of the normal recuperative process.
1. Incisional discomfort (i.e., itching, burning, or mild pain)	
2. Fatigue	
3. Transient hematuria (after prostatic surgery)	

NURSING OBJECTIVE 4. Explanation of instructions concerning postdischarge activities

Plan for implementation	Rationale
Provide the patient with instructions prescribed by his physician concerning postdischarge activities. In general, these include:	
1. If the patient had surgery: a. Avoid heavy lifting for 6 weeks.	The increase in intraabdominal pressure induced by lifting may result in an incisional hernia or, after transurethral surgery, may precipitate bleeding.
b. Participate in mild exercise (e.g., walking) as tolerated. c. Bathe normally (bath or shower) if there is no drainage from the surgical wound. If the wound is still draining, avoid tub baths; showers are permitted, followed by application of a clean dressing.	
2. Consume at least 2 L of fluid per day (unless this is contraindicated by a coexisting medical condition).	A rapid flow of urine through the urinary tract reduces the incidence of infection, urolithiasis, and urethral obstruction by clot formation.
3. Refrain from sexual activity until after the follow-up appointment with the physician.	
4. Follow diet limitations (if any). a. If the patient was treated for urolithiasis, he may be required to eliminate certain foods, depending on the composition of the stone.	
b. If the patient was treated for a prostate condition, he may be advised to limit his intake of alcohol and highly spiced foods.	Some physicians feel that alcohol consumption following a prostatectomy might increase the risk of prostatic bleeding. It is also considered by some physicians to be an irritant to the prostate, as are highly spiced foods. Medical data confirming this are very limited.

NURSING OBJECTIVE 5. Explanation of symptoms that constitute a reason to contact the physician

Plan for implementation	Rationale
Provide the patient with information concerning symptoms that may indicate complications and warrant medical attention. (See individual care plans for warning signs of specific complications associated with a particular condition.) In general, these include:	Some patients are so distressed by the possibility of having to return to the hospital for more treatment that they occasionally ignore potentially serious symptoms and postpone notifying the physician. If this occurs, the health of the patient may be seriously jeopardized.
1. Chills, fever, flank pain, hematuria	These may indicate a urinary tract infection.
2. Severe pain and/or increasing redness at the incision site	These may indicate a wound infection.
3. Inability to void	This may indicate obstruction of the lower urinary tract.
4. Skin eruptions (if the patient has been given medication to take after discharge)	Although the physician should be notified if **any** drug reactions occur, it is unlikely that the patient will develop the more common ones (e.g., gastrointestional disturbances) after he is discharged, since he will usually be given a prescription for a medication he had been receiving during his hospitalization, and any untoward effects will have already occurred and been handled appropriately. However, skin eruptions (an indication of **drug toxicity)** commonly occur after the first week of therapy and therefore may not appear until after discharge. This type of reaction is often associated with sulfonamides[2], which are frequently used in urology.

NURSING OBJECTIVE 6. Review of admitting diagnosis and mode of treatment

Plan for implementation	Rationale
1. Determine the level of understanding the patient has regarding his condition on admission and the treatment that was provided.	
2. Provide information when necessary.	The patient should know enough about his condition and treatment to be able to provide basic information to health care providers if, at some time in the future, he is required to furnish his health history.

CHAPTER 11

The patient with an indwelling urethral catheter

The indwelling urethral catheter is probably the most common piece of urologic equipment used in hospitals. Its purpose is to drain the bladder of urine for one or more of the following reasons: the normal voiding process has been disturbed by a pathologic condition; voiding would interfere with healing; precise monitoring of urine output is required.

The catheter's specific uses are numerous, but its serious potential hazards must also be considered. Thorton and Andriole[4] and Maki et al.[3] have shown that indwelling urethral catheters readily promote ascending infection of the urinary tract and that catheters are a leading cause of nosocomial infections. However, when preventative measures are taken, the incidence of infection can be considerably reduced.[1,2] Other complications arising from incorrect use or care of these catheters is the development of severe inflammation of the urethra, scarring, and stricture formation.

There are many types of indwelling urethral catheters. The variations exist in the material of which the catheter is made, the number of lumens, the structure of the retention mechanism, and the shape of the tip (Fig. 11-1). Each type has a specific function, but the Foley catheter is probably the most frequently used model.

Because almost all urologic patients require an indwelling urethral catheter for at least part of their hospitalization, the following master care plan has been included to provide the nurse with a comprehensive approach to this important aspect of patient care. It presents general guidelines for meeting the basic needs of any patient with an indwelling urethral catheter. Subsequent care plans provide information pertinent only to the particular condition discussed in the chapter.

THE PATIENT WITH AN INDWELLING URETHRAL CATHETER
Care after Insertion of the Catheter
NURSING DIAGNOSIS: NEED FOR MANAGEMENT OF INDWELLING URETHRAL CATHETER

Objectives of nursing intervention
1. Appropriate care of catheter and equipment
2. Prevention or early detection of infection
3. Care of tissue surrounding catheter
4. Maintenance of accurate records of urine output
5. Appropriate administration of hand-irrigation of catheter
6. Management of discomfort or pain caused by catheter
7. Satisfactory collection of urine specimens from catheter

Expected outcomes
Absence of severe bladder spasms and suprapubic distention
Urine draining freely through system
Absence of fever, chills, and foul-smelling urine
Absence of urethral discharge and tissue inflammation
Minimal discomfort caused by the catheter
Urine specimens in optimum condition for all necessary tests

Care after Removal of Catheter
NURSING DIAGNOSIS: POTENTIAL FOR VOIDING COMPLICATIONS FOLLOWING REMOVAL OF INDWELLING URETHRAL CATHETER

Objectives of nursing intervention
1. Appropriate management of accidental ejection of catheter
2. Prevention or early detection of voiding complications following removal of catheter

Expected outcomes
Resumption of normal voiding pattern
Absence of dysuria

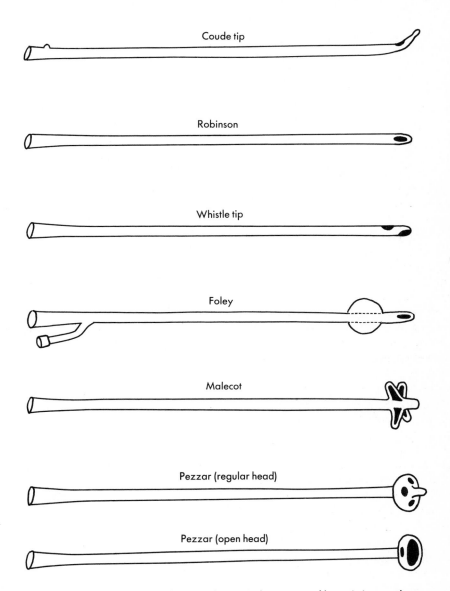

Coude tip

Robinson

Whistle tip

Foley

Malecot

Pezzar (regular head)

Pezzar (open head)

Fig. 11-1. Commonly used catheters; bottom four are self-retaining catheters.

Care after insertion of the catheter

NURSING OBJECTIVE 1. Appropriate care of catheter and equipment

Plan for implementation	Rationale
1. Prevent kinks and loops in the tubing.	These might restrict the flow of urine.
2. Keep the collecting container below the level of the patient's bladder at all times.	This promotes drainage by gravity. Elevating the collecting container will cause urine to flow from the tubing back into the bladder.
3. Tape the tubing securely to the thigh or abdomen of a male patient and to the thigh of a female patient. The catheter should remain slack once it is taped to prevent pressure on any portion of the urethra or bladder neck.	Taping the tubing prevents inadvertent traction on the catheter. If prolonged, such traction may cause irritation, necrosis, and possible stricture formation, especially in a male patient. Securing the tubing to the thigh or abdomen also prevents fecal contamination of the external portion of the tubing.
4. "Milk" the tubing (i.e., exert pressure on the tubing with thumb and forefinger while moving the hand along the tubing away from the patient) if clots or tissue particles appear to be blocking it.	This will facilitate the passage of particles through the lumen and help to avoid obstruction of the catheter.
5. Encourage the patient to drink enough fluid so that his total intake (including intravenous fluid) is approximately 3000 ml per day (unless contraindicated by a coexisting medical condition).	Internal irrigation (i.e., a liberal fluid intake) is considered the safest way to maintain patency of the catheter. A brisk flow of urine not only discourages infection but also decreases the incidence of clot formation and thus reduces obstruction of the drainage system.

NURSING OBJECTIVE 2. Prevention or early detection of infection

Plan for implementation	Rationale
1. Maintain a fluid intake of approximately 3000 ml per day.	Continual flushing of urine through the urinary tract is one of the best methods of preventing infection. It eliminates stagnation of urine, so it reduces the multiplication of pathogens in the urinary tract.
2. Cleanse the catheter and meatus three times a day and after bowel movements. (Cleansing should be done even more often if there is a considerable amount of exudate.) Encrustations can be removed easily with a gauze pad soaked in hydrogen peroxide or soap and water. Most patients can be taught to do this themselves, but the nurse must encourage the patient to do it and check that it is done.	Irritation of the urethral wall by the catheter may result in an increase in mucus secretion. Some bleeding may also be present within the urethra after prostatic or urethral surgery. Both these conditions cause drainage to accumulate on the catheter near the meatus. This material, when dried, is a source of irritation to the urethral tissue and an ideal site for the multiplication of pathogens.
3. Apply antimicrobial solutions or ointments as ordered.	Povidone-iodine preparations or antibiotic ointments are used in some hospitals as prophylaxis against ascending infection. The efficacy of this procedure has not been established.
4. If the catheter requires irrigation, use guidelines presented in nursing objective 5, p. 80.	
5. Do not open any portion of the drainage system unless absolutely necessary. If tubing must be disconnected (e.g., for irrigation), prevent contamination of open ends of the tubing, and reconnect the system as soon as possible.	Once it is opened to the air, the system is potentially contaminated.
6. Notify the physician if: a. The urine develops a strong odor or becomes cloudy. b. The patient develops chills, fever, and/or flank pain.	These may be indications of a urinary tract infection. A urine and blood specimen will probably be ordered for culture and sensitivity tests.
7. If the catheter is to remain in the bladder for more than 1 week: a. Change the tubing and collecting container weekly and the catheter every 2 weeks. b. Administer prophylactic antibiotics as ordered.	The longer the drainage system remains in place, the more likely it is to become contaminated. Because the risk of infection increases considerably if the catheter is in place for more than a few days, prophylactic antibiotics are frequently ordered.

NURSING OBJECTIVE 3. Care of tissue surrounding the catheter

Plan for implementation	Rationale
1. Provide routine cleansing of catheter and meatus (see nursing objective 2, no. 2).	
2. Be certain that the foreskin of an uncircumcised patient is not left in the retracted position after cleansing.	Paraphimosis might develop if the foreskin is left in a retracted position.
3. Check the skin around the meatus of male patients. If swelling is observed, notify the physician.	Edema of the foreskin sometimes occurs after urethral instrumentation. It can be very painful and can result in decreased circulation to the tip of the urethra. Sitz baths or cold compresses may be ordered.
4. Avoid the use of a red rubber catheter if the catheter is to be left indwelling.	Red rubber is very irritating to tissue.
5. Use only latex or silicone-coated catheters for indwelling catheter drainage.	These substances are biologically inert and do not give rise to tissue reaction.
6. Use the smallest possible caliber for an indwelling catheter: males, nos. 16 to 18 French; females, nos. 16 to 22 French.	The catheter should fit loosely in the urethral lumen so mucus and exudate have space through which to drain.

NURSING OBJECTIVE 4. Maintenance of accurate records of urine output

Plan for implementation	Rationale
1. Record volume of urine output for each shift.	Thorough documentation of drainage characteristics helps maintain continuity of care from one shift to the next. It also prevents indications of impending complications from being overlooked.
2. Record character of output (e.g., clear, cloudy, blood tinged, clots or mucus shreds, bright red).	

NURSING OBJECTIVE 5. Appropriate administration of hand-irrigation of catheter

Plan for implementation	Rationale

1. Perform hand-irrigation of the catheter for the following reasons only:
   a. The physician has specifically ordered periodic hand-irrigation.
   b. The catheter is obstructed.

Unless otherwise ordered, irrigation should be done only for obstruction because it requires opening a closed sterile system, thus potentially contaminating the urinary tract.

2. Be alert for indications of catheter obstruction, most commonly manifested by scanty urine output (less than 30 ml per hour) combined with one or more of the following conditions:
   a. Severe, persistent bladder spasms
   b. Urine leaking around catheter
   c. Suprapubic distention noted on palpation or percussion
   d. Blood clots or tissue shreds adhering to the lumen of the tubing

Catheter obstruction may occur from any solid matter passed in the urine (e.g., blood clots, mucus shreds, tissue particles, urinary calculi).

3. If the catheter is obstructed, irrigate it with sterile normal saline using the guidelines described in no. 5.

4. If the urine output is scanty **without** the accompanying conditions usually associated with obstruction, consider some of the causes of oliguria, such as dehydration, hypotension, shock, renal failure, or bilateral ureteral obstruction, which require the attention of the physician. If there is no indication that any of these conditions exist, have the patient drink 300 to 400 ml of fluid.

   If drainage does not increase within 30 minutes, irrigate the catheter, regardless of the absence of any other symptoms. However, unless an obstruction is aspirated and identified as the cause of scanty output, notify the physician.

Plan for implementation	**Rationale**

5. Use the following guidelines when performing hand-irrigation of the catheter:
   a. Reduce the risk of infection.
   (1) Use a sterile set of irrigation equipment each time a series of irrigations is performed. Be aware that the cost of treating a urinary tract infection with regard to money, time, and **patient discomfort** is far greater than using a new set each time the catheter requires irrigation.

   Once the equipment has been used, reuse after exposure to the air in the room invites contamination of the urinary tract. The new, disposable irrigation sets facilitate adherence to sterile technique.

   (2) Use sterile normal saline only, unless a specific medication is ordered. Do not use tap water or distilled water.

   Normal saline is isotonic to the body fluids, and it contains no bacterial contamination (provided it has not been left open to the air or been in contact with contaminated equipment).

   (3) Avoid contamination of open ends of the tubing while performing irrigation. Many irrigation sets provide a sterile cap that can be placed over the distal opening of the tubing while irrigation is in progress.
   (4) Wipe open ends of tubing with alcohol before rejoining them.

   This is an extra precaution against contamination of the lumen.

   b. Avoid excessive distention of the bladder while irrigating.
   (1) Do not instill more than 100 ml of irrigant at one time into a normal bladder.
   (2) Identify patients known to have a small bladder capacity by making a note on the Kardex so that any nurse providing care for the patient will take the appropriate precautions.

   More than this amount would cause discomfort and after surgery might damage the surgical site by overdistention. Shrinkage of the bladder may occur after radiation therapy for malignant conditions of the bladder and adjacent organs. Other causes of small bladder capacity include interstitial cystitis, segmental resection of the bladder, and hyperreflexive neurogenic bladder.

   (3) Be certain that the amount of fluid aspirated is equivalent to that which was instilled.
   c. In most cases, continue irrigation until the return solution is clear.

   This ensures removal of all debris.

   d. In the event that the irrigant cannot be aspirated but, instead, trickles out of the catheter by itself:
   (1) Do not continue instilling more fluid.

   This will cause overdistention and considerable discomfort for the patient.

   (2) Apply gentle pressure over the suprapubic area or have the patient cough or turn from side to side.

   Sometimes this facilitates obtaining an adequate return flow.

   (3) If the catheter contents still cannot be aspirated, reconnect the catheter and for the next few hours carefully observe the patient for additional signs of catheter obstruction. Sometimes the fluid will drain out by gravity, indicating that the catheter is indeed patent.

   Rapid aspiration of fluid may be difficult or impossible if the patient is having bladder spasms or if the eye of the catheter is pressing against the bladder mucosa. Although these conditions may not prevent adequate drainage, they complicate the picture because a partial obstruction will manifest itself in the same way. A partial obstruction may easily develop into a full obstruction, so close observation of the patient is essential.

   e. Attempt the following procedures if the obstruction is not relieved by the aforementioned methods and the physician is not immediately available:
   (1) Use a piston syringe instead of a bulb syringe. (The nurse should check hospital policy before irrigating with a piston syringe. Considerable pressure can be generated, which may cause damage if irrigation is not done skillfully.)

   This increases the amount of negative pressure while aspirating.

Plan for implementation	**Rationale**

(2) If adequate return flow cannot be obtained with a piston syringe, thoroughly cleanse the external portion of the catheter and meatus with hydrogen peroxide or povidone-iodine and apply sterile lubricant. Then, while gently rotating and advancing the catheter into the urethra, attempt to aspirate. This procedure takes four hands, and the nurse handling the catheter should wear sterile gloves once the catheter has been cleansed.

This procedure sometimes reestablishes adequate drainage, especially if the "obstruction" occurred because the catheter slipped into the prostatic fossa (following prostatectomy) where the eye of the catheter is easily occluded. It is a potentially dangerous procedure because it inevitably forces microorganisms past the proximal urethra. It should be approved by the physician before it is attempted. However, since the alternative may be the removal of the catheter and then recatheterization, it is usually considered a worthwhile risk if done with care. Recatheterization could be harmful (if not impossible) if the patient has had recent prostatic or bladder neck surgery.

f. Check the patient's temperature within 2 hours after any difficult irrigation during which manipulation of the catheter was required. If there is an elevation of more than 101°:
(1) Notify the physician.
(2) Be prepared to obtain urine and blood specimens for culture, if ordered.

The possibility of a "urethral chill" is always present after any instrumentation or manipulation within the urethra. This occurs as a result of absorption of bacteria into the bloodstream through the urethral mucosa. Transient bacteremia might occur, producing a high fever and sometimes a shaking chill. Blood and urine cultures are often ordered and should be obtained while the fever is spiking. Antibiotic therapy is usually started (in addition to any prophylactic antibiotics the patient may already be receiving).

NURSING OBJECTIVE 6. Management of discomfort or pain caused by the catheter

Plan for implementation	**Rationale**

Question and observe the patient for information about what he is experiencing.

The characteristics of the patient's discomfort will provide clues to its source and thus indicate ways to relieve it. Pain may be caused by an obstructed catheter or the catheter's irritating effect on the bladder wall. There may also be psychologic factors because discomfort associated with the genitalia may trigger fears of loss of function or mutilation.

PERSISTENT, SEVERE, INCREASING PAIN IN SUPRAPUBIC AREA

1. Check for obstruction of the catheter (see p. 79) and, if necessary, hand-irrigate the catheter with normal saline.

Pain with the aforementioned characteristics is usually caused by an obstructed catheter.

2. If the obstruction cannot be aspirated:
a. Notify the physician at once.

Either the obstruction or the catheter itself will have to be removed or other causes of the pain identified.

b. Administer analgesic only as a stopgap measure until the source of the pain (i.e., the obstructed catheter) is corrected.

Analgesic medication will not provide much relief from pain caused by catheter obstruction. Furthermore, if the obstruction is not quickly corrected, the increasing bladder distention may disrupt a suture line if the patient had recent bladder or prostatic surgery.

Plan for implementation	Rationale
SPASMODIC, INTERMITTENT PAIN IN SUPRAPUBIC AREA (MAY RADIATE TO URETHRAL AREA)	
1. Check the catheter for patency.	Bladder spasms caused by catheter irritation may be quite uncomfortable for the patient and difficult to distinguish from spasms caused by an obstructed catheter. Generally, these "normal" spasms do not increase in intensity or frequency. If, however, the catheter is obstructed, spasms become increasingly painful as the bladder distends with urine.
2. If no obstruction is present, administer analgesic or antispasmodic medication as ordered, or suggest that such medications be ordered. Opium and belladonna suppositories are considered the treatment of choice for patients with bladder spasms, with the exception of those who have had prostatic surgery within the last 72 hours.	Analgesics will reduce the pain associated with bladder spasms **provided that the catheter is patent.** Antispasmodics will reduce the intensity of the spasms. Opium and belladonna suppositories have both analgesic and antispasmodic properties and therefore provide the most complete relief. However, these suppositories (or **any** suppositories) are contraindicated immediately after a prostatectomy because of the risk of disruption of the surgical site. (See Appendix A for other contraindications for the use of opium and belladonna suppositories.)
3. Reassure the patient that this pain is not abnormal and will be relieved by medication.	The psychologic aspects of pain management are a major factor in its control. Eradication of the fear that "something has gone wrong" is often sufficient to relieve the discomfort.
4. Assist the patient with slow, abdominal breathing if spasms are severe.	Deep breathing promotes general relaxation. Whether it has a relaxing effect on the bladder itself has not been proved, but it does seem to relieve some of the discomfort, and it provides a distraction from the pain.
5. If a male patient has pain radiating to his penis, apply witch hazel compresses to the area.	Bladder pain is often referred to the penis. These compresses provide moderate relief for some patients, probably because of the astringent effect on the urethral mucosa.
6. If there is no relief after these procedures, inform the physician and suggest aspiration of some of the fluid from the balloon portion of the catheter.	This will decrease the size of the balloon and thus reduce its irritating effect. This procedure should not, however, be done without the physician's consent because of the risk of accidental ejection of the catheter.

Plan for implementation	Rationale

VAGUE, GENERALIZED COMPLAINTS OF DISCOMFORT, **NOT** ACCOMPANIED BY ANY PHYSICAL
MANIFESTATIONS OF PAIN (e.g., GRIMACES, DIAPHORESIS, AND INCREASED BLOOD PRESSURE,
PULSE, AND RESPIRATORY RATES)

Plan for implementation	Rationale
1. Determine the patient's understanding of the function of the catheter and how it is retained in the bladder.	Sometimes ignorance of the mechanics of the catheter gives rise to anxiety. The patient may experience this as physical discomfort in the area.
2. Provide an explanation of the catheter's function and correct any misconceptions the patient might have.	Fear that the catheter might fall out if the patient does not limit his activities and fear that the catheter will not be able to be removed without causing considerable pain are common sources of anxiety.
3. In simple terms, explain the reason for the bladder spasms (i.e., the bladder is trying to rid itself of a foreign object—the catheter). Patients often refer to spasms as "burning" or simply "when I urinate through the catheter. . . ." Reassure the patient that what he is feeling is normal and no cause for alarm. (See previous implementation plans if there is any chance that these spasms are causing more than the minimal, expected discomfort.)	Usually reassurance is sufficient to relax the patient and reduce the distress he may be feeling.
4. Provide comfort measures such as a back rub or repositioning the patient.	These activities are additional methods to facilitate relaxation.

NURSING OBJECTIVE 7. Satisfactory collection of urine specimens from the catheter

Plan for implementation	Rationale
1. Obtain specimens for most tests from the distal opening of the collecting container. (See further for tests that require urine directly from the catheter.) The procedure follows: a. Empty the container and discard the urine. b. Collect the urine that drains during the next hour as the specimen. (See Chapter 8 for collection of timed specimens.) c. Send specimen to the laboratory at once or refrigerate it.	
2. For tests that must be done on freshly produced urine, obtain specimens from the self-sealing, rubber window provided on most brands of drainage tubing. Specimens that must be collected in this manner include urine for: a. Sugar and acetone tests	The most recently produced urine is the most accurate

Plan for implementation	Rationale
	indicator of the patient's serum glucose level at a particular time. It is especially important to know this if insulin coverage is to be determined by the amount of sugar and acetone in the urine. Furthermore, if the amount of glucose (and other reducing sugars) in the urine is not determined at once, bacterial action will alter it and invalidate the test. Obtaining the specimen from the collecting container would be completely inappropriate for both these reasons.
b. Culture and sensitivity tests	Urine for this test must not be in contact with any potentially contaminated portion of the drainage system, since a urinary tract infection is determined by the quantity of a microorganism found in the culture specimen. Since the collection container is the portion of the system that is least likely to be sterile, urine taken from there will probably produce inaccurate culture readings.
3. Obtain specimens from the rubber window in the following way: a. Cleanse the rubber thoroughly with an alcohol wipe.	This removes microorganisms from the surface of the rubber so they are not introduced into the lumen by the syringe.
b. Aspirate the specimen through the rubber using a sterile syringe. Sometimes the tubing may have to be clamped for a few minutes, distal to the window, to accumulate enough urine for the specimen.	
4. If no window exists in the tubing, aspirate the specimen through the wall of the catheter, not the tubing.	Puncturing the plastic tubing with a syringe may cause it to leak; it will also produce a portal of entry for microorganisms.
However, if the catheter is the type that is retained by an inflated balloon, take precautions not to aspirate the fluid from the balloon. This hazard can be avoided if the aspirating needle is inserted **distal** to the arm of the catheter that communicates with the balloon (Fig. 11-2).	Inadvertent removal of the inflating fluid will not only cause the catheter to be ejected but will also provide a totally inaccurate and misleading specimen.

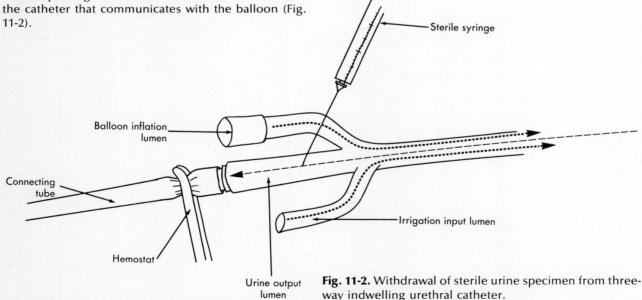

Fig. 11-2. Withdrawal of sterile urine specimen from three-way indwelling urethral catheter.

Care after removal of the catheter

NURSING OBJECTIVE 1. Appropriate management of accidental ejection of the catheter

Plan for implementation	Rationale
1. If the catheter is accidentally ejected within 4 days after bladder neck, prostatic, or urethral surgery, notify the physician at once. Do not attempt to replace the catheter.	The catheter may require replacement quickly if there is a possibility that edema will occlude the urethra. However, this should be done by the physician. Catheterization of patients with certain types of urologic disorders may be extremely difficult and sometimes hazardous if not done with adequate skill.
2. Handle other instances in which a catheter is ejected on an individual basis, depending on the physician's evaluation of the patient and hospital regulations concerning catheterization by a nurse.	

NURSING OBJECTIVE 2. Prevention or early detection of voiding complications following removal of the catheter

Plan for implementation	Rationale
1. Do not remove a catheter without a physician's order.	The replacement of a prematurely removed catheter subjects the patient to unnecessary discomfort.
2. After removal of the catheter, give the patient the following information:	
a. There may be some discomfort while voiding for the first 24 hours.	Catheters often cause urethritis. If the urine is highly concentrated, it may cause a burning sensation on the inflamed tissue.
b. The patient should consume at least eight 8-ounce glasses of fluid daily, preferably before 6 P.M.	Much of the aforementioned discomfort will be relieved if the patient's urine is dilute. However, effort should be made to prevent nocturia so that the patient can have adequate rest at night.
3. Assess the patient's voiding ability.	
a. Record the time and volume of each voiding for 48 to 72 hours. Most patients can be taught to do this themselves.	
b. Note the character of the urine.	
c. Inform the physician if the patient has not voided for more than 6 hours, despite adequate fluid intake.	Obstruction of the urethra occasionally occurs, necessitating recatheterization.

CHAPTER 12

The patient receiving intravenous therapy

The care of a patient with an intravenous (IV) infusion is hardly unique to urology. This topic, however, has been included as a master care plan because almost every urology patient will have an IV during his hospitalization. Therefore IV therapy must be considered in the patient's nursing care plan, and nursing care must be aimed at prevention of the serious complications that might result from intravenous infusions.

Furthermore, urology patients may require special considerations concerning volume of fluid intake. Patients undergoing nephrectomies may have strict limitations on the amount of fluid they receive. Patients with an indwelling urethral catheter may require a fluid intake greater than what they normally are accustomed to, to prevent infection. Patients who have a tendency to form stones may also require an unusually high fluid intake. Finally, urology patients, the majority of whom are part of an older population, may have cardiac problems that require careful fluid maintenance.

The most commonly used IV solutions are those containing electrolytes, dextrose, plasma expanders, and antibiotics, and certain guidelines must be considered in the administration of each of these fluids. Although blood transfusions and hyperalimentation may also be part of the IV therapy for a urology patient, these are not routinely provided and therefore are not included in the master care plan. For the same reason, nursing care involving infusions through central lines has also been omitted.

The following master care plan presents general guidelines for intravenous therapy for the urology patient. Subsequent care plans provide information relating to IV therapy that is pertinent only to the particular condition being discussed in the chapter.

THE PATIENT RECEIVING INTRAVENOUS THERAPY
NURSING DIAGNOSIS: NEED FOR MANAGEMENT OF INTRAVENOUS INFUSION

Objectives of nursing intervention
1. Appropriate administration of specific types of intravenous solutions
2. Prevention or early detection of local complications
3. Prevention or early detection of systemic complications
4. Management of discomfort caused by the intravenous infusion
5. Maintenance of proper function of intravenous equipment
6. Maintenance of accurate records of the patient's hydration status

Expected outcomes
Normal hydration status
Normal electrolyte status
Absence of thrombophlebitis, infiltration, infection, fluid overload, and pulmonary embolism
Absence of discomfort caused by the intravenous infusion

NURSING OBJECTIVE 1. Appropriate administration of specific types of intravenous solutions

Plan for implementation	Rationale
1. Administer dextrose solutions as ordered, using the following guidelines:	These solutions are used to maintain adequate fluid volume, provide calories, and spare protein breakdown. Hypertonic dextrose solutions act as a diuretic and are used to reduce central nervous system edema.
a. Flush the IV line with normal saline before and after the administration of blood.	Blood will coagulate in the tubing if mixed with a solution containing sugar.
b. Avoid using solutions containing dextrose for administration of piggyback medications if the patient is a diabetic.	Standard piggyback bottles usually contain dextrose and water. This is a hidden source of sugar that should be avoided when the patient has strict limitations placed on his carbohydrate intake.
c. Check for drug incompatibilities before diluting a medication in a dextrose solution.	A few medications cannot be administered in a dextrose solution because of potentially harmful chemical reactions that occur when they are mixed.
2. Administer electrolyte solutions as ordered, using the following guidelines:	These solutions are used for electrolyte maintenance and/or for correcting electrolyte deficiencies.
a. Check laboratory values for serum levels of potassium before administering a solution containing this electrolyte.	The normal range for serum potassium levels is very narrow. Levels higher or lower than normal may result in severe cardiac arrhythmias and other serious disturbances. Patients receiving digitalis preparations are particularly vulnerable to complications arising from hypokalemia.
b. If a potassium solution is to be administered, explain to the patient beforehand that he might feel a mild burning sensation at the IV site.	Potassium solutions are frequently irritating to venous tissue. Prior knowledge avoids unnecessary anxiety.
3. Administer plasma expanders as ordered, using the following guidelines:	These solutions (e.g., Plasmanate, dextran, albumin) are used to treat depleted plasma volume and shock. They are frequently given after lymphadenectomies because there is often a considerable loss of plasma from the surgical site.
a. Use these solutions as soon as possible after opening.	These solutions provide an excellent medium for bacterial multiplication.
b. When administering dextran:	
(1) Report any hypersensitive reactions (e.g., itching, urticaria, joint pain).	Dextran is a potent antigen, and therefore allergic reactions are not uncommon. However, when they do occur, they are generally mild.
(2) Flush IV line with normal saline before and after administering blood.	Blood will coagulate in the tubing if mixed with dextran.
(3) If any crystals are present, submerge the bottle in warm water to dissolve the particles before administration.	Crystallization can occur at low temperatures.
c. Maintain adequate fluid input from other sources.	Tissue dehydration might occur as a result of the osmotic action of these solutions.
d. Notify the physician if there are any indications of fluid overload. These include: (1) Pulmonary congestion (dyspnea, rales) (2) Neck venous distention	Hypervolemia may occur, necessitating rapid reevaluation of the patient's hydration status and changes in the IV fluid management.

Plan for implementation	Rationale
4. Administer antibiotics as ordered, using the following guidelines:	These solutions are frequently used to treat or prevent infection. Patients with infected urine (whether or not they manifest symptoms) are usually given antibiotics prophylactically after urologic surgery to prevent wound sepsis.
a. Be alert for side effects of antibiotics, and report indications of allergies or toxicity at once (see Appendix A).	
b. Be certain any medication given intravenously has been reordered for oral, intramuscular, or subcutaneous administration once the IV infusion has been discontinued.	On a busy floor, it is not unusual for changes in IV medication to be overlooked when the IV providing fluid and electrolyte maintenance has been discontinued. When the nurse is alert to this possibility, difficulties arising from missed doses of medication can be prevented.

NURSING OBJECTIVE 2. Prevention or early detection of local complications

Plan for implementation	Rationale
SUPERFICIAL VEIN THROMBOPHLEBITIS	
1. Change the infusion site every 48 to 72 hours.	An IV needle or cannula may irritate the walls of the vein, producing a thrombophlebitis reaction that can be very painful and progress rapidly. Steel needles are the least likely to cause such a reaction.
2. Anchor IV needle securely to prevent its motion within the vein.	Shifting of the IV needle position within the vein may have an irritating effect on the wall of the vein.
3. Use a vein large enough to adequately dilute any infusion that is known to be irritating.	Venous inflammation may occur from the infusion of certain drugs, such as hypertonic glucose and solutions with a relatively high or low pH.
4. Be alert for the following indications of thrombophlebitis: redness, warmth, and hardness along the known course of the affected vein; extreme tenderness near infusion site; slowed rate of infusion; generalized symptoms such as fever, rapid pulse, and malaise.	
5. If any of these conditions are present: a. Remove the IV at once. b. Apply warm soaks to the inflamed area. c. Restart the IV in a different vein. d. Do not rub or massage affected area.	Local heat reduces inflammation. This could dislodge part of the thrombus, sending it into the general circulation and risking a pulmonary embolism.

Plan for implementation	Rationale
INFILTRATION OF IV FLUID INTO SURROUNDING TISSUE	

Plan for implementation	Rationale

1. Be alert for the following evidence of infiltration:
  a. Marked slowing of rate of infusion despite readjustment of drop regulator
  b. Swelling, pallor, pain, and coldness around infusion site
  c. IV fluid leaking around infusion site
  d. Continuation of infusion after placement of a tourniquet proximal to the injection site
	Dislodgement of the IV needle out of the vein and into the surrounding tissue is relatively frequent. It can result in damage to the surrounding tissue if the IV solution is irritating and will cause an unpredictable absorption rate of any infused medication.
	
	A tourniquet will occlude the vein and therefore stop the infusion if the needle is in the vein. It will not, however, stop the flow if the needle has perforated the vessel.

2. If any of these conditions are present, remove the IV and restart it in a different vein.	

LOCALIZED INFECTION

Plan for implementation	Rationale
1. Keep the insertion site clean and dry.	An infection at the insertion site is always a possibility, since any area of broken skin permits microbial invasion. Furthermore, the constant irritation by the needle or catheter may result in thrombus formation, which is an excellent medium for microbial growth.
2. If the dressing requires changing, apply antimicrobial ointment over insertion site.	
3. Tape needle securely to the skin to avoid an in-out motion.	

NURSING OBJECTIVE 3. Prevention or early detection of systemic complications

Plan for implementation	Rationale
FEBRILE REACTION CAUSED BY INVASION OF MICROORGANISMS	
1. Inspect solution for any abnormal cloudiness or particles.	This could indicate bacteria or fungi in the solution.
2. Examine all containers for any cracks or defects. Plastic bags containing IV solution should also be squeezed to detect any holes in the bag.	

Plan for implementation	Rationale
3. If the method of sterilization of the solution produces a vacuum, do not use any bottle that does not make the characteristic sound of air rushing in when opened.	The absence of a vacuum may indicate loss of sterility of of the solution.
4. In general, use any solution within 24 hours after the seal is broken.	
5. All protein solutions or solutions with a high sugar content should be used immediately on opening.	These solutions are a particularly good medium for bacterial growth.
6. Protect all open bottles of solution that are not in use with a sterile cap to prevent contamination.	

7. Avoid contamination of IV infusion while it is in progress by the following measures:
  a. Disconnect tubing only if necessary (i.e., to change bottles or add medication).
  b. Keep infusion site clean and dry.
  c. When using piggyback infusions:
    (1) Thoroughly cleanse area before inserting piggyback needle.
    (2) Keep piggyback needle securely taped in place to prevent in-out motion during infusion.
	Any opening in the system provides a portal for contamination.
	
	Motion of the needle could introduce microorganisms into the system.

8. Reconstitute all drugs using sterile technique.	
9. Be alert for the following symptoms of bacteremia: sudden onset of chills and fever, sudden changes in pulse rate, facial flushing, malaise, headache, backache, nausea, and vomiting.	Microorganisms in the bloodstream may be transient, or they may be overwhelming and lead to septic shock unless early intervention is implemented. Symptoms would occur within 30 to 90 minutes of contact with a contaminated infusion.

10. If any of these symptoms occur:
  a. Remove container of suspect solution and replace with an isotonic dextrose or saline solution.
 	
  b. Monitor the patient's vital signs.
  c. Notify the physician.
  d. Provide verbal reassurance.
 	
  e. Save the IV solution for culture.
 	
  f. Make preparations to obtain a blood specimen for culture.
	It is not recommended that the IV be completely terminated because, in the event that the patient goes into shock, it may be difficult to locate another vein.
	
	The suddenness of these reactions can be very frightening.
	The presence and type of contamination must be determined.

Plan for implementation	Rationale

FLUID OVERLOAD

Plan for implementation	Rationale
1. Maintain infusion at the prescribed rate.	Circulatory overload, and its potential progression to pulmonary edema, can be a serious hazard of IV therapy. It is most likely to occur in elderly patients and/or those with cardiac or renal conditions.
2. Do not attempt to make up for any considerable deficiency in fluid input from the previous shift without notifying the physician.	Certain patients may not be able to tolerate a rapid rate of infusion.
3. Be alert for the following indications of fluid overload: a. Pulmonary congestion (dyspnea, rales) b. Neck venous distention	
4. If these symptoms occur: a. Place the patient in an upright position. b. Slow the infusion to a minimum rate. c. Notify the physician. d. Keep the patient calm. e. Have a fast-acting diuretic (e.g., furosemide) on hand for rapid administration if the physician should request it.	This facilitates breathing by reducing the pressure of the abdomen against the diaphragm.

PULMONARY EMBOLISM

Plan for implementation	Rationale
1. Use a filter for all blood and plasma infusions.	Any particles permitted to infuse into the patient's bloodstream could result in a pulmonary embolism.
2. Avoid the use of positive pressure to dislodge any clot formation at the tip of the IV needle or cannula.	Irrigation of an IV needle by nurses is prohibited in most hospitals. In principle it is considered unsafe. However, if the alternative is to restart the IV in a different vein and the patient has only a limited number of available veins, flushing 2 ml of normal saline through an IV needle is occasionally done without adverse effects. A clot small enough to be dislodged by the positive pressure of 2 ml of fluid would probably be too small to cause serious consequences.
3. Reconstitute drugs completely before administering them.	Undissolved particles are a potential cause of emboli.
4. Check all solutions for particles before administration.	

Plan for implementation	Rationale

5. Prevent the possibility of an air embolism by taking the following precautions:
  a. Keep all connections of the infusion system tightly sealed.
  b. Empty the air from the tubing before starting an infusion.
  c. Do not allow the container of solution to run dry, since this would result in air in the tubing.
	In principle, air in the bloodstream could result in the same life-threatening condition as an embolism formed by solid particles. In practice, however, it is highly unlikely that enough air could enter the system through a peripheral line to harm the patient. (This is, however, an important consideration with subclavian or jugular vein infusions.) But, since the minimum lethal quantity of air in the human bloodstream has not been established, these precautions are considered good nursing practice. Furthermore, from the point of view of the patient's **psychologic** well-being, air should be removed from the line. A patient may become extremely apprehensive as he watches a bubble of air descend through the line toward his vein.

NURSING OBJECTIVE 4. Management of discomfort caused by an IV

Plan for implementation	Rationale
1. Explain to the patient the purpose of his IV infusion.	Many patients harbor the incorrect notion that intravenous therapy is needed only if one is seriously ill. This may be a source of anxiety for the patient who fears he is not being told the truth about his condition.
2. When possible, use a relatively large vein for the administration of any solution that is known to be irritating to the veins (e.g., potassium chloride).	This allows for more rapid dilution of the fluid, since there is a greater amount of blood in a larger vein.

3. If the patient is receiving a solution known to be irritating and he complains of pain (without the accompanying signs and symptoms of thrombophlebitis):
  a. Slow the infusion rate (if the physician's orders permit).
  b. Apply a warm compress over the infusion site.
	This dilates the vein and permits more rapid dilution of the fluid in the bloodstream.

NURSING OBJECTIVE 5. Maintenance of proper function of IV equipment

Plan for implementation	Rationale
1. Keep the IV tubing free from kinks.	
2. Prevent external obstruction of the infusion, such as the patient lying on the tubing.	
3. Avoid the use of a blood pressure cuff on the area proximal to the infusion.	Occlusion of the vein by an inflated blood pressure cuff will cause venous stasis at the infusion site. In some cases this will result in the development of a clot at the tip of the needle.
4. Prevent accidental acceleration or deceleration of the infusion rate by the following measures:	
a. Readjust drop rate when the height of the bottle has been changed in relation to the site of infusion.	The velocity of flow at the needle is determined by the hydrostatic pressure at that point. If the relative position of the bottle is changed (e.g., if the patient is transferred onto a stretcher) the rate of infusion will also change.
b. Check the drop rate periodically.	Positional changes of the patient's extremity may interfere with a steady rate of flow. Furthermore, as the bottle empties, hydrostatic pressure within the bottle will slightly decrease, and therefore the rate will also diminish.
c. Apply an arm board if the IV is in a vein that becomes partially occluded by positional changes.	This will provide relative immobility at the infusion site.
d. If the drop regulator has been incorrectly adjusted, determine whether the patient has been handling it, and discourage him from doing so.	It is not uncommon for a patient to assume that a very slow drop rate indicates that he is not getting enough IV solution. Many an IV has run dry long before its time after the patient has "corrected" it.
e. If it is essential that the volume of the infusion be strictly monitored:	
(1) Place a piece of tape over the drop regulator to prevent unintentional rate changes.	
(2) Place a vertical strip of tape on the bottle with markings to correlate the level of fluid remaining in the bottle with each hour of the duration of the infusion.	This enables the nurse to determine instantly whether the IV is infusing on schedule.

NURSING OBJECTIVE 6. Maintenance of accurate records of the patient's hydration status

Plan for implementation	Rationale

1. Label all solutions with the following information:
  a. The patient's name, room, and bed number
  b. The type of solution, the prescribed rate of infusion, and the time the solution began infusing
  c. The name of the nurse who prepared and started the particular container of solution
	This provides staff on subsequent shifts with information necessary to the appropriate continuation of IV therapy.

2. Record in the patient's chart the type, volume, and rate of infusion.	
3. If fluid input requires strict monitoring, maintain records of oral intake as well as IV infusion.	
4. Whenever a patient is receiving an IV infusion, record volume of urine output.	This enables rapid assessment of the patient's hydration status, so it helps to prevent any serious fluid imbalances.

CHAPTER 13

The patient at risk for deep
vein thrombosis

Deep vein thrombosis is a serious complication of urologic surgery, although its incidence is also associated with a variety of other conditions. It usually occurs in conjunction with an acute inflammation of the affected vein(s), known as thrombophlebitis, in which pain, local swelling, redness, and fever are frequently present. It may, however, develop without local signs or symptoms, in which case the condition is known as phlebothrombosis.

Regardless of the early pathologic changes associated with deep vein thrombosis, the dangers it poses to the patient are an important consideration for the urology nurse. The thrombus usually causes varying degrees of obstruction to the venous circulation, which, if not treated, may develop into venous gangrene. Furthermore, thrombi may break loose (embolization) and be swept into the general circulation and eventually lodge in the lungs (pulmonary embolism).

The most common sites of deep vein thrombosis are the veins of the calf, and the femoral, iliac, and pelvic veins. Deep vein thrombosis of the upper extremities does not occur as frequently, although thrombophlebitis of the superficial veins (often caused by IV infusions) is not uncommon (see Chapter 12). This condition, however, does not usually give rise to the serious complications associated with deep vein thrombosis.

Factors that predispose a urology patient to deep vein thrombosis include stasis of blood and injury to a vessel wall. Although these conditions may exist to some extent in many hospitalized patients, and especially postsurgical ones, the urology patient is particularly at risk for the following reasons:

1. The lithotomy position used for many urologic procedures may place an unusual amount of pressure on the popliteal vessels, resulting in injury and inflammation of these veins.

2. The large vessels in the pelvis are frequently manipulated during ureteral, bladder, and prostatic surgery.

3. These same vessels may be subjected to considerable irritation during pelvic and retroperitoneal lymphadenectomies.

4. A large portion of urologic patients are elderly and therefore may require a longer period of relative immobility in the early postoperative period, predisposing them to venous stasis.

Treatment for deep vein thrombosis is aimed at prevention of new thrombus formation and prevention of embolization of the original thrombus(i). However, the nurse's role is considerably more significant in the prevention and early detection of the condition.

It is for these reasons that the following master care plan has been formulated. Prevention and early detection of deep vein thrombosis are virtually the same for all urologic patients, so in the subsequent chapters all references concerning this aspect of nursing care will be made to the following care plan.

THE PATIENT AT RISK FOR DEEP VEIN THROMBOSIS
NURSING DIAGNOSIS: POTENTIAL FOR DEEP VEIN THROMBOSIS

Objectives of nursing intervention
1. Explanation and implementation of precautions against deep vein thrombosis (preoperative period)
2. Maintenance of precautions against deep vein thrombosis (postoperative period)
3. Early detection of deep vein thrombosis

Expected outcomes
Cooperation with regimen to prevent deep vein thrombosis
Absence of local pain, swelling, and redness of a lower extremity
Absence of fever

NURSING OBJECTIVE 1. Explanation and implementation of precautions against deep vein thrombosis (preoperative period)

Plan for implementation	Rationale
1. Apply antiembolic stockings (or Ace bandages) as ordered by the physician.	Although conflicting data exist in regard to an association between elastic support of the legs and reduction of the incidence of deep vein thrombosis, many physicians will order elastic support to be worn during surgery and in the early postoperative period.
2. Obtain a baseline measurement of the circumference of the patient's calves and record it in the patient's chart. (This can be done when the patient is being measured for stockings or just before wrapping the patient's legs in Ace bandages.)	An increase in the girth of the affected extremity is the most reliable physical finding in the diagnosis of deep vein thrombosis. The additional minutes required to obtain a record of the patient's calf measurements are well worth the rapid diagnostic aid it might provide.
3. Explain to the patient the importance of changing positions frequently while in bed and the value of getting out of bed as soon as it is permitted by his physician.	Muscular activity reduces venous stasis by providing a pumping action against the veins. Patients should be told beforehand that they will be expected to get out of bed soon after surgery. In most cases they will not want to do it when the time comes, and prior knowledge makes them more cooperative postoperatively.

NURSING OBJECTIVE 2. Maintenance of precautions against deep vein thrombosis (postoperative period)

Plan for implementation	Rationale
1. Encourage range of motion exercises.	This improves venous circulation and thus reduces pooling of the blood in the veins.
2. Encourage the patient to change his position frequently while he is in bed.	
3. If necessary, teach the patient to use the siderails on the bed while changing positions.	A patient's reliance on staff to turn and reposition him should be discouraged unless it is deemed necessary. In most cases the patient will benefit by the additional exertion, since it will increase ventilation and promote circulation in the patient's arms.
4. Discourage the use of the knee-elevating mechanism on the bed.	Sitting in bed with the knees flexed and elevated for prolonged periods may cause blood to pool in the deep veins of the calves. Propping the legs in this position may also place excessive pressure on the popliteal vessels.
5. Discourage any position in which one leg is resting on the other.	This may impede venous circulation and may also damage underlying vessels.
6. Avoid massage of calf and popliteal areas on all postoperative patients regardless of absence of any symptoms of deep vein thrombosis.	Massage could embolize a silent thrombosis condition.

Plan for implementation	Rationale
7. If antiembolic stockings or Ace bandages are ordered: a. Remove and reapply them each shift.	The condition of the patient's skin must be periodically evaluated.
b. Keep them free from wrinkles and rolls.	Uneven distribution of pressure from the elastic may cause skin breakdown. Rolled stockings may also impede circulation.
c. Encourage the patient to wear them until he is ambulating well.	While the patient is relatively immobile, elastic support of the legs is considered useful in reducing venous stasis.

8. Assist the patient out of bed as soon as the physician permits. Take the following precautions the first time the patient is out of bed:
  a. Have the patient sit on the side of the bed for a few minutes before ambulating.
  b. Check his vital signs.
  c. Assist with ambulation.	

d. If there are any untoward effects (e.g., dyspnea, tachypnea, pleuritic chest pain or pain radiating to the shoulder, hemoptysis) help the patient back to bed at once and take the following actions: (1) Notify the physician.	These are symptoms of pulmonary embolism.
(2) Keep head of bed elevated 30 degrees or more.	This position facilitates breathing.
(3) Start oxygen.	This will relieve some of the dyspnea.
(4) Start an IV line.	This provides the most rapid route for medications and fluids.
(5) Keep the patient calm.	Dyspnea can be very frightening for the patient, and any agitation will make adequate ventilation more difficult.

NURSING OBJECTIVE 3. Early detection of deep vein thrombosis if it occurs

Plan for implementation	Rationale

1. If the patient is rubbing his leg or limping, investigate the cause.
  a. Check the patient's temperature and examine for swelling and/or redness of the affected area. Measure the calf and thigh girth and compare with preoperative measurements or the other extremity.
  b. If any of these signs and symptoms are present, notify the physician.
	The patient may not complain of pain but may be suffering nonetheless. Furthermore, deep vein thrombosis may only cause a feeling of heaviness around the affected area.

2. If the patient complains of severe pain behind the knee or in the calf area:
  a. Do **not** massage the area.
  b. Keep the patient in bed.
  c. Elevate the patient's legs, but take care not to elevate the knee above the calf.
 	
  d. Notify the physician.
	Massage or activity could throw the thrombus into the general circulation and result in a pulmonary embolism. This decreases pressure in the veins and will relieve some of the pain and edema. However, blood should not be permitted to pool in the calf veins.

CHAPTER 14

The patient at risk for respiratory complications

Any patient who undergoes major surgery is predisposed to various respiratory conditions postoperatively. The two most common complications are atelectasis (collapse of part or all of a lung) and pneumonia (inflammation of either or both lungs with consolidation of exudate).

Factors that contribute to the development of these conditions during surgery include the irritating effects of anesthesia, oxygen, and endotracheal tubes; stasis of secretions from prolonged positioning of the patient; and possible vomiting and aspiration of foreign matter. Predisposing factors in the postoperative period include pain, which inhibits adequate lung expansion and coughing, and limited mobility, which contributes to stasis of secretions and consolidation of alveoli.

Prevention and/or early detection of respiratory complications in urology patients will involve different nursing actions, depending on the type of surgery involved. The following master care plan has been divided into nursing objectives according to four general categories of urologic surgery. In most cases the nurse will use only one particular section when formulating a care plan for a patient undergoing a particular procedure, and many of the principles discussed are repeated in each section. The extent of nursing care ranges from the relatively basic measures for a patient who has had transurethral surgery (presented in nursing objective 1) to the continuous surveillance, assessment, and assistance for a patient who has had renal or unusually extensive abdominal surgery (presented in nursing objectives 4 and 5).

THE PATIENT AT RISK FOR RESPIRATORY COMPLICATIONS

NURSING DIAGNOSIS: POTENTIAL FOR RESPIRATORY COMPLICATIONS RELATED TO SURGICAL INTERVENTION

Objectives of nursing intervention
1. Prevention or early detection of atelectasis and/or pneumonia following transurethral, penile, scrotal, or perineal surgery
2. Prevention or early detection of atelectasis and/or pneumonia following surgery involving an abdominal incision at or below the level of the bladder
3. Prevention or early detection of atelectasis and/or pneumonia following surgery involving an abdominal incision above the level of the bladder
4. Early detection of pneumothorax
5. Prevention or early detection of atelectasis and/or pneumonia following renal surgery

Expected outcomes

Cooperation with therapeutic respiratory regimen

Absence of fever or audible lung congestion

Sputum clear or white and easily mobilized

Absence of dyspnea and other symptoms of pneumothorax (for renal surgery only)

NURSING OBJECTIVE 1. Prevention or early detection of atelectasis and/or pneumonia following transurethral, penile, scrotal, or perineal surgery

Plan for implementation	Rationale
1. Encourage turning, coughing, and deep breathing every 2 to 4 hours for the first 24 hours.	Anesthesia, endotracheal tubes, and oxygen are irritants to the tracheobronchial tree and cause increased mucous secretions. Stasis of these secretions and shallow respirations are thought to be contributing factors in the development of atelectasis and pneumonia.
2. Maintain adequate fluid intake.	Sufficient hydration aids in the thinning of mucous secretions, enabling them to be coughed up more easily.
3. Note character of respirations, presence of productive cough, and color, odor, and amount of sputum.	
4. If the patient will not cough **and his lungs sound clear,** at least encourage him to sigh and yawn a few times every hour.	These maneuvers help to inflate the alveoli and expand the lungs to total capacity. They do not, however, mobilize secretions as does coughing.
5. Notify the physician if any of the following conditions are present: 　a. The patient is unable to cough and his lungs sound congested. 　b. Sputum volume is copious. 　c. Sputum color is other than clear or white. 　d. There is a rise in the patient's temperature. 　e. Breath sounds are diminished.	These conditions require additional treatment. The physician may order therapies such as incentive spirometry, nasotracheal suctioning, postural drainage, or intermittent positive pressure breathing, depending on the extent of the respiratory embarrassment.

NURSING OBJECTIVE 2. Prevention or early detection of atelectasis and/or pneumonia following surgery involving an abdominal incision at or below the level of the bladder

Plan for implementation	Rationale
1. Encourage turning, coughing, and deep breathing every 2 to 4 hours for the first 24 hours.	Anesthesia, endotracheal tubes, and oxygen are irritants to the tracheobronchial tree and cause increased mucous secretions. Stasis of these secretions and shallow respirations are thought to be contributing factors in the development of atelectasis and pneumonia.
2. Maintain adequate fluid intake.	Sufficient hydration aids in the thinning of mucous secretions, enabling them to be coughed up more easily.
3. Note character of respirations, presence of productive cough, and color, odor, and amount of sputum.	
4. Use an additional pillow to splint the incision if the patient is unable to cough adequately because of pain.	Counterpressure against the incision relieves some of the discomfort of increased intraabdominal pressure while coughing. However, the incision is so low in the pelvic area that these patients usually do not have problems with coughing. Although intraabdominal pressure is transmitted equally throughout the abdomen, lung expansion is not affected by the incision, and therefore these patients generally are not reluctant to cough.
5. If the patient is unwilling to cough **and his lungs sound clear,** at least encourage him to sigh and yawn a few times every hour.	These maneuvers help to inflate the alveoli and expand the lungs to total capacity. They do not, however, mobilize secretions as does coughing.
6. Notify the physician if any of the following conditions are present: 　a. The patient is unable to cough and his lungs sound congested. 　b. Sputum volume is copious. 　c. Sputum color is other than clear or white. 　d. There is a rise in the patient's temperature. 　e. Breath sounds are diminished.	These conditions require additional treatment. The physician may order therapies such as incentive spirometry, nasotracheal suctioning, postural drainage, or intermittent positive pressure breathing, depending on the extent of the respiratory embarrassment.

NURSING OBJECTIVE 3. Prevention or early detection of atelectasis and/or pneumonia following surgery involving an abdominal incision above the level of the bladder

Plan for implementation	Rationale
1. Encourage turning, coughing, and deep breathing every 2 to 4 hours for the first 24 to 48 hours.	Anesthesia, endotracheal tubes, and oxygen are irritants to the tracheobronchial tree and cause increased mucous secretions. Stasis of these secretions and shallow respirations are thought to be contributing factors in the development of atelectasis and pneumonia.
2. Maintain adequate fluid intake.	Sufficient hydration aids in the thinning of mucous secretions, enabling them to be coughed up more easily.
3. Note character of respirations, presence of productive cough, and color, odor, and amount of sputum.	
4. Use additional pillow to splint the incision if the patient is unable to cough effectively because of pain.	Counterpressure against the incision relieves the discomfort of increased intraabdominal pressure while coughing.
5. Explain the reason for coughing and deep breathing.	If the patient understands that there is a risk of complications if he does not cough, he will usually cooperate with the regimen.
6. Provide reassurance that the patient will not "break his stitches" from coughing; many patients fear this.	Although there is always a possibility that wound dehiscence will occur (especially if the patient is obese or his nutritional status is poor), the incidence of respiratory complications in the early postoperative period is considerably greater. It should be remembered that during the first 48 hours after surgery the sutures are strongest. However, if coughing exercises are neglected and respiratory complications set in, the patient will be required to cough once the internal sutures begin to dissolve. At this time, if the healing process is delayed, there is a risk of wound disruption.
7. When appropriate, plan coughing sessions to coincide with the time when there is a high level of pain medication in the patient's bloodstream. Intramuscular meperidine HCl (Demerol) reaches its peak in the bloodstream in approximately 30 to 50 minutes. Subcutaneous morphine reaches its peak in approximately 50 to 90 minutes.*	When there is a high level of pain medication in the patient's system, the discomfort caused by coughing is reduced. Unfortunately, however, the patient is often strongly sedated at this time and usually just wants to sleep. Furthermore, narcotic analgesics suppress the cough reflex and physiologic sigh, both of which are extremely beneficial in the prevention of atelectasis. So the nurse must determine priorities with regard to narcotic administration in each particular case.
8. If the patient will not cough **and his lungs sound clear,** at least encourage him to sigh and yawn a few times every hour.	These maneuvers help to inflate the alveoli and expand the lungs to total capacity. They do not, however, mobilize secretions as does coughing.

*For peak levels of other analgesics see Silman, J.: The management of pain—reference guide to analgesics, Am. J. Nurs. **79:**74-78, Jan. 1979.

Plan for implementation	Rationale

9. Notify the physician if any of the following conditions are present:
  a. The patient is unable to cough and his lungs sound congested.
  b. Sputum volume is copious.
  c. Sputum color is other than clear or white.
  d. There is a rise in the patient's temperature.
  e. Breath sounds are diminished.
	These conditions require additional treatment. The physician may order therapies such as incentive spirometry, nasotracheal suctioning, postural drainage, or intermittent positive pressure breathing, depending on the extent of the respiratory embarrassment.

NURSING OBJECTIVES 4 AND 5. Early detection of pneumothorax; prevention or early detection of atelectasis and/or pneumonia following renal surgery

Plan for implementation	Rationale
PNEUMOTHORAX	

1. Be alert for the following signs and symptoms of pneumothorax:
  a. Sudden chest pain
  b. Dyspnea
  c. Decreased breath sounds on affected side
  d. Asymmetric chest expansion
  e. Symptoms of shock
  f. Feelings of extreme apprehension
	Because of the proximity of the kidneys to the base of the lungs, the diaphragmatic pleura may have been accidentally perforated during surgery. This might result in pneumothorax and would manifest itself within the first 24 hours after surgery.

2. If any of the above conditions occur:
  a. Inform the physician at once.
  b. Place the patient in an upright position.
  c. Keep the patient as calm as possible.
  d. Administer oxygen.
  e. Prepare for possible chest tube insertion.
	Air in the pleural space compromises lung expansion and therefore gas exchange. The situation can deteriorate rapidly, and prompt recognition and appropriate treatment can be life saving.

ATELECTASIS AND PNEUMONIA	
1. Encourage turning, coughing, and deep breathing every 2 to 4 hours for the first 24 to 48 hours after surgery.	Anesthesia, endotracheal tubes, and oxygen are irritants to the tracheobronchial tree and cause increased mucous secretions. Stasis of these secretions and shallow respirations are thought to be contributing factors in the development of atelectasis and pneumonia.
2. Encourage the patient to lie on the affected side, as well as on his back and unaffected side, even if he is not as comfortable in this position.	The lung on the **unaffected** side is particularly vulnerable to atelectasis because the patient will choose to lie on this side rather than on the operative side. This will result in an accumulation of secretions in the inferior lung and possible development of atelectasis and pneumonia.
3. Maintain adequate fluid intake.	Sufficient hydration aids in the thinning of mucous secretions, enabling them to be coughed up more easily.

Plan for implementation	Rationale
4. Note characteristics of respirations, presence of productive coughing, and color, odor, and amount of sputum.	
5. Use additional pillow to splint the incision if the patient is unable to cough adequately because of pain.	Counterpressure against the incision relieves the discomfort of increased intraabdominal pressure while coughing.
6. Explain the reason for coughing and deep breathing. Patients who have undergone renal surgery are particularly apprehensive about coughing because the proximity of the diaphragm to the incision makes it especially painful.	If the patient understands that there is a risk of complications if he does not cough, he will usually cooperate with the regimen.
7. Provide reassurance that the patient will not "break his stitches" from coughing; many patients fear this.	Although there is always a possibility that wound dehiscence will occur (especially if the patient is obese or his nutritional status is poor), the incidence of respiratory complications in the early postoperative period is considerably greater. It should be remembered that during the first 48 hours after surgery the sutures are strongest. However, if coughing exercises are neglected and respiratory complications set in, the patient will be required to cough once the internal sutures begin to dissolve. At this time, if the healing process is delayed, there is a risk of wound disruption.
8. When appropriate, plan coughing sessions to coincide with a time when there is a high level of pain medication in the patient's bloodstream. Intramuscular meperidine HCl (Demerol) reaches its peak in the bloodstream in approximately 30 to 50 minutes. Subcutaneous morphine reaches its peak in approximately 50 to 90 minutes.*	When there is a high level of pain medication in the patient's system, the discomfort caused by coughing is reduced. Unfortunately, however, the patient is often strongly sedated at this time and usually just wants to sleep. Furthermore, narcotic analgesics suppress the cough reflex and physiologic sigh, both of which are extremely beneficial in the prevention of atelectasis. So the nurse must determine priorities with regard to narcotic administration in each particular case.
9. If the patient will not cough **and his lungs sound clear,** at least encourage him to sigh and yawn a few times every hour.	These maneuvers help to inflate the alveoli and expand the lungs to total capacity. They do not, however, mobilize secretions as does coughing.
10. Notify the physician if any of the following conditions are present: a. The patient is unable to cough and his lungs sound congested. b. Sputum volume is copious. c. Sputum color is other than clear or white. d. There is a rise in the patient's temperature. e. Breath sounds are diminished.	These conditions require additional treatment. The physician may order therapies such as incentive spirometry, nasotracheal suctioning, postural drainage, or intermittent positive pressure breathing, depending on the extent of the respiratory embarrassment.

*For peak levels of other analgesics see Silman, J.: The management of pain—reference guide to analgesics, Am. J. Nurs. **79:**74-78, Jan. 1979.

References and bibliography

REFERENCES
Chapter 9

1. Atkinson, R.S., Rushman, G.B., and Alfred Lee, J.: A synopsis of anesthesia, ed. 8, Chicago, 1977, Year Book Medical Publishers, Inc.
2. Boore, J.R.P.: Pre-operative care of patients, Nurs. Times **73:**409-411, 1977.
3. Felton, G., et al.: Preparative nursing intervention with the patient for surgery: outcomes of three alternative approaches, Int. J. Nurs. Stud. **13:**83-96, 1976.
4. Levine, D.C.: Fears, facts, and fantasies about pre- and post-operative care, Nurs. Outlook **18:**26-28, 1970.
5. Marks, R.N., and Sachar, E.J.: Undertreatment of medical inpatients with narcotic analgesics, Ann. Intern. Med. **78:**173-181, 1973.
6. McCaffery, M., et al.: Undertreatment of acute pain with narcotics, Am. J. Nurs. **76:**1586-1591, 1976.
7. Meyers, F.H., Jawetz, E., and Goldfein, A.: Review of medical pharmacology, ed. 5, Los Altos, Calif., 1976, Lange Medical Publications.
8. Redman, B.K.: The process of patient teaching in nursing, ed. 3, St. Louis, 1976, The C.V. Mosby Co.
9. Schmitt, F.E., and Wooldridge, P.J.: Psychological preparation of surgical patients, Nurs. Res. **22:**108-116, 1973.
10. Shader, R.I.: Manual of psychiatric therapeutics, Boston, 1975, Little, Brown & Co.
11. Wade, A.: Martindale: the extra pharmacopoeia, ed. 27, London, England, 1977, The Pharmaceutical Press.
12. Wilson, R.E.: Symposium on pain, New York, 1979, Appleton-Century-Crofts.
13. Wong, J.W.: An exploration of patient-centered nursing in the admission of surgical patients—a replicated study, J. Adv. Nurs. **4:**611-619, 1979.

Chapter 10

1. Department of Health, Education, and Welfare: P.S.R.O. Program Manual, chapter 7, p. 13, section 705.29, Chicago, March 15, 1974, American Hospital Association.
2. Goodman, L.S., and Gilman, A.: The pharmacological basis of therapeutics, ed. 5, New York, 1975, Macmillan Publishing Co. Inc.

Chapter 11

1. De Groot, J.: Urethral catheterization—observing the niceties prevents infection, Nurs. 76 **6:**51-55, Nov. 1977.
2. Garabaldi, R.A., et al.: Factors predisposing to bacteriuria during indwelling catheterization, N. Engl. J. Med. **291:**215, 1974.
3. Maki, D.G., Hennekens, C.H., and Bennett, J.V.: Prevention of catheter-associated urinary tract infection, J.A.M.A. **221:**1270, 1972.
4. Thorton, G.F., and Andriole, V.T.: Bacteriuria during indwelling catheter drainage. II. Effect of a closed sterile drainage system, J.A.M.A. **214:**339, 1970.

BIBLIOGRAPHY

Abels, L.F.: Mosby's manual of critical care, St. Louis, 1979, The C.V. Mosby Co.

Brunner, L.S., and Suddarth, D.S.: The Lippincott manual of nursing practice, ed. 2, Philadelphia, 1978, J.B. Lippincott Co.

Collins, V.J.: Principles of anesthesiology, ed. 2, Philadelphia, 1976, Lea & Febiger.

Duma, R.J., Warner, J.F., and Dalton, H.P.: Septicemia from intravenous infusions, N. Engl. J. Med. **284:**257-260, 1961.

Gahart, B.L.: Intravenous medications: a handbook for nurses, ed. 2, St. Louis, 1977, The C.V. Mosby Co.

Goodman, L.S., and Gillman, A.: The pharmacological basis of therapeutics, ed. 6, New York, 1980, Macmillan Publishing Co., Inc.

Guyton, A.: A textbook of medical physiology, ed. 5, Philadelphia, 1977, W.B. Saunders Co.

Hushower, G., Gamberg, D., and Smith, N.: The nursing process in discharge teaching, Superv. Nurs. **9:**55-58, Sept. 1978.

Jennings, C.: Discharge planning and the government, Superv. Nurs. **8:**48-52, March 1977.

Joint Commission of Accreditation of Hospitals: Accreditation manual for hospitals, Chicago, 1980, Nursing Services.

Keywood, O.: Preparing the elderly patient to return home, Nurs. Mirror **147:**42-44, Sept. 7, 1978.

Luckman, J., and Sorensen, K.C.: Medical-surgical nursing—a psychophysiologic approach, ed. 2, Philadelphia, 1980, W.B. Saunders Co.

Mandler, G.: Helplessness—theory and research in anxiety. In Speilberger, C.D., editor: Anxiety: current trends in theory and research, New York, 1972, Academic Press, Inc.

Mitchell, P.H.: Concepts basic to nursing, ed. 2, New York, 1977, McGraw-Hill Book Co., Inc.

Painter, M.R., et al.: Urethral reaction to foreign objects, J. Urol. **106**:227-230, 1971.

Phipps, W.J., Long, B.C., and Woods, N.F.: Medical-surgical nursing, St. Louis, 1979, The C.V. Mosby Co.

Plummer, A.L.: Principles and practice of intravenous therapy, ed. 2, Boston, 1975, Little, Brown & Co.

Quimby, C.W., Jr.: Anesthesiology—a manual of concept and management, ed. 2, New York, 1979, Appleton-Century-Crofts.

Redman, B.K.: The process of patient teaching in nursing, ed. 3, St. Louis, 1976, The C.V. Mosby Co.

Schwartz, S.I., et al.: Principles of surgery, ed. 3, New York, 1979, McGraw-Hill Book Co., Inc.

Silman, J.: The management of pain—reference guide to analgesics, Am. J. Nurs. **79**:74-78, Jan. 1979.

Steagall, B.: How to prepare your patients for discharge, Nurs. 77 **7**:14, Nov. 1977.

Strand, M.M., and Elmer, L.A.: Clinical laboratory tests—a manual for nurses, ed. 2, St. Louis, 1980, The C.V. Mosby Co.

Sturdevant, B., Patterson, R.: Helping patients do their homework, Superv. Nurs. **8**:72-73, April 1977.

Thorn, G.W., et al.: Harrison's principles of internal medicine, ed. 8, New York, 1977, McGraw-Hill Book Co., Inc.

Winter, C.C., and Morel, A.: Nursing care of patients with urologic diseases, ed. 4, St. Louis, 1977, The C.V. Mosby Co.

Zander, K., et al.: Practical manual for patient teaching, St. Louis, 1978, The C.V. Mosby Co.

UNIT IV

PSYCHOSOCIAL AND PSYCHOPHYSICAL FACTORS AFFECTING THE UROLOGY PATIENT

CHAPTER 15

The pediatric urology patient

In any large institution, pediatric patients with a urologic condition will be in the pediatric unit among all other hospitalized children. They will be treated by their pediatrician (unless urologic surgery is required), and their nurse will specialize in pediatric nursing. However, an understanding of the urologic conditions that commonly occur in children enhances the urology nurse's general knowledge of the field. Furthermore, an awareness of the psychosocial aspects of patient care throughout the life cycle enables the nurse to provide better understanding of the adult patient's psychosocial needs, particularly since adolescents are frequently placed among the adults on the urology unit.

Therefore a description of the most common pediatric urologic conditions has been included. It is followed by a care plan for the psychosocial needs of each of the different stages of growth and development. Emphasis has been placed on the psychosocial considerations because this aspect of nursing care is the major difference between caring for a child and caring for an adult. The physical care associated with each surgical procedure appears elsewhere in the book. It can be combined with the appropriate psychosocial considerations of the patient's particular age group to form a care plan for the pediatric urology patient. (Modifications to suit the physiologic needs of the very young child and infant will have to be added to the care plan. The reader is advised to consult a pediatric nursing textbook for this information.)

Urologic birth defects are the most common of all anomalies. It is estimated that as many as 10% of the babies born in the United States have some degree of structural abnormality affecting the urologic organs[1], although a vast majority of the conditions are either asymptomatic throughout life or spontaneously resolve during childhood.

Of the anomalies that will cause illness, many are not detected until after the first year of life. Others are identified shortly after birth, although surgery may be deferred until the child is older. Whenever possible, surgery is postponed to allow the affected organ(s) an opportunity to grow and become more amenable to surgical correction. In some cases structural abnormalities may resolve spontaneously. The psychologic effect of hospitalization and separation from parents is also an important factor in delaying surgery until the child is older. Urologic surgery is considered least traumatic when the child is over 5 years of age, since many of the castration and mutilation anxieties have been resolved by this age. However, some authorities believe correction of visible abnormalities should be done earlier to prevent the child from feeling stigmatized or deformed, especially when the defects involve the genitalia. But in cases where the child's life is endangered or function of an organ is severely compromised, there is no dispute: surgery is performed as soon as the condition is diagnosed.

Most urologic infections in male children are associated with congenital structural abnormalities that cause obstruction of the urinary flow and thus urinary stasis and bacterial multiplication. In young females the short urethra often accounts for ascending infection from fecal contamination. It should be noted that symptoms of urinary tract infection in children under 6 or 7 are less specific than the "classic" signs and symptoms in the adult. Infants develop fever, do not eat well, have strong-smelling urine, and are irritable. Toddlers and preschoolers have fever, abdominal pain, vomiting, strong-smelling urine, enuresis, dysuria, and frequency. Older children have symptoms similar to those of the adult (see Chapter 27).

Abdominal masses in children may be of urologic origin. A common cause is **hydronephrosis,** which often results from an obstruction of the ureteropelvic junction. The obstruction may be caused by fibrous bands, aberrant blood vessels, or an intrinsic defect at the junction. Urinary tract infection is often present. The condition may be corrected by means of a pyeloplasty (see Chapter 25), but usually surgery is postponed until the child is over 2 years of age, unless recurrent infection cannot be controlled by antibiotic medication or if renal function is severely compromised.

Another cause of an abdominal mass is **Wilms' tumor,** a highly malignant tumor of the kidney that is usually not palpable at birth but appears within the first 6 years of life (usually before the age of 3). It characteristically presents as a nontender mass, often discovered by the child's parents. Nephrectomy is performed as soon as the diagnosis is confirmed (see Chapter 22). The surgical approach is abdominal to enable visualization of the abdominal cavity. Prior to surgery care is taken not to manipulate the mass, since this may result in dissemination of cancer cells into adjacent organs. Radiotherapy is started shortly after surgery, and courses of chemotherapy (actinomycin D) are administered periodically during the next year or longer. The disease can be controlled for substantial periods of time in approximatley 80% of the cases.[2]

Anomalies of the ureter include various forms of ureteral duplication. The position of the ureteral orifices will determine the manifestation of the condition. If they terminate in the bladder without reflux of urine or obstruction, the condition is of little concern. However, a condition often associated with ureteral duplication is **ectopic ureter,** which will cause incontinence if the orifice is in the vagina or lower urethra in the female. Obstruction is also frequently present, giving rise to hydronephrosis. The condition is corrected by ureteral reimplantation (see Chapter 31), which is usually done before the age of 3 or 4 so the psychologic hazards of incontinence can be avoided.

Ureteral reimplantation may also be employed for **vesicoureteral reflux** (retrograde reflux of urine from the bladder into the ureter). This condition is associated with a high incidence of urinary tract infection and hydronephrosis. However, if the condition can be controlled medically, surgery is usually postponed until adolescence, when the condition often resolves spontaneously as the child reaches his full growth potential.

Exstrophy of the bladder is a serious anomaly often associated with other defects in the urinary tract. It occurs when the embryonic mesoderm fails to close over the lower anterior wall of the abdomen. This causes the bladder to remain open, lying on the external surface of the lower abdomen with the ureteral orifices exposed. The result is constant spillage of urine onto the abdomen. In some institutions, primary closure of the bladder and abdominal wall may be attempted shortly after birth. Usually, however, the condition must be corrected by urinary diversion such as conduit diversion or ureterosigmoidostomy (see Chapter 38).

Posterior urethral valves are the most common cause of urinary obstruction in the male infant. They are thought to be caused by vestigial embryonic structures in the prostatic urethra. Symptoms include decrease in force of the urinary stream, bladder distention, urinary tract infection, and, in extreme cases, uremia. Transurethral resection is usually done at the time of diagnosis.

Hypospadias is an anomaly in which the urethra terminates on the ventral surface of the penis or in some cases at the penoscrotal junction or the perineum. It is usually accompanied by chordee (ventral curvature of the penis). The condition is corrected surgically by means of urethroplasty (see Chapter 48), usually between the ages of 4 and 6. Circumcision should not be performed on a child with hypospadias because the skin of the prepuce is used in the surgery to correct the condition.

Cryptorchidism (undescended testicle) is a common condition affecting 3% of term male newborns and 20% of premature males at birth. In approximately 80% of the cases the testicle descends spontaneously during the first year of life.[1] If it fails to do so, hormonal therapy (human chorionic gonadotropin) sometimes brings about descent. Otherwise orchidopexy (see Chapter 54) is performed, usually around the age of 5 for cosmetic reasons and to prevent the adverse effect of the body temperature on spermatogenesis. If the testicle remains in the abdominal cavity after puberty, spermatogenesis will be permanently impaired. However, the incidence of testicular neoplasms is higher in individuals with undescended testicles, so orchidopexy may be performed on an adult with bilateral cryptorchidism to maintain appropriate surveillance of the testicles throughout the patient's life. If the condition is unilateral, the undescended testicle is usually removed prophylactically, since testosterone production will not be compromised by the removal of one testicle.

If bilateral cryptorchidism occurs in conjunction with hypospadias, the true sex of the child must be investigated, since these anomalies, when combined, frequently indicate hormonal or chromosomal abnormalities. Diagnostic studies to determine the true sex of the child should be begun early so that appropriate sexual designation can be made as soon as possible.

THE PEDIATRIC UROLOGY PATIENT
NURSING DIAGNOSES FOR PSYCHOSOCIAL NEEDS:

1. Potential psychosocial disturbances in the infant (ages 1 to 12 months) related to hospitalization
2. Potential psychosocial disturbances in the toddler (ages 1 to 3 years) related to hospitalization
3. Potential psychosocial disturbances in the preschooler (ages 3 to 6 years) related to hospitalization
4. Potential psychosocial disturbances in the school-aged child (ages 6 to 12 years) related to hospitalization
5. Potential psychosocial disturbances in the adolescent (ages 12 to 18 years) related to hospitalization

---

1. NURSING DIAGNOSIS: Potential psychosocial disturbances in the infant (ages 1 to 12 months) related to hospitalization

Objectives of nursing intervention
- Provision of an environment that promotes trust
- Provision of an environment that enables the mother* maximum contact with the infant
- Provision of sensory-motor stimulation
- Provision of psychosocial stimulation

Expected outcomes
- Absence of prolonged crying
- Alertness, responsiveness, frequent smiling
- Progression of sensory-motor and psychosocial development at a normal rate

Plan for implementation	Rationale
1. Promote an attitude of trust in the child by reducing **parental** anxiety in the following ways:	Anxiety is highly contagious, particularly between parent and child and especially during the first year of life, when the mother-child relationship is intimately connected to feelings rather than words.
a. When possible, maintain consistency in the personnel assigned to the patient.	When care is provided by only a few nurses, the development of trust and continuity of care is facilitated.
b. Chose words carefully when giving information and be certain the parents understand any medical terminology used.	The vocabulary used by medical personnel can be very confusing, and, if the parents are already anxious, they will be even less likely to comprehend what is being said. Seeking information and striving to understand what is happening is a common coping mechanism parents use to reduce their anxiety, and care should be taken that they do not misinterpret information and become more anxious.
c. Encourage the mother to participate in the care of the child as much as she is able.	The act of doing for the child is another parental coping mechanism that should be encouraged. It alleviates the frequent sense of helplessness and frustration the parents often feel, and it is particularly useful if the parents feel guilty (consciously or unconsciously) about the child's illness.

---

*The term *mother* is used loosely. It applies to any person—mother, father, grandparent, etc.—who provides the child with the physical contact and affection traditionally associated with the mother.

Plan for implementation	Rationale
d. Maintain consistency among caregivers regarding how a procedure is to be performed.	Frequently the same procedure is done slightly differently by different nurses, although they may each attain the same results. However, the untrained onlooker may misinterpret these differences and think that one way is superior to another.
e. Maintain a calm, confident, unhurried attitude when providing patient care.	This conveys to the parents that the child is in competent hands and that anxiety is unwarranted.
f. Provide the parents with an opportunity to express their feelings about their child's condition, hospitalization, and treatment, and provide as much emotional support as possible.	The stress of the child's hospitalization and treatment has many ramifications, depending on the gravity of the child's condition, the parents' additional responsibilities with other children, jobs, or travel requirements, and various other factors. All their coping mechanisms must be supported for them to function in an optimum way, for the child's sake as well as for their own.
2. Encourage rooming-in or rooming-by for the mother whenever possible.	This enables the child to have maximum contact with the mother. It is especially important after 6 months because separation anxiety can occur at this age.
3. If the mother is unable to be present for considerable lengths of time each day:	
a. Make a special effort to provide the infant with one primary caregiver (mother substitute).	This helps to establish continuity of care and enables the infant to develop a sense of trust in the mothering figure.
b. Allow additional time for cuddling, rocking, and physical contact with the infant.	This is extremely important for the infant's psychosocial and motor development. It provides him with sensory stimulation, motor stimulation, and, most important, physical affection.
c. Talk, sing, or make other vocal sounds to the infant.	Rudimentary speech is an important developmental task, especially after the first 6 months of life.
4. Make initial contact with the infant in the mother's presence, especially an infant over 6 months of age.	This helps the infant to associate the nurse with the safety and trust he feels from his mother.
5. Determine the parents' methods of comforting the infant, as well as the eating habits and other home routines they have established. Attempt to simulate these conditions as much as possible within the limits of the hospital setting.	Simulation of home activities will provide the infant with continuity of experiences, reducing the new and often frightening effects of the hospital environment.
6. Provide the infant with comfort and pleasure experiences, especially when food is being withheld prior to tests and/or surgery.	
7. Encourage the parents to leave toys or a "security blanket" with the child.	These provide the infant with at least some familiar elements in a new and totally foreign environment.

Plan for implementation	Rationale
8. Provide the patient with sensory and motor stimulation with the judicious use of toys. For example, music boxes, rattles, stuffed toys with contrasting textures, and mobiles provide appropriate sensory stimulation for an infant. Toys that reward motor behavior, such as rattles, or toys that make a noise when squeezed provide appropriate motor stimulation.	
9. If the patient must be restrained, use the following guidelines:	
a. Use the least amount of restraint required. Often elbow or knee splints are adequate to keep the child from pulling catheters or dressings.	Aside from the psychologic hazards imposed on the infant when he is physically restrained, prolonged restraining will retard his motor development, a vital developmental task.
b. Prevent injuries from occurring by the following measures: (1) Keep ankle and wrist restraints well padded. (2) Release the restraints every 2 to 4 hours, day and night, for 5 to 10 minutes under supervision. (3) Inspect skin adjacent to the restraints for redness or other signs of irritation, and readjust as necessary.	

2. **NURSING DIAGNOSIS:** Potential psychosocial disturbances in the toddler (ages 1 to 3 years) related to hospitalization

Objectives of nursing intervention
{ Provision of an environment that promotes trust and autonomy
{ Maintenance of familiar vocabulary and routines used at home

Expected outcomes
{ Absence of despair or denial when reacting to separation from parents
{ Minimal or absent regression to behavior from earlier developmental level
{ Interest in environment, toys, and games
{ Cooperation with treatments and procedures

Plan for implementation	Rationale
1. Promote an attitude of trust in the patient by reducing parental anxiety (see p. 111, no. 1)	
2. Encourage rooming-in or rooming-by for the mother whenever possible.	The mother's presence provides the child with a sense of security. This is especially important at this age because separation anxiety is usually intense.

Plan for implementation	Rationale
3. Reduce the effects of separation from the parents by promoting the following measures:	Since the child cannot be with the parents at all times, it is essential that he develop a sense of trust that they will return. Otherwise, he will feel abandoned each time they leave, and the entire hospitalization will be a devastating experience.
	The concept of time is not well understood by the toddler.
a. When informing the child of their return, the parents should associate it with an activity (e.g., "I will be back after dinner.").	
b. Suggest that the parents leave a personal article with the patient (e.g., a key or a glove) each time they leave.	This usually helps to convince the child that his parents will return.
c. Suggest that the parents bring from home the patient's favorite toy or blanket. Photographs of family and pets are also helpful reminders of home.	
d. Encourage honesty with regard to parental visits. The nurse should not promise that the parents are coming soon when they are not, and the parents should leave and return when they say they will.	This promotes the childs sense of trust. Once he knows that he can rely on his parents to return as they say they will, it makes separation easier.
e. Once the parents say they are leaving, do not permit them to stay just because the patient is protesting loudly. (It sometimes helps the parents if they are reassured that the nurse will stay with the patient and comfort him, and that usually the negative behavior stops shortly after they leave.)	If the parents were to do this, it would reinforce a negative behavior pattern and reduce the chances of the child's acceptance of the parent's absence.
f. Discourage the parents from sneaking out when the patient is asleep or is not looking.	This is damaging to the child's sense of trust.
g. Stay with the patient after the parents leave if he appears to be having difficulty adjusting to the separation. Hold him, soothe him, and reassure him that his parents still love him and that they will be back.	
h. Divert the patient's attention by the judicious use of story-telling, toys, or cuddling.	
i. Place a note on the patient's chart or care plan stating when the parents will return.	This enables those who care for the patient to provide him with accurate information. The consistency in the answers will also promote a sense of trust.
4. Explain to the parents that separation anxiety is normal in this age group and negative behavior (i.e., screaming and crying) is expected.	
5. Be alert for the following indications that the patient is experiencing a severe emotional reaction to the separation: a. The patient stays in his room and cries for prolonged periods. b. The patient refuses to eat.	The degree to which the child reacts to separation is based on various factors, including his overall relationship with his parents, the extent of the hospitalization, and the amount of separation required. The initial response is usually signified by extreme protest in which crying and screaming are expected. The child can usually be distracted from these reactions once his parents have left, and then he copes with his parents' short-term absence. However, the child who is severely affected by the separation will despair for prolonged periods. This reaction may progress to a complete denial of his feelings for his parents so that, when they do return, he ignores them.

Plan for implementation	Rationale
c. The patient reaches for the nurse instead of his parents.	Although on the surface it appears that the child has made a healthy adjustment to the hospital, this is usually not the case. This type of behavior indicates that his relationship with his parents has been so badly impaired by his despair over their absence that he is unwilling or unable to relate to them altogether.
6. If any of the aforementioned behavior is observed: a. Increase efforts to provide one staff member as the primary caregiver and make every effort to develop a trusting relationship between the patient and that individual. b. Explain to the parents what is happening and encourage them to spend more time with the patient if this is possible.	Every effort should be made to reestablish the parent-child relationship so that in the future the child's ability to form intimate, trusting relationships with significant others is not impaired.
7. Obtain information from the patient's parents concerning his habits and routines and, when possible, incorporate them into his care.	Children of this age are preoccupied with routines and rituals, especially those involved with eating, sleeping, bathing, and elimination. It provides them with a sense of security because they know what to expect. Any interuption in these newly formed habits is highly stressful and should be avoided whenever possible.
8. Allow the patient to wear his own clothes whenever possible.	This fosters the child's sense of normalcy.
9. Inform the parents that they should not be alarmed if the patient regresses to some behavior patterns he appeared to have outgrown. This may include reduction of bowel and bladder control and resumption of behavior from a more infantile stage of development.	Regression is very common when a child is placed in the stressful atmosphere of a hospital. Usually it is the most recently achieved behavior patterns that are the first to be lost, but this is temporary and self-limiting.
10. Promote adequate nutrition by the following measures: a. Allow the patient to feed himself, if he wishes. b. Do not force-feed the patient. c. Have a familiar person help with the meal. d. Chart what was eaten at each meal.	A child of this age usually has somewhat erratic eating habits. Extra efforts should be made to ensure that he is eating adequately. This provides a frame of reference for the child's general eating habits and is the only way to determine the amount of food he consumes in a 24-hour period.
11. Provide the patient with frequent rest periods.	The child may not be sleeping well at night because of the unfamiliar environment.
12. Encourage the patient to have as much independence as possible. a. Allow the child to dress himself. b. Keep a potty chair near his bed. c. Let him explore his environment.	Achievement of a sense of autonomy is an important developmental task of this age group.

Plan for implementation	**Rationale**

13. Reduce the effects of the patient's limited ability to communicate by the following measures:
    a. Find out from his parents what words he is accustomed to using for his daily routines.
    b. Give one direction at a time.
    c. Use a positive approach by stating what he **should** do rather than what he should **not** do.
    d. Be gentle but firm.
    e. Avoid talking about the patient's condition (or that of any other patient) within his range of hearing.

In addition to the child's limited use of language, negativism dominates much of the behavior in this age group.

Toddlers often understand considerably more than what we would expect, judging from their limited vocabulary. Furthermore, they may easily misinterpret what has been said and become excessively fearful.

14. Include the following actions in preparing the patient for treatments or surgery:
    a. Explain all procedures by using anatomic references to body surfaces.

    b. Allow the patient to play with any equipment used in his care (after removing any needles or other potentially dangerous parts).
    c. Encourage the parents to provide explanations and reassurance about a procedure (after first determining that they have an appropriate understanding of what is to occur).
    d. If a painful procedure is to be performed, tell the patient that it will hurt but the nurse will be there to help him.
    e. Tell the young toddler he is to have surgery shortly before it commences. The older toddler may be told a day before or earlier if a great deal of preparation is required.
    f. Use simple explanations like: "The doctor will fix . . ." or "You will have a special tube . . ." Anesthesia may be described as: "A special medicine so it won't hurt."
    g. Reassure the patient that only the specific part of his body that was discussed will be operated on, and that the operation will make it better.

    h. Tell the patient where his parents will be waiting if they cannot be with him during the procedure.
    i. Answer any questions the patient might have as simply and honestly as possible.

The child of this age understands names for external parts of the body, but internal organs are not easy for him to conceptualize.
Handling the equipment often reduces the child's anxiety about unfamiliar objects.

The child will be reassured if he knows that somebody he trusts understands and approves of what will happen to him, even if he cannot fully understand what he is being told.
It is essential not to lie about pain, or the child's sense of trust will be destroyed.

Fears of mutilation and castration are prevalent at this age. Since much of urologic surgery performed on toddlers involves the genitalia, the child usually requires considerable reassurance that his body integrity will not be harmed.

Plan for implementation	**Rationale**
15. Take the patient's favorite toy or blanket with him when he goes to the operating or treatment room.	
16. Comfort the patient after any painful procedure, and divert his attention from the pain by getting him in-interested in a toy or story.	

17. After surgery, assist the parents in providing care and comfort for the patient.
  a. Explain all drains and dressings.
  b. Show them how the patient can be held and as-sisted out of bed.
 	
  c. Inform them when and what the patient may eat.
  d. Tell them who they can call for assistance.
	Often parents are unnecessarily apprehensive about touching the child when he is connected to a lot of equipment.

18. If the patient must be restrained, use the guidelines listed on p. 113.	
19. During periods of relative immobility, provide the patient with diversions such as picture books, soft stuffed toys, clay, or Play-Doh.	
20. Prior to discharge, explain to the parents that the patient might have some temporary anxiety reactions such as bed-wetting or night fears. This is a fairly common response to hospitalization and is usually self-limiting.	Prior knowledge of possible behavioral regression helps the parents to cope better with it. Their understanding that this is not abnormal will reduce their anxiety and thus make it easier for the child to work through his anxiety reactions.

3. NURSING DIAGNOSIS: Potential psychosocial disturbances in the preschooler (ages 3 to 6) related to hospitalization

Objectives of nursing intervention
{ Provision of an environment that promotes trust, autonomy, and initiative
Anticipation and correction of distorted perceptions related to hospitalization

Expected outcomes
{ Absence of despair or denial when reacting to separation from parents
Minimal or absent regression to behavior from earlier developmental level
Willingness to communicate feelings and ask appropriate questions
Absence of indications of guilt and fear of punishment
Interest in environmental toys and games
Cooperation with treatments and procedures

Plan for implementation	Rationale
1. Provide the patient with an orientation tour of the areas in the hospital in which he will receive treatment. Omit showing the patient any areas that would require him to see other children in pain or connected to frightening equipment, such as the intensive care unit.	This will reduce the child's anxiety, since most children of this age group fear unfamiliar environments, sounds, and equipment. Once they are given an explanation of where things are and what they are seeing, they often relax considerably.
2. Promote an attitude of trust in the patient by reducing **parental** anxiety (see p. 111, no. 1).	
3. Encourage rooming-in or rooming-by for the mother whenever possible.	The continued presence of the mother provides the child with a sense of security in an environment filled with unfamiliar sounds, smells, and activities.
4. Reduce the effects of separation from parents (see p. 114, no. 3).	
5. Reassure the patient that he is not to blame for his condition and that he is not being punished.	Children in this age group frequently have vengeful wishes and fantasies, which instill a sense of guilt and thus a fear (and expectation) of punishment. Illness, hospitalization, and surgery are often misinterpreted as such punishment.
6. Obtain information from the patient's parents concerning his habits and routines and, whenever possible, incorporate them into his care.	Familiarity of routines is very reassuring for children of this age, since they have just begun to rely on predictability in their environment and activities.

Plan for implementation	Rationale
7. If possible, allow the patient to wear his own clothes.	This fosters a sense of normalcy.
8. Inform the parents that they should not be alarmed if the patient regresses to some behavior patterns he appeared to have outgrown. This may include reduction of bowel and bladder control and resumption of behavior from a more infantile stage of development.	Regression is common when a child is placed in the stressful atmosphere of the hospital setting. Usually it is the most recently achieved behavior patterns that are the first to be lost, but this is temporary and self-limiting.
9. If the patient should have an "accident" and soil his clothing, reassure him that he will not be punished.	The preschooler is often preoccupied with guilt and fears of punishment.
10. Encourage the patient to have as much independence as possible. a. Allow him to feed and dress himself and perform any self-care functions he has already mastered. b. Allow him to explore his environment. c. Allow him choices within the framework of his treatment; for example: Would he prefer to ride to the operating room in a stretcher or a wheelchair? or Which arm would he like his IV in?	Although regression to a more dependent level of functioning may be expected in a hospitalized child, it should by no means be encouraged. Performing tasks he has already mastered and being permitted to make choices give the child a sense of security.
11. Use the following principles in patient teaching: a. Determine the patient's understanding of the reason for his hospitalization. b. Find out from his parents what words the patient is accustomed to using for body functions and anatomy, and continue to use these words when communicating with the patient. c. Explain the reason for any procedures and/or surgery by discussing the presence of distressing symptoms (e.g., fevers, vomiting, flank pain, dysuria, incontinence). If the child has been asymptomatic, provide a simple description of the condition and the need to correct it before the child becomes ill. d. Use a body outline or doll and give simple anatomic information. For a boy the word "dummy" may be substituted for "doll" if the idea of playing with dolls is unsatisfactory to him. e. If a painful procedure is to be performed, tell the patient that it will hurt but that the nurse will be there to help him, and it is OK if he cries. f. Encourage the patient to play with equipment used in his care (after removing any needles or dangerous parts).	This provides the nurse with a basis on which to begin patient teaching. It is essential not to lie about pain, or the child's sense of trust will be quickly destroyed. Giving the child permission to cry removes the additional burden often imposed by well-meaning family: "Big boys (girls) don't cry" or "Good boys (girls) don't cry." When the child is familiar with the equipment, it is less frightening. Furthermore, it enables him to work out his fears and frustrations through constructive play.

Plan for implementation	**Rationale**
g. If the patient is to have surgery, inform him of it it 1 or 2 days before it is to be done (or earlier if much preparation is required).	
h. Use nonthreatening vocabulary such as "repair" rather than "cut out" or "cut into." Older preschoolers have some concept of internal organs, so they can be told: "The doctor will make a small opening here [point to area on a doll] so he can reach the part to be fixed."	Fear of castration and mutilation may still be present, particularly in the young preschooler. The choice of words can make a considerable difference in the way the child envisions the forthcoming procedure.
i. Reassure the male patient that his penis (use whichever word with which he is familiar) will not be harmed by the surgery.	
j. Describe the indwelling urethral catheter as a special tube for urine that will not hurt. Explain that the patient might feel the urge to urinate although urine is flowing through the tube.	The catheter may cause bladder spasms, which the child will interpret as an urge to void.
k. When describing general anesthesia: (1) Avoid the use of the word "sleep," if possible. (2) Tell the patient the doctor will given him a special medicine so he will not feel the surgery or remember it. (3) If the word "sleep" has already been introduced (e.g., by the parents), be certain that the patient understands that it is different from normal nighttime sleep.	Children who are told they will be put to sleep for the surgery sometimes associate anesthesia "sleep" with normal sleep and they develop frightening notions. For example, they might fear waking up during the surgery. Postoperatively they might resist going to bed for fear that more surgery will be performed when they are asleep.
l. Tell the patient where his parents will be waiting if they cannot be with him during the procedure.	
m. Answer any questions the patient might have as simply and honestly as possible.	
12. Take the patient's favorite toy or blanket with him when he goes to the operating or treatment room.	
13. Comfort the patient after any painful procedure and divert his attention from the pain by getting him interested in a toy or story.	
14. After surgery, help the parents provide care and comfort for the patient. a. Explain all drains and dressings. b. Show them how the patient can be held and assisted out of bed. c. Tell them when and what the patient may eat. d. Tell them who they can call for assistance.	

Plan for implementation	Rationale
15. If the patient must be restrained, use the guidelines listed on p. 113. However, it is usually possible to reason with children in this age group, and often they will obey if they are told not to pull at a tube or dressing.	
16. During periods of relative immobility, provide the patient with diversions such as dolls, simple books, clay, Play-Doh, and television.	
17. Prior to discharge, explain to the parents that the patient might have some temporary anxiety reactions such as bed-wetting, soiling of clothing, bad dreams, and reverting to "baby talk." This is a fairly common response to hospitalization and is usually self-limiting.	Prior knowledge that the child might go through a period of behavioral regression will help the parents cope if it occurs. Their understanding that this is not abnormal will reduce their own anxiety and thus make it easier for the child to work through his anxiety reactions.

4. NURSING DIAGNOSIS: Potential psychosocial disturbances in the school-age child (ages 6 to 12) related to hospitalization

Objectives of nursing intervention
- Provision of an environment that promotes trust, autonomy, initiative, and industry
- Promotion of communication with peers
- Provision of instructions and explanations of procedures

Expected outcomes
- Absence of evidence of severe anxiety
- Constructive interaction with peers
- Willingness and ability to communicate feelings and ask questions
- Cooperation with procedures

Plan for implementation	Rationale
1. When possible, maintain consistency in the personnel caring for the patient.	When care is provided by only a few nurses, it is easier for the child to develop a sense of trust.
2. When possible, assign the patient to a room with children his age.	Peer relationships are very meaningful to children of this age group. They provide much of the security and emotional support that the family provided throughout earlier stages of development.

Plan for implementation	Rationale
3. Encourage socialization with other hospitalized children in the playroom. However, be sure to explain to the patient the difference between his condition and that of patients who are having more extensive procedures.	Socialization is an important developmental task of this age group. However, seeing children who are extremely ill or connected to complicated equipment can be a source of anxiety for the child who already has fears about what is to occur during his hospitalization.
4. Use the following principles in patient teaching: a. Have the patient verbalize his perception of his condition and correct any misconceptions.	This provides the nurse with a basis on which to begin patient teaching. Inaccurate notions and the vocabulary with which the child is familiar can be identified.
b. Explain the reason for procedures and/or surgery by discussing the presence of distressing symptoms (e.g., fevers, vomiting, flank pain, dysuria, incontinence). If the patient has been asymptomatic, provide a simple description of the condition and the need to correct it before the patient becomes ill. c. Use basic scientific terminology for anatomy and medical procedures.	Children of this age group usually adapt quite easily to a scientific approach, even if they are not accustomed to some words. They are also able to conceive of internal organs.
d. Use drawings of body outlines for explanations. Dolls may also be used, but some children of this age will not want to be seen with a doll. e. If a painful procedure is to be performed, tell the patient that it will hurt but that the nurse will be there to help him.	It is essential not to lie about pain, or the child's sense of trust will be destroyed.
f. Reassure the patient that there will not be any other children in the room during the procedure. g. Reassure the patient that his genitalia will not be harmed by the surgery.	One of the biggest concerns of children of this age group is peer opinion, and they may be particularly fearful of ridicule if their peers were to see them cry. Young school-age children may still be preoccupied with fears of castration and mutilation. However, in general, urologic surgery is less traumatic during this period than during the toddler, preschool, and adolescent periods.
h. Describe an indwelling urethral catheter as a tube through which urine will flow out of his body automatically. Reassure the patient that it will not hurt, but he might feel an urge to urinate even though urine is flowing through the tube. i. Encourage the patient to play with equipment used in his care (after removing any needles or dangerous parts).	
5. Encourage the patient to ask any questions and express any feelings he might have.	
6. Comfort the patient after any painful procedure and divert his attention from the pain by getting him interested in a story or toy or game. It might help to distract him if he is taken into the playroom.	

Plan for implementation	Rationale

7. Convey respect for the patient's sense of modesty:
  a. Draw bed curtains for any examinations.
  b. Drape the patient so that exposure is minimal.
  c. Reassure the patient that nobody will walk into the room while he is bathing or using the bedpan (and ensure that nobody does).
	It is during this age that concern for modesty and a desire for privacy begin to develop.

8. During periods of relative immobility, provide the patient with items such as books, board games, and television. If possible, permit him to visit the playroom on a stretcher, even if he cannot actively participate in the activities.	This enables the child to be with his peers and derive some pleasure out of the activities by watching.
9. If the patient is to be hospitalized for more than 2 weeks, determine from the local board of education in the community if a visiting teacher is available. If the parents or patient is interested, make appropriate arrangements.	Because of the importance of peer relationships in this period, the child may become anxious if he feels he will not be able to keep up in school. A visiting teacher will help alleviate some of his concerns and will also provide some diversion for him.

5. **NURSING DIAGNOSIS:** Potential psychosocial disturbances in the adolescent (ages 12 to 18) related to hospitalization

Objectives of nursing intervention
- Provision of an environment that promotes trust, autonomy, initiative, industry, and identity
- Continuation of peer group interaction
- Provision of instructions and explanations of procedures

Expected outcomes
- Constructive interaction with peers
- Absence of evidence of severe anxiety
- Willingness and ability to communicate feelings and ask questions
- Cooperation with procedures

Plan for implementation	Rationale
1. When possible, arrange staffing assignments so that the nurse providing most of the patient's care is of the same sex as the patient and not close to him in age.	Children of this age group tend to be very self-conscious about their bodies, particularly concerning development of secondary sexual characteristics. A nurse of the opposite sex or one who is practically within the patient's peer group may make the patient even more self-conscious.

Plan for implementation	**Rationale**
2. When possible, assign the patient to a room with others his age. If he is on an adult unit, at least try to place him in a room with a patient who has somewhat similar interests.	Peer relationships are important to the adolescent, who is in the process of developing social skills and a sense of identity.

3. Be aware that frequently there are conflicts (conscious or unconscious) between patients of this age and their parents. If this appears to be the case:
  a. Reassure the patient that any conversations with him are strictly confidential, unless the patient's safety is in jeopardy.
  b. Plan teaching sessions for periods when the parents are absent.
	The adolescent's attempt to develop his own identity and emancipation from the dependent role in his family may manifest itself in hostility and strong opinions that are very different from those of his parents. In other cases he may simply want to exercise his need for privacy about certain matters.

4. Use the following principles in patient teaching:
  a. Determine the patient's degree of knowledge regarding his condition and/or impending surgery.
  b. Correct any misconceptions.
  c. Use body diagrams and scientific terminology to explain procedures.
	This provides the nurse with a basis on which to begin patient teaching.
	
	The adolescent is usually quite comfortable with a scientific approach. This is particularly useful when the topics of sexual function and sexual organs are discussed (as they frequently are on a urology unit). The slang terms to which the patient may be accustomed are sometimes associated with emotional conflicts he may be experiencing, whereas the scientific term becomes impersonal and easier to relate to objectively.

d. Guard against being deceived by the patient's **seeming** lack of concern for his condition.	Adolescents are usually preoccupied with their bodies, any physical changes they are experiencing, and how they compare to others. However, they may not want to reveal their concern for their physical condition, and this attitude is easily misinterpreted as disinterest.

e. Use the same manner of conversation as that used when talking to an adult.
  f. When describing a surgical procedure, tell him where the scar will be and, when appropriate, reassure him that within a few months it will hardly show.
  g. Reassure the patient that the procedure will not adversely affect sexual function (unless, of course, this information is inaccurate).
	This will flatter the adolescent and usually promote his cooperation.
	Because the appearance of their bodies is so important to adolescents, the location and appearance of the scar is often a major source of anxiety.
	
	Any procedure involving the genitalia will result in considerable anxiety in the adolescent, who may just be becoming aware of his own sexuality. Even an indwelling urethral catheter may be a source of concern.

h. Encourage the patient to ask any questions and express his thoughts. If the patient appears to be having difficulty verbally expressing what he is feeling, suggest that he write his feelings or that he try to express them with a drawing or some other art form in which he is interested.	Verbalizing of feelings may be extremely difficult for the adolescent, who at one minute feels like an adult and the next minute feels like a child. This rapid vacillation between opposing emotions and behavior patterns may be so confusing for the adolescent that he is simply unable to say what is going on inside him. Other means of emotional expression may be extremely helpful for him.

Plan for implementation	**Rationale**
5. Provide the patient with a sense of autonomy by including him in the planning of his care. Some of the choices he may certainly be permitted to make are: a. When to bathe b. What he wants to eat c. When he wants his bed made	Adolescents have a strong need to feel they are in control of a situation. Unfortunately a hospital setting is hardly a place that fosters such feelings, and every effort should be made to compensate for this in the patient's treatment regimen.
6. Convey respect for the patient's sense of modesty. a. Draw the bed curtains for any examinations. b. Drape the patient so that exposure is minimal. c. Reassure the patient that nobody will walk into the room when he is bathing or using the bedpan (and ensure that nobody does).	Adolescents are frequently extremely modest and apprehensive about exposure of their bodies, often because they are concerned about how their bodies are maturing.
7. Be alert for the possibility that the patient is developing a crush on a staff member of the opposite sex. If this should become evident: a. Do not tease or belittle the patient. b. Do not flirt with the patient. c. Maintain a friendly "I-like-you-too" attitude toward the patient.	This is very common among adolescents, and on a urology floor it will probably be a young male patient taking a special liking to a female nurse. She can help him gain self-confidence and still keep his feelings under control by graciously accepting his behavior, being warm and friendly, but still maintaining her professional manner.
8. Promote peer group contact by the following measures: a. If possible, set aside an area where adolescents can socialize, listen to music, and play games that are not disturbing to others on the unit. b. Provide facilities so that the patient can talk with friends on the telephone in relative privacy. c. Encourage the patient to have visitors. If there is an age limit (most hospitals do not permit visitors under 16 years of age) make arrangements for the patient to visit with friends in the lobby.	
9. If the patient is to be hospitalized for more than a few weeks, suggest that he contact his school and make plans for ways to continue his school work.	Continuation of school work is a useful diversion from the hospital environment and also helps the patient remain in the same class with his peers.

CHAPTER 16

The adult urology patient

Specific psychosocial considerations have been incorporated into almost all the care plans for the urology patient undergoing a particular surgical or medical treatment. The following nursing diagnoses are very general and may apply to any patient who is undergoing treatment affecting the genital area.

THE ADULT UROLOGY PATIENT
POTENTIAL NURSING DIAGNOSES:

1. Anxiety about communicating information related to the genitalia
2. Embarrassment related to exposure of the genitalia
3. Fear of changes in body image or body function

---

1. NURSING DIAGNOSIS: Anxiety about communicating information related to the genitalia

Objectives of nursing intervention	Maintenance of an attitude that conveys respect for the patient's privacy Achievement of effective verbal communication
Expected outcomes	Ability and willingness to express feelings and information related to the genitalia Absence of verbal and nonverbal indications of anxiety

Plan for implementation	Rationale
1. Be aware that any condition which directly or indirectly affects the genitalia may be a source of anxiety for the following reasons:	
a. The patient may feel a sense of shame concerning his genitalia.	This is often an unconscious psychologic mechanism.
b. The patient may lack knowledge of terminology about the genitalia and is therefore unable to formulate questions.	
c. The patient may lack accurate knowledge about the function of the organs involved and is therefore subject to incorrect and often frightening notions.	Knowledge of the internal organs related to reproduction is often vague, inaccurate, or only partially accurate.
d. The patient may have been raised to believe that discussion of sexual function and/or related organs is taboo.	Until recent years sex was not an appropriate topic of discussion. Many patients have difficulty discussing related subjects simply because they are not accustomed to doing so.

Plan for implementation	Rationale
2. Investigate one's own feelings about discussing problems related to the genitalia.	Often embarrassment or anxiety is transmitted. Unless the nurse feels relaxed in these circumstances, the patient will not feel so either.
3. Provide the patient with basic knowledge concerning the anatomy and physiology of the genitourinary tract.	
4. Use simple diagrams whenever possible.	
5. Use basic scientific terminology.	Simple but correct terminology is usually accepted. For example, "sexual intercourse" is well understood, whereas "coitus" may be too technical. Slang terms are inappropriate and prevent the patient from relating to the discussion in an objective way.
6. Maintain a professional, objective approach.	This helps the patient concentrate on the problem and not his embarrassment.
7. Convey having had prior experience in caring for patients with similar conditions.	Often patients feel their problems are unique because conditions of the genital organs are infrequently discussed. Knowing the nurse has seen similar problems reduces the patient's anxiety and increases his confidence in the nurse.

8. Provide as much privacy as circumstances permit.
  a. Choose a time to talk when other patients are out of the room.
  b. Pull the bed curtain around the bed and speak softly.
	Most patients share a room with others, so this may be difficult. The patient will be much more relaxed if any discussions take place at a time when other patients are out of the room or if he is certain they are not able to hear what is being said.

9. When possible, arrange staffing assignments so that the patient's primary caregiver is of whichever sex he appears to be the least self-conscious with.	In some cases it may be easier for the patient to relate to a nurse of the same sex. Other patients may feel more at ease with a nurse of the opposite sex.
10. Maintain an accepting, nonjudgmental attitude toward a patient whose sexual behavior, preferences, or philosophy differs considerably from one's own.	If the patient senses that he will experience disapproval from the nurse if he communicates openly, he will be less likely to reveal any information about himself. Important nursing problems may remain undetected and thus unresolved.

2. NURSING DIAGNOSIS: Embarrassment related to exposure of genitalia

Objective of nursing intervention	Promotion of patient comfort by reducing causes of embarrassment
Expected outcome	Reduction or absence of embarrassment

Plan for implementation	Rationale
1. Draw bed curtain completely around bed when performing any procedures or examinations that require genital exposure.	
2. Drape the patient to ensure minimal exposure.	
3. Maintain a professional attitude for any treatment involving the genitalia (e.g., catheter care).	
4. Reassure the patient that nobody will walk into the room during the procedure or while he is using the bedpan (and ensure that nobody does).	
5. When possible, arrange staffing assignments so that the patient's primary caregiver is of whichever sex he appears least self-conscious with.	Some patients are less embarrassed about genital exposure with somebody of the same sex. Others may be more comfortable in the presence of somebody of the opposite sex.

3. NURSING DIAGNOSIS: Fear of changes in body image or body function

Objectives of nursing intervention
{ Elimination of unrealistic fear by providing accurate information
Reduction of realistic fear by providing supportive information related to management of the changes

Expected outcome   Behavioral or verbal indications that fear is absent or adequately reduced

Plan for implementation	Rationale
1. Encourage the patient to share his feelings and convey willingness to answer all questions.	In only a few instances will urologic surgery result in permanent deleterious changes in body appearance and/or function. However, it is common for patients to harbor numerous unrealistic fears, especially when surgery involves the genitalia. The nurse should be aware of the long-term effects of any procedure and be able to provide factual reassurance if no permanent change in the patient's physical appearance or sexual function is anticipated. This is particularly important in relation to sexual function, where mind and emotions play an integral role in the physiologic function. For example, if the patient **thinks** he will be impotent after a simple prostatectomy, he may well become so, although there should be no physiologic basis for this.
2. Provide accurate information regarding the treatment and its expected effects.	
3. If no changes in body image or body function are anticipated, provide the patient with thorough reassurance of this.	
4. If changes are anticipated*: a. Be aware that grief is a normal reaction to the loss(es) the patient faces. b. Provide emotional support. c. Provide supportive information regarding management of the changes. d. Determine the need for additional supportive measures (e.g., psychiatric consultation, sex counseling, visit by an ostomate) and make the appropriate arrangements.	

*For interventions related to specific procedures involving significant changes in body image or body function, see Chapters 38, 44, 49, and 55.

CHAPTER 17

The elderly urology patient

It is not unusual for the majority of patients on a urology unit to be over 65 years of age. These patients have unique physical and psychologic needs that must be considered in planning their care. Some of the physiologic changes associated with aging are included in Table 1. Nursing interventions for problems most frequently encountered among elderly urology patients are provided in the following care plan.

THE ELDERLY UROLOGY PATIENT
POTENTIAL NURSING DIAGNOSES:

1. Potential for adverse reactions to medication
2. Impaired communication because of hearing disability
3. Reluctance to ambulate after treatment
4. Depression related to loneliness, loss of independence, and/or financial circumstances

Table 1. Anatomic changes to consider in care of aged

	Functional change	Outcome
Heart	Decreased stroke volume; slower heart rate	Drop in cardiac output
	Estimated left ventricular work declines at rest	
	Blood flow through the coronary arteries decreases	
	Myocardial ability to use oxygen decreases[1]	Heart less well equipped to handle stress; with coexisting heart disease, cardiac failure and death may result
Blood vessels	Smooth muscle replaced by fibrous and hyaline tissue causing decreased vascular elasticity	Increased pulse pressure and systolic blood pressure
Kidney	Renal blood flow drops at a steady rate, starting at age 40[2]	Proportional reduction in glomerular filtration rate (usually measured as creatinine clearance)
	Decreased fluid intake leads to decreased ability to concentrate urine	Normal GFR at age 40 of 120 ml/min falls to 60 or 70 ml/min at age 85[3]
	Ability to dilute urine decreases	BUN rises from a normal value of 9.5 mg/100 ml at age 20 to 15-20 mg/100 ml at age 70-80[3]
Lungs	Reduction in vital capacity and increase of residual volume; reduction of pulmonary diffusion; loss of lung recoil; and maldistribution of pulmonary ventilation/perfusion ratios—all due to change in type or quantity of fibrous proteins, collagen, and elastin in lung matrix[4]	Decrease in arterial oxygen tension, less respiratory reserve in major illnesses, surgery, or trauma
	Progressive weakening of respiratory muscles	Reduced negative and positive intrathoracic pressure on forced inspiration and expiration; this plus reduced expiratory flow rates account for decrease in maximum breathing capacity
GI tract	Decreased motility of stomach and intestines	Constipation
	Reduction in intestinal blood flow[5]	Possible delay or slight reduction in drug absorption
	Increase in gastric pH	Affects solubility of some drugs
	Number of absorbing cells may be decreased and active transport systems may be modified	No data to support major change in drug absorption[6]
Musculoskeletal system	Decrease in number and bulk of muscle fibers; muscle fibers are replaced by nonmuscular fibrous tissue	Decrease in muscular strength, endurance, and agility
	Density of bone decreases; in women after middle age may be related estrogen deficiency, insufficient dietary intake, and perhaps abnormalities in calcium, protein, and amino acid metabolism[7,8]	Osteoporosis, osteoarthritis
Hematological system	Iron deficiency anemia, probably caused by malnutrition and malabsorption[9]	Iron and folate deficiency and a change in oxygen-carrying capacity
	Anemia due to chronic diseases such as infection, arthritis, malignant disease	Mild, normocytic and normochromic anemia
Endocrine system	Insulin response or peripheral sensitivity to insulin release may be reduced	Return to fasting level in glucose tolerance test is slower[3]

Reproduced with permission from American Journal of Nursing, vol. 78, no. 8, p. 70, 1978. Copyright © 1978 American Journal of Nursing Company.
[1]Harris, R.: Special features of heart disease in the elderly patients. In Chinn, A.R., editor: Working with older people—a guide to practice, vol. 4, Public Health Service Publ. No. 1459, Washington, D.C., 1971, U.S. Government Printing Office, pp. 81-102.
[2]Papper, S.: The effects of aging in reducing renal function, Geriatrics **28**:83-87, May 1973.
[3]Cole, W.H.: Medical differences between the young and the aged, J. Am. Geriatr. Soc. **18**:589-614, Aug. 1970.
[4]Williams, M.H.: Special problems in respiratory diseases, Geriatrics **29**:67-71, June 1974.
[5]Bender, A.D.: Effects of age on intestinal absorption: implications for drug absorption in the elderly, J. Am. Geriatr. Soc. **16**:1331-1339, Dec. 1968.
[6]Crooks, J., et al.: Pharmacokinetics in the elderly, Clin. Pharmacokinet. **1**(4):280-296, 1976.
[7]Trotter, M., et al.: Densities of bones of white and Negro skeletons, J. Bone Joint Surg. **42**(A):50-58, Jan. 1960.
[8]Yoshikaw, M., et al.: Osteoporosis in Japan, a clinical and experimental study. In Proceedings of the Eighth International Congress on Gerontology, vol. 1, Washington, D.C., 1969, Federation of American Societies for Experimental Biology, p. 225.
[9]Evans, D.M.: Hematological aspects of iron-deficiency in the elderly, Gerontol. Clin. (Basel) **13**:12-30, 1971.

1. NURSING DIAGNOSIS: Potential for adverse reactions to medication

Objective of nursing intervention	Prevention and/or early detection and correction of adverse reactions to medication
Expected outcome	Absence of confusion, respiratory depression, disorientation, agitation, and other untoward effects of medication

Plan for implementation	Rationale
1. Be especially alert for adverse reactions to any medication administered to an elderly patient.	The risk of adverse drug reactions in the elderly is considerably higher than in younger adults.[2,3] This is attributed to a decrease in renal function, which often accompanies aging, and thus a decrease in the rate of clearance of drugs excreted by the kidneys.[1,4]
2. Verify with the physician any order for barbiturates for a patient over 65 years of age.	Many elderly patients become severely disoriented from barbiturates and may be more safely sedated with chloral hydrate.[1]
3. Verify with the physician any order for narcotic analgesia in an unusually high dosage (even if it is within the accepted dosage range) when it is ordered for a patient over 65 years of age.	An elderly patient is more likely than a younger adult to experience respiratory depression, urinary retention, and gastrointestinal disturbances form narcotics, and he may not require as much analgesia to produce the same degree of comfort.
4. If any adverse reactions are observed: a. Inform the physician at once. b. Do not give subsequent doses of the medication unless it is reordered by the physician. c. Place a conspicuous note in the patient's chart (and on the medication sheet if it is separate from the chart) stating the patient's reaction to the medication at the particular dose given. d. Record measures taken to alleviate the reaction.	This will reduce the possibility of subsequent inadvertent administration.
5. If the patient is confused or agitated, take the following measures, in addition to those mentioned above:	Confusion in the elderly is not uncommon, particularly when they are under the stress of the unfamiliar hospital environment and physical pain. Changes in mental status are particularly common in the early postoperative period due to the effects of anesthesia and narcotic analgesia.
a. If the patient is only mildly confused and appears to understand simple statements, explain to him what is happening with slow, short, deliberate statements, such as: "You are confused. It is from the pain medication. I have seen this happen before. You will be all right in a few hours. Lie still for now." b. Have the patient repeat what has been said to him and, if necessary, repeat any of the statements until he appears to understand. c. Obtain an order for restraints but use them only if absolutely necessary, for instance, if the patient tries to get out of bed or pulls at tubes or dressings.	Restraining the patient may contribute to his disorientation and make him more frightened and agitated.

Plan for implementation	**Rationale**
d. If it is night, keep a light on in the room.	This helps the patient to be oriented.
e. Observe the patient frequently.	
f. If the family is present, reassure them that the disorientation is transient (if this is the case) and enlist their cooperation in helping to orient the patient.	

2. NURSING DIAGNOSIS: Impaired communication because of hearing disability

Objective of nursing intervention   Achievement of effective verbal and nonverbal communication with the patient

Expected outcome   Ability to communicate effectively with staff

Plan for implementation	**Rationale**
1. Use the following guidelines when communicating with the patient:	
a. Face the patient when addressing him.	This enables the patient to use lip-reading.
b. Speak clearly, loudly, and slowly, but do not shout.	An increase in volume will help the patient hear better, but shouting may be offensive to him and to other patients.
c. Enunciate words carefully, using maximum lip movement.	This helps the patient to use lip-reading as he listens, which generally increases his ability to understand what is being said.
2. Label the intercom system to the patient's room with appropriate instructions to whomever uses the system (e.g., "This patient is hard of hearing.")	This prevents inadvertent use of the intercom system to communicate with the patient.
3. If the patient wears a hearing aid, leave it in his ear when he goes to the operating room (unless hospital policy will not allow this).	A hearing aid is one of the few personal items a patient is allowed to wear in the operating room. It enables the anesthesiologist to assess more precisely the patient's level of consciousness by providing him with auditory stimuli.
4. If the patient does not have a hearing aid:	
a. Label his chart to indicate that he has a hearing impairment.	This alerts any caregiver to the patient's problem. It is especially important if the patient has general anesthesia because the anesthesiologist will be asking him questions postoperatively to assess his level of consciousness.
b. If the patient hears better with either ear, place this information on a conspicuous part of his chart.	

133

Plan for implementation	Rationale

5. If a hearing impairment is suspected but not confirmed (i.e., there is no indication of it on the patient's chart and he does not volunteer the information), confirm or refute the suspicion in the following ways:
   a. Address the patient in a soft voice or face away from him when asking him a question to which he must respond with more than a yes or no.
   b. Ask the patient if he has any problems with his hearing.

This is the least reliable method to detect minor hearing deficits because many patients do not realize they are suffering from a loss of hearing until it is well advanced.

---

3. NURSING DIAGNOSIS: Reluctance to ambulate after treatment

    Objective of nursing   Promotion of optimum mobility
         intervention

    Expected outcome   Rapid return to the level of activity existing prior to hospitalization

Plan for implementation	Rationale

1. Determine the patient's level of mobility on admission and the ease with which he ambulates.

Arthritis, circulatory problems, slowed coordination, and other factors make ambulation more difficult for an elderly patient. It is extremely important for the nurse to determine **prior** to surgery or medical treatment how well the patient ambulates to know the extent of assistance he will need during convalescence and the degree of verbal pressure the nurse can safely apply in encouraging him to ambulate. The fear of falling is often one of the greatest factors inhibiting the patient from resuming his optimal level of mobility and is often responsible for self-imposed mobility restrictions in the early postoperative period. Only if the nurse knows the patient's capabilities can the patient's reluctance to ambulate be appropriately handled.

2. Maintain a safe environment (i.e., nothing on the floor on which the patient might slip or trip, easy access to the bathroom, adequate lighting, etc.)

3. Encourage range of motion and isometric exercises while the patient is in bed.

This tones the muscles so that the patient does not experience muscular weakness once he begins to ambulate.

4. Help the patient get out of bed.

Plan for implementation	Rationale
5. Encourage him to allow his legs to dangle over the side of the bed for a few minutes if he has been lying in bed prior to getting up.	This allows for changes to occur in the vascular bed and reduces the chances of orthostatic hypotension.
6. Encourage the patient to use street shoes or slippers with a sturdy back while ambulating in the room.	Shoes that fit securely provide support and stability.
7. Show the patient how to ambulate while pushing the IV pole in front of him.	
8. If the patient normally uses a cane or walker, keep these items close to the patient at all times.	
9. If the patient appears to be unstable on his feet, make arrangements for him to use a walker.	
10. If the patient is still reluctant to ambulate or appears unable to walk alone, ensure that either a staff or family member walk with him at least three times a day.	
11. Reassure the patient that moderate activity (within his particular limitations) will promote recuperation faster than if he remains in bed.	Many elderly patients think that if they stay in bed and rest they will get stronger. They often need to be convinced that just the opposite is true and that bed rest results in disuse atrophy of the muscles and a decreased tolerance to activity once it is resumed.

4. NURSING DIAGNOSIS: Depression related to loneliness, loss of independence, or financial circumstances

Objectives of nursing intervention
{ Achievement of effective verbal and nonverbal communication
Promotion of independence
Provision of a supportive environment

Expected outcomes
{ Absence or adequate reduction of indications of depression
Expression of positive feelings and a sense of optimism

Plan for implementation	Rationale
1. Be alert for behavior that may indicate depression (e.g., withdrawal, weeping, insomnia, refusal to eat).	
2. Rule out or correct other causes of the above behavior (e.g., fear, pain, nausea).	
3. Encourage the patient to verbalize his feelings.	
4. Convey acceptance of crying by statements such as "Many patients cry when they experience similar events. . . ." Or describe the benefits of crying.	Many patients feel ashamed about expressing their unhappiness and need reassurance that it is not only all right, but it has the beneficial effects of releasing tension and clearing the mind for constructive thinking.
5. Determine the source of the depression by asking the patient directly or by seeking clues in the patient's conversation.	
6. If the depression appears to be caused mainly by loneliness: a. Allow additional time to sit and talk with the patient. b. Encourage socialization among other patients with similar interests. c. Encourage reminiscence.	Listening to the frequent (and sometimes tedious) reminiscences of the elderly can be extremely therapeutic for the following reasons: 1. It conveys the nurse's interest in what is meaningful to the patient. 2. It provides information about the patient's strengths and coping mechanisms, which may be applied to the present. 3. It often reflects a current situation, although it may be presented in terms of a past experience (e.g., the patient recalls an early memory of being a helpless child, which has been reactivated by a present feeling of helplessness).

Plan for implementation	Rationale
7. If the depression appears to be caused by a loss of independence and autonomy:	Illness and the effects of aging impose limits on the patient's physical abilities. An individual who is accustomed to being highly self-sufficient may find dependence on others to be humiliating and demoralizing.
a. Allow the patient as much decision-making as possible, within the limits of his condition, physician's orders, and nurse's schedule. This might include: (1) Diet substitutions (2) Choices about when the patient's bed is to be made (3) Choices about when the patient will ambulate b. Promote as much independence as possible. (1) Place all necessary items within easy reach of the patient. (2) Provide an over-bed trapeze and side rails if these items help the patient move more independently. (3) Provide the patient with a sturdy chair with arms. (4) Provide a bedside commode rather than a bedpan. c. Encourage the patient to perform as many tasks as he is capable of doing, regardless of how long it might take.	
8. If the depression appears to be caused by financial problems: a. Encourage the patient to verbalize his fears and concerns despite any reluctance he might have about doing so. b. Contact the hospital social service department if deemed necessary.	Like many elderly people in today's society, the patient may be on a fixed income that is only barely adequate for survival. However, he may not want to talk about his financial difficulties, since this subject is often considered personal. Pride may also be a factor in the patient's unwillingness to reveal his financial situation. Community resources or other means of financial assistance may be available for the patient. A social worker can best determine the type of services for which the patient might be eligible.

CHAPTER 18

The patient with a venereal disease

The patient with a venereal disease is rarely hospitalized for the condition, except when cases of gonorrhea develop into epididymoorchitis (Chapter 59) or if the patient requires surgery for venereal warts (Chapter 60). Furthermore, patients suffering from a venereal disease are usually treated by their primary physician and not a urologist (unless surgery is required). Therefore a nurse on the urology unit may not see many cases of venereal diesase, although these conditions do affect the male genitourinary tract and thus are within the domain of urology.

However, it is not unusual for a venereal disease to be discovered incidentally in a patient who is hospitalized for another condition, and nursing interventions will be required in such instances. The most common venereal diseases are discussed briefly, and a care plan concentrating on the psychosocial problems related to the condition follows.

GONORRHEA

The infecting agent in gonorrhea is *Neisseria gonorrhoeae*. It is a highly communicable disease and is almost always spread by sexual contact. The disease primarily affects the urethra, although it frequently spreads to other organs of the genital tract and may, in such instances, result in infertility. Occasionally it progresses to arthritis and endocarditis. Symptoms include a purulent urethral discharge 4 to 10 days after exposure, accompanied by burning during urination and urethral itching. It may be asymptomatic in women. It is treated with penicillin or tetracycline.

SYPHILIS

The infecting agent in syphilis is *Treponema pallidum*. The disease is almost always spread by sexual contact. In its initial stage the disease affects the external genitalia. A painless indurated ulcer, usually on the glans penis, develops 2 to 4 weeks after exposure. If it is untreated, the lesion will heal spontaneously, but the disease will progress to serious systemic manifestations and possibly death unless treatment is instituted. (Consult a medical textbook for information on advanced syphilis.) The disease is treated with penicillin.

CHANCROID (SOFT CHANCRE)

The infecting agent in chancroid is *Haemophilus ducreyi*. The disease is spread by sexual contact, initially affecting the external genitalia in the form of one or more painful ulcers on the penis 3 to 10 days after exposure. Fever and enlarged inguinal lymph nodes may also be present. It is treated with tetracycline or sulfonamides.

HERPES PROGENITALIS

The infecting agent in herpes progenitalis is herpesvirus type 2. The disease is spread by sexual contact. One or more superficial vesicles appear on the genitalia, with slight local pain or itching within a week after exposure. These vesicles heal spontaneously, usually within a week, but have a tendency to recur. No successful cure has been identified. Emphasis is on prevention of spread, and the patient is encouraged to abstain from sexual contact or use a condom when vesicles are present. There are some indications that herpes infection of the cervix is associated with an increased incidence of cervical cancer.[1] If vesicles are present in the vagina at the time of labor, a cesarean section is usually performed to prevent potential fatal infection of the newborn.[1]

CONDYLOMATA ACUMINATA (VENEREAL WARTS)

See Chapter 60.

THE PATIENT WITH A VENEREAL DISEASE
POTENTIAL NURSING DIAGNOSES:

1. Anxiety related to the presence of a venereal disease
2. Inadequate information about transmission, cure, and prevention of venereal disease

1. NURSING DIAGNOSIS: Anxiety related to the presence of a venereal disease

Objective of nursing intervention	Provision of an atmosphere of acceptance
Expected outcome	Willingness to discuss the disease and identify contacts

Plan for implementation	Rationale
1. Investigate one's own emotions about venereal disease and confront any feelings of prejudice toward the patient.	Venereal diseases have traditionally been a taboo subject —something that "nice" people do not talk about and certainly never contract. Although recent changes in sexual mores have dispelled this myth, there are still many emotional reactions to these diseases that keep them from being discussed like any other infectious disease.
2. Be aware that the patient will probably be psychologically distressed about the following: a. Fear that family and friends will find out	This fear is especially prevalent among teenagers who live at home and do not want their family to know they are having sexual relations. They are also very conscious of what their peer group will say or think of them.
b. Anxiety about naming numerous sexual contacts	Guilt about considerable sexual activity may be present.
3. If the patient is a minor, reassure him that his family need not know he has a venereal disease. (Only if surgery is required, as in the case of large venereal warts, would parental consent be necessary.)	
4. Convey an attitude of acceptance.	This will promote a sense of trust in the patient, which is a prerequisite for open communication and effective patient teaching.
5. Assure the patient that his privacy will be respected. a. Discuss details of the patient's condition at a time when there are no others present in the room. b. Be particularly careful to avoid discussion of the patient's condition with other staff members if visitors are present.	

2. NURSING DIAGNOSIS: Inadequate information about transmission, cure, and prevention of venereal diseases

Objectives of nursing intervention
{ Provision of information regarding transmission, cure, and prevention of the disease
Maintenance of appropriate infection precautions

Expected outcome   Accurate return verbalization of information

Plan for implementation	Rationale

1. Provide the patient with the following information:
  a. The patient will be treated with an antibiotic that usually cures the disease. (See discussion on the particular disease for the drug of choice.)
  b. The patient **must** return to the physician's office for a follow-up examination at the prescribed time (usually 2 weeks after treatment and then again in 6 weeks).
  c. Once the patient is cured, there is no immunity from future infections.
  d. To prevent future infections, the patient should do the following:
    (1) Check sex partners for signs of infection (e.g., lesions, discharge).
    (2) Encourage any partner suspected of infection to seek medical attention.
    (3) Abstain from sexual activity until the infection is cured, or use a condom.
	Treatment failures do occur, and reinfection rates are high. To be certain the infection is eradicated, a laboratory analysis for the specific organism is required.

2. Maintain the following precautions to prevent cross-contamination of others and protect self.
 	
  a. When emptying the urinal or catheter drainage container of a patient with newly diagnosed gonorrhea, take special precautions to avoid splashing the urine into the eyes.
  b. If the patient has syphilis, be certain to dispose of all needles carefully so that there is no danger of a puncture wound by a contaminated needle.
  c. Use double-bagging technique when disposing of any material in contact with contaminated secretions.
  d. Wash hands thoroughly before and after any patient contact.
  e. If there is any broken skin on the hands of the caregiver, wear gloves during catheter care or other treatments that require direct contact with the lesion or urethral secretions.
	Although these diseases are almost entirely transmitted through sexual contact, certain routine hospital activities may promote spread of the disease.
	The urethra is heavily contaminated with the infectious organism, and the conjunctivae are susceptible to infection by this organism.
	
	Because the infectious organism invades the bloodstream, the possibility of contracting syphilis from a contaminated needle must be considered.
	These are general precautions for **any** infected drainage. Their value in prevention of the spread of a venereal disease has not been established, but common sense and good nursing habits will probably dictate that they be observed.

CHAPTER 19

The patient with infertility

Infertility is a problem that affects approximately 15% of couples in the United States. The male partner is thought to be responsible in about 30% of these cases.[1]

The causes of infertility are complex and in some cases not well understood. They include systemic diseases such as mumps orchitis, diabetes, and renal disease; endocrine disorders that involve pituitary, adrenal, thyroid, and testicular function; venereal diseases, especially gonorrhea, which may cause fibrosis and occlusion of the sperm transport system; sexual problems such as impotence; and, according to some authorities, conditions that raise the temperature of the testicles, such as prolonged hot baths, constricting underwear, and varicocele.

Most of the diagnostic studies are performed in the physician's office. They begin with a complete physical examination and health and sexual histories. A semen specimen may be obtained to determine the morphology, motility, and concentration of sperm, fructose content, and the presence of sperm antibodies. A blood specimen may be obtained for serum levels of gonadotropin hormones and androgens, and a testicular biopsy and vasogram may be performed.

Hospitalization is required only for testicular biopsy (Chapter 58), but the nurse on the urology unit may also provide care for the patient with infertility if he is to have a varicocelectomy (Chapter 53) or a vasovasotomy (Chapter 57). The following care plan focuses on the psychosocial aspects of infertility, which may apply to almost all male patients who are unable to father a child.

NURSING DIAGNOSIS: Psychologic distress related to infertility

Objective of nursing intervention	Provision of a supportive environment
Expected outcomes	Willingness and ability to verbalize feelings Absence of prolonged depression Realistic decision-making

Plan for implementation	Rationale
1. Be aware that the patient with infertility has been under considerable emotional stress for a prolonged period. Sources of this stress include: a. Unsuccessful attempts at impregnation for a considerable length of time	An investigation of infertility usually does not begin until a couple has had at least 1½ years of unprotected intercourse at a frequency of 2 or 3 times per week.

Plan for implementation	Rationale
b. Repeated tests that involve abstinence and then production on demand of semen specimens	Although most patients are not unduly upset about masturbating in a physician's office to produce a specimen, it creates certain emotional and/or religious conflicts among some.
c. Considerable financial expenditures	The series of tests to determine the cause of infertility may be expensive, depending on the types and number of tests performed.
d. Possible conscious or unconscious feelings of threat to the patient's sense of manhood and even uncertainties about his marriage if he finds he cannot have children	The psychologic effect of a diagnosis of infertility may, in some cases, be devastating, particularly if both the husband and wife are extremely eager to have children.
e. Inability to plan for the future because of uncertainty about the presence of children	
2. Encourage the patient to verbalize his feelings.	
3. When possible, include the patient's wife in any discussions.	Communication of feelings between husband and wife on this highly sensitive topic can often lead to a better understanding of their mutual needs and anxieties.
4. If the prognosis looks bleak, explore with the couple their feelings about other options, such as adoption and artificial insemination by donor.	Although adoption is a relatively well-known alternative, artificial insemination by donor has only recently been gaining popularity. It provides the couple with a child who is half their own in terms of genetic structure, and it allows the woman to experience pregnancy, childbirth, and the development of a maternal bond with her own baby. It also enables the couple to exercise control over the environmental factors affecting prenatal life (e.g., they can ensure that the fetus is not exposed to toxic drugs or chemicals).
5. If necessary, explain that artificial insemination by donor is performed by the physician by instilling a semen specimen from a donor into the woman's vagina or cervix. In most instances the donor's identity is not revealed, although he is carefully screened for genetic abnormalities. Usually donors are medical students and interns. Sometimes the height and hair and eye color of the husband are matched.	

CHAPTER 20

The patient with cancer

Throughout this book, care plans for patients with different types of cancer are included. However, certain aspects of the care of these patients depends on the circumstances surrounding their hospitalization and the reactions of each specific patient to his illness. How a patient reacts to the diagnosis of cancer and how he copes with the changes in his life-style later in the disease process are highly individual responses.

The following care plan provides interventions for cancer patients anywhere on this continuum of adjustment. The nurse will have to determine which interventions are appropriate for the specific patient.

THE PATIENT WITH CANCER
POTENTIAL NURSING DIAGNOSES:

1. Psychologic distress related to diagnosis of cancer
2. Dependence on assistance in coping with changes in life-style imposed by advanced cancer

---

1. NURSING DIAGNOSIS: Psychologic distress related to the diagnosis of cancer

Objectives of nursing intervention
{ Provision of an emotionally supportive environment
  Achievement of effective communication between patient, family, and staff

Expected outcomes
{ Verbalization by the patient of feelings about the diagnosis
  Realistic decision-making
  Absence of severe or protracted depression

Plan for implementation	Rationale
1. Be aware of one's own attitudes toward cancer and attempt to maintain as positive an approach as possible.	Any negative attitude such as fear, defeat, or hopelessness is easily conveyed to the patient, even if it is not openly expressed. Conversely, looking at the disease as a highly interesting and challenging illness can alter some of the patient's negative ideas.
2. Encourage the patient to express his feelings.	Verbalization of fears often makes them easier to deal with and gives the nurse the opportunity to identify and correct any inaccurate notions. The diagnosis of cancer is often interpreted as a death sentence.
a. Appoint a specific time to talk.	This will help the patient consolidate his thoughts and prevents haphazard discussions that may wander off the topic.

Plan for implementation	Rationale
b. Verify the patient's concerns as they are verbalized.	This clarifies (for the patient as well as for the nurse) what has been expressed by the patient.
3. Convey willingness to answer any of the patient's questions.	
4. Give emotional support and encouragement (within realistic limits).	No matter how bleak the prognosis, mentioning that aggressive research is constantly in progress can be a source of hope for the patient, since nobody can predict when a big breakthrough or discovery will occur. It might also be encouraging to remind the patient that over 2 million people are alive today after a diagnosis of cancer more than 5 years ago.[1]
5. Convey to the patient that expression of grief is expected and not something to be ashamed of.	Patients sometimes feel embarrassed if they are unable to control weeping, particularly if they are with a relatively unfamiliar nurse.
6. Recognize the covert signs of grief (withdrawal, decreased appetite, difficulty in concentrating) and interpret the behavior to the patient's family, who may misunderstand some of the patient's responses and feel rejected.	
7. Determine the need for psychiatric consultation.	Usually it is the patient's attending physician who makes the official request that the patient be seen by a psychiatrist during his hospitalization. However, since nurses are with the patient on a more continual basis, they may be the first to recognize the need.
8. Suggest spiritual counseling and make appropriate arrangements if the patient expresses interest.	Whether or not the patient considers himself religious, spiritual guidance may be extremely supportive and beneficial.
9. When appropriate, involve the family in any discussions, and encourage open communication between family members.	The support of the patient's loved ones can be the most valuable psychologic therapy available. However, this is not always possible, particularly if there has not been emotional closeness in the past. Careful observation and judgment must be exercised by the nurse to know how much family interaction to encourage.

2. NURSING DIAGNOSIS: Dependence on assistance in coping with changes in life-style imposed by advanced cancer

Objectives of nursing intervention
- Promotion of activity that enables optimum level of patient function
- Achievement of effective verbal and nonverbal communication
- Maintenance of an emotionally supportive environment
- Provision of information regarding supportive community organizations

Expected outcomes
- Maximum participation in activities that are within the patient's ability
- Ability and willingness to communicate feelings
- Absence of severe or protracted depression

Plan for implementation	Rationale
DECREASING ACTIVITY STATUS	
1. Plan frequent rest periods for the patient throughout the day.	The debilitating effects of metastatic disease cause a progressive decrease in the patient's activity capabilities.
2. Encourage as much activity as the patient can tolerate.	Provided that the patient does not become exhausted, maintaining his maximum level of activity is extremely important for the patient's psychologic well-being as well as his physical condition.
3. Provide diversional activities, such as reading, television, radio, and playing cards, that require only limited physical activity.	These activities provide a relief from boredom and are often a distraction from physical and/or psychologic pain.
4. Plan frequent contact with the patient, other than for routine care.	Even if time permits the nurse to stop at the patient's bedside for only a few minutes at intervals throughout the day, this alleviates some of the patient's boredom and isolation resulting from decreased activity status.
5. Keep any items the patient might need within easy reach.	This promotes the patient's sense of independence.
FINANCIAL PROBLEMS	
1. Observe the patient for indications of depression or worry.	Prolonged illness places considerable monetary burdens on a patient and his family. The patient may be unwilling to express his concerns, since the condition of one's finances is often considered personal.
2. Encourage the patient to verbalize his fears and concerns.	
3. Contact the hospital social service department if deemed necessary.	Community resources or other financial assistance may be available to the patient. A social worker can best determine the type of services for which the patient may be eligible.

Plan for implementation	Rationale

FACING THE REALITY OF DEATH

See Chapter 21.

STRESS ON FAMILY MEMBERS

1. Encourage the family to share their feelings and provide them with emotional support.

In many cases the family members are making considerable sacrifice to be with the patient on a daily basis. The hospital may not be close to home, and other aspects of their lives may be severely neglected. These factors, combined with the despair of seeing a loved one suffer, can result in extreme distress for the family.

2. Encourage them to participate in patient care whenever appropriate.

Active participation helps the family in the following ways:
1. It gives them something useful to do for the patient, thereby reducing their sense of powerlessness in a situation that often makes them feel increasingly helpless.
2. It increases their contact with the patient, laying the groundwork for sharing of feelings and constructive communication.

3. Do not take hostile behavior directed at staff members at face value. Instead:
   a. Investigate for any realistic cause of the negative behavior.
   b. If possible, correct any situation that may be triggering the behavior.
   c. If behavior appears ungrounded in reality, be aware of the following possible causes:

Hostility, especially when it appears to be unwarranted, is extremely difficult to deal with, without becoming angry oneself. Recognition that the source of the hostility is based on an internal conflict helps the nurse to deal with it in a more constructive way.

   (1) This may be the family's only outlet for repressed anger at the patient, at themselves, or at their concept of a supreme being.

Unconscious anger is very common when people are suffering and unable to control a situation. They may not permit themselves to direct the anger toward loved ones, so the hospital and staff become a safe target for their feelings.

   (2) The family may be going through the "anger" stage of the grieving process.

Like the patient who is dying, the loved ones go through stages in their adjustment to the impending loss. One of these stages involves anger, which manifests itself in various forms.

   d. If the behavior of the family is unacceptable (i.e., it is interfering with patient care), set firm guidelines without instilling guilt.

4. If family members appear to be having difficulty coping with the stress, convey to them that it is all right for them to take a day off now and then so they can have some time for themselves.

The psychologic stress of seeing a loved one suffer throughout the last stages of a terminal illness can be devastating. Guilt often prevents family members from taking necessary time for themselves. They can be reassured if the nurse explains that they will be **more** helpful and supportive if they are rested and able to tend to their own needs.

Plan for implementation	**Rationale**

NEED FOR COMMUNITY ASSISTANCE

Provide the patient and/or family with information concerning services within the community that can help them cope with this difficult period in their lives. These include:

1. Services either coordinated or directly provided by the American Cancer Society*
   a. Programs to assist the patient and family with emotional and social problems ("I Can Cope"; "Can Surmount")
   b. Programs to help defray the cost of appliances, medical supplies, and medication, if funds are not available from other sources
   c. Programs to assist parents of children with cancer ("Candlelighters")
   d. Arrangement of transportation for medical care
   e. Numerous informative publications designed to provide valuable instruction and emotional support for the cancer patient

   The American Cancer Society† has divisions throughout the United States that either directly provide numerous services or have information about where these services are available. The organization is an extremely valuable liaison uniting the specific care provided in the hospital with the many other aspects of the patient's daily life, including his home life and his emotional and social problems. The phone number for any local unit can be obtained by calling the toll-free information operator and asking for the toll-free number for Cancer Information Service or by checking the local telephone directory.

2. Services offered by the United Ostomy Association
   a. Contact with others who have made a successful adjustment to life with an ostomy and are trained in counseling new ostomates
   b. Education in proper ostomy care and management

   The United Ostomy Association‡ provides the ostomy patient with valuable current information and continued psychologic support. There are numerous chapters throughout the country.

---

*All of these services may not be available in each community.
†American Cancer Society, 777 Third Ave., New York, N.Y. 10017.
‡United Ostomy Association, 2001 W. Beverly Blvd., Los Angeles, Calif. 90057.

CHAPTER 21

The patient facing death

There are few generalizations one can make regarding death from a urologic disease. The causes are varied, elderly patients are not exclusively susceptible, and the subjective experience of the dying process is considerably different depending on the type and location of the disease. Most patients with a urologic condition can be cured either medically or surgically. However, for a sizable number there is no cure.

The most common cause of death from a urologic condition is cancer, most notably bladder and prostatic carcinoma. Because cancer is more common in the later decades of life, the dying urology patient is usually over the age of 60. However, there are exceptions, such as a young man in his 20s or 30s dying of testicular cancer.

Death from causes other than malignancies is not common, although a fatal pulmonary embolism from deep vein thrombosis following urologic surgery does occasionally occur. Furthermore, a patient hospitalized for a urologic condition (and therefore on the urology unit) may die of an unrelated cause, since most urology patients are over 60 and therefore may have diabetes, hypertension, a heart condition, or other health problems.

The events experienced by the dying urology patient vary considerably. A patient with prostatic cancer may be perfectly alert but in agonizing bone pain for months. A patient whose bladder tumor has metastasized to his brain may be incoherent and confused most of the time. A patient whose tumor has severely impaired his renal function will slowly drift into the stupor caused by uremia.

Thus there can be no one care plan for the dying urology patient. The following care plan has been included as a general guide with the emphasis on the psychosocial aspects of death. It comprises seven nursing diagnoses, which cover the topics of communication, stages of dying, self-concept, emotional support, and physical comfort.

The first nursing diagnosis involves a problem frequently encountered by the hospitalized dying patient—inadequate communication with staff. However, the root of the problem is often found to be poor communication between staff members. Interventions to alleviate this problem are provided at the beginning of the care plan. Inadequate communication between patient and family may also occur, and actions to resolve this problem are aimed at improvement of the communication between staff and family.

The second nursing diagnosis, based on the work of Kübler-Ross,[4] postulates that a patient goes through five psychologic stages in the dying process. A particular patient may not go through all the stages or experience them in the sequence presented. In fact, some patients do not appear to go through any stages at all.[9] However, Kübler-Ross's concept of stages is useful for nurses because it provides a broad definition of various coping behavior patterns. Some of the conflicts triggering the behavior can often be resolved by specific interventions in the attempt to provide the patient with an anxiety-free, peaceful death—what Kübler-Ross calls the stage of acceptance, and what caregivers generally recognize as the ultimate goal for the dying patient.* The concept of stages also provides a tool useful in helping the family work through their grief and in explaining to them the reason for some of the patient's unexpected behaviors.

The next nursing diagnosis concerns the patient who has poor self-esteem as death approaches. Un-

---

*A word of caution is required here regarding the term "goal." We, as caregivers, must not impose our idea of an ideal death onto a patient. A sad illustration of this is a patient who died recently after having become superficially familiar with these stages; but he interpreted them as rigid goals he had to reach. However, he was unable to resolve his anger and was therefore not only unable to find peace and acceptance regarding his death but also felt he was a failure in not achieving this final goal.

fulfilled dreams and aspirations and the disfigurement of illness are examples of common causes, and nursing care is aimed at helping the patient be more accepting of himself and his life.

The following two nursing diagnoses involve emotional support from one or more "significant others." When this cannot be achieved adequately with a friend or family member, sometimes a nurse can be the one with whom the patient finds solace by sharing some of his final and meaningful feelings.

The next nursing diagnosis deals with control of the severe chronic pain often experienced by patients with advanced urologic cancers. Adequate management of pain includes an appropriate medication regimen as well as management of various psychologic components.

The last nursing diagnosis addresses physical care of the dying patient and the promotion of a pleasant environment for him. Like all the preceding nursing diagnoses, it is sufficiently general to apply to almost any dying patient. The nurse will have to adapt the diagnosis and its corresponding interventions to meet the needs of the particular patient.

THE PATIENT FACING DEATH
POTENTIAL NURSING DIAGNOSES:

1. Inadequate communication between staff, patient, and family
2. Difficulty working through the psychologic stages of dying
3. Absence of positive self-concept as a result of illness and hospitalization
4. Insufficient emotional support from the family
5. Dependence on staff for emotional support
6. Dependence on control of disease-related pain
7. Dependence on maintenance of bodily and environmental comfort during the last days or weeks of life

---

1. NURSING DIAGNOSIS: Inadequate communication between staff, patient, and family

Objectives of nursing intervention
{
Ability to provide all information requested by the patient

Provision of an environment in which information and feelings can be shared between patient, family, and staff
}

Expected outcomes
{
Verbal and/or behavioral indications that the patient is receiving as much information as he wants

Effective communication between patient, family, and staff
}

Plan for implementation	Rationale
STAFF-STAFF COMMUNICATION	
1. Discuss with the patient's physician what information he has given him and the words he has used to describe the patient's condition.	When nurses fear that they are liable to reveal information that the patient is not supposed to hear, they are likely to avoid communicating with the patient on anything but superficial levels.
2. If the physician has chosen to deny important information to the patient (e.g., the presence of incurable disease), ask him his reasons.	Most authorities agree that it is better to tell the patient that he has only limited time to live. Some reasons behind this relatively recent approach are that, if the patient is not told the truth, he will be less inclined to trust the staff, he will not participate as well in his treatment, and he may deeply regret (too late) that he was not given ample opportunity to put his affairs in order. However, the physician may have overriding reasons for not being candid with the patient, and the nursing staff should strive to understand the reasons and act accordingly.

Plan for implementation	Rationale
3. If there is considerable difference of opinion among the nursing and medical staffs regarding the amount of information the patient should be given, discuss it in a joint meeting.	Traditionally the physician decides what information should be given the patient concerning his medical diagnosis and prognosis, and the nursing staff must abide by the decision. Differences of opinion sometimes arise if the patient has been hospitalized for a long time and the nurses have become well acquainted with the patient, often better than the physician. Their input in the decision regarding how much should be told to the patient may be extremely beneficial. If done diplomatically, it also facilitates better communication among staff members in the future.
4. If the physician has denied basic information to the patient, discuss with him options as to how to handle the situation if the patient directly asks for information or reveals that he already knows that he is dying.	Usually a patient's direct questions indicate that he suspects his condition is terminal and that he is emotionally ready to hear the truth. Although in cases like this it is generally agreed that honesty should prevail, if the physician still believes that the patient should not know the truth, his wishes must be considered orders. (This can be extremely difficult for the nurse, emotionally as well as ethically.)
5. Hold periodic meetings among those staff members who are providing most of the patient's care to determine the patient's psychologic status and his progress in accepting his condition.	
6. Be aware that those providing direct patient care may have difficulty communicating with the patient openly if they deny their **own** feelings about death. Such problems can be alleviated to some extent by the following measures: a. Provide opportunities for staff to express their feelings in a supportive atmosphere. b. Include members of the psychiatric team for discussions whenever possible (provided that the particular psychiatrist is at ease with the subject of death). c. Include members of the hospital clergy in the discussions. d. Be nonjudgmental about others' feelings, as well as one's own.	If nurses have many unresolved emotions about their own deaths, they will be less likely to recognize the patient's subtle needs and hear what he is **really** saying when he speaks.[3] Often they will only hear what makes **them** feel comfortable, and the entire communication process becomes distorted. The most common pitfalls in such instances are the nurses' conscious or unconscious avoidance of the patient and their projecting onto the patient what they would **like** him to be communicating rather than what he really feels. It is much easier to live and function with one's feelings (regardless of what they are) if energy is not being wasted to suppress or mask them from oneself. Fear, revulsion, anger, sorrow, and so-called negative emotions are normal. They are only likely to stand in the way of therapeutic communication with the patient if they are overwhelming to the nurse; or, if the nurse is so busy trying to cover them up, there is no attention left to focus on the **patient's** feelings.[3]

STAFF-PATIENT COMMUNICATION

1. Maintain open communication between staff members (see preceding).

Plan for implementation	**Rationale**
2. Encourage the patient to express his feelings.	
3. Convey willingness to listen. This includes nonverbal clues such as: a. Maintaining an unhurried attitude b. Sitting down with the patient c. Maintaining eye contact d. Leaning closer to the patient e. Touching the patient f. Nodding at suitable moments when the patient is talking	
4. Answer all questions as simply and honestly as possible.	Often anxiety of the unknown is more difficult to cope with than painful truth. Facts such as where the tumor is, why the patient has his particular symptoms, and what he can expect from the treatment are often appreciated.
5. Give painful information gently and without destroying all hope.	
6. Convey willingness to answer all questions, no matter how many times they are asked.	Anxiety often limits the patient's ability to absorb information. A patient manner on the part of the nurse reduces anxiety and enables the patient to ask for information he wants to have.
7. Suggest a consultation with a psychiatrist or member of the clergy if deemed appropriate.	

PATIENT-FAMILY COMMUNICATION

1. Provide the patient and family with private time together.	Often this simple convenience is overlooked when treatments and continuous activity in a multi-bed room keep the environment filled with distractions and interruptions. It makes sharing of meaningful feelings difficult.
2. Determine the willingness and ability of family members to participate in the nontechnical care of the patient (e.g., feeding, bathing, ambulating) and, if appropriate, encourage them to participate in the patient's care.	Participation in the patient's care can be therapeutic for the family in the following ways: 1. It enables the patient and family to be together without feeling the **need** to keep a conversation going (i.e., another activity is taking the place of verbal communication, which is sometimes difficult in the face of grief). 2. It provides the family with a sense of helping at a time when the patient's illness often makes them feel increasingly helpless.
3. Teach simple skills to one or more of the family members, and provide supervision until he or she feels comfortable with the activity.	

Psychosocial and psychophysical factors affecting the urology patient

Plan for implementation	Rationale
4. When appropriate, encourage the patient to discuss any feelings he has revealed to the staff with his family.	Sometimes a staff member is a "safe" object with whom to communicate feelings because there is no emotional involvement. The patient may not want to burden his family with his troubles. However, when there can be an honest exchange of feelings between family members, the impending death of a loved one can bring a profound experience of sharing and closeness.

FAMILY-STAFF COMMUNICATION (BEFORE DEATH OF PATIENT)

Plan for implementation	Rationale
1. Convey willingness to answer any questions the family might have. 2. Answer all questions as simply and honestly as possible. 3. Provide a nonjudgmental environment for expression of feelings.	The family usually goes through a preparatory grieving process that may include feelings of shock, denial, anger, guilt, and sorrow. They require considerable support, not only so that they can live their lives at an optimal level of psychologic health throughout the patient's illness, but also so that they can provide the necessary emotional support the patient needs.
4. Give painful information gently and without destroying all hope, but do not foster false hope.	Hope is a vital coping mechanism. To destroy it before the family is ready to let go can be devastating. But it is equally unkind to encourage false hopes when a realistic appraisal of the patient's condition demonstrates only deterioration.
5. Help the family convert realistic hope into short-term goals, such as pleasurable activities, and the sharing of positive feelings together.	
6. Prepare the family for sudden changes in the patient's condition before they enter his room.	
7. When possible, convey information regarding impending or actual death to the entire family rather than one individual.	Sharing bad news **together** provides the family with valuable emotional support.

FAMILY-STAFF COMMUNICATION (AFTER DEATH OF PATIENT)

Plan for implementation	Rationale
1. Provide an opportunity for the family to be together in private to express their feelings.	
2. Answer all questions as simply and honestly as possible.	

Plan for implementation	Rationale
3. Foster sharing of feelings and support among family members.	The family will need each other more than ever in the period of adjustment that follows. Sharing of feelings and the ensuing sense of closeness are usually the most healing aspects of the rehabilitation process.
4. If circumstances permit the nurse to spend additional time with the family, explain some of the emotional changes they might experience over the next few months. Reassure them that these feelings are normal and are part of their psychologic adjustment to the loss of their loved one. Although the grieving process is highly individual, the following are some relatively common experiences:	Occasionally the nurse will have developed a close rapport with the patient's family. This is relatively common if the patient had a long illness. Since there is usually little opportunity to give continued emotional support to the family after the patient's death, a discussion of some of the psychologic changes the family members might experience may help the family in the transition period when when they can no longer rely on emotional support from the nurse.
a. Shock and numbness	No matter how well prepared the family is for the patient's death, the reality and finality of it are almost always difficult to accept fully at first.
b. Relief that the ordeal is over	This reaction is very common when there has been a long period of suffering. The family must be helped not to feel guilty about such thoughts and feelings.
c. Anger and indignation at the suffering endured by the patient and the entire family	These feelings are also quite common. They are frequently a source of guilt, particularly if the anger is directed at their concept of a supreme being. It helps to know that this, too, is normal.
d. A sense of being overwhelmed by the adjustment to new roles in life	Experiences that may simply appear challenging under normal circumstances may appear impossible when compounded by extreme loneliness and loss. Actually the new responsibilities can be a source of strength and support, forcing family members to continue with their own lives rather than dwelling in the past.
e. The feeling that the grief and sense of loss will never end	It is very difficult to anticipate recovering from a deeply painful experience. The family must trust that time does heal even the greatest of wounds.

2. **NURSING DIAGNOSIS:** Difficulty working through the psychologic stages of dying: denial, anger, bargaining, depression, and acceptance[4]

Objectives of nursing intervention
- Provision of a nonjudgmental environment
- Maintenance of therapeutic communication that encourages expression of feelings
- Provision of necessary information at appropriate time

Expected outcomes
- Patient able to express feelings with significant other(s) and/or staff member
- Patient reaches stage of acceptance

Plan for implementation	Rationale
DENIAL	
1. Be alert for indications of denial, such as the following: a. The patient makes statements such as, "I don't believe it!"	Denial is a normal defense mechanism that is vital in shielding the patient from information he is not yet ready to face. It may, however, be so extreme that it prevents adequate expression of feelings and the often comforting

Plan for implementation	Rationale
b. The patient blames symptoms on a less serious condition. c. The patient uses euphemisms such as "my bad back." d. The patient refuses follow-up treatment. e. The patient asks no questions about his condition. f. The patient avoids talking about dying. g. The patient makes long-range plans for the future.	activities of attending to any unfinished business and verbalizing feelings that may have gone unexpressed for too long. Periods of denial may occur throughout the patient's illness, but ideally they become shorter as death approaches.
2. Be aware of one's own potential to avoid confronting death. Denial on the part of the nurse cannot always be eliminated, but recognizing its presence enables one to deal with it rather than be handicapped by it.	In our society very few people are totally at ease with the idea of death or are willing to deal with a patient's (as well as their own) feelings on the subject. If the nurse's denial is mostly unconscious, it may reinforce the patient's denial and thus impede his progress in acceptance of his death. But to recognize that one does tend to avoid thinking about death begins the process of working through ones feelings on the subject and thus greatly diminishes the need to continue denying.
3. Find out what the physician has told the patient (i.e., what words were used, what kind of hope was offered) before communicating with the patient regarding his condition. Attempt to pattern any additional information given to the patient along the same lines. (It is assumed that the patient's physician has told him the truth about his condition. If not, the likelihood of the patient working through denial is diminished, since denial anywhere along the lines of communication [from physician to nurse to family to patient] will serve to reinforce the patient's own denial mechanisms).	Restating what the physician has said serves these functions: 1. It reinforces what the patient has already heard, so the information is more readily retained. 2. It prevents confusion of terminology and opinions. 3. It establishes, in the patient's mind, a sense of continuity regarding his care. 4. It conveys that the nurse can be relied on to give accurate information.
4. Recognize that the patient needs a period of denial to adapt to the information and mobilize his coping mechanisms.	
5. Do not insist that a patient face a situation he clearly is not psychologically ready to accept.	Forcing the truth on a patient is cruel. Furthermore, it usually **strengthens** his denial mechanisms as well as fosters mistrust of the nurse.
6. Be alert for clues in the patient's conversation that indicate he is ready to face the reality of impending death. When such clues occur: a. Refrain from providing any false reassurances. b. Encourage the patient to discuss what he is feeling. c. Provide any information the patient requests with gentleness. d. Above all, do not close the door to all hope.	

Plan for implementation	**Rationale**

7. Assist the patient who is trying to overcome denial used by family members. Some ways this can be done are:
  a. Role-play with the patient to allow him to try out what he wants to say to his family, with the nurse playing the role of a family member.
  b. Offer to act as a temporary liaison with the family to convey that the patient realizes that he is dying and that their lack of acceptance is making him feel more isolated.
	Sometimes the patient is able to accept the reality of his condition, whereas loved ones are either unable or unwilling to do so. Instead, they maintain the mistaken belief that a cheery facade is better for the patient than a realistic discussion of his condition and their feelings about it. But the strain of pretense is exhausting and emotionally unrewarding for all involved. Instead, open, honest communication of feelings should, if possible, be established so that the last period of the patient's life can include emotional sharing and closeness.

8. Do not assume that the patient is in the stage of denial just because he does not discuss his feelings about his condition and he exhibits none of the other reactions to death (anger, bargaining, depression) that frequently appear after the denial stage has, to some extent, been worked through.	Lack of discussion and other emotional responses may be due to any number of reasons, including: 1. A basically shy, inexpressive personality 2. Feelings of distrust for the caregivers 3. Profound religious convictions that enable him to view death as simply a transition from one plane of existence to another

ANGER

1. Refrain from responding to the overt reason for the patient's anger. Instead, attempt to explore with the patient his **feelings** so that he can gain insight into the actual source of his anger.	Once the patient has accepted the reality of his condition, there is often considerable anger and resentment at the irrevocable situation. Sometimes these emotions are displaced onto staff and family. Although, intellectually, the staff may recognize that they are not really the target, it often takes tremendous self-restraint not to react in kind to angry, irrational outbursts, which are common at this stage of psychologic adjustment. Recognizing that envy plays a considerable role in certain patients' anger (envy of those who are young, healthy, and appear to have a long life ahead of them) sometimes helps the staff deal realistically with this difficult stage.
2. Explain and interpret to the patient's family any expressions of anger that are directed at them. The positive side is that at least he is accepting the reality of his condition, which is a significant emotional step.	Once the family realizes that they are not at fault for the patient's behavior, they can better understand what the patient is experiencing and remain supportive of him.
3. Maintain limits to the extent that angry outbursts are permitted. Hospital regulations, the functioning of the floor, and the psychologic well-being of the staff must be considered.	There is often a tendency to go overboard with pity for a dying patient and to permit abusive behavior that is incompatible with the routines of the hospital unit. This is of no value to the patient himself, to other patients, or to the staff. Kind but firm limits must be established.

4. Provide the patient with avenues through which he can exert some control by giving him choices such as:
  a. When his bed will be made
  b. What he would like to eat
  c. What position he wants to lie in (provided precautions against decubitus ulcers are maintained)
	This enables the patient to retain a sense of autonomy in a situation that is forcing him gradually to relinquish **all** control.

Plan for implementation	Rationale

5. Encourage the family to provide the patient with as many choices as are reasonable, such as:
  a. When family members should visit
  b. How long they should stay
  c. What foods they should bring from home	

6. In the event that the **family** is expressing anger at hospital personnel or policies, be aware that this may be a displacement of their anger at the situation. There may even be unconscious anger at the patient himself for bringing the tragedy on them; or their anger may be due to their frustration at being relatively helpless in the situation.	Loved ones frequently go through stages similar to those of the patient as their reaction to the patient's illness progresses. They need as much support as the patient in dealing with their anger and frustration and working through it constructively.
7. Encourage the family to explore the source of their feelings and reassure them that negative emotions are normal among the loved ones of someone who is dying.	

BARGAINING

1. Be alert for indications that the patient is going through a period of attempting to alter the inevitable by various psychologic maneuvers. They make take various forms:
  a. The patient may begin to talk about radical changes in his life-style, usually involving some sort of sacrifice.
  b. The patient may offer huge sums of money to organizations. (This may not **necessarily** indicate that the patient is bargaining. He may simply want to make a monetary contribution to a cause he believes in.)
  c. The patient may assert new religious faith.
	A period of bargaining frequently occurs as a last effort to change the forecast of impending death. It is actually a form of magical thinking, i.e., "If I am good, this terrible thing won't happen." It does not occur as regularly as the other psychologic reactions to death and is usually short-lived.

2. Be aware that sometimes this behavior indicates a sense of guilt at how the patient has lived his life.	It stands to reason that, if the patient thinks that changing his behavior will change the course of events, he feels that his behavior in some way precipitated the "punishment" because it was "bad."
3. If appropriate, encourage the patient to verbalize what it is he does not like about himself that he desires to change.	Insight into the underlying reasons for making a particular bargain may be helpful. For example, does the patient feel his previous life-style was not a worthy one? Does he feel guilty about not having more religious faith?
4. Recognize that the family may also be experiencing this pattern of behavior and encourage them to explore their feelings.	

DEPRESSION

1. Be aware that this is considered a necessary stage for the patient in the psychologic adjustment to his im-	There is nothing pathologic or abnormal about this depression. The patient is grieving over the impending loss

Plan for implementation	**Rationale**
pending death, and refrain from attempting to cheer him up by changing the subject or offering false hope.	of all he knows and loves. Unless he experiences this grief, it is unlikely that he will reach the stage of emotional acceptance of his death.[4]
2. Encourage the patient to verbalize his feelings only if he appears in need of talking.	The patient should not feel that he has to talk to "earn" the nurse's presence.
3. Convey empathy by a touch or simply silent presence.	Silence is often more meaningful at this time than conversation.
4. Reassure the family that, although this is deeply painful for the patient, it is important in helping him separate himself from this world.	The family may be tempted to try to lift the patient's spirits with jokes, stories, and various diversions. Although this may provide him with some welcome relief from his feelings of depression, if done in the extreme, it will delay the patient's progress and may become burdensome to him if he feels that he must maintain a happy facade for their benefit.

ACCEPTANCE

1. Be alert for indications of emotional acceptance of impending death, characterized by behavior such as:
  a. Prolonged periods of sleep (this may also be due to the physiologic aspects of dying)
  b. Diminished sphere of interests
  c. Relative disinterest in most visitors except those who are very close
	When a patient reaches this stage, he is no longer depressed or angry and has, in a way, reached a sense of peace regarding his death. He is ready to disengage himself from the world he has known.

2. Refrain from encouraging conversation unless the patient appears to want to talk.	Usually the patient will prefer silence, a touch of the hand, or perhaps a prayer read aloud.
3. Use nonverbal communication with the patient, such as sitting with him or holding his hand.	This conveys that he will not be abandoned and that he is still being cared for even though he cannot be cured.
4. Observe the patient for clues regarding how much company he wants, and limit the number of visitors accordingly.	Usually the patient will prefer the presence of only one or two people to whom he has been very close during his his life.
5. Explain to loved ones what the stage of acceptance means and that they should not encourage the patient to "keep fighting," since he has finally reached a point where there is relatively little psychic pain.	Often the patient is ahead of the family in accepting that his death is imminent. It can be very reassuring for the family to realize that this is a relatively pain-free state and reassuring for the patient to know that his loved ones are also ready to accept the inevitable.

3. NURSING DIAGNOSIS: Absence of positive self-concept as a result of illness and hospitalization

Objective of nursing intervention	Promotion of an environment and activities which help the patient feel good about himself

Expected outcomes

- Verbal and/or behavioral indications by the patient that his life has been meaningful
- Absence of depression, guilt, or regret
- Participation (to capacity) in activities from which the patient obtains some pleasure

Plan for implementation	Rationale

1. Convey to the patient an interest in him as an individual. This can be done in various ways.
  a. Make frequent visits to the patient's room when nursing tasks are **not** required.
  b. Encourage the patient to talk about his interests and feelings.
  c. Use nonverbal listening devices (see p. 151).
	Often nursing functions focus primarily on physical care, especially when the patient is very weak and has many physical needs. With such concentration on the patient's body, the nurse must not forget to relate to the person as a whole—an individual with unique interests, concerns, ideas, and personality characteristics.

2. Help the patient to focus on the productive aspects of his life rather than dwelling on what he might consider to be his shortcomings.	People who have not been able to fulfill certain aspirations or live by a specific value system often feel a sense of failure, guilt, and/or meaninglessness about their lives.
3. If appropriate, discuss with the patient's family aspects of the patient's life where he feels he has failed. When possible, encourage them to help him see a different, more positive point of view.	Sometimes a patient may feel he has not achieved certain goals when, in fact, he has. This is particularly true in relation to emotional attachments where the people involved simply have not given adequate feedback. This can sometimes be overcome by reassurance from loved ones, verbal expression of feelings, and reminders of the good the patient has done in his life.

4. Help the patient feel content with whatever religious beliefs give him a sense of peace. This can be done in the following ways:
  a. Express interest in the patient's beliefs.
  b. Refrain from expressing ones own beliefs particularly if they differ greatly from those of the patient.
  c. Maintain a nonjudgmental attitude.
  d. Encourage the patient to talk about his beliefs.
	Many patients will find comfort in talking about their religion. Sometimes a nurse is seen as a less threatening figure with whom to discuss these beliefs than a clergyman. This is especially true if the patient feels he has not adequately participated in a religious organization and if the nurse maintains a nonjudgmental approach.
	
	Most religions deal with events and awarenesses that are not limited to biologic life. Such thoughts often diminish the importance of the world the patient knows he will soon he leaving while giving him something permanent to hold onto.

5. When possible, suggest opportunities in which the patient can have a sense of giving or doing something meaningful for another person. Although the patient's level of strength may prevent any physical activity, something as effortless as a prayer for another person may lift the patient's own spirits.	Helplessness and uselessness are potent inhibitors of self-esteem, whereas doing something for another person often makes one feel better about himself.

Plan for implementation	Rationale
6. Encourage the patient to maintain a sense of autonomy by providing him with choices whenever possible; e.g., what and when he wants to eat, when to do a treatment, how he wants his pain relieved (see p. 162).	This conveys to the patient that his opinions are valued and that he can, and is expected to, play a role in his care.
7. When possible, encourage the patient to wear his own articles of clothing (e.g., a favorite cap or a robe from home) rather than only hospital attire.	Clothing is a personal expression of oneself. Patients who are hospitalized for a long time often develop a sense of anonymity. Their own clothing may help them retain a sense of their individuality, a reminder that they still are who they once were.
8. Encourage the patient to participate in activities he enjoys that are not taxing to his strength (e.g., playing cards or chess, reading, watching television).	
9. When appropriate, encourage the patient to communicate with other patients. When possible, match roommates with similar interests or arrange visits with other patients.	The support system among patients can be extremely strong. Even if the patient is too weak to engage actively in much conversation, listening to others and feeling included can be diverting and comforting.
10. Promote good hygiene. Unpleasant odors from drainage or incontinence should be eliminated or reduced as much as possible.	Perhaps the foremost psychosocial barrier for a patient is odor. Unfortunately the purulent drainage, necrotic tissue sloughing, and/or incontinence that frequently are present as death approaches produce such a barrier. Today's highly deodorized standard of living makes these factors a strong deterrent to socialization. The staff, family, and other patients will respond much more favorably to the patient if foul odors are not present.
11. Encourage the patient to maintain good grooming. A haircut and a shave or a touch of lipstick and some light cologne are just a few familiar practices that help one feel better.	Although this may lift the spirits of any patient, it is particularly important for the patient whose body is undergoing visible changes.
12. Reassure the patient that physical disfigurement does not detract from the person himself.	Many patients experience shock and self-rejection as they become aware of their physical deterioration. The extent of this reaction depends on the degree to which the patient defines himself in terms of his physical body.

4. NURSING DIAGNOSIS: Insufficient emotional support from family*

Objective of nursing intervention	Promotion of an emotionally supportive atmosphere for the family so they can function at an optimum level (emotionally and physically) with the patient
Expected outcome	Patient able and willing to share meaningful feelings with at least one family member

Plan for implementation	Rationale
1. Promote optimum communication between patient and family and staff and family (see nursing diagnosis 1).	

2. If lack of patient-family interaction is observed:
  a. Question the family about their needs, problems, fears and other concerns. For example, ask how they are managing and what could be done to help them through this difficult period.
  b. Make appropriate referrals (e.g., psychiatric, medical, or social service consultations) and/or adjustments (e.g., modifications in visiting hours) when deemed necessary.
  c. Maintain a nonjudgmental attitude if the family expresses dislike for the patient.
	Often the family members are preoccupied with financial worries, concerns about children and other responsibilities, and their own failing health. The extra concern expressed by the patient's nurse is often welcomed by the family and provides useful information for the nurse with regard to how the patient's situation may be improved. Providing the family with emotional support generally enhances their ability to be more supportive of the patient.

3. Be ready to handle the reaction of family members if the patient exhibits a decline of interest in family matters and conversation as death approaches. They may see it as a rejection and then begin to withdraw themselves. If this occurs:
  a. Explain that this is a normal step in the patient's emotional acceptance of his death.
  b. Encourage them not to feel rejected.
  c. If appropriate, suggest the following modifications of their activities:
    (1) Sit quietly with the patient and wait for him to initiate any conversation.
    (2) Convey their presence and caring by touch.
    (3) Limit the number of visitors at one time to one or two people who are very close to the patient.
	As death approaches, the patient may begin to disengage himself from the people and interests he has loved during his life. This is an important step for him because it indicates he has worked through much of his grief and is becoming emotionally ready to die. However, it is common for loved ones to misinterpret this behavior and feel rejected. Their immediate reaction is often withdrawal from the situation. Instead, they should be encouraged to remain with the patient and convey to him that they understand his needs and will not abandon him.

4. If the patient has no close relationships and is still relatively active, encourage interaction among other patients with similar interests.	

*The term "family" is used loosely. It includes any person who plays a significant role in the patient's emotional life.

5. NURSING DIAGNOSIS: Dependence on staff for emotional support

Objective of nursing intervention   Availability of a surrogate significant other when the patient appears to have no friends or family readily available

Expected outcome   Patient able and willing to share meaningful feelings with a member of the staff

Plan for implementation	Rationale
1. Arrange staff assignments so the patient has most contact with one primary caregiver and allot sufficient time for nurse-patient interaction (for reasons other than treatments and tasks).	
2. Promote optimum communication between staff and patient (see nursing diagnosis 1, under staff-patient communication).	Good communication fosters trust, a prerequisite for an emotional bond between two human beings.
3. Promote a positive self-concept (see nursing diagnosis 3).	Those who help a person feel better about himself are generally liked and often relied on for assistance in dealing with emotional conflicts.
4. Convey to the patient that he is important to the staff by making frequent visits to his room (for reasons other than nursing tasks).	Even if these visits are short (and they usually have to be on a busy floor), they demonstrate to the patient that the staff is available and concerned about his well-being.
5. Provide reassurance by conveying to the patient that he will be cared for throughout his illness, even if cure is no longer possible.	
6. Determine if the patient would like to see a psychiatrist or clergyman and make appropriate referrals.	
7. Recognize that some patients may not wish to share their private feelings with anybody.	The decision to communicate feelings must be left to the patient. All the nurse can do is be available.

6. NURSING DIAGNOSIS: Dependence on control of disease-related pain

Objective of nursing intervention	Maintenance of patient comfort by reducing or eliminating perception of pain
Expected outcome	Verbal and/or behavioral indications that the pain is absent or adequately reduced

Plan for implementation	Rationale
1. Be aware that medication alone is often insufficient in providing optimum comfort for a patient who suffers from chronic pain.	Many factors play a role in the patient's perception of pain. These include his anxiety about disfigurement and death and the extent of psychologic support he is receiving.
2. Discuss the pain with the patient and find out how **he** thinks it can best be controlled. Whenever possible, follows the patient's suggestions.	By allowing the patient to take an active role in the control of his pain, he is more likely to respond to the measures taken.[2] This also fosters trust, conveys concern, and reinforces his coping mechanisms.
3. When administering narcotic analgesics: a. Do not withhold p.r.n. medication or wait for the pain to become severe because you think that the patient will become addicted.	Fear of addiction in the terminal patient with severe chronic pain is inappropriate, although common among nurses.[11] If anything, it is **undertreatment** with narcotic analgesics that may contribute to the craving and psychologic dependence associated with addiction.[7]
b. Respond to the patient's request for p.r.n. medication at once.	It is easier to control severe pain at its onset rather than once it is established. This is thought to be due to the mode of action of narcotic analgesics, which is to alter the emotional response to pain at the cerebral level. Once pain is severe, the anxiety and fear response makes it harder to control.[8]
c. If the pain is severe and continuous, suggest that the physician order administration of analgesia at regular intervals (e.g., every 4 hours) rather than on a p.r.n. basis.	Waiting for pain to reappear accentuates the difficulties in controlling it. Conversely, once the anxious anticipation and memory of it diminishes, the amount of required analgesia often decreases.[7]
d. Tell the patient when the medication is expected to take effect, and express confidence that it will adequately control the pain.	The power of suggestion is a strong influence in pain relief.[1]
e. Determine the speed, the degree, and the duration of relief obtained by the medication.	
f. If the pain is not adequately relieved at the prescribed dosage, do not be reluctant to suggest to the physician that the dosage be raised.	The notion that patients suffering from severe chronic pain will develop tolerance to the medication and require escalating doses is being proved erroneous. Many patients with severe chronic pain can be maintained on the same dosage for long periods of time **once the adequate dosage is determined and the pain is under control.**[6,10]

Plan for implementation	**Rationale**
4. Use nursing measures, in addition to the administration of analgesic medication, to control the patient's pain: a. Resposition the patient. b. Give a back rub. c. Teach slow, abdominal breathing and other relaxation and diversional techniques.[5] d. Provide gentle stroking or firm pressure on the painful area.	The chronic pain cycle involves not only the pain itself but also fearful anticipation of its recurrence, anxiety, and depression. Therefore, in addition to analgesic administration, these measures often bring about considerable relief by providing relaxation and emotional support.

7. **NURSING DIAGNOSIS:** Dependence on maintenance of bodily and environmental comfort during the last days or weeks of life

Objective of nursing intervention	Provision of cleanliness, physical comfort, and a pleasant environment
Expected outcomes	Absence of eye, nose, or mouth discomfort Nutritional intake maintained as desired Absence of adverse effects from incontinence Absence of skin breakdown Absence of unpleasant odors

Plan for implementation	**Rationale**
HYGIENE	
1. Provide mouth care as needed.	As the patient's condition deteriorates, his mouth may become dry and sore. This may be caused by various factors, including moniliasis or other infections and cancer medications.
a. Offer water with increasing frequency, especially if the patient is only able to tolerate a few sips at a time.	Thirst is often present, even if the patient refuses food.
b. If the patient is unable to drink from a cup, allow him to suck cool water from a water-soaked gauze pad.	The coordination of drinking may be difficult, but the sucking reflex usually enables swallowing without choking.
c. Apply petroleum jelly to dry, cracked lips.	
d. Aspirate secretions with suction if the patient cannot swallow.	
e. Cleanse teeth, gums, tongue, and inside of cheeks with a soft toothbrush or a piece of gauze wrapped around a tongue blade.	
f. If mouth pain is present, suggest that the physician order a topical anesthetic such as 2% lidocaine (Xylocaine 2% Viscous) mouthwash.	

163

Plan for implementation	**Rationale**

2. Provide nose care as needed.
   a. Keep nares free from encrustations with gauze or cotton-tipped applicator dipped in saline.
   b. Lubricate nares with water-soluble jelly.

3. Provide eye care as needed.
   a. Cleanse eyelids and remove mucous secretions with gauze or cotton-tipped applicator dipped in saline.
   b. Apply artificial tear solution (e.g., Tearisol) into conjunctival sac as needed.

NUTRITION AND ELIMINATION

1. Promote food intake by the following measures:
   a. Suggest that the physician order an antiemetic to be administered before meals if the patient is nauseated.
   b. Find out what the patient's favorite foods are and, when possible, provide them. (Family may be encouraged to bring special food items from home.)
   c. Feed the patient in an unhurried manner.

2. Maintain care of the patient's elimination by the following measures:
   a. Keep accurate records of the patient's fecal and urinary output.
   b. If urinary incontinence occurs:
      (1) Use a condom catheter for a male patient (see p. 432).
      (2) Keep rolled combines between the legs and under the buttocks of a female patient.
      (3) Avoid the use of plastic bed shields directly against the patient's skin.

      (4) Use an indwelling urethral catheter only as a last resort (i.e., skin breakdown cannot be controlled).

   c. If fecal incontinence occurs:
      (1) Clean the patient after every episode of incontinence.

      (2) Examine the skin around the rectal area for evidence of breakdown (blanched, red, or broken skin).
      (3) Keep the room well ventilated.
      (4) Be alert for symptoms of impaction, such as:
         (a) Constant seepage of stool

         (b) Absence of stool for more than 3 days

These prevent evaporation of moisture and therefore predispose the patient to skin breakdown.
An indwelling urethral catheter predisposes the patient to numerous problems (see master care plan for the patient with an indwelling urethral catheter).

Unless the patient is cleaned immediately, the excreta contributes to skin breakdown, especially around the coccygeal area.

Fecal impaction is sometimes manifested by incontinence. What actually happens is that liquid stool seeps out around the impaction in small amounts.

Plan for implementation	**Rationale**

(5) If the patient appears to have impacted stool, a digital examination and disimpaction are required (these may or may not be nursing functions, depending on hospital policy), and the physician should be notified.

    d. If any incontinence occurs, maintain an accepting attitude and convey to the patient that he need not feel embarrassed.

To lose control of the most basic body functions is psychologically devastating to a conscious patient. He usually feels helpless, infantile, and depressed by the situation, since it only emphasizes his progressive loss of control over **all** his body functions, and eventually life itself.

SKIN CARE

1. Keep linen clean, dry, and unwrinkled.

2. Massage pressure points with lotion.

This keeps the skin lubricated and promotes circulation to the area.

3. Maintain a regimen of range of motion exercises (active or passive) at least twice a day.

4. Teach isometric exercises if the patient is alert and able to perform them.

5. For the bedridden patient:
    a. Provide water bed, lamb's-wool pad, silicone pad, or alternating pressure mattress as needed.
    b. Turn the patient every 2 hours and alternate the height of the head of the bed.
    c. Pad bony prominences with lamb's wool or cotton.

All these measures are aimed at reducing pressure on specific parts of the body that are prone to skin breakdown from decreased peripheral circulation. The areas at risk are those where the bone is close to the surface of the skin (e.g., heels, coccyx, scapula, greater trochanter).

6. If skin breakdown has occurred, use the following measures as well as those just listed:
    a. Use a heat lamp on the area three times a day for 30 minutes; use a 40-watt bulb, 18 to 24 inches away.

The exposure to light and air promotes healing.

    b. Keep the area clean and dry.
    c. Irrigate the area with normal saline.
    d. Suggest to the physician that he order topical medication such as:
       (1) Sutilains ointment (Travase Ointment) for biochemical debridement
       or

This substance digests necrotic soft tissue by proteolytic action.

       (2) Dextranomer (Debrisan) granules to drain the wound of exudate and accelerate the normal healing process

These hydrophilic beads promote healing by drawing exudate and bacterial particles to the surface of the wound, thus reducing edema, inflammation, and pain. This cleansing action speeds up the formation of granulation tissue so healing is accelerated.

Plan for implementation	**Rationale**
7. If the patient is diaphoretic: a. Change the linens more frequently. b. Keep only a light cover or sheet over the patient. c. Provide tepid sponge baths. d. Keep the room well ventilated.	As death approaches, diaphoresis is common, and the patient may feel (subjectively) very warm although his skin might feel cool to the touch. Keeping him dry and not overly covered promotes comfort.

ENVIRONMENTAL CONSIDERATIONS

1. Control environmental odors by the following measures: a. Keep the room well ventilated. b. Keep the patient clean. c. Irrigate draining wounds and change dressings frequently. d. Remove soiled linen and dressings at once. e. Place powdered charcoal in dressings to absorb foul-smelling drainage. f. Deodorize necrotic wounds with potassium permanganate solution 1:2000 or activated zinc peroxide.	Odors are frequently a problem when the patient's condition is considerably deteriorated. They may be caused by sloughing of necrotic tissue, purulent drainage, incontinence, or other factors. The effect on staff and visitors alike is often repulsion and avoidance. Every effort should be made to eliminate odor so that others will not be deterred from spending time with the patient.
g. Use commercially prepared room deodorizers, preferably of the nonspray variety, such as those with a wick.	An aerosol spray deodorant may contain a scent that is offensive to the patient. Spraying the room is also a blatant reminder to the patient that he is causing an unpleasant odor.
2. Maintain other aspects of a pleasant environment by the following measures: a. Keep the room well lighted and cheerful.	Vision usually begins to fail as death approaches. The patient will see better if the room is not dark.
b. Place personal photographs and/or other memorabilia within the patient's line of vision.	These familiar items may be very comforting to the patient.
c. When possible, place the patient in a private room or keep the bed curtains partially drawn.	The patient should be provided with enough privacy so that he is not unduly disturbed. This also enables him to have some privacy with his loved ones and enhances more meaningful communication.
however d. Avoid accentuating the patient's sense of isolation by the following measures: (1) If he is in a private room and does **not** have family or friends:	
(a) Place him in a room close to the nursing station. (b) Keep his door open. (c) Make frequent visits.	This enables him to see some activity if he is interested. The proximity also favors more frequent visits by the staff.
(2) Keep the shades of his window open (unless the patient requests otherwise or is no longer able to see).	
e. Keep the room neat and orderly. This includes any nursing equipment that is kept near the patient's bed.	An orderly room not only helps nurses provide well-organized care but also conveys to the patient's family that those who are caring for the patient have neat, orderly habits and thus are probably providing superior care.
f. Refrain from saying anything within hearing distance of the patient that would be distressing for him to hear, even if he is unresponsive to verbal stimuli.	One cannot be certain whether the patient is able to hear what is being said around him. There is the possibility that he simply cannot respond to what is being said to him and yet does hear and understand.

UNIT IV

References and bibliography

REFERENCES
Chapter 15

1. Kempe, C.H., Silver, H.K., and Donough, O.: Current pediatric diagnosis and treatment, ed. 5, Los Altos, Calif., 1978, Lange Medical Publications.
2. Schwartz, S.I., et al.: Principles of surgery, ed. 3, New York, 1979, McGraw-Hill Book Co., Inc.

Chapter 17

1. Bender, A.D.: Working with older people: a guide to practice. Section B. Clinical problems closely related to multiple organ systems—drug therapy in the aged, Public Health Service Publication no. 1459, Washington, D.C., 1971.
2. Hurwitz, N.: Predisposing factors in adverse reactions to drugs, Br. Med. J. **1:**536-539, 1969.
3. Melmon, K.L.: Preventable drug reactions, N. Engl. J. Med. **284:**1361, 1981.
4. Papper, S.: The effects of age on renal function, Geriatrics **28:**83, May 1973.

Chapter 18

1. Hawkins, G.P., and Thomlinson, J.: Herpesvirus hominis infection of the female genital tract, Obstet. Gynecol. **40:**878, 1972.

Chapter 19

1. Lapides, J.: Fundamentals of urology, Philadelphia, 1976, W.B. Saunders Co.

Chapter 20

1. Cancer facts and figures, New York, 1980, American Cancer Society.

Chapter 21

1. Billars, K.S.: You have pain? I think this will help, Am. J. Nurs. **70:**2143, 1970.
2. Castles, M.R., and Murray, R.B.: Dying in an institution: nurse/patient perspectives, New York, 1979, Appleton-Century-Crofts.

3. Epstein, C.: Nursing the dying patient—learning processes for interaction, Reston, Va., 1975, Reston Publishing Co., Inc.
4. Kübler-Ross, E.: On death and dying, New York, 1970, Macmillan Publishing Co.
5. McCaffery, M.: Relieving pain with noninvasive techniques, Nursing 80 **80:**55, 1980.
6. Melzak, R., Ofiesh, J.G., and Mount, B.M.: The Brompton mixture: effects on pain in cancer patients, CMA J. **115:**125, July 17, 1976.
7. Mount, B.M., Ajemian, I., and Scott, J.F.: Use of Brompton mixture in treating chronic pain of malignant disease, CMA J. **115:**122-124, July 17, 1976.
8. O'Connor, A.B.: Dying and grief: nursing interventions, Contemporary Nursing Series, New York, 1976, American Journal of Nursing Co.
9. Schulz, R., and Aderman, D.: Clinical research in the stages of dying, Omega **5**(2):137, 1974.
10. Shimm, D.S., et al.: Medical management of chronic cancer pain, J.A.M.A. **241:**2408, 1979.
11. Valentine, A.S., Stickel, S., and Weintraub, M.: Pain relief for cancer patients, Am. J. Nurs. **78:**2054, 1978.

BIBLIOGRAPHY

Billings, D.M., and Stokes, L.G.: Medical-surgical nursing: common health problems of adults and children across the life span, St. Louis, 1982, The C.V. Mosby Co.

Brown, E.A.: Care of the terminal patient. 2. Personal experience in the professional care of the dying, Nurs. Times, March 29, 1979, p. 545.

Earle, N.T.A., and Kutscher, A.H.: The nurse as caregiver—for the terminal patient and his family, New York, 1976, Columbia University Press.

Eckstein, H.B., Hohenfellner, R., and Williams, D.I.: Surgical pediatric urology, Philadelphia, 1977, W.B. Saunders Co.

Giaquinta, B.: Helping families face the crisis of cancer, Am. J. Nurs., Oct. 1977, p. 1585.

Jones, P.G., editor: Clinical paediatric surgery—diagnosis and management, ed. 2, London, 1976, Blackwell Scientific Publications.

McLaughlin, M.F.: Grief—who helps the living? Am. J. Nurs., March 1978, p. 422.

Mount, B.M.: Pilot Project Report (January 1975-1977, Palliative Care Service, Royal Victoria Hospital, Montreal, Quebec), presented at Symposium on Urology and Psychosocial Aspects of Chronic, Critical, and Terminal Illness, by the Foundation of Thanatology, New York, 1980.

Murphy, J.C.: Communicating with the dying patient, Am. J. Nurs., June 1979, p. 1084.

O'Connor, A.B.: Nursing of children and adolescents, New York, 1975, American Journal of Nursing Co.

Petrillo, M.P., and Sanger, S.: Emotional care of hospitalized children, ed. 2, Philadelphia, 1980, J.B. Lippincott Co.

Physician's desk reference, ed. 35, Oradell, N.J., 1981, Medical Economics Co.

Scholler, A.: Grief (letter), Am. J. Nurs., March 1978, p. 424.

Scipien, G., et al.: Comprehensive pediatric nursing, ed. 2, New York, 1979, McGraw-Hill Book Co., Inc.

Smith, D.R.: General urology, ed. 9, Los Altos, Calif., 1978, Lange Medical Publications.

Whaley, L.F., and Wong, D.L.: Nursing care of infants and children, St. Louis, 1979, The C.V. Mosby Co.

UNIT V

PROCEDURES FOR DISORDERS
OF
THE KIDNEY

CHAPTER 22

Nephrectomy

The most common indication for a nephrectomy is a renal tumor or a nonfunctioning kidney that is causing pain, infection, or hematuria (such as a kidney with a large staghorn calculus).

For the procedure the patient is placed on his side (Fig. 22-1) and a flank incision is made, or he is placed in a supine position for an abdominal approach. The renal artery, renal vein, and ureter are carefully defined, and each in turn is ligated and cut. If a **simple nephrectomy** is being performed, the kidney is shelled out of the perinephric fat. If, however, a **radical nephrectomy** is being performed, both the kidney and surrounding fat are removed. If the nephrectomy is for a tumor in the renal pelvis, the entire ureter is removed along with the kidney and perinephric fat. This procedure is called a **nephroureterectomy.**

After removal of the kidney, a Penrose drain is usually inserted into the operative site for drainage of serosanguineous fluid. The wound is then closed and a dressing is applied. An indwelling urethral catheter may be inserted to provide rapid evaluation of the remaining kidney's function.

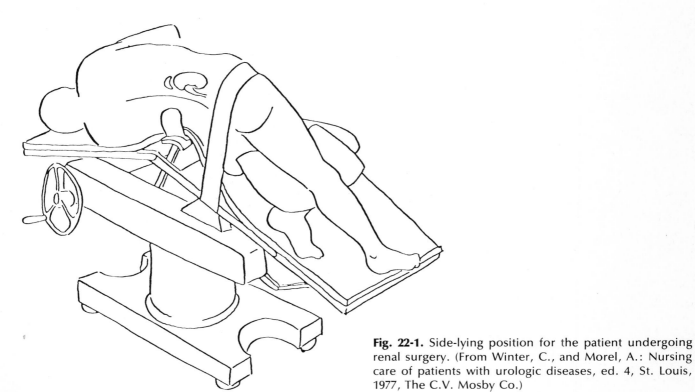

Fig. 22-1. Side-lying position for the patient undergoing renal surgery. (From Winter, C., and Morel, A.: Nursing care of patients with urologic diseases, ed. 4, St. Louis, 1977, The C.V. Mosby Co.)

NEPHRECTOMY
Outline of Care Plan
ANTICIPATED NURSING DIAGNOSES:

Preoperative period
1. Need for preoperative teaching.
2. Psychologic distress related to the diagnosis of cancer.*
3. Need for discharge planning.

Early postoperative period
4. Potential for shock.
5. Potential for respiratory complications related to surgical intervention.
6. Potential for wound complications.

---

*Only applies to the patient having a nephrectomy for a malignant tumor.

7. Need for management of indwelling urethral catheter.
8. Postoperative pain.
9. Need for management of intravenous infusion.
10. Potential for fluid and electrolyte imbalance.
11. Alterations in gastrointestinal function.
12. Potential for deep vein thrombosis.

Late postoperative period
13. Potential for gastrointestinal complications related to resumption of oral intake.
14. Potential for voiding complications following removal of indwelling urethral catheter.

Convalescent period
15. Potential for late postoperative complications (pulmonary embolism and hemorrhage).
16. Need for discharge teaching.

NURSING CARE PLAN FOR THE PATIENT UNDERGOING NEPHRECTOMY

1. NURSING DIAGNOSIS: Need for preoperative teaching

Objectives of nursing intervention

If necessary, clarification of reason for hospitalization and type of surgery to be performed

Elimination of any negative or inaccurate notions regarding the forthcoming surgery

Explanation of preoperative tests and procedures

Psychologic preparation for general anesthesia

Explanation of events expected in the early postoperative period

Explanation of body conditions expected in the early postoperative period

Identification of any known allergies

Expected outcomes

Verbal indications that explanations are understood

Verbal indications of optimistic expectations (within realistic limits) related to forthcoming surgery

Cooperation during preoperative tests and procedures

Verbal or behavioral indications of reduction of anxiety

Absence of postoperative complications

Absence of allergic reactions

Preoperative period

Plan for implementation	Rationale
See master care plan for the patient receiving preoperative teaching.	
In addition to the topics covered in the master care plan, include the following items in the preoperative teaching:	
1. Be aware that, in addition to routine preoperative tests, the following diagnostic studies may have been performed, and answer any questions the patient has regarding them.	
a. If the patient was suspected of having a tumor:	
(1) Intravenous pyelogram	This is done to provide information about any anatomic abnormalities.

172

Plan for implementation	Rationale
(2) Sonogram	This is done to differentiate between a cyst and a tumor.
(3) CT scan	This is done to provide information on the type of tumor by evaluating different tissue densities. In this way a benign tumor (e.g., angiomyolipoma) may be differentiated from a malignant one (e.g., hypernephroma).
(4) Renal angiogram	This may be done to provide information about the kidney's vascular structure and the presence of abnormal vessels.
(5) Bone and liver scans	These are done to determine the presence of metastatic disease.
b. If the patient was suspected of having a renal stone	
(1) Plain tomography of kidney	This series of films is similar to a plain film of the abdomen (KUB) because no contrast medium is required. However, these x-ray examinations focus on different planes of the kidney so the location of the stone can be more precisely determined.
(2) Intravenous pyelogram	This is done to provide information about anatomic abnormalities and the location of any radiolucent stones.
(3) Sonogram	This is done to differentiate between radiolucent stones and tumor tissue.
2. Provide reassurance that the patient's remaining kidney will be able to carry out the work of both kidneys (provided it is a normal kidney) without compromising the patient's health.	Some patients harbor the unfounded fear that they will be seriously incapacitated after a nephrectomy. This would occur only if the kidney to be removed is the patient's only functioning one, in which case the patient would require hemodialysis, and his life-style would change considerably. Otherwise the patient's general health would not be affected.
3. The preoperative shave is from the nipple line to mid-thigh on the affected side.	
4. Oral intake will probably be withheld for 24 to 48 hours after surgery or until bowel sounds are heard and the patient passes flatus.	There is usually a period of intestinal atony following nephrectomy due to irritation of the peritoneum. It generally resolves itself within 1 or 2 days, but premature oral intake would cause severe abdominal discomfort, distention, and vomiting.
5. The patient will have an incision either in his flank or abdomen (depending on the approach used). It will be covered with a dressing, which will require frequent changing for the first few postoperative days.	
6. There may be an indwelling urethral catheter in place for 24 to 72 hours.	This is to provide precise measurement of urinary output from the remaining kidney.

Preoperative period

2. NURSING DIAGNOSIS: Psychologic distress related to the diagnosis of cancer*

Objectives of nursing intervention
Provision of an emotionally supportive environment
Achievement of effective communication between patient, family, and staff

Expected outcomes
Verbalization by the patient of feelings about the diagnosis
Realistic decision-making
Absence of severe or protracted depression

Plan for implementation	Rationale
See Chapter 20, nursing diagnosis 1.	

*Only applies to the patient undergoing nephrectomy for a malignant tumor.

3. NURSING DIAGNOSIS: Need for discharge planning

Objectives of nursing intervention
Early commencement of discharge planning
Accurate estimate of time required for all discharge teaching

Expected outcome
Smooth transition of care after discharge

Plan for implementation	Rationale

See master care plan for the patient requiring discharge preparations: discharge planning.
 	
In addition to the topics covered in the master care plan, the following items should be considered:
1. The duration of hospitalization for this procedure is approximately 7 to 10 days.
 	
2. Required teaching includes:
  a. General postoperative discharge teaching
  b. Possible diet restrictions
  c. Possible fluid restrictions
  d. The need for periodic check-ups	

Preoperative period

4. NURSING DIAGNOSIS: Potential for shock

Objective of nursing intervention   Prevention or early detection of shock

Expected outcomes { Vital signs normal, skin dry, color normal
Absence of bright red drainage

Plan for implementation	Rationale

1. Check the patient's vital signs every 2 to 4 hours once stable (every 15 minutes if unstable).
 	
2. Be alert for any indications of shock. These include:
  a. Increasing pulse and respiratory rates
  b. Decreasing blood pressure
  c. Diaphoresis, pallor, and cold clammy skin
  d. Feelings of apprehension
	Hemorrhagic shock is a potential complication in the early postoperative period following nephrectomy. If the sutures in the renal arteries should slip, a considerable amount of blood might be lost very rapidly. Internal as well as external hemorrhage may occur. Therefore careful observation of the patient is essential.

3. Check the dressing for excessive bleeding at least every 4 hours. Be certain to check under the patient's back if he has a flank incision.	Drainage will flow with gravity. If the patient has a flank incision, the side of the dressing may remain dry while the inferior portion becomes saturated.
4. Notify the physician at once if there are any signs or symptoms of impending shock.	

5. NURSING DIAGNOSIS: Potential for respiratory complications related to surgical intervention

Objectives of nursing intervention { Early detection of pneumothorax
Prevention or early detection of atelectasis and/or pneumonia

Expected outcomes { Cooperation with therapeutic respiratory regimen
Absence of dyspnea and other symptoms of pneumothorax
Absence of fever or audible lung congestion
Sputum clear or white and easily mobilized

Plan for implementation	Rationale
See master care plan for the patient at risk for respiratory complications, nursing objectives 4 and 5.	

Early postoperative period

6. NURSING DIAGNOSIS: Potential for wound complications

| Objective of nursing intervention | Prevention or early detection of complications arising from the incisional area |

Objective of nursing intervention Prevention or early detection of complications arising from the incisional area

Expected outcome Absence of fever, purulent exudate, erythema, edema, dehiscence, hematoma, and other abnormal wound conditions

Plan for implementation	Rationale
1. Check the dressing every 4 hours during the first 24 to 48 hours and then every shift. Change it when it becomes wet and use sterile technique for the procedure.	These dressings usually require changing at least once a shift in the early postoperative period. The drainage is serosanguineous fluid.
2. Use caution when removing soiled dressings to prevent the inadvertent removal of the incisional drain(s). (A Penrose drain, tube drain, or Hemovac will be used. See pp. 492 and 634 for nursing management of tube drains and Hemovacs.)	Premature removal of a drain may result in prolonged healing.
3. Cut and arrange gauze pads around the incisional drain(s).	This prevents the dressings from flattening the drain(s) and possibly obstructing the flow of drainage from the wound.
4. If the dressing requires frequent changing, use Montgomery straps instead of adhesive tape.	This eliminates the need to remove the adhesive tape from the patient's skin each time the dressing is changed. Skin irritation and patient discomfort can be considerably reduced by this method.
5. Note the condition of the suture line. Chart its appearance and the presence of edema, erythema, ecchymosis, hematoma, or other abnormal conditions.	This provides a frame of reference for other staff members caring for the patient.
6. Notify the physician if there is any evidence of dehiscence.	
7. If there is purulent drainage: a. Notify the physician. b. Obtain a wound culture specimen.	This indicates a wound infection. This will facilitate identification of the infecting organism so that appropriate treatment can be instituted quickly.
8. Check the patient's temperature every 4 hours, and notify the physician if there is an elevation above 101°.	Wound infection must always be suspected when the patient runs a fever postoperatively. Other causes include respiratory complications and pharmacologic intervention.

Early postoperative period

7. NURSING DIAGNOSIS: Need for management of indwelling urethral catheter

Objectives of nursing intervention

Appropriate care of catheter and equipment
Prevention or early detection of infection
Care of tissue surrounding catheter
Maintenance of accurate records of urine output
Appropriate administration of hand-irrigation of catheter
Management of discomfort or pain caused by the catheter
Satisfactory collection of urine specimens from catheter

Expected outcomes

Absence of severe bladder spasms and suprapubic distention
Urine draining freely through system
Absence of fever, chills, and foul-smelling urine
Absence of urethral discharge and tissue inflammation
Minimal discomfort caused by the catheter
Urine specimens in optimum condition for all necessary tests

Plan for implementation	Rationale
See master care plan for the patient with an indwelling urethral catheter: care after insertion of the catheter.	
In addition to the topics covered in the master care plan, the following interventions are required: 1. Notify the physician if the urine turns bright red.	After a simple nephrectomy the urine is usually clear amber. It may be blood tinged if additional surgery was done (e.g., nephroureterectomy).
2. Notify the physician if there is a major increase or decrease in the volume of urine that cannot be accounted for by changes in the patient's fluid intake or lack of patency of the drainage equipment.	This may be an indication that the patient's remaining kidney is not functioning properly. An unusually high or low volume may be an early warning of acute tubular necrosis.

Early postoperative period

8. NURSING DIAGNOSIS: Postoperative pain

Objective of nursing intervention   Appropriate management of pain or discomfort

Expected outcome   Behavioral and/or verbal indications that pain is adequately reduced or absent

Plan for implementation	Rationale
Determine the source of the pain. It may be related to the catheter, the surgical wound, the gastrointestinal tract, or the musculoskeletal system.	Pain from different sources usually requires different intervention.
1. Question and observe the patient to obtain information about the pain.	
2. Be aware that pain is a unique and individual experience. Although the different sources of pain can usually be determined by their characteristics, there are also many variations.	
3. Be alert for indications (verbal or behavioral) that the patient is experiencing discomfort other than physical pain, and attempt to resolve the problem.	Fear, loneliness, depression, and numerous other conditions may be sources of extreme discomfort for the patient who may unconsciously translate these feelings into "pain."

PERSISTENT, SEVERE, INCREASING PAIN IN SUPRAPUBIC AREA

See Chapter 11, part one, nursing objective 6.	This pain is probably caused by an obstructed catheter.

SPASMODIC, INTERMITTENT PAIN IN SUPRAPUBIC AREA, OR PAIN RADIATING TO URETHRAL AREA

See Chapter 11, part one, nursing objective 6.	This pain is probably caused by the catheter's irritating effect on the bladder.

MODERATE TO SEVERE PAIN AT SURGICAL SITE, USUALLY AGGRAVATED BY PHYSICAL ACTIVITY

1. Be certain the catheter is not obstructed. Although pain with these characteristics is usually of incisional origin, which is expected, the patient may not be able to identify accurately the precise location of the pain.	Catheter obstruction must be ruled out first because it cannot remain untreated. However, after this type of surgery it is unlikely for the catheter to become obstructed because there is rarely enough blood in the drainage for clots to form, and there are no tissue particles normally passed in the urine.
2. Administer analgesics as ordered.	Analgesic medication usually provides considerable relief from incisional pain.

Early postoperative period

178

Plan for implementation	**Rationale**
3. Plan the patient's activities to coincide with a time when there is a high level of pain medication in the patient's bloodstream.	The patient will cooperate better with coughing exercises, ambulating, bathing, etc. when the pain is well under control.
4. Notify the physician if the patient's requests for pain medication do not decrease within 48 to 72 hours.	Although the intensity of postoperative pain varies enormously between patients, there should be a marked decrease in the apparent severity of the pain within 2 or 3 days. If this does not occur, it may indicate the development of wound complications.

COLICKY, INTERMITTENT VISCERAL PAIN, USUALLY ACCOMPANIED BY ABDOMINAL DISTENTION

1. Check the patient's abdomen for the presence and extent of distention.	Because some areas of the intestines regain function before others, abdominal distention and gas pains often occur. General activity may help to relieve the discomfort.
2. Encourage ambulation as soon as possible.	
3. Administer neostigmine methylsulfate (Prostigmin) as ordered.	Neostigmine is a cholinergic drug that occasionally relieves postoperative distention.
4. Suggest that a rectal tube be ordered for insertion 2 to 4 times per day for approximately 30 minutes.	This may provide some relief from flatus.
5. Check laboratory values for the patient's serum potassium level, and if it is lower than normal: a. Notify the physician. b. Monitor the patient's pulse and cardiac status.	Hypokalemia may contribute to distention and decreased intestinal motility. However, there are more important reasons for correction of deficient serum potassium as soon as possible (e.g., cardiac arrhythmias).

MUSCULAR DISCOMFORT IN NECK, SHOULDERS, EXTREMITIES, ETC.

1. Provide the patient with an explanation for the pain and reassurance that it is transient.	Because of the positioning during nephrectomy (Fig. 22-1) the patient may feel stiffness or soreness in various parts of his body. For the first few days after surgery the administration of narcotic analgesics and the presence of severe incisional pain may mask this discomfort. Generally, reassurance that it does not indicate complications is sufficient to take the patient's mind off it.
2. Apply warm compresses to affected area.	
3. Provide back rubs as needed.	

Early postoperative period

9. NURSING DIAGNOSIS: Need for management of intravenous infusion

Objectives of nursing intervention

Appropriate administration of specific types of intravenous solutions

Prevention or early detection of local complications

Prevention or early detection of systemic complications

Management of discomfort caused by the intravenous infusion

Maintenance of proper function of intravenous equipment

Maintenance of accurate records of the patient's hydration status

Expected outcomes

Normal hydration status

Normal electrolyte status

Absence of thrombophlebitis, infiltration, infection, fluid overload, and pulmonary embolism

Absence of discomfort caused by the intravenous infusion

Plan for implementation	Rationale
See master care plan for the patient receiving intravenous therapy.	
In addition to the items covered in the master care plan, the following interventions are required:	
1. Monitor **carefully** the prescribed rate, volume, and type of intravenous fluids. Fluid and electrolyte replacement will depend on the function of the remaining kidney.	Mistakes in carrying out intravenous orders may have particularly hazardous consequences for the patient with only one kidney.
2. If, for any reason, the intravenous fluids have not been infusing as ordered, notify the physician.	The physician may choose to compensate for deficits or overloads by temporarily changing the intravenous orders. Even minor changes in rate should not be made without the physician's knowledge.

Early postoperative period

10. NURSING DIAGNOSIS: Potential for fluid and electrolyte imbalance

Objective of nursing intervention	Prevention or early detection of fluid and electrolyte imbalance
Expected outcomes	Absence of signs and symptoms of fluid and electrolyte imbalance Normal laboratory values for serum electrolytes

Plan for implementation	Rationale
1. Notify the physician if there are any indications of electrolyte imbalances. **In general** these include: a. Changes in level of consciousness (from somnolence to agitation) b. Changes in respiratory rate and depth c. Cardiac irregularities d. Abnormalities in muscle tone (from flaccidity to convulsions)	After nephrectomy, careful monitoring of the patient's kidney function is essential. Any evidence of abnormalities requires the physician's immediate attention to prevent or treat deterioration in the patient's remaining kidney.
2. Notify the physician if there are any indications of fluid overload. These include: a. Pulmonary congestion (dyspnea, rales) b. Elevation of central venous pressure, which may be manifested by prominent jugular veins when the patient is in a semi-Fowler or upright position	
3. Check laboratory values for abnormalities in blood chemistry, and notify the physician if any are present.	
4. If ordered: a. Check the patient's weight daily (at the same time, on the same scale, and with the same amount of clothing) and report increases of more than 1 pound per day. b. Weigh dressings and record weight of saturated dressings (minus the weight of dry dressings) as output.	These are extra precautions, which are only ordered in special cases.
5. In general, keep strict records of the patient's fluid input and output for the first week after surgery.	This facilitates rapid assessment of the patient's hydration status.

Early postoperative period

11. NURSING DIAGNOSIS: Alterations in gastrointestinal function

Objectives of nursing intervention { Prohibition of oral intake as ordered
Promotion of patient comfort

Expected outcome   Return of bowel sounds and passage of flatus within 24 to 48 hours

Plan for implementation	Rationale
1. Inform the patient that he is to have no oral intake. Notify the auxiliary staff as well so that nobody inadvertently gives the patient something to eat or drink.	There is often a period of intestinal atony following this type of surgery. Within 48 hours it usually resolves itself, but premature oral intake will cause severe abdominal discomfort, distention, and vomiting. Although most patients will not feel like eating at this time, the nurse cannot rely on this alone as a deterrent to oral intake. If water is left at the patient's bedside, he may drink it.
2. Provide mouth care as needed.	Lack of salivary stimulation often causes dryness and an unpleasant taste in the patient's mouth.
3. Check periodically for bowel sounds and passage of flatus, and notify the physician when they occur.	These are indications that the intestines are regaining their function.

12. NURSING DIAGNOSIS: Potential for deep vein thrombosis

Objectives of nursing intervention { Explanation and maintenance of precautions against deep vein thrombosis
Early detection of deep vein thrombosis

Expected outcomes { Cooperation with regimen to prevent deep vein thrombosis
Absence of local pain, swelling, and redness of a lower extremity
Absence of fever

Plan for implementation	Rationale
See master care plan for the patient at risk for deep vein thrombosis.	These patients are at considerable risk for deep vein thrombosis because the operative site is near the vena cava and other large veins.

Early postoperative period

182

13. NURSING DIAGNOSIS: Potential for gastrointestinal complications related to resumption of oral intake

Objective of nursing intervention
Early detection of gastrointestinal complications

Expected outcomes
{ Absence of abdominal distention, tympany, nausea, or vomiting
Return to normal bowel function

Plan for implementation	Rationale
1. Permit oral intake of fluids and food only on the physicians's orders.	The physician will usually wait until bowel sounds are heard and the patient passes flatus before permitting him to have anything by mouth.
2. Note the presence of distention, tympany, nausea, or vomiting. Otherwise, if ordered, advance the diet as tolerated.	
3. Inform the physician if the patient has not had a bowel movement for more than 2 days after resumption of oral intake.	A cathartic is usually indicated at this stage in the patient's recuperation if he has not moved his bowels spontaneously.

14. NURSING DIAGNOSIS: Potential for voiding complications following removal of indwelling urethral catheter

Objective of nursing intervention
Prevention or early detection of complications

Expected outcomes
{ Resumption of normal voiding pattern
Absence of dysuria

Plan for implementation	Rationale
See master care plan for the patient with an indwelling urethral catheter: care after removal of the catheter.	

Late postoperative period

15. NURSING DIAGNOSIS: Potential for late postoperative complications (pulmonary embolism and hemorrhage)

Objective of nursing intervention   Early detection and treatment of pulmonary embolism or hemorrhage

Expected outcome   Normal respirations, blood pressure, and pulse

Plan for implementation	Rationale

PULMONARY EMBOLISM

1. Be alert for symptoms of pulmonary embolism:
   a. Dyspnea
   b. Tachypnea
   c. Pleuritic chest pain or pain radiating to the shoulder
   d. Hemoptysis

Although pulmonary embolism is a potential complication after any kind of major surgery, the patient undergoing most types of renal surgery is at greater risk because the operative site is close to the vena cava and other large vessels. It might occur at any time in the postoperative period, but its incidence is highest 5 to 10 days after surgery. Depending on its size and location, a pulmonary embolism can be lethal or essentially asymptomatic. When symptoms do occur, they may indicate a serious ventilation-perfusion imbalance, and prompt recognition and treatment are imperative.

2. If any of these symptoms occur, notify the physician at once, and institute the following measures:
   a. Keep the patient in bed with the head elevated more than 30 degrees.
   b. Start oxygen.
   c. Start an intravenous line.
   d. Keep the patient calm.

LATE POSTOPERATIVE HEMORRHAGE

Check the patient's vital signs every shift, and observe the patient for signs of impending hypovolemic shock due to internal bleeding.

The risk of hemorrhage increases between the eighth and twelfth day after surgery because this is the period during which tissue sloughing occurs. Although the patient is often going home toward the end of this time, the nurse should still be aware that late postoperative hemorrhage is a potential, but rare, complication after certain types of renal surgery, and appropriate observations must be continued throughout this period.

Convalescent period

16. NURSING DIAGNOSIS: Need for discharge teaching

Objectives of nursing intervention

Explanation of basic information about medications to be taken at home
Explanation of information regarding follow-up care
Explanation of residual effects of the condition and/or treatment
Explanation of instructions concerning postdischarge activities
Explanation of symptoms that constitute a reason to contact the physician
Review of admitting diagnosis and mode of treatment

Expected outcomes

Accurate return verbalization and/or demonstration of all material learned
Smooth transition of care after discharge
Absence or early detection of complications arising after discharge
Ability to provide future health care practitioners with important data about health history

Plan for implementation	Rationale
See master care plan for the patient requiring discharge preparations: discharge teaching.	
In addition to the topics covered in the master care plan, include the following items in the discharge teaching:	
1. At the follow-up office visit, the physician will check the incision for adequate healing and obtain a urine specimen for culture.	Urine cultures are particularly important for patients who are stone formers. Urinary tract infection must be completely eradicated if the patient is to remain free from urinary calculi in the future.
2. If the patient had a malignant tumor, he will be expected to return for periodic check-ups, which may include intravenous pyelograms, chest x-ray examinations, and bone scans.	The purpose of these follow-up visits is to check for any metastatic spread of the disease as well as to assess the function of the remaining kidney.
3. If the patient had a renal calculus, he will also require periodic check-ups, which may include intravenous pyelograms, plain films of the abdomen, urine analyses, urine cultures, and evaluation of serum electrolytes.	A patient who has developed one urinary calculus is likely to develop another. Since he now has only one kidney, close observation of his urinary tract will be required so that any new stones can be detected early, before renal damage occurs.
4. During the next few weeks, expected residual effects of the surgery include fatigue and incisional discomfort.	

Convalescent period

Plan for implementation	Rationale
5. The patient should follow the guidelines prescribed by his physician regarding fluid intake and diet restrictions.	The nurse will have to ask the physician what type of regimen the patient requires; it is highly individual. A patient who is a stone former might be required to drink at least 2.5 L of fluid per day. However, if the remaining kidney has limited function, fluid restrictions may be ordered. A low-sodium diet might be ordered if the patient has limited function in the remaining kidney, if he has hypertension, or if there is impaired cardiac function. If he is a stone former, he may also have diet restrictions according to the stone composition.
6. The patient should notify his physician if any of the following occur:	
a. Chills, fever, hematuria, flank pain	These may indicate a urinary tract infection.
b. Sudden decrease in urinary output despite adequate intake	This may indicate renal failure or the presence of an obstruction. In either case, prompt intervention by the physician is essential to prevent further renal damage.
c. If the patient had a malignant tumor, weight loss or bone pain	These symptoms may indicate metastatic spread of the tumor.

Convalescent period

CHAPTER 23

Nephrolithotomy

A nephrolithotomy is performed to remove a staghorn calculus. The procedure is relatively complicated because, if any of the major blood vessels within the kidney are damaged, renal function will be impaired. The following surgical description is of a particular version of nephrolithotomy employed to reduce the incidence of bleeding and renal atrophy; hence the name **anatrophic nephrolithotomy.**

For the procedure that patient is either positioned on his side (see Fig. 22-1) and a flank incision is made, or he is placed in a supine position for an abdominal approach. After the incision is made, the area around the kidney is packed with ice and remains this way throughout the procedure to reduce the metabolic rate of the kidney cells. Methylene blue is used to delineate the renal segments, and for this reason the urine may have a bluish color postoperatively.*

The incision into the kidney is then performed, and all parts of the stone are carefully extracted (Fig. 23-1). Sometimes a ureteral catheter is inserted to prevent fragments of stones from being dislodged

---

*Methylene blue is used only in an anatrophic nephrolithotomy. Therefore, unless this type of nephrolithotomy is performed, mention of it in the nursing care plan should be omitted.

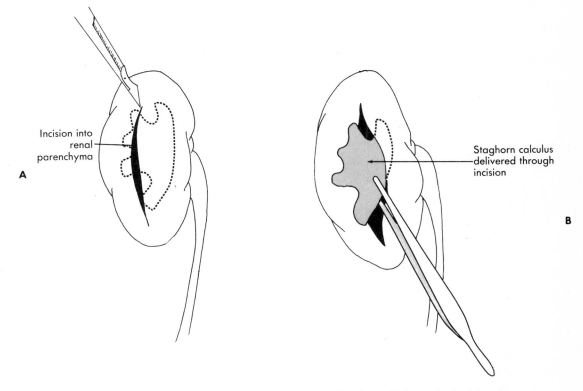

Incision into renal parenchyma

A

Staghorn calculus delivered through incision

B

Fig. 23-1. A and **B,** Extraction of staghorn calculus from kidney via incision into renal parenchyma.   *Continued.*

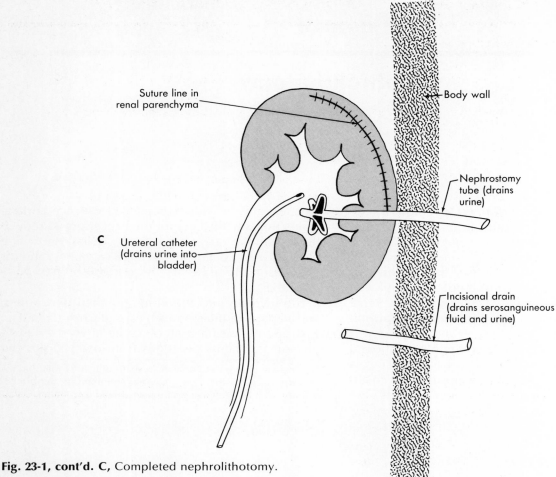

Suture line in renal parenchyma

Body wall

Nephrostomy tube (drains urine)

C Ureteral catheter (drains urine into bladder)

Incisional drain (drains serosanguineous fluid and urine)

Fig. 23-1, cont'd. C, Completed nephrolithotomy.

into the ureter. The removal of all stone particles is then confirmed by x-ray examination.

The ureteral catheter may be left in place to facilitate drainage of urine from the affected kidney. An incisional drain is inserted near the kidney and brought out through the skin. Sometimes a nephrostomy tube is also inserted. The wound is then closed and a dressing is applied. An indwelling urethral catheter may be inserted to provide accurate monitoring of urinary output.

NEPHROLITHOTOMY
Outline of Care Plan
ANTICIPATED NURSING DIAGNOSES:
Preoperative period
1. Need for preoperative teaching.
2. Need for discharge planning.
Early postoperative period
3. Potential for shock.
4. Potential for respiratory complications related to surgical intervention.

5. Potential for wound complications.
6. Need for management of nephrostomy tube.*
7. Need for management of indwelling urethral catheter.*
8. Need for management of ureteral catheter.*
9. Postoperative pain.
10. Need for management of intravenous infusion.
11. Alterations in gastrointestinal function.
12. Potential for deep vein thrombosis.
Late postoperative period
13. Potential for gastrointestinal complications related to resumption of oral intake.
14. Potential for voiding complications following removal of indwelling urethral catheter.*
15. Potential for complications related to termination of nephrostomy drainage system.*
Convalescent period
16. Potential for late postoperative complications (pulmonary embolism and hemorrhage).
17. Need for discharge teaching.

_____

*May not apply.

NURSING CARE PLAN FOR THE PATIENT UNDERGOING NEPHROLITHOTOMY

1. NURSING DIAGNOSIS: Need for preoperative teaching

Objectives of nursing intervention

If necessary, clarification of reason for hospitalization and type of surgery to be performed

Elimination of any negative or inaccurate notions regarding the forthcoming surgery

Explanation of preoperative tests and procedures

Psychologic preparation for general anesthesia

Explanation of events expected in the early postoperative period

Explanation of body conditions expected in the early postoperative period

Identification of any known allergies

Expected outcomes

Verbal indications that explanations are understood

Verbal indications of optimistic expectations (within realistic limits) related to forthcoming surgery

Cooperation during preoperative tests and procedures

Verbal or behavioral indications of reduction of anxiety

Absence of postoperative complications

Absence of allergic reactions

Plan for implementation	Rationale
See master care plan for the patient receiving preoperative teaching.	
In addition to the topics covered in the master care plan, include the following items in the preoperative teaching:	
1. Be aware that in addition to the routine preoperative tests, the following diagnostic studies may have been performed prior to this surgery, and answer any questions the patient has regarding them:	
a. Plain tomography of the kidney	This series of films is similar to a plain film of the abdomen (KUB) because no contrast medium is required. However, these x-ray films focus on different planes of the kidney so that the location of the stone can be more precisely determined.
b. Intravenous pyelogram	This is done to provide information about anatomic abnormalities and the location of any radiolucent stone(s).
c. Sonogram	This is done to differentiate a radiolucent stone from a tumor.
d. Renal angiogram	This is done to provide information about the vascular structure of the affected kidney.
2. The preoperative shave will be from the nipple line to midthigh on the affected side.	
3. Oral intake will probably be withheld for 24 to 48 hours after surgery or until bowel sounds are heard and the patient passes flatus.	There is usually a period of intestinal atony following nephrolithotomy due to irritation of the peritoneum. It generally resolves itself within 1 or 2 days, but premature oral intake would cause severe abdominal discomfort, distention, and vomiting.

Preoperative period

Plan for implementation	Rationale
4. The patient will have an incision in his flank or abdomen, depending on the approach used. It will be covered with a dressing, which will require frequent changing for the first few postoperative days.	
5. There may be a tube coming from the patient's kidney. It will drain urine into a bedside collecting container and will remain in place for approximately 10 days.	The purpose of the nephrostomy tube is to prevent extravasation of urine from the suture line in the kidney by providing an unobstructed pathway. It is not always used, and the nurse should be aware of the particular surgeon's preference prior to the preoperative teaching session.
6. The patient may have an indwelling urethral catheter in place to drain urine from his bladder for 1 or 2 days. There may also be a ureteral catheter connected to separate drainage equipment for approximately 4 days.	The catheter in the bladder ensures adequate emptying of the bladder and decreases the risk of back-pressure in the affected ureter and kidney. The ureteral catheter facilitates drainage of urine from the affected kidney. The use of these catheters is also at the surgeon's discretion.
7. The patient should not be alarmed if the urine draining through any of the tubes is blood tinged. It may also have a bluish color in the immediate postoperative period because of the use of methylene blue dye during the surgery (if anatrophic nephrolithotomy is performed).	

Preoperative period

2. NURSING DIAGNOSIS: Need for discharge planning

Objectives of nursing intervention   { Early commencement of discharge planning
Accurate estimate of time required for all discharge teaching

Expected outcome   Smooth transition of care after discharge

Plan for implementation	Rationale
See master care plan for the patient requiring discharge preparations: discharge planning.	

In addition to the topics covered in the master care plan, the following items should be considered:
1. The duration of hospitalization for this procedure is approximately 10 to 14 days.

2. Required teaching includes:
   a. General postoperative discharge teaching
   b. Possibly instructions on stone prevention regimen

3. NURSING DIAGNOSIS: Potential for shock

Objective of nursing intervention Prevention or early detection of shock

Expected outcomes
{ Vital signs normal, skin dry, color normal
{ Absence of bright red drainage

Plan for implementation	Rationale
1. Check the patient's vital signs every 2 to 4 hours once stable (every 15 minutes if unstable).	Hemorrhagic shock is a potential complication in the early postoperative period following nephrolithotomy because the kidney is highly vascular, and numerous blood vessels must be cut.

2. Be alert for any indications of shock. These include:
  a. Increasing pulse and respiratory rates
  b. Decreasing blood pressure
  c. Diaphoresis, pallor, and cold clammy skin
  d. Feelings of apprehension	

3. Check the dressing (and nephrostomy tube, if present) for excessive bleeding at least every 4 hours. Be certain to check under the patient's back if he has a flank incision.	Drainage will flow with gravity. If the patient has a flank incision, the side of the dressing may remain dry while the inferior portion becomes saturated.
4. Notify the physician at once if there are any signs or symptoms of impending shock.	

4. NURSING DIAGNOSIS: Potential for respiratory complications related to surgical intervention

Objectives of nursing intervention
{ Early detection of pneumothorax
{ Prevention or early detection of atelectasis and/or pneumonia

Expected outcomes
{ Cooperation with therapeutic respiratory regimen
{ Absence of dyspnea and other symptoms of pneumothorax
{ Absence of fever or audible lung congestion
{ Sputum clear or white and easily mobilized

Plan for implementation	Rationale
See master care plan for the patient at risk for respiratory complications, nursing objectives 4 and 5.	

Early postoperative period

5. NURSING DIAGNOSIS: Potential for wound complications

<table>
<tr><td>**Objective of nursing intervention**</td><td>Prevention or early detection of complications arising from the incisional area</td></tr>
<tr><td>**Expected outcome**</td><td>Absence of fever, purulent exudate, erythema, edema, dehiscence, hematoma, and other abnormal wound conditions</td></tr>
</table>

Plan for implementation	Rationale

1. Check the dressing frequently (every 2 to 4 hours during the first 24 to 48 hours after surgery). Change it when it becomes wet and use sterile technique for the procedure.	The dressing may become saturated rapidly with serosanguineous fluid and urine from the incision. This is because the suture line in the kidney may not become watertight for at least 48 hours after surgery. A wet dressing must be changed as soon as possible for the following reasons:
	1. It is a source of infection
	   a. It acts as a wick, enabling microorganisms on the skin to move toward the incision.
	   b. It provides a good medium for bacterial multiplication.
	2. It is highly irritating to the skin because of the presence of urine in the drainage.

2. Note the odor of the drainage. The characteristic odor of urine is not abnormal, but if it is foul smelling: a. Notify the physician. b. Obtain a wound culture specimen.	This would indicate a wound infection. This will facilitate identification of the infecting organism so that appropriate treatment can be instituted quickly.
3. Use caution when removing soiled dressings to prevent inadvertent removal of the incisional drain (and nephrostomy tube, if present).	Premature removal of a drain may result in the development of a urinoma and prolonged healing.
4. Cut and arrange gauze pads around the nephrostomy tube (if present) and incisional drain. Usually a Penrose drain is used.	This prevents the dressings from flattening the drainage mechanisms and possibly obstructing the flow of drainage from the wound and through the nephrostomy tube.
5. If the dressing requires frequent changing, use Montgomery straps instead of adhesive tape.	This eliminates the need to remove the adhesive tape from the patient's skin each time the dressing is changed. Skin irritation and patient discomfort can be considerably reduced by this method.
6. Note the condition of the suture line. Chart its appearance and the presence of edema, erythema, hematoma, ecchymosis, or other abnormal conditions.	This provides a frame of reference for other staff members caring for the patient.
7. Notify the physician if there is any evidence of dehiscence.	

Early postoperative period

Plan for implementation	Rationale
8. Check the patient's temperature every 4 hours and notify the physician if there is an elevation above 101°.	Wound infection must always be suspected when the patient runs a fever postoperatively. Other causes include respiratory complications and pharmacologic intervention.

6. NURSING DIAGNOSIS: Need for management of nephrostomy tube*

Objective of nursing intervention Prevention or early detection of complications related to the nephrostomy tube

Expected outcome Urine draining freely through system
Absence of fever, chills, or foul-smelling drainage

Plan for implementation	Rationale

1. Maintain satisfactory function of nephrostomy drainage system.
    a. Tape tubing **securely** to the patient's flank to prevent inadvertent displacement of the nephrostomy tube.
    b. If the patient is confused, obtain an order for hand restraints. They should be used if there is **any** indication that the patient might pull at the tube.
    c. If the tube becomes dislodged, notify the physician **at once.**
 	
    d. Keep the collecting container below kidney level and the tubing free from kinks.
	The nephrostomy tube is usually a retention catheter placed directly into the kidney through the flank incision. The catheter's distal end is attached to bedside drainage. It is frequently held in place with only one or two sutures, and, if accidentally removed, it may be very difficult to replace.
	The tube must be replaced promptly. If it is not reinserted within 1 to 2 hours, it may be impossible to replace. However, this is not a nursing function. It requires precise anatomic knowledge of the internal suture lines and the structure of the affected kidney.
	If urine is not permitted to flow freely through the system, structural damage to the kidney can occur.

2. Reduce the risk of infection associated with the tube:
    a. Use sterile technique when changing the dressing around the tube.
    b. Remove exudate from around the tube with hydrogen peroxide when changing the dressing.
    c. Maintain a fluid intake of 2 or 3 L per day unless contraindicated by a coexisting medical condition.
    d. Do not disconnect the tubing unless absolutely necessary.
    e. If tubing must be disconnected, avoid contamination of any openings in the system.
	Because this tube goes directly into the renal collecting system, it poses a considerable risk of pyelonephritis unless strict precautions are maintained.
	Exudate causes irritation of the tissue surrounding the tube and is a good medium for bacterial growth.
	A brisk flow of urine through the urinary tract discourages bacterial growth.
	Once the system is open to the air, it is potentially contaminated.

Early postoperative period

*May not apply; a nephrostomy tube is used at the surgeon's discretion.

Plan for implementation	Rationale
3. Keep accurate records of the character and volume of the drainage. The color of the drainage is normally pink to amber within 48 hours. It may be bluish for the first few hours following anatrophic nephrolithotomy.	
4. Notify the physician if any of the following conditions occur:	
a. Bright red drainage	This indicates abnormal bleeding.
b. Scanty drainage	This may indicate that the tubing is displaced or obstructed, or that kidney function is impaired.
c. Excessive drainage from **around** the tubing (rather than through it)	This may indicate that the tubing is obstructed or displaced.
5. If the patient has an indwelling urethral catheter as well, label both collecting containers accordingly.	This is a precaution against mistakes in recording sources of output when urine is draining through more than one external system.
6. Observe the following precautions regarding hand-irrigation of the nephrostomy tube:	
a. Do not irrigate unless specifically ordered to do so by the physician.	The benefits of irrigation must be weighed against the risk of introducing pathogens into the kidney. This is not a nursing judgment.
b. Maintain strict sterile technique when irrigating.	
c. Do not instill more than 5 ml of irrigant at one time unless specifically ordered to do so.	The normal renal pelvis can hold only 2 to 5 ml of fluid. Overdistention of the pelvis can cause renal damage.
7. If ordered, maintain Renacidin irrigation through the nephrostomy tube. This is usually a continuous drip.	Renacidin is occasionally used postoperatively to dissolve any retained particles of calculi.

Early postoperative period

7. NURSING DIAGNOSIS: Need for management of indwelling urethral catheter*

Objectives of nursing intervention

Appropriate care of catheter and equipment

Prevention or early detection of infection

Care of tissue surrounding catheter

Maintenance of accurate records of urine output

Appropriate administration of hand-irrigation of catheter

Management of discomfort or pain caused by the catheter

Satisfactory collection of urine specimens from the catheter

Expected outcomes

Absence of severe bladder spasms and suprapubic distention

Urine draining freely through system

Absence of fever, chills, and foul-smelling urine

Absence of urethral discharge and tissue inflammation

Minimal discomfort caused by the catheter

Urine specimens in optimum condition for all necessary tests

Plan for implementation	Rationale
See master care plan for the patient with an indwelling urethral catheter: care after insertion of the catheter. In addition to the topics covered in the master care plan, the following intervention is required: Notify the physician if the urine turns bright red.	The urine is normally pink to amber within 48 hours after surgery and bluish immediately after surgery from methylene blue dye (if anatrophic nephrolithotomy was performed). Abnormal bleeding must be investigated at once. The kidneys are highly vascular, and a considerable amount of blood may be lost in a short time.

Early postoperative period

*May not apply; an indwelling urethral catheter is used at the surgeon's discretion.

8. NURSING DIAGNOSIS: Need for management of ureteral catheter*

Objective of nursing intervention	Prevention or early detection of complications caused by the ureteral catheter

Expected outcomes	Urine draining freely through system
	Absence of fever, chills, or foul-smelling urine

Early postoperative period

Plan for implementation	Rationale
1. Irrigate the catheter only if specifically ordered and only after the technique has been previously mastered.	Unless done with extreme care and skill, irrigation of a ureteral catheter could cause serious damage to the ureter and kidney.
2. Keep the catheter securely taped to the patient's thigh.	This helps to prevent inadvertent traction on the catheter. Often it is tied to the urethral catheter at the point where they both emerge from the urethra. Both drainage tubes can then be taped together on the patient's thigh.
3. Maintain accurate records of output. This may vary considerably from patient to patient, depending on the diameter of the ureter in relation to the catheter and the presence of a nephrostomy tube.	The drainage from the ureteral catheter is the urine produced by the affected kidney minus the drainage from the nephrostomy tube (if present) and the drainage flowing through the ureter **around** the catheter.
4. If scanty or nonexistent output is noted: a. Milk the catheter and tubing. b. If no results, notify the physician.	The catheter may be obstructed. However, this is not as critical a situation as obstruction of a urethral catheter since urine can usually drain around the ureteral catheter (and through the nephrostomy tube, if one is used).
5. Disconnect the tubing only if absolutely necessary. Maintain sterile technique and prevent contamination of open ends of tubing.	Any break in the closed system may result in contamination of the urinary tract.
6. If the physician has ordered that the patient remain in bed while the catheter is in place: a. Explain to the patient that he must remain in bed to prevent accidental displacement of the catheter. b. The patient may not sit in a completely upright position. c. The patient may sit in a semiupright position and turn from side to side while lying in bed. (See p. 232 for additional interventions for the patient confined to bed.)	Bed rest may be ordered unless the catheter is held in place with sutures. Understanding the reason for a specific regimen increases patient cooperation. The patient should be aware that if he assumes an erect position, gravity may cause the ureteral catheter to become dislodged and slip into the bladder. It may then require replacement, which is a complicated procedure.

*May not apply; a ureteral catheter is used at the surgeon's discretion.

Plan for implementation	Rationale

7. If the catheter is to be irrigated, use the following guidelines:
  a. Use a syringe with an appropriate size needle that fits snugly into the ureteral catheter.
  b. Aspirate **before** irrigating to relieve distention.
  c. With a different syringe, instill no more than 3 ml of irrigant at one time.
  d. Irrigate very gently.
  e. Maintain sterility throughout the procedure.
	Irrigation may be required if there is no drainage from the catheter **and** if the patient is in pain. The absence of drainage indicates obstruction. Pain, in this case, indicates ureteral distention proximal to the obstruction because urine cannot drain through the ureter. Lack of drainage **without** pain is usually not an indication for irrigation because, in this case, urine is draining around the catheter, and the obstruction is not causing structural damage to the urinary tract.

9. NURSING DIAGNOSIS: Postoperative pain

Objective of nursing intervention   Appropriate management of pain or discomfort

Expected outcome   Behavioral and/or verbal indications that pain is adequately reduced or absent

Plan for implementation	Rationale
Determine the source of the pain. It may be related to the catheter(s) (if used), the surgical wound, the gastrointestinal tract, or the musculoskeletal system.	Pain from different sources usually requires different intervention.
1. Question and observe the patient to obtain information about the pain.	
2. Be aware that pain is a unique and individual experience. Although the difference sources of pain can usually be determined by their characteristics, there are also many variations.	
3. Be alert for indications (verbal or behavioral) that the patient is experiencing discomfort other than physical pain, and attempt to resolve the problem.	Fear, loneliness, depression, and numerous other conditions may be sources of extreme discomfort for the patient, who may unconsciously translate these feelings into pain.

PERSISTENT, SEVERE, INCREASING PAIN IN SUPRAPUBIC AREA

See Chapter 11, part one, nursing objective 6.	This pain is probably caused by an obstructed urethral catheter.

Early postoperative period

Plan for implementation	Rationale

SPASMODIC, INTERMITTENT PAIN IN SUPRAPUBIC AREA, OR PAIN RADIATING TO URETHRAL AREA

See Chapter 11, part one, nursing objective 6.	This pain is probably caused by the urethral catheter's irritating effect on the bladder.

SPASMODIC PAIN IN FLANK; MAY RADIATE TO SCROTUM OR LABIA

1. Check the ureteral catheter for obstruction. If it is not draining properly despite milking of the catheter, notify the physician and obtain an order for hand-irrigation of the catheter. (Do not irrigate a ureteral catheter without an order.)	The pain may be due to an obstructed ureteral catheter that is occluding the ureteral lumen and causing distention in the urinary tract proximal to the catheter.
2. If the catheter is draining well:	The presence of the ureteral catheter sometimes causes an increase in ureteral peristaltic activity as the ureter attempts to rid itself of the foreign object (i.e., the catheter). This can occur even if the catheter is draining well.
a. Provide analgesic or antispasmodic medication as ordered.	Analgesics reduce the perception of pain; antispasmodics decrease ureteral peristaltic activity.
b. Encourage slow, abdominal breathing during spasms.	Deep breathing promotes general relaxation. Concentrating on breathing during spasms may also provide temporary distraction from pain.
c. Reassure the patient that the pain is from the catheter and will disappear after the catheter is removed.	

MODERATE TO SEVERE PAIN AT SURGICAL SITE, USUALLY AGGRAVATED BY PHYSICAL ACTIVITY

1. Be certain the catheter(s) is (are) not obstructed. Although pain with these characteristics is usually of incisional origin, which is expected, the patient may not be able to identify accurately the precise location or quality of the pain.	Catheter obstruction must be ruled out first because it cannot remain untreated.
2. Administer analgesics as ordered.	Analgesic medication usually provides considerable relief from incisional pain.
3. Plan the patient's activities to coincide with a time when there is a high level of pain medication in the patient's bloodstream.	The patient will cooperate better with coughing exercises, ambulating, bathing, etc. when the pain is well under control.
4. Notify the physician if the patient's requests for pain medication do not decrease within 48 to 72 hours.	Although the intensity of postoperative pain varies enormously between patients, there should be a marked decrease in the apparent severity of the pain within 2 or 3 days. If this does not occur, it may indicate the development of wound complications.

Early postoperative period

Plan for implementation	Rationale

COLICKY, INTERMITTENT VISCERAL PAIN, USUALLY ACCOMPANIED BY ABDOMINAL DISTENTION

Plan for implementation	Rationale
1. Check the patient's abdomen for the presence and extent of distention.	Because some areas of the intestines regain function before others, abdominal distention and "gas" pains often occur. General activity may help to relieve the discomfort.
2. Encourage ambulation as soon as possible.	
3. Administer neostigmine methylsulfate (Prostigmin) as ordered.	Neostigmine is a cholinergic drug that occasionally relieves postoperative distention.
4. Suggest that a rectal tube be ordered for insertion 2 to 4 times per day for approximately 30 minutes.	
5. Check laboratory values for the patient's serum potassium level, and, if it is lower than normal: a. Notify the physician. b. Monitor the patient's pulse and cardiac status.	Hypokalemia may contribute to distention and decreased intestinal motility. However, there are more important reasons for correction of deficient seurm potassium levels as soon as possible (e.g., cardiac arrhythmias).

MUSCULAR DISCOMFORT IN NECK, SHOULDERS, EXTREMITIES, ETC.

Plan for implementation	Rationale
1. Provide the patient with an explanation for the pain and reassurance that it is transient. 2. Apply warm compresses to affected area. 3. Provide back rubs as needed.	Because of the positioning during the surgery (see Fig. 22-1), the patient may feel stiffness or soreness in various parts of his body. For the first few days after surgery the administration of narcotic analgesics and the presence of severe incisional pain may mask this discomfort. Generally, reassurance that it does not indicate complications is sufficient to take the patient's mind off it.

Early postoperative period

10. NURSING DIAGNOSIS: Need for management of intravenous infusion

Objectives of nursing intervention

Appropriate administration of specific types of intravenous solutions

Prevention or early detection of local complications

Prevention or early detection of systemic complications

Management of discomfort caused by the intravenous infusion

Maintenance of proper function of intravenous equipment

Maintenance of accurate records of the patient's hydration status

Expected outcomes

Normal hydration status

Normal electrolyte status

Absence of thrombophlebitis, infiltration, infection, fluid overload, and pulmonary embolism

Absence of discomfort from the intravenous infusion

Plan for implementation	Rationale
See master care plan for the patient receiving intravenous therapy.	These patients usually receive isotonic dextrose and saline solutions. They may also receive antibiotics, particularly if their urine was infected prior to surgery.

11. NURSING DIAGNOSIS: Alterations in gastrointestinal function

Objectives of nursing intervention

Prohibition of oral intake as ordered

Promotion of patient comfort

Expected outcome   Return of bowel sounds and passage of flatus within 24 to 48 hours

Plan for implementation	Rationale
1. Inform the patient that he is to have no oral intake. Notify the auxiliary staff as well, so that nobody inadvertently gives the patient something to eat or drink.	There is often a period of intestinal atony following this type of surgery. Within 48 hours it usually resolves itself, but premature oral intake will cause severe abdominal discomfort, distention, and vomiting. Although most patients will not feel like eating at this time, the nurse cannot rely on this alone as a deterrent to oral intake. If water is left at the patient's bedside, he may drink it.
2. Provide mouth care as needed.	Lack of salivary stimulation often causes dryness and an unpleasant taste in the patient's mouth.
3. Check periodically for bowel sounds and passage of flatus, and notify the physician when they occur.	These are indications that the intestines are regaining their function.

Early postoperative period

200

12. NURSING DIAGNOSIS: Potential for deep vein thrombosis

Objectives of nursing intervention
- Explanation and maintenance of precautions against deep vein thrombosis
- Early detection of deep vein thrombosis

Expected outcomes
- Cooperation with regimen to prevent deep vein thrombosis
- Absence of local pain, swelling, and redness of a lower extremity
- Absence of fever

Plan for implementation	Rationale
See master care plan for the patient at risk for deep vein thrombosis.	These patients are at considerable risk for deep vein thrombosis because the operative site is near the vena cava and other large veins.

Early postoperative period

13. NURSING DIAGNOSIS: Potential for gastrointestinal complications related to resumption of oral intake

Objective of nursing intervention
- Early detection of gastrointestinal complications

Expected outcomes
- Absence of abdominal distention, tympany, nausea, or vomiting
- Return of normal bowel function

Plan for implementation	Rationale
1. Permit oral intake of fluids and food only on physician's orders.	The physician will usually wait until bowel sounds are heard and the patient passes flatus before permitting him to have anything by mouth.
2. Note the presence of distention, tympany, nausea, or vomiting. Otherwise, if ordered, advance the diet as tolerated.	
3. Inform the physician if the patient has not had a bowel movement for more than 2 days after resumption of oral intake.	A cathartic is usually indicated at this stage in the patient's recuperation if he has not moved his bowels spontaneously.

Late postoperative period

14. NURSING DIAGNOSIS: Potential for voiding complications following removal of indwelling urethral catheter (if used)

Objective of nursing intervention   Prevention or early detection of complications

Expected outcomes { Resumption of normal voiding pattern
Absence of dysuria

Plan for implementation	Rationale
See master care plan for the patient with an indwelling urethral catheter: care after removal of the catheter.	
Be aware that the volume of urine the patient voids will be less than normal if a nephrostomy tube is present. This is because a portion of the urine produced by the affected kidney will drain through the nephrostomy tube.	

Late postoperative period

15. NURSING DIAGNOSIS: Potential for complications related to termination of nephrostomy drainage system (if used)

Objectives of nursing intervention
Explanation of test(s) to determine patency of the ureter
Early detection of ureteral obstruction

Expected outcomes
Absence of flank pain or fever
Urinary output in adequate proportion to fluid input

Plan for implementation	Rationale
1. If a nephrostogram is ordered, explain the procedure.	Before removing the nephrostomy tube the physician will usually order this x-ray examination to determine the patency of the ureter (see Chapter 3).
2. If pressure/flow studies are ordered, explain the procedure. (Fluid is infused into the nephrostomy tube, and the degree of patency of the ureter is indicated by the rate at which the fluid is able to flow.)	This test may be ordered in addition to the nephrostogram for the same reason.
3. After the above test(s), check the physician's orders concerning clamping of the tube.	If adequate patency of the ureter is confirmed, the physician will usually order the tube to be clamped for 24 hours before its removal.
4. If ordered, clamp the nephrostomy tube and for the next 24 hours do the following: a. Check for flank pain and/or fever. b. Maintain accurate records of urine output. c. Notify the physician at once if pain, fever, or significant decrease in urinary output occurs.	Pain, fever, or unusually low urinary output may indicate obstruction and/or leakage of urine into the retroperitoneal space. This requires medical or surgical intervention as quickly as possible.
5. Check the dressing at least every 4 hours for the first 24 hours after the removal of the nephrostomy tube, and change it when it becomes wet.	The sutures (or staples) are usually removed on the sixth or seventh postoperative day. However, until the sinus created by the nephrostomy tube has an opportunity to close, there may be considerable drainage from the wound. Since it is mostly urine draining onto the skin, the dressing must not be allowed to remain wet, or skin irritation and breakdown will occur.

Late postoperative period

16. NURSING DIAGNOSIS: Potential for late postoperative complications (pulmonary embolism and hemorrhage)

Objective of nursing intervention   Early detection and treatment of pulmonary embolism or hemorrhage

Expected outcome   Normal respirations, blood pressure, and pulse

Plan for implementation	Rationale

PULMONARY EMBOLISM

1. Be alert for symptoms of pulmonary embolism:
  a. Dyspnea
  b. Tachypnea
  c. Pleuritic chest pain or pain radiating to the shoulder
  d. Hemoptysis
	Although pulmonary embolism is a potential complication after any kind of major surgery, the patient undergoing most types of renal surgery is at greater risk because the operative site is close to the vena cava and other large vessels. It might occur at any time in the postoperative period, but its incidence is highest 5 to 10 days after surgery. Depending on its size and location, a pulmonary embolism can be lethal or essentially asymptomatic. When symptoms do occur, they may indicate a serious ventilation-perfusion imbalance, and prompt recognition and treatment are imperative.

2. If any of these symptoms occur, notify the physician at once, and institute the following measures:
  a. Keep the patient in bed with the head elevated more than 30 degrees.
  b. Start oxygen.
  c. Start an intravenous line.
  d. Keep the patient calm.	

LATE POSTOPERATIVE HEMORRHAGE

Check the patient's vital signs every shift, and observe the patient for signs of impending hypovolemic shock due to internal bleeding.	The risk of hemorrhage increases between the eighth and twelfth day after surgery because this is when tissue sloughing occurs. Although the patient is often going home toward the end of this time, the nurse should still be aware that late postoperative hemorrhage is a potential, but rare, complication after certain types of renal surgery, and appropriate observations must be continued throughout this period.

17. NURSING DIAGNOSIS: Need for discharge teaching

Objectives of nursing intervention
- Explanation of basic information about medications to be taken at home
- Explanation of information regarding follow-up care
- Explanation of residual effects of the condition and/or treatment
- Explanation of instructions concerning postdischarge activities
- Explanation of symptoms that constitute a reason to contact the physician
- Review of admitting diagnosis and mode of treatment

Convalescent period

Expected outcomes
- Accurate return verbalization and/or demonstration of all material learned
- Smooth transition of care after discharge
- Absence or early detection of complications arising after discharge
- Ability to provide future health care practitioners with important data about health history

Plan for implementation	Rationale
See master care plan for the patient requiring discharge preparations: discharge teaching.	
In addition to the topics covered in the master care plan, include the following items in the discharge teaching:	
1. At the follow-up office visit, the physician will check the incision for adequate healing and obtain a urine specimen for culture.	Urinary tract infection must be completely eradicated if the patient is to remain free from urinary calculi in the future.
2. The physician may prescribe periodic x-ray examinations to check for recurrence of calculi because an individual who has a history of stone formation is likely to develop another.	Detection of calculi before they become symptomatic may prevent serious renal damage.
3. During the next few weeks the expected residual effects of the surgery include fatigue and incisional discomfort.	
4. The patient should notify the physician if any of the following occur: a. Chills, fever, flank pain b. Severe pain and/or increasing redness at the incisional site c. Bright red urine	These may indicate a urinary tract infection. This may indicate a wound infection. This may indicate a late postoperative hemorrhage.
5. Unless contraindicated by a coexisting medical condition, the patient should maintain a fluid intake of at least 2.5 L per day for the rest of his life. (See p. 249 for details on hydration regimen.)	A rapid flow of urine through the urinary tract reduces the incidence of infection and precipitation of urinary elements. Therefore it retards the development of urinary calculi.
6. If medication, dietary limitations, or pH monitoring has been prescribed, provide the patient with all necessary information. (See pp. 250 to 251 for complete stone prevention regimen.)	Depending on the composition of the stone, the physician may place the patient on a regimen aimed at reducing the development of urolithiasis in the future.

Convalescent period

CHAPTER 24

Pyelolithotomy

A pyelolithotomy is performed to remove one or more stones from the renal pelvis. For the procedure the patient is positioned on his side (see Fig. 22-1) and a flank incision is made, usually through the bed of the eleventh rib. The renal pelvis is then exposed and incised with a U-shaped incision. The stone is removed (Fig. 24-1), and the incision is closed. An incisional drain may be inserted for leakage of urine. The wound is then closed, and a dressing is applied. An indwelling urethral catheter may be inserted to ensure adequate drainage of the bladder.

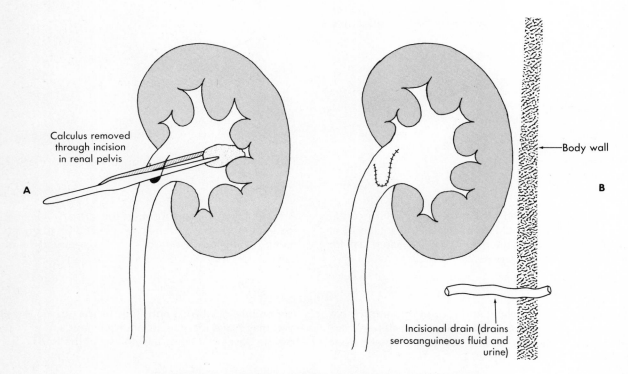

Fig. 24-1. A, Pyelolithotomy. **B,** Completed pyelolithotomy.

PYELOLITHOTOMY
Outline of Care Plan
ANTICIPATED NURSING DIAGNOSES:

Preoperative period
1. Need for preoperative teaching (See p. 189. Diagnostic tests may include plain film of the abdomen, intravenous pyelogram, and sonogram if the stone is radiolucent. Omit discussion of a nephrostomy tube and uteral catheter.)*
2. Need for discharge planning. (See p. 190.)*

Early postoperative period
3. Potential for shock. (See p. 191. The risk of hemorrhage is less after pyelolithotomy.)*
4. Potential for respiratory complications related to surgical intervention. (See p. 191.)*
5. Potential for wound complications. (See p. 192.)*

6. Need for management of indwelling urethral catheter. (See p. 195.)*
7. Postoperative pain. (See p. 197. Omit material concerning spasmodic pain in flank, scrotum, or labia.)*
8. Need for management of intravenous infusion. (See p. 200.)*
9. Alterations in gastrointestinal function. (See p. 200.)*
10. Potential for deep vein thrombosis. (See p. 201.)*

Late postoperative period
11. Potential for gastrointestinal complications related to resumption of oral intake. (See p. 201.)*
12. Potential for voiding complications following removal of indwelling urethral catheter (See p. 202.)*

Convalescent period
13. Need for discharge teaching. (See p. 204.)*

---

*Nursing care is the same as for the patient undergoing nephrolithotomy.

*Nursing care is the same as for the patient undergoing nephrolithotomy.

CHAPTER 25

Pyeloplasty

A pyeloplasty is indicated when there is obstruction at the ureteropelvic junction. There are numerous causes of such an obstruction, the most common ones being of congenital origin. Occasionally the obstruction may be due to a urinary calculus.

For the procedure the patient is usually positioned on his side (Fig. 22-1), and an oblique flank incision is made either in the space between the eleventh and twelfth ribs or in the subcostal area, depending on the position of the kidney.* The redundant portion of the renal pelvis and the upper portion of the ureter are excised, and anastomosis is performed. A ureteral stent and a nephrostomy tube, which is connected to bedside drainage, may be inserted. An additional drain is usually placed inferior to the anastomosis for any urinary leakage Fig. 25-1). The wound is then closed and a dressing is applied.

---

*When the procedure is performed on an infant, an abdominal approach is used.

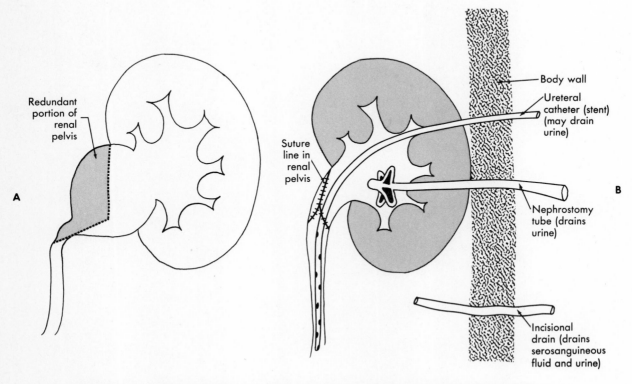

Fig. 25-1. A, Hydronephrotic kidney and line of excision before pyeloplasty. **B,** Completed pyeloplasty.

PYELOPLASTY
Outline of Care Plan
ANTICIPATED NURSING DIAGNOSES:

Preoperative period

1. Need for preoperative teaching. (See p. 189. Diagnostic tests may include intravenous pyelogram and retrograde pyelogram to detect the location and extent of the obstruction. Omit discussion of ureteral and indwelling urethral catheters.)*

2. Need for discharge planning. (See p. 190. Possible diet restrictions only apply to a patient with urolithiasis.)*

Early postoperative period

3. Potential for shock. (See p. 191. The risk of hemorrhage is less after pyeloplasty.)*

4. Potential for respiratory complications related to surgical intervention. (See p. 191.)*

5. Potential for wound complications. (See p. 192.)*

6. Need for management of nephrostomy tube. (See p. 193. The patient may have a ureteral stent next to the nephrostomy tube. Care of this stent is included in the care of the nephrostomy tube and wound. The stent is usually coiled up under the dressing, and the small amount of drainage from it drains into the dressing.)*

7. Postoperative pain. (See p. 197. Omit material concerning suprapubic pain and pain in the flank, scrotum, or labia.)*

8. Need for management of intravenous infusion. (See p. 200.)*

9. Alterations in gastrointestinal function. (See p. 200.)*

10. Potential for deep vein thrombosis. (See p. 201.)*

Late postoperative period

11. Potential for gastrointestinal complications related to resumption of oral intake. (See p. 201.)*

12. Potential for complications related to termination of nephrostomy drainage system. (See p. 203.)*

Convalescent period

13. Need for discharge teaching. (See p. 204. Omit references to urolithiasis unless applicable. Follow-up care may include periodic intravenous pyelograms or renal scans to check for recurrence of obstruction.)*

---

*Nursing care is the same as for the patient undergoing nephrolithotomy.

CHAPTER 26

Nephrostomy

The purpose of a nephrostomy is to provide an alternative route for urinary drainage when obstruction exists in the upper urinary tract. There are numerous conditions for which a nephrostomy might be performed. It is usually employed in conjunction with additional surgical procedures to correct an obstructive condition. It may, however, be done to provide permanent urinary drainage when an abdominal malignancy is causing an obstruction of the ureters.* It is occasionally done as an emergency procedure if the patient is uremic.

For the surgery the patient is positioned on his side (see Fig. 22-1), and a flank incision is made. Once the kidney has been partially separated from the surrounding fat tissue, a suitable calyx is approached via an incision through the renal pelvis. The area of the renal capsule adjacent to the calyx is then incised, and the nephrostomy tube is inserted through the opening in the renal capsule and positioned in the calyx or the renal pelvis. It is then brought to the surface of the body through a small stab incision and anchored to the skin with a suture. A Penrose drain is usually brought out through the main incision. The wound is then closed and a dressing is applied.

---

*Many surgeons consider it inadvisable to perform a nephrostomy on a terminal patient because it causes considerable discomfort for the patient and increases management problems. In these cases, percutaneous placement of a ureteral stent may sometimes be done instead (see p. 37).

NEPHROSTOMY
Outline of Care Plan
ANTICIPATED NURSING DIAGNOSES:

Preoperative period
1. Need for preoperative teaching.
2. Need for discharge planning.

Early postoperative period
3. Potential for shock.
4. Need for management of nephrostomy tube.
5. Potential for wound complications.
6. Postoperative pain.
7. Potential for urinary retention.
8. Need for management of intravenous infusion.
9. Potential for deep vein thrombosis.
10. Potential for respiratory complications related to surgical intervention.

Late postoperative period
11. Potential for complications related to termination of nephrostomy drainage system.*
12. Dependence on long-term care of nephrostomy drainage system.*

Convalescent period
13. Need for discharge teaching.

---

*May not apply.

NURSING CARE PLAN FOR THE PATIENT UNDERGOING NEPHROSTOMY

1. NURSING DIAGNOSIS: Need for preoperative teaching

Objectives of nursing intervention

- If necesssary, clarification of reason for hospitalization and type of surgery to be performed
- Elimination of any negative or inaccurate notions regarding the forthcoming surgery
- Explanation of preoperative tests and procedures
- Psychologic preparation for general anesthesia
- Explanation of events expected in the early postoperative period
- Explanation of body conditions expected in the early postoperative period
- Identification of any known allergies

Expected outcomes

- Verbal indication that explanations are understood
- Verbal indication of optimistic expectations (within realistic limits) related to forthcoming surgery
- Cooperation during preoperative tests and procedures
- Verbal or behavioral indication of reduction of anxiety
- Absence of postoperative complications
- Absence of allergic reactions

Plan for implementation	Rationale
See master care plan for the patient receiving preoperative teaching.	
In addition to the topics covered in the master care plan, include the following items in the preoperative teaching:	
1. Be aware that, in addition to routine preoperative tests, the following diagnostic studies may have been performed, and answer any questions the patient has regarding them:	
a. Intravenous pyelogram	This is done to provide information about anatomic abnormalities.
b. Cystoscopy	This is done to check the patency of the ureteral orifices.
c. Retrograde pyelogram	This is done to localize the site of obstruction in the ureter.
d. Antegrade pyelogram	This is done if renal function is poor and the retrograde pyelogram is unsuccessful.
2. The preoperative shave will be from nipple line to mid-thigh on the affected side.	
3. The patient will probably be permitted a light supper in the evening after surgery and will resume his normal diet in the morning.	Because the peritoneal cavity is not entered during this surgery, the incidence of postoperative gastrointestinal disturbances is relatively low.

Preoperative period

Plan for implementation	Rationale

4. The patient will have an incision on his flank. It will be covered by a dressing that will require frequent changing in the early postoperative period.

5. The patient will have a tube coming from the kidney. It will drain urine into a bedside collecting container.

6. The patient should not be alarmed if the urine is blood tinged.

---

2. NURSING DIAGNOSIS: Need for discharge planning

Objectives of nursing intervention { Early commencement of discharge planning
Accurate estimate of time required for all discharge teaching

Expected outcome Smooth transition of care after discharge

Plan for implementation	Rationale

See master care plan for the patient requiring discharge preparations: discharge planning.

In addition to the topics covered in the master care plan, the following items should be considered:
1. Duration of hospitalization for this procedure is approximately 1 week, but often the patient is hospitalized for additional procedures, since a nephrostomy is usually a temporary form of urinary diversion.

2. If the patient is to be discharged with the nephrostomy tube in place, nursing actions include:
   a. Assess the patient's general health and activity levels with regard to his ability to perform nephrostomy care. Bear in mind that this will also depend on the location of the nephrostomy site and his ability to reach it easily.
   b. Determine the existence of a significant other who might be willing and able to provide nephrostomy care.

Although some of these actions cannot be completed in the preoperative period, they should be commenced during this time so that they may be completed well in advance of the patient's scheduled discharge date. This prevents unnecessary last-minute delays in discharging the patient and thus spares the patient additional expense and psychologic distress.

Preoperative period

Plan for implementation	Rationale
c. Consult with the hospital social service department if it appears that professional care will be needed, such as Visiting Nurse Service or transferring the patient to an extended care facility.	If the patient is to be seen by a visiting nurse, the necessary documents must be completed in time to be mailed and processed by the Visiting Nurse Service so that the nurse's first visit can take place on the patient's first or second day home. (Thereafter the visits are usually scheduled two or three times a week.)
d. Plan adequate time during the postoperative period for teaching sessions if the patient or significant other will be providing nephrostomy care.	
3. If the patient is to be discharged after the tube is removed, required teaching will include general postoperative discharge teaching only.	

Preoperative period

3. NURSING DIAGNOSIS: Potential for shock

Objective of nursing intervention   Prevention or early detection of shock

Expected outcomes $\left\{\begin{array}{l}\text{Vital signs normal, skin dry, color normal}\\ \text{Absence of bright red drainage}\end{array}\right.$

Plan for implementation	Rationale
1. Check the patient's vital signs every 2 to 4 hours once stable (every 15 minutes if unstable).	Hemorrhagic shock is a potential complication in the early postoperative period following nephrostomy because the kidney is a highly vascular organ, and blood vessels may have been inadvertently severed during placement of the nephrostomy tube.
2. Be alert for indications of impending shock. These include: a. Increasing pulse and respiratory rates b. Decreasing blood pressure c. Diaphoresis, pallor, and cold clammy skin d. Feelings of apprehension	
3. Check the dressing and nephrostomy tube for excessive bleeding at least every 4 hours. Be certain to check under the patient's back.	Drainage will flow with gravity. If the patient is lying on his back, the side of the dressing may remain dry while the inferior portion becomes saturated.
4. Notify the physician at once if there are any signs or symptoms of impending shock.	

Early postoperative period

4. NURSING DIAGNOSIS: Need for management of nephrostomy tube

Objective of nursing intervention

Prevention or early detection of complications related to the nephrostomy tube

Expected outcomes { Urine draining freely through system
Absence of fever, chills, or foul-smelling drainage

Plan for implementation	Rationale

1. Maintain satisfactory function of nephrostomy drainage system.
  a. Tape tubing **securely** to the patient's flank to prevent inadvertent displacement of the nephrostomy tube.
  b. If the patient is confused, obtain an order for hand restraints. They should be used if there is **any** indication that the patient might pull at the tube.
  c. If the tube becomes dislodged, notify the physician **at once.**
	The nephrostomy tube is usually a retention catheter placed directly into the kidney through the flank incision. The catheter's distal end is attached to bedside drainage. It is frequently held in place with only one or two sutures and if accidentally removed, it may be very difficult to replace.
	The tube must be replaced promptly. If it is not reinserted within 1 or 2 hours, it may be impossible to replace. However, this is not a nursing function. It requires precise anatomic knowledge of the internal suture lines and the structure of the affected kidney.

d. Keep the collecting container below kidney level and the tubing free from kinks.	If urine is not permitted to flow freely through the system, structural damage to the kidney may occur.

2. Reduce the risk of infection associated with the tube:
  a. Use sterile technique when changing the dressing around the tube.
  b. Remove exudate from around the tube with hydrogen peroxide when changing dressing.
  c. Maintain a fluid intake of 2 to 3 L per day (unless contraindicated by a coexisting medical condition).
  d. Do not disconnect the tubing unless absolutely necessary.
  e. If tubing must be disconnected, avoid contamination of any openings in the system.
	Because this tube goes directly into the renal collecting system, it poses a considerable risk of pyelonephritis unless strict precautions are maintained.
	Exudate causes irritation of the tissue surrounding the tube and is a good medium for bacterial growth.
	A brisk flow of urine through the urinary tract discourages bacterial growth.
	Once the system is open to the air, it is potentially contaminated.

Early postoperative period

Plan for implementation	Rationale
3. Keep accurate records of the character and volume of the drainage. The color of the drainage is normally pink to amber within 48 hours.	
4. Notify the physician if any of the following conditions occur:	
a. Bright red drainage	This indicates abnormal bleeding.
b. Scanty drainage	This may indicate that the tubing is displaced or obstructed or that kidney function is impaired.
c. Excessive drainage from **around** the tubing (rather than through it)	This may indicate that the tubing is obstructed or displaced.
5. Observe the following precautions regarding hand-irrigation of the nephrostomy tube:	
a. Do not irrigate unless specifically ordered to do so by the physician.	The benefits of irrigation must be weighed against the risk of introducing pathogens into the kidney. This is not a nursing judgment.
b. Maintain strict sterile technique when irrigating.	
c. Do not instill more than 5 ml of irrigant at one time unless specifically ordered to do so.	The normal renal pelvis can hold only 2 to 5 ml of fluid. Overdistention of the pelvis can cause renal damage.

Early postoperative period

5. NURSING DIAGNOSIS: Potential for wound complications

Objective of nursing intervention	Prevention or early detection of complications arising from the incisional area
Expected outcome	Absence of fever, purulent exudate, erythema, edema, dehiscence, hematoma, and other abnormal wound conditions

Early postoperative period

Plan for implementation	Rationale

1. Check the dressing frequently (every 2 to 4 hours during the first 24 to 48 hours after surgery). Change it when it becomes wet, and use sterile technique for the procedure.	The dressing may become saturated rapidly with serosanguineous fluid and urine from the incision. This is because the suture line in the kidney may not become watertight for at least 48 hours after surgery. A wet dressing must be changed as soon as possible for the following reasons:
	1. It is a source of infection.
	  a. It acts as a wick, enabling microorganisms on the skin to move toward the incision.
	  b. It provides a good medium for bacterial multiplication.
	2. It is highly irritating to the skin because of the presence of urine in the drainage.

2. Note the odor of the drainage. The characteristic odor of urine is not abnormal, but if it is foul smelling: a. Notify the physician. b. Obtain a wound culture specimen.	This would indicate a wound infection. This will facilitate identification of the infecting organism so that appropriate treatment can be instituted quickly.
3. Use caution when removing soiled dressings to prevent inadvertent removal of the incisional drain and nephrostomy tube.	Premature removal of a drain may result in the development of a urinoma and prolonged healing. Accidental removal of the nephrostomy tube may necessitate more surgery.
4. Cut and arrange gauze pads around the nephrostomy tube and incisional drain (usually a Penrose drain is used).	This prevents the dressings from flattening the drainage mechanisms and possibly obstructing the flow of drainage from the wound and through the nephrostomy tube.
5. If the dressing requires frequent changing, use Montgomery straps instead of adhesive tape.	This eliminates the need to remove the adhesive tape from the patient's skin each time the dressing is changed. Skin irritation and patient discomfort can be considerably reduced by this method.
6. Note the condition of the suture line. Chart its appearance and the presence of edema, erythema, hematoma, ecchymosis, or other abnormal conditions.	This provides a frame of reference for other staff members caring for the patient.
7. Notify the physician if there is any evidence of dehiscence.	

Plan for implementation	Rationale
8. Check the patient's temperature every 4 hours and notify the physician if there is an elevation above 101°.	Wound infection must always be suspected when the patient runs a fever postoperatively. Other causes include respiratory complications and pharmacologic intervention.

6. NURSING DIAGNOSIS: Postoperative pain

Objective of nursing intervention   Appropriate management of pain or discomfort

Expected outcome   Behavioral and/or verbal indications that pain is adequately reduced or absent

Plan for implementation	Rationale
1. Question and observe the patient to obtain information about the pain.	
2. Be alert for indications (verbal or behavioral) that the patient is experiencing discomfort other than physical pain, and attempt to resolve the problem.	Fear, loneliness, depression, and numerous other conditions may be sources of extreme discomfort for the patient, who may unconsciously translate these feelings into pain.
3. Administer analgesic as ordered.	Moderate incisional pain is expected after this type of surgery. It is usually well controlled by analgesic medication.
4. Plan the patient's activities to coincide with a time when there is a high level of pain medication in the patient's bloodstream.	The patient will cooperate better with coughing exercises, ambulating, bathing, etc. when the pain is well under control.
5. Notify the physician if the patient's requests for pain medication do not begin to decrease within 48 to 72 hours.	Although the intensity of postoperative pain varies enormously between patients, there should be some decrease in the apparent severity of the pain within 2 or 3 days. If this does not occur, the possibility of wound complications should be considered.

Early postoperative period

7. NURSING DIAGNOSIS: Potential for urinary retention*

Objectives of nursing { Maintenance of accurate records of urinary output
intervention { Early detection of retention

Expected outcome   Normal voiding pattern resumed within 6 hours after surgery

Plan for implementation	Rationale
1. Instruct the patient to notify the nurse when he needs to void for the first time after surgery, and leave urinal by the bedside.	The effects of the anesthesia may cause temporary urinary retention; a blood clot or tissue particle might cause urethral obstruction. In either case, early detection and correction of the problem will prevent discomfort and possible renal damage.
2. Keep accurate records of the volume, frequency, and character of each voiding for at least 72 hours, or as long as the patient is on intravenous infusion. Be aware that the amount voided will be approximately half the normal amount because of the drainage from the nephrostomy tube.	
3. If the patient has not voided within 6 hours after surgery: a. Be certain he is receiving adequate fluids. b. Palpate the suprapubic area for distention. c. Depending on the condition of the patient, assist a male patient to a standing position with a urinal, and help a female patient to sit on a commode by the bedside. d. Provide the patient with adequate privacy. e. If the patient still cannot void, notify the physician.	Occasionally dehydration may be the cause of anuria. If the patient is in severe retention, the suprapubic area will be hard and distended. Assuming the accustomed position for voiding will help the patient to void if the retention is caused by psychologic factors. Catheterization may be necessary.

Early postoperative period

*May not apply; some patients have an indwelling urethral catheter after nephrostomy is performed.

8. NURSING DIAGNOSIS: Need for management of intravenous infusion

Objectives of nursing intervention

Appropriate administration of specific types of intravenous solutions
Prevention or early detection of local complications
Prevention or early detection of systemic complications
Management of discomfort caused by the intravenous infusion
Maintenance of proper function of intravenous equipment
Maintenance of accurate records of the patient's hydration status

Expected outcomes

Normal hydration status
Normal electrolyte status
Absence of thrombophlebitis, infiltration, infection, fluid overload, and pulmonary embolism
Absence of discomfort caused by the intravenous infusion

Plan for implementation	Rationale
See master care plan for the patient receiving intravenous therapy.	The type(s) of solution(s) and duration of intravenous therapy depends on the patient's general physical condition.

9. NURSING DIAGNOSIS: Potential for deep vein thrombosis

Objectives of nursing intervention

Explanation and maintenance of precautions against deep vein thrombosis
Early detection of deep vein thrombosis

Expected outcomes

Cooperation with regimen to prevent deep vein thrombosis
Absence of local pain, swelling, and redness of a lower extremity
Absence of fever

Plan for implementation	Rationale
See master care plan for the patient at risk for deep vein thrombosis.	

Early postoperative period

10. NURSING DIAGNOSIS: Potential for respiratory complications related to surgical intervention

Objectives of nursing intervention { Early detection of pneumothorax
Prevention or early detection of atelectasis and/or pneumonia

Expected outcomes { Cooperation with therapeutic respiratory regimen
Absence of dyspnea and other symptoms of pneumothorax
Absence of fever or audible lung congestion
Sputum clear or white and easily mobilized

Plan for implementation	Rationale
See master care plan for the patient at risk for respiratory complications, nursing objectives 4 and 5.	

11. NURSING DIAGNOSIS: Potential for complications related to termination of nephrostomy drainage system*

Objectives of nursing intervention { Explanation of test(s) to determine patency of the ureter
Early detection of ureteral obstruction

Expected outcomes { Absence of flank pain or fever
Urinary output in adequate proportion to fluid input

Plan for implementation	Rationale
1. If a nephrostogram is ordered, explain the procedure.	Before removing the nephrostomy tube, the physician will usually order this x-ray examination to determine the patency of the ureter (see Chapter 3).
2. If pressure/flow studies are ordered, explain the procedure. Fluid is infused into the nephrostomy tube, and the degree of patency of the ureter is indicated by the rate at which the fluid is able to flow.	This test may be ordered in addition to the nephrostogram for the same reason.
3. After the above test(s), check the physician's orders concerning clamping on the tube.	If adequate patency of the ureter is confirmed, the physician will usually order the tube to be clamped for 24 hours before its removal.
4. If ordered, clamp the nephrostomy tube and for the next 24 hours: a. Check for flank pain and/or fever. b. Maintain accurate records of the volume of urine output. c. Notify the physician at once if pain, fever, or significant decrease in urinary output occurs.	Pain, fever, or unusually low urinary output may indicate obstruction and/or leakage of urine into the retroperitoneal space. This requires medical or surgical intervention as quickly as possible.

*May not apply.

Early postoperative period

Late postoperative period

Plan for implementation	Rationale
5. Check the dressing at least every 4 hours for the first 24 hours after the removal of the nephrostomy tube, and change it when it becomes wet.	The sutures (or staples) are usually removed on the sixth or seventh postoperative day. However, until the sinus created by the nephrostomy tube has an opportunity to close, there may be considerable drainage from the wound. Since it is mostly urine draining onto the skin, the dressing must not be allowed to remain wet, or skin irritation and breakdown will occur.

12. NURSING DIAGNOSIS: Dependence on long-term care of nephrostomy drainage system*

Objectives of nursing intervention {
Prevention or early detection of complications arising from drainage system

Explanation and demonstration of nephrostomy care to patient and/or significant other

Expected outcomes {
Urine draining freely through system

Absence of chills, fever, flank pain

Bacterial colony count below 10^5 in urine cultures

Accurate return verbalization and demonstration of all material learned

Plan for implementation	Rationale

1. Maintain satisfactory function of nephrostomy drainage system:
   a. Check for accumulation of encrustation within the tube by rolling it between the fingers.
   b. Notify the physician if the tube feels gritty when checked in this manner, and suggest that the tube be changed. A nurse should not attempt to change a nephrostomy tube. It is a highly delicate procedure that can result in considerable damage if not done skillfully.
   c. Keep tubing securely anchored to the patient's flank with adhesive tape.
   d. Keep collecting container below kidney level and the tubing free from kinks.
	The nephrostomy tube and all parts of the drainage system should be changed by the physician when there is obstruction within the tubing and on a monthly basis, even if tubing remains free from debris.
	
	This is to prevent inadvertent displacement of the tube.
	
	Urine must be permitted to flow freely through the system, or structural damage to the kidney may occur.

2. Reduce the risk of infection:
 	
   a. Maintain a fluid intake of 2 to 3 L per day unless contraindicated by a coexisting medical condition.
   b. Do not disconnect the tubing unless absolutely necessary.† If it must be disconnected, do it quickly and avoid contamination of the inner surfaces of the system.
	Infection is the most common complication associated with long-term nephrostomy drainge.
	A rapid flow of urine through the urinary tract discourages multiplication of bacteria.
	Once the system is open to the air, it is potentially contaminated.

*May not apply.
†Some authorities encourage the use of a leg bag during the day for the ambulatory patient. Although this greatly enhances the patient's psychosocial comfort, it means frequent opening of the system and thus an increased risk of infection. If a leg bag is used, it must be thoroughly disinfected daily.

Late postoperative period

Plan for implementation	Rationale
c. Administer prophylactic antimicrobial medication as ordered.	Patients on long-term nephrostomy drainage usually require medication to help reduce the incidence of infection.
d. Cleanse nephrostomy site daily. If the patient is able to shower, he should wash the area thoroughly with soap and water. Otherwise, hydrogen peroxide can be used to cleanse the area.	
e. Change the dressing around the nephrostomy tube daily or more often if needed (eventually there may be only scant drainage from around the tubing).	
f. Empty drainage bag at least three times a day.	

Late postoperative period

3. If the patient and/or significant other is to be taught nephrostomy care:
   a. Provide demonstration and explanation of all procedures.
   b. Obtain a satisfactory return demonstration and verbalization.

---

13. NURSING DIAGNOSIS: Need for discharge teaching

Convalescent period

Objectives of nursing intervention
- Explanation of basic information about medications to be taken at home
- Explanation of information regarding follow-up care
- Explanation of residual effects of the condition and/or treatment
- Explanation of instructions concerning postdischarge activities
- Explanation of symptoms that constitute a reason to contact the physician
- Review of admitting diagnosis and mode of treatment

Expected outcomes
- Accurate return verbalization and/or demonstration of all material learned
- Smooth transition of care after discharge
- Absence or early detection of complications arising after discharge
- Ability to provide future health care practitioners with important data about health history

Plan for implementation	Rationale
See master care plan for the patient requiring discharge preparations: discharge teaching.	
In addition to the topics covered in the master care plan, include the following items in the discharge teaching:	

Plan for implementation	**Rationale**

PATIENT GOING HOME WITH NEPHROSTOMY TUBE IN PLACE

1. At the follow-up office visit the physician will check the incision for adequate healing, check the placement of the tube, and take a urine specimen for culture.

2. During the next few weeks, residual effects of the surgery include mild incisional discomfort and fatigue.

3. The patient may shower. It should be followed by nephrostomy care and dressing change.

4. The patient should be given a list of the items he will need for nephrostomy care and for replacement of parts of the drainage system. The location of places where these items are available must also be on the list.

5. The patient or significant other must give satisfactory return verbalization and demonstration of nephrostomy care.

6. The patient should be told of any arrangements with the Visiting Nurse Service (or other community organization), and these arrangements must be finalized before the patient is discharged.

7. The patient should notify the physician if any of the following occur:
   a. Chills, fever, flank pain
   b. Bright red drainage in the tubing

   c. Sudden cessation of drainage through the tube

These are symptoms of urinary tract infection.
Any bleeding is abnormal if it occurs after the early postoperative period, and it warrants immediate medical attention. Sloughing of tissue may occur, resulting in hemorrhage.
This indicates either obstruction or displacement of the tube.

PATIENT GOING HOME AFTER REMOVAL OF NEPHROSTOMY TUBE

1. At the follow-up office visit the physician will check the incision for adequate healing and obtain a urine specimen for culture.

Convalescent period

Plan for implementation	Rationale
2. During the next few weeks the expected residual effects of the surgery are fatigue and mild incisional discomfort.	
3. The patient should notify the physician if any of the following occur:	
a. Chills, fever, flank pain	These are symptoms of urinary tract infection.
b. Hematuria	This may also be a symptom of a urinary tract infection, or it may be a result of tissue sloughing and can signify hemorrhage.

Convalescent period

CHAPTER 27

Management of the patient with
acute pyelonephritis

Acute pyelonephritis is a fulminating urinary tract infection affecting the kidneys. Symptoms of the disease include chills, fever, and flank pain, often accompanied by nausea, vomiting, hematuria, urgency, and urinary frequency. The diagnosis is based on the patient's symptoms, the presence of infected urine, and structural abnormalities apparent on an intravenous pyelogram.

The organisms responsible for the infection are those normally found in the colon (e.g., *E. coli, Proteus, Klebsiella,* and *Pseudomonas*). Most commonly these bacteria ascend from the distal part of the urethra to the bladder, ureters, and then the kidneys. However, spread by way of the bloodstream or lymphatics may also occur. Host resistance is a major factor in the etiology of the disease, and obstruction anywhere in the urinary tract must be corrected before the patient is free from infection.

The duration of acute symptoms may be only a few days. However, the disappearance of symptoms does not necessarily mean that the infection has been eradicated. In fact, it is the low-grade, asymptomatic infection (chronic pyelonephritis) that re-

sults in the most serious consequences.* Therefore it is essential that the patient continue antimicrobial medication for the prescribed length of time and have follow-up care for 1 year or more, during which periodic urine cultures are obtained.

ACUTE PYELONEPHRITIS
Outline of Care Plan
ANTICIPATED NURSING DIAGNOSES:

Period of acute symptoms
1. Need for reduction of symptomatic discomfort (pain, nausea, urgency, dysuria, fever).
2. Potential for septic shock.
3. Potential for renal failure.
4. Need for psychologic and physical preparation for diagnostic procedures.
5. Need for management of intravenous infusion.
6. Potential for complications related to bed rest.
7. Need for discharge planning.
Convalescent period
8. Need for discharge teaching.

---

*Nursing care for the patient with chronic pyelonephritis has not been included in this book because the patient is rarely hospitalized for this condition. The recurrent infections that characterize chronic pyelonephritis are usually treated with antibiotics after the patient's condition is evaluated by the physician during an office visit. In acute pyelonephritis, however, the diagnostic workup and the management of renal colic and high fever are best carried out within the hospital setting.

NURSING CARE PLAN FOR THE PATIENT WITH ACUTE PYELONEPHRITIS

1. NURSING DIAGNOSIS: Need for reduction of symptomatic discomfort (pain, nausea, urgency, dysuria, fever)

Objective of nursing intervention	Appropriate management of discomfort

Expected outcomes
- Absence or adequate reduction of pain
- Absence of nausea and vomiting
- Absence of voiding discomfort
- Fever maintained below 101°

Plan for implementation	Rationale
PAIN IN FLANK, ABDOMEN, OR BACK	
1. Medicate with analgesics as ordered.	Pain in these areas is a common symptom of acute pyelonephritis and is caused by the inflammation of renal tissue. It can usually be adequately controlled with analgesics and local heat.
2. Provide local heat or, if the patient is permitted out of bed, a warm tub bath.	
NAUSEA AND VOMITING	
1. Administer an antiemetic such as trimethobenzamide (Tigan) or prochlorperazine (Compazine) as ordered or suggest that such medication be ordered **before** the symptoms become severe.	Since nausea and vomiting frequently accompany acute pyelonephritis, anticipation and early treatment may spare the patient considerable discomfort.
2. Encourage slow abdominal breathing if the nausea is severe.	Concentration on deep breathing promotes general relaxation and may provide distraction from the nausea.

3. If the patient is vomiting:
  a. Prohibit oral intake.
  b. Keep the patient lying on his side or sitting up.
  c. Provide frequent mouth care.
  d. Maintain accurate records of volume and character of vomitus.
	This prevents aspiration of vomitus.
	
	If vomiting is severe, the patient may become dehydrated and develop electrolyte imbalances, since sodium, potassium, and hydrogen ions are lost in the gastric juices. Fluid and electrolyte replacements may be ordered to correct losses before they become severe.

Period of acute symptoms

Management of the patient with acute pyelonephritis

Plan for implementation	Rationale
URINARY FREQUENCY AND URGENCY	
1. Administer antispasmodic medication such as oxybutynin chloride (Ditropan) or propantheline (Pro-Banthine) as ordered or suggest that such medication be ordered, provided that the patient does not have glaucoma or a cardiac condition. See Appendix A for details on these medications.	Antispasmodics are effective in reducing the intensity of bladder spasms, which occur if the infection involves the bladder as well as the upper tract. These spasms result in urinary frequency and urgency.
2. Provide the patient with easy access to the bathroom, urinal, or bedpan.	
3. Avoid the use of strong sleeping medications.	If the patient has nocturia, he might fall and injure himself under the effects of a strong sedative.
DYSURIA	
1. Administer a urinary tract analgesic such as phenazopyridine hydrochloride (Pyridium) or antispasmodic medication (as above) or suggest that these medications be ordered.	Phenazopyridine exerts a topical analgesic effect on the urinary tract. Antispasmodics reduce the intensity of bladder spasms and the pain associated with them.
FEVER AND CHILLS	
1. Medicate with an antipyretic as ordered.	Measures to reduce fever are usually ordered for temperatures above 101° or 102°. However, this is controversial, since the exact role of fever in fighting infection has not yet been explained.
2. Provide alcohol sponge baths, hypothermia blanket, or tepid bath as ordered.	
3. Be alert for symptoms of septic shock (see further).	

Period of acute symptoms

2. NURSING DIAGNOSIS: Potential for septic shock

Objective of nursing intervention

Prevention or early detection and treatment of septic shock

Expected outcomes

Vital signs normal, extremities warm, color normal

Patient alert and oriented

Urinary output approximately 60 ml per hour

Plan for implementation	Rationale
1. Check the patient's vital signs every 4 hours (or more often if unstable).	Septic shock, as with other forms of shock, occurs as a result of inadequate tissue perfusion. However, in septic shock, unlike hypovolemic shock, which has been discussed in relation to most surgical procedures, the syndrome is a result of abnormalities in the vascular bed rather than in the volume of circulating blood, and it occurs in the setting of a preexisting infection. Endotoxins released from gram-negative bacteria are implicated in the pathogenesis of the syndrome, sometimes referred to as endotoxic shock. The condition progresses rapidly, resulting in severe tissue anoxia, coagulation defects, and respiratory, renal, and cardiac failure. **Prompt recognition and treatment are essential or the condition is irreversible.** The patient is usually started on aggressive antibiotic and steroid therapy. The administration of massive doses of corticosteroids is controversial but appears to be effective. Changes in the type of antibiotic may be made after the results of the culture are known, but broad spectrum antibiotics, effective against gram-negative bacteria, are given initially.
2. Be alert for the following signs of septic shock (keeping in mind that there may be other causes for some of these signs): a. Decreasing blood pressure b. Cool, pale extremities, often with peripheral cyanosis c. Increasing pulse and respiratory rates d. Chills and fever (not always present) e. Mental obtundation f. Oliguria	
3. Be aware that in the elderly or debilitated patient septic shock may not be readily detectable, and the only clues may be the following signs: a. Unexplained hypotension b. Increasing confusion and disorientation c. Hyperventilation	
4. Notify the physician **at once** if septic shock is suspected.	
5. Obtain blood and urine specimens for cultures.	

Period of acute symptoms

3. NURSING DIAGNOSIS: Potential for renal failure

Objectives of nursing intervention
{ Accurate monitoring of fluid intake and output
Early detection of deteriorating renal function as revealed on laboratory tests

Expected outcomes
{ Urine output approximately 60 ml per hour
Normal blood urea nitrogen and creatinine levels
Normal creatinine clearance

Plan for implementation	Rationale
1. Maintain precise records of fluid intake and output. Fluid output includes: a. Volume and character of each voiding b. Volume of abnormal fluid output such as vomitus or loose stool c. Estimate of volume of observable perspiration (i.e., excessive, moderate, light)	This provides the physician with fundamental information about the patient's hydration status. Normally the amount of fluid lost in perspiration is approximately 600 ml/24 hours. This is referred to as insensible output, since it is not actually seen. When perspiration can be observed (as in febrile states), the amount of fluid lost is considerably higher and, like other abnormal losses, will affect the patient's fluid and electrolyte needs.
2. Notify the physician if the patient's urine output is less than 30 ml per hour.	This may signify numerous conditions such as dehydration, shock, obstruction of the lower urinary tract, or renal failure, all of which require prompt attention by the physician.
3. Notify the physician if the following abnormalities are noted in the patient's laboratory tests: a. Elevated blood urea nitrogen and creatinine levels b. Depressed creatinine clearance	Abnormalities in these tests indicate deteriorating renal function. Acute pyelonephritis is one of numerous disease states that may result in renal failure, particularly if it is bilateral or if the affected kidney is the patient's only functioning one. Renal failure is a complex spectrum of conditions that affect the kidney's excretory mechanisms. Thus water and electrolyte metabolism, acid metabolism, urea and organic acid metabolism, and drug metabolism will, to a lesser or greater extent, be jeopardized when some degree of renal failure exists.

Period of acute symptoms

4. NURSING DIAGNOSIS: Need for psychologic and physical preparation for diagnostic procedures

Objectives of nursing intervention

Reduction of patient anxiety

Provision of description and explanation of purpose for the procedures

Provision of physical preparation for the procedures

Expected outcomes

Absence of anxiety related to tests and procedures

Cooperation during tests and procedures

Specimens and x-ray film in satisfactory condition for diagnosis

Plan for implementation	Rationale
1. Provide information and physical preparation for whichever of the following procedures are ordered: a. Intravenous pyelogram b. Voiding cystourethrogram c. Cystourethroscopy* d. Retrograde pyelogram*	Some or all of these procedures may be required to to determine the presence of conditions contributing to the infection, such as obstruction or reflux of urine within the urinary tract. The patient may need considerable support and reassurance that these tests are necessary, since there is some discomfort associated with some of them, and the patient is already in considerable discomfort from his illness.
2. Obtain specimens for urine and blood cultures as ordered. a. Urine should be a midstream specimen from a cleansed orifice. b. Blood specimens should be obtained before the administration of any antibiotics.	These will be ordered to determine the type and sensitivity of the infecting organism. This prevents contamination by bacteria on the skin and in the distal urethra. Antibiotics in the bloodstream might interfere with the growth of the culture.

Period of acute symptoms

*Although these procedures are not usually performed in the presence of an active infection, they may be done in this case, provided effective antibiotic coverage has been given beforehand.

5. NURSING DIAGNOSIS: Need for management of intravneous infusion

Objectives of nursing intervention

Appropriate administration of specific types of intravenous solutions

Prevention or early detection of local complications

Prevention or early detection of systemic complications

Management of discomfort caused by the intravenous infusion

Maintenance of proper function of intravenous equipment

Maintenance of accurate records of the patient's hydration status

Precautions against adverse effects of nephrotoxic and ototoxic antibiotics*

Expected outcomes

Normal hydration status

Normal electrolyte status

Absence of thrombophlebitis, infiltration, infection, fluid overload, and pulmonary embolism

Absence of discomfort caused by the intravenous infusion

Normal blood urea nitrogen and creatinine levels*

Normal audiometry tests*

Plan for implementation	Rationale
See master care plan for the patient receiving intravenous therapy.	
In addition to the items mentioned in the master care plan, the following interventions may be required:	
1. If the patient is receiving an aminoglycoside (e.g., gentamicin, kanamycin, tobramycin), be certain laboratory studies are being performed for blood urea nitrogen and serum creatinine at least three times per week.	These drugs may be nephrotoxic. However, they are highly effective in the treatment of infections caused by gram-negative organisms. They are most commonly given via the intravenous route. If they are given intramuscularly, instead, the same precautions apply.
2. If the patient is scheduled for audiometric studies during the period of aminoglycoside administration, explain the purpose.	These drugs are also ototoxic, and the patient's physician may want the patient to have his hearing tested initially for a baseline reading and then periodically throughout the period that he is receiving aminoglycoside therapy. However, this adverse effect does not commonly occur unless the dosage is unusually high, the duration of treatment is prolonged, or if renal impairment exists.

Period of acute symptoms

*Applies to patients receiving intravenous nephrotoxic and ototoxic antibiotics.

6. NURSING DIAGNOSIS: Potential for complications related to bed rest*

Objective of nursing intervention	Prevention or early detection of complications associated with bed rest

Expected outcomes

- Absence of adverse psychologic effects of bed rest (boredom, depression, frustration, etc.)
- Normal bowel function and respiratory function
- Good skin integrity
- Absence of deep vein thrombosis and disuse atrophy of the muscles

Period of acute symptoms

Plan for implementation	Rationale
1. Place all necessary items within easy reach of the patient.	This encourages the patient to remain in bed without causing him to feel overly dependent on others.
2. Provide the patient with diversional activities (e.g., books, television, newspapers).	Boredom and depression are not unusual reactions when a normally active individual is confined to bed.
3. Promote adequate bowel function by encouraging fruit juices and high-residue foods.	Constipation is a common complication of immobility. If the patient is taking narcotic analgesics, such as codeine, it is even more likely to occur.
4. Keep accurate records of the patient's bowel movements and provide a cathartic or stool softener as needed.	
5. Check the integrity of the patient's skin daily; massage reddened areas over bony prominences, and avoid the use of plastic bed shields (e.g., Chux) in direct contact with the patient's skin.	Skin breakdown may occur on areas where there is prolonged pressure. Promoting circulation and keeping the areas as dry as possible will reduce the incidence of pressure necrosis.
6. Encourage periodic abdominal breathing, yawning, and sighing.	These maneuvers are considered to be a deterrent to atelectasis and pneumonia by helping to inflate the alveoli and expand the lungs to total capacity.
7. Encourage frequent changing of position, flexing and relaxing of leg muscles, range of motion exercises, and isometric exercises.	These activities help to prevent venous stasis (a predisposing factor in deep vein thrombosis), disuse atrophy of the muscles, joint contractures, skin breakdown, and respiratory congestion.

*In most cases these patients will not be required to remain in bed for more than a week. Therefore many of the hazards resulting from immobility will not be a threat. However, if the patient is elderly or debilitated or if for some reason bed rest must be prolonged, related complications are a major nursing consideration.

7. NURSING DIAGNOSIS: Need for discharge planning

Objectives of nursing intervention
{ Early commencement of discharge planning
Accurate estimate of time required for all discharge teaching

Expected outcome   Smooth transition of care after discharge

Plan for implementation	Rationale

See master care plan for the patient requiring discharge preparations: discharge planning.
 	
In addition to the topics covered in the master care plan, the following items should be considered:
1. The duration of hospitalization for the treatment of acute pyelonephritis is approximately 1 week.
 	
2. Required teaching includes elements of the patient's discharge regimen:
  a. High fluid intake
  b. Only light to moderate exercise until after the follow-up physician's appointment
  c. Importance of diligent antibiotic administration	

Period of acute symptoms

8. NURSING DIAGNOSIS: Need for discharge teaching

Objectives of nursing intervention

Explanation of basic information about medications to be taken at home
Explanation of information regarding follow-up care
Explanation of residual effects of the condition and/or treatment
Explanation of instructions concerning postdischarge activities
Explanation of symptoms that constitute a reason to contact the physician
Review of admitting diagnosis and mode of treatment

Expected outcome

Accurate return verbalization and/or demonstration of all material learned
Smooth transition of care after discharge
Absence or early detection of complications arising after discharge
Ability to provide future health care practitioners with important data about health history

Plan for implementation	Rationale
See master care plan for the patient requiring discharge preparations: discharge teaching.	
In addition to the topics covered in the master care plan, include the following items in the discharge teaching:	
1. It is extremely important that the patient continue the antibiotic medication for the entire length of time prescribed, despite absence of symptoms.	Medication is usually prescribed for approximately 10 to 14 days to decrease the risk of resistant microorganisms.
2. At the initial follow-up appointment the physician will obtain a urine specimen for culture.	
3. Additional check-ups and x-ray examinations will be scheduled periodically for at least a year to detect asymptomatic recurrence of the infection and prevent the development of chronic pyelonephritis.	
4. There should be no residual effects from the condition.	
5. The patient should notify the physician if he has any recurrence of symptoms.	
6. Until the patient's follow-up appointment with the physician he should maintain the following regimen:	
a. Fluid intake should be 2 to 3 L per day.	A high fluid intake discourages the recurrence of infection.
b. Heavy exercise should be avoided.	Heavy exercise reduces host resistance and retards the healing process.

Convalescent period

References and bibliography

BIBLIOGRAPHY

Atkins, E., and Bodel, P.: Physiology in medicine: fever, N. Engl. J. Med. **286:**27-34, 1972.

Davis-Sharts, J.: Mechanisms and manifestations of fever, Am. J. Nurs. **78:**1874-1877, 1978.

Goodman, L.S., and Gilman, A.: The pharmacologic basis of therapeutics, ed. 6, New York, 1980, Macmillan Publishing Co., Inc.

Harvey, A.M., et al.: The principles and practice of medicine, ed. 20, New York, 1980, Appleton-Century-Crofts.

Lapides, J.: Fundamentals of urology, Philadelphia, 1976, W.B. Saunders Co.

Luckmann, J., and Sorensen, K.C.: Medical-surgical nursing: a psychophysiologic approach, ed. 2, Philadelphia, 1980, W.B. Saunders Co.

Mitchell, P.H.: Concepts basic to nursing, ed. 2, New York, 1977, McGraw-Hill Book Co., Inc.

Phipps, W.J., Long, B.C., and Woods, N.F.: Medical-surgical nursing: concepts and clinical practice, St. Louis, 1979, The C.V. Mosby Co.

Schumann, D.: How to help wound healing in your abdominal surgery patient, Nurs. '80 **10**(4):34-40, 1980.

Smith, D.R.: General urology, ed. 9, Los Angeles, 1978, Lange Medical Publications.

Smith, R.B., and Skinner, D.G.: Complications of urologic surgery: prevention and management, Philadelphia, 1976, W.B. Saunders Co.

Thorn, G.W., et al.: Harrison's principles of internal medicine, ed. 8, New York, 1977, McGraw-Hill Book Co., Inc.

Williams, S.R.: Nutrition and diet therapy, ed. 4, St. Louis, 1981, The C.V. Mosby Co.

Winter, C.C., and Morel, A.: Nursing care of patients with urologic diseases, ed. 4, St. Louis, 1977, The C.V. Mosby Co.

UNIT VI

PROCEDURES FOR DISORDERS
OF
THE URETER

CHAPTER 28

Conservative management of acute
ureteral (renal) colic

Acute ureteral colic* is a common urologic condition that is most frequently caused by urolithiasis. It is estimated that approximately 200,000 Americans are hospitalized each year for this problem, but its incidence is considerably higher, since small stones frequently are passed spontaneously without necessitating a hospital admission.

Calcium is the major component of urinary tract stones, with phosphate, oxalate, uric acid, cystine, and xanthine following in decreasing order of frequency. Most stones are a combination of these elements.

The pathophysiology is highly varied and complex, and many aspects of it are not well understood. Stone formation may be secondary to many diseases, including hyperparathyroidism, sarcoidosis, Cushing's disease, gout, leukemia, renal tubular acidosis, chronic diarrhea, and urinary tract infection with urea-splitting organisms. These conditions (as well as others) must be ruled out or treated if the pattern of stone formation is to be corrected. In many cases the reason for the development of a stone remains unexplained.

Unlike renal calculi (discussed in the preceding unit), which are often "silent," excruciating pain is the most immediate adverse effect associated with ureteral calculi. However, the most serious long-term hazards are obstruction and chronic infection, which eventually lead to irreversible renal damage. For these reasons, prompt surgical relief of obstruction is often the treatment of choice.

However, some stones (those under 1 cm in diameter) may be passed out of the urinary tract spontaneously. If there are any indications that this will occur and that ureteral and renal distention are not serious enough to cause permanent renal damage,

the patient is usually managed conservatively with medical relief of symptoms and careful monitoring of urinary function. Some stones (e.g., those composed of uric acid and cystine) can sometimes be dissolved with medication.

Although acute ureteral colic is usually caused by the passage of a urinary calculus, occasionally it may be caused by other materials, such as a blood clot or a sloughed papilla. Either of these conditions requires further diagnostic investigation, but the symptoms of ureteral colic are similar, regardless of the nature of the obstructive material.

During the period that the obstruction is passing through the ureter is when the patient is usually seen in the emergency room and is often admitted to the hospital. He is frequently in excruciating pain, which may be in the area of the flank or lower abdomen, or it may radiate to the groin area. Nausea, vomiting, and paralytic ileus are often present because of peritoneal irritation and the common innervation of the ureter and the gastrointestinal tract. Since these are nonspecific symptoms, the precise source of the pain may take a while to confirm. Fever and hematuria may also be present, and, if it is the patient's first experience with a stone, he is usually in a state of considerable anxiety because of the sudden onset of his condition.

Nursing care is aimed at control of the symptomatic distress and, later, educating the patient about a stone prevention regimen, once the particular stone has passed.

ACUTE URETERAL COLIC
Outline of Care Plan
ANTICIPATED NURSING DIAGNOSES:

Period of acute symptoms
1. Need for reduction of symptomatic discomfort (pain, nausea, vomiting).

---

*Often referred to as renal colic.

239

2. Need for psychologic and physical preparation for diagnostic procedures.
3. Need for management of intravenous infusion.
4. Potential for passage of abnormal constituents in the urine.
5. Dependence on regulation of activity level.
6. Need for management of ureteral catheter.*
7. Need for discharge planning.
Convalescent period
8. Need for discharge teaching.

---

*May not apply.

NURSING CARE PLAN FOR THE PATIENT WITH ACUTE URETERAL COLIC

1. NURSING DIAGNOSIS: Need for reduction of symptomatic discomfort (pain, nausea, vomiting)

| **Objective of nursing intervention** | Appropriate management of discomfort |

Expected outcomes { Behavioral and/or verbal indication that pain is adequately reduced or absent
Absence of nausea and vomiting

Plan for implementation	Rationale
PAIN	
1. Medicate with analgesics as ordered.	The pain caused by the passage of a urinary stone has been described as the most excruciating pain a person can experience. It may be in the flank, abdomen, or back and may radiate to the groin, labia, or scrotum. Narcotic analgesia is usually required.
and/or	
2. Medicate with antispasmodics as ordered.	Antispasmodic medication will reduce the intensity of ureteral spasms, which are a major source of pain.
3. Chart location, duration, and quality of pain.	This provides a frame of reference for subsequent pain evaluation and control.
4. Chart the effects of the analgesic and/or antispasmodic. These include: a. When the patient obtained relief from the pain b. The degree of pain reduction c. The duration of pain reduction d. Side effects of the medications (see Appendix A)	This enables the physician to evaluate dosage and type of medication required.

Period of acute symptoms

240

Plan for implementation	Rationale
NAUSEA AND VOMITING	
1. Do not allow oral intake if there is any evidence of nausea, vomiting, or abdominal distention.	Nausea and vomiting frequently accompany ureteral colic. Abdominal distention due to paralytic ileus is also usually present.
2. Administer an antiemetic such as trimethobenzamide (Tigan) or prochlorperazine (Compazine) as ordered, or suggest that such medication be ordered, **before** the symptoms become severe.	Once vomiting is established, it is more difficult to control.
3. Encourage slow abdominal breathing if nausea is severe.	Concentration on slow deep breathing promotes general relaxation and may provide some distraction from the nausea.
4. If vomiting occurs: a. Keep the patient lying on his side or sitting up. b. Maintain accurate records of amount and character of vomitus. c. Chart frequency of episodes of vomiting. Note any relationship to medication the patient has recently received. d. Provide mouth care. e. Maintain adequate ventilation in the room.	This prevents aspiration of vomitus. If vomiting is severe, the patient may become dehydrated and develop electrolyte imbalances. Sodium, potassium, and hydrogen ions are lost in gastric juices. Fluid and electrolyte replacements will be ordered to correct losses. Narcotic analgesics may cause vomiting in certain individuals.

Period of acute symptoms

2. NURSING DIAGNOSIS: Need for psychologic and physical preparations for diagnostic procedures

Objectives of nursing intervention
{ Reduction of patient anxiety
Provision of description and explanation of purpose for the procedures
Provision of physical preparation for the procedures

Expected outcomes
{ Absence of anxiety
Cooperation during procedures
Specimens and x-ray films in satisfactory condition for diagnosis

Plan for implementation	Rationale
1. Ask the patient whether he has ever passed a stone before and, if so, what kind it was.	If the patient has a history of urolithiasis, this information may be useful in determining the type of stone from which he is currently suffering.

2. Provide information regarding which ever of the following urine tests have been ordered:
a. Urinalysis
b. Culture and sensitivity
  (1) This should be a midstream specimen.
  (2) The urethral orifice should be cleansed prior to voiding.
c. pH
	Frequently, patients with urolithiasis have infected urine.
	
	The acidity of urine plays an important role in the formation of some urinary tract stones and may provide a clue as to the type of stone from which the patient is currently suffering. For example, calcium ammonium phosphate stones form more readily in an alkaline medium. Uric acid precipitates in an acid medium.

(1) Check the urine pH after each voiding and maintain accurate records.	This enables the physician to determine the particular patient's typical urinary pH range.
(2) Take the pH reading as soon as the specimen is voided.	If the specimen is permitted to stand at room temperature, bacterial metabolism of urea will increase its alkalinity.

Period of acute symptoms

Plan for implementation	Rationale
d. Twenty-four-hour specimens for specific constituents, such as calcium, uric acid, oxalate, or cystine	These tests determine the total excretion of a substance during a 24-hour period.
(1) Collect these specimens sequentially. Usually a container with an appropriate preservative is provided by the hospital biochemistry laboratory.	
(2) Be certain that all voided urine during the 24-hour period is included in the specimen.	The test is inaccurate if any urine voided during the 24 hours is not included.
(3) If the patient must leave the unit (e.g., for an x-ray examination), he should either bring the collection bottle with him or start the specimen collection when he returns.	
3. Explain to the patient that blood specimens are necessary to determine the concentration of certain urinary stone-forming elements in his blood and to check his kidney function.	Specimens will be drawn to test for serum calcium, uric acid, creatinine, and BUN (blood urea nitrogen). Some patients become upset when frequent blood specimens are drawn unless they understand how it relates to their treatment.
4. Provide information concerning whichever radiologic procedures are ordered:	
a. Plain film of the abdomen (KUB) and intravenous pyelogram	These are done to determine the location of the stone, the extent of anatomic damage it may be causing, and in some instances the content of the stone (e.g., calcium stones are radiopaque; uric acid stones are radiolucent).
b. Cystoscopy and retrograde pyelogram	This may be done if there is any uncertainty as to whether the obstruction of the ureter is caused by a stone or a tumor.

Period of acute symptoms

243

3. NURSING DIAGNOSIS: Need for management of intravenous infusion

Objectives of nursing intervention

Appropriate administration of specific types of intravenous solutions

Prevention or early detection of local complications

Prevention or early detection of systemic complications

Management of discomfort caused by intravenous infusion

Maintenance of proper function of intravenous equipment

Maintenance of accurate records of the patient's hydration status

Expected outcomes

Normal hydration status

Normal electrolyte status

Absence of thrombophlebitis, infiltration, infection, fluid overload, and pulmonary embolism

Absence of discomfort caused by the intravenous infusion

Plan for implementation	Rationale
See master care plan for the patient receiving intravenous therapy.	
In addition to the topics covered in the master care plan, the following interventions are often required:	
1. Keep the patient well hydrated by maintaining a urine output of 2000 to 3000 ml/24 hours.	A brisk flow of urine through the system greatly assists passing a stone through the ureter.
2. Notify the physician if the patient is losing a considerable amount of fluid from sources other than urine (i.e., perspiration, vomiting).	The rate and electrolyte content of the intravenous infusion may need to be adjusted to compensate for these losses.
3. If ordered, administer intravenous sodium bicarbonate solutions.	Sodium bicarbonate may be ordered for a patient with a small uric acid stone. Sodium bicarbonate raises the pH of urine, and sometimes these stones can be dissolved in a relatively alkaline medium.
4. If ordered, administer intravenous antibiotic solutions.	Patients with urinary calculi frequently have infected urine. The infection may be a result of stasis of urine proximal to the stone or irritation of the ureteral wall from the stone. However, it is more likely to have been a predisposing factor in the formation of the stone. Many pathogens that infect the urinary tract split the urea molecules in the urine, creating an alkaline environment in which calcium ammonium phosphate may precipitate out of solution. Furthermore, clumped bacteria and inflammatory debris are thought to act as a nidus to which precipitants in the urine can adhere.

Period of acute symptoms

4. NURSING DIAGNOSIS: Potential for passage of abnormal constituents in the urine (blood, calculi, tissue particles, etc.)

Objective of nursing intervention	Precise monitoring of visible elements in the urine
Expected outcome	Cooperation with regimen of straining urine or saving it for observation

Plan for implementation	Rationale
1. Note the color of the patient's urine.	Dark, concentrated urine may indicate the patient's fluid intake is inadequate and requires further evaluation. Blood-tinged urine may indicate that the stone is moving through the ureter; rough edges of the stone often cause capillaries in the ureter wall to rupture.
2. If the patient expresses anxiety about the presence of blood in his urine, provide reassurance that this is not unusual and is no cause for alarm.	See preceding rationale.
3. Strain all urine before disposal. Most patients can be taught to do this themselves.	Very small stones may be passed without the patient knowing it unless the urine is strained.
4. Send all solid matter passed in the urine to the laboratory for analysis.	The chemical content of the stone must be known before a preventative medical and dietary regimen can be formulated. Occasionally the material passed will be a sloughed papilla or a blood clot rather than a stone. If this is the case, further diagnostic studies will be required.

Period of acute symptoms

Period of acute symptoms

5. NURSING DIAGNOSIS: Dependence on regulation of activity level

Objective of nursing intervention Provision of instructions concerning the patient's activity

Expected outcomes { Safe ambulation when appropriate
Early passage of ureteral obstruction

Plan for implementation	Rationale
1. Unless ordered otherwise, encourage the patient to ambulate as much as possible, except under the following conditions:	It is thought that activity enhances the passage of a stone through the ureter.
a. The patient has recently been medicated with a narcotic analgesic.	One of the side effects of narcotics is dizziness. Therefore the patient should stay in bed after being medicated for pain to avoid accidental injury.
b. The patient is in severe pain.	Usually the patient himself can be the judge as to how much pain he can endure and still walk around safely. Sometimes patients feel **more** comfortable if they can ambulate. However, a severe attack of ureteral colic is usually too incapacitating for almost any activity.
2. Unless the patient appears completely steady on his feet, provide supervision for ambulation.	

6. NURSING DIAGNOSIS: Need for management of ureteral catheter*

Objective of nursing intervention Prevention or early detection of complications related to ureteral catheter

Expected outcomes { Urine draining freely through system
Absence of fever, chills, or foul-smelling urine
Reduction of pain
Spontaneous passage of stone out of ureter

Plan for implementation	Rationale
1. Irrigate the catheter only if specifically ordered and only after the technique has been previously mastered.	Unless done with extreme care and skill, irrigation of a ureteral catheter could cause serious damage to the ureter and kidney.

---

*This may not apply. The use of a ureteral catheter (inserted beyond the location of the obstruction) is at the urologist's discretion. It is sometimes employed to drain a hydronephrotic kidney and distended ureter when obstruction is severe and infection is present. It usually brings about some relief from pain after the distention is reduced, it helps in the resolution of the infection, and it sometimes facilitates the spontaneous passage of the obstruction after the catheter is removed. Occasionally it is used as an irrigating catheter to dissolve calculi.

246

Plan for implementation	Rationale
2. Keep the catheter securely taped to the patient's thigh.	This helps to prevent inadvertent traction on the catheter. Often an indwelling urethral catheter is inserted into the bladder to help prevent dislodgement of the ureteral catheter. They are usually tied together with suture material at the point where they both emerge from the distal portion of the urethra.
3. Maintain accurate records of output. If an indwelling urethral catheter is used as well, label both collecting containers accordingly and record outputs separately.	This enables assessment of the catheter's patency.
4. If scanty or nonexistent output is noted: a. Milk the catheter and tubing. b. If no results, notify the physician.	The catheter may be obstructed.
5. Disconnect the tubing only if absolutely necessary. Maintain sterile technique and prevent contamination of open ends of the tubing.	Any break in the closed system may result in contamination of the urinary tract.
6. If the physician has ordered that the patient remain in bed while the catheter is in place: a. Explain to the patient that he must remain in bed to prevent accidental displacement of the catheter. b. The patient may not sit in a completely upright position. c. The patient may sit in a semiupright position and turn from side to side while lying in bed. (See p. 232 for additional interventions for the patient on bed rest.)	Bed rest may be ordered, depending on the type of ureteral catheter being used. Understanding the reason for a specific regimen increases patient cooperation. The patient should be aware that, if he assumes an erect position, gravity may cause the ureteral catheter to become dislodged and slip into the bladder. It may then require replacement, which is a complicated procedure.
7. If the catheter is to be irrigated, use the following guidelines: a. Use a syringe with an appropriate size needle that fits snugly into the ureteral catheter. b. Aspirate **before** irrigating to relieve distention. c. With a different syringe, instill no more than 3 ml of irrigant at one time. d. Irrigate very gently. e. Maintain sterility throughout the procedure.	Irrigation may be ordered if there is no drainage from the catheter or if the physician is attempting to dissolve the calculus with sodium bicarbonate solution (for a uric acid stone) or Renacidin (for a calcium oxalate stone).

Period of acute symptoms

Period of acute symptoms

7. NURSING DIAGNOSIS: Need for discharge planning

| Objectives of nursing intervention | Early commencement of discharge planning |
| | Accurate estimate of time required for all discharge teaching |

Expected outcome   Smooth transition of care after discharge

Plan for implementation	Rationale
See master care plan for the patient requiring discharge preparations: discharge planning.	
In addition to the topics covered in the master care plan, the following items should be considered:	
1. Duration of hospitalization for acute ureteral colic varies considerably from a few hours to several days.	If the patient becomes pain free and afebrile, the physician may discharge him with instructions to strain his urine and to save the stone when it is passed. However, if pain and fever persist and extravasation of urine occurs, surgery will probably be required. (See Chapters 29 and 30.)
2. Discharge teaching will also vary considerably. If the patient is a habitual stone former, he may be placed on on a stone prevention regimen.	Instructions on diet, medication, and urine pH testing may be required, and teaching should be begun as soon as possible.

Convalescent period

8. NURSING DIAGNOSIS: Need for discharge teaching

Objectives of nursing intervention	Explanation of basic information about medications to be taken home
	Explanation of information regarding follow-up care and stone prevention regimen
	Explanation of symptoms that constitute a reason to contact the physician
	Review of admitting diagnosis and mode of treatment

Expected outcomes	Accurate return verbalization and demonstration of all information
	Absence or early detection of complications arising after discharge
	Ability to provide future health care practitioners with important data about health history

Plan for implementation	Rationale
See master care plan for the patient requiring discharge preparations: discharge teaching.	
In addition to the topics mentioned in the master care plan, some or all of the following information should be included in the discharge teaching, depending on the composition of the stone and how the physician intends to manage the patient. The nurse should obtain this information from the physician before commencing discharge teaching.	The extent of discharge teaching for the patient who has passed a urinary calculus will vary considerably. If he is a chronic stone former and a complete investigation has been carried out, he may be placed on a specific stone prevention regimen, including diet and medication. If the patient has had only an isolated incident of urolithiasis, he may not be required to follow any particular regimen except, perhaps, to maintain good hydration.

Plan for implementation	Rationale
1. At the follow-up office visit the physician will obtain a urine specimen for culture and will review the particular stone prevention regimen the patient is to be following. (See further.)	Urinary tract infection must be eradicated if future stone formation is to be prevented.
2. The physician may prescribe periodic x-ray examinations to check for recurrence of calculi if the patient is a chronic stone former.	Detection of calculi before they become symptomatic may prevent serious renal damage.
3. The patient should notify the physician if any of the following occur: chills, fever, hematuria, flank pain.	These symptoms are indications of a urinary tract infection, which should be treated as soon as possible.
4. The patient should contact the physician if he has any questions or problems with his stone prevention regimen. The important aspects of whichever regimen he is to follow should be given to him in writing before he leaves the hospital. The plan may be based on one or more of the following stone prevention principles.	

ROLE OF HYDRATION IN STONE PREVENTION

Convey to the patient the importance of maintaining a high fluid intake and suggest ways to help him comply with the regimen:	Unless contraindicated by a coexisting medical condition, these patients should drink a **minimum** of 2.5 L of fluid per day. A brisk flow of dilute urine through the urinary tract discourages the development of urolithiasis.
1. The patient should keep a large supply of his favorite beverages on hand.	
2. He should establish the habit of drinking approximately one 8-ounce glass of fluid every 2 hours (or more often, depending on the total amount of intake prescribed.)	
3. If possible, he should awaken once during the night and drink two glasses of fluid at this time.	This helps to prevent concentration of urine, which normally occurs at night.
4. If climate or strenuous exercise causes the patient to perspire excessively, the amount of fluid intake should be increased accordingly.	Even mild dehydration should be avoided at all times, since crystallization of various constituents of the urine is more likely to occur in a concentrated solution.

Convalescent period

Plan for implementation	Rationale
ROLE OF MEDICATION IN STONE PREVENTION	
If the patient is given medication to control the incidence of future urolithiasis, explain the dosage and any possible side effects. (See Appendix A.) The type of medication will depend on the composition of the stone.	Certain types of stones can often be prevented by specific medications.
1. Uric acid stones	
a. Allopurinol (Zyloprim)	This reduces uric acid production.
b. Sodium bicarbonate; potassium citrate, sodium citrate, and citric acid (Polycitra Syrup)	These alkalinize the urine.
2. Calcium stones	
a. Vitamin C (ascorbic acid), ammonium chloride	These acidify the urine.
b. Potassium acid phosphate (K-Phos), neutral sodium and potassium phosphate (Neutra-Phos)	These are thought to increase urine solubilizers.
c. Hydrochlorothiazide	This reduces urinary calcium.
3. Cystine stones	
a. Penicillamine (Cuprimine)	This lowers urinary cystine.
ROLE OF MONITORING URINARY pH IN STONE PREVENTION	
If the patient is to maintain his urine at a specific pH:	If the patient has a history of forming uric acid stones, he should maintain a relatively alkaline urine. In contrast, an acid urine may help prevent the development of calcium phosphate stones.
1. Demonstrate the procedure for testing urine with Nitrazine paper.	
2. Have the patient give a return demonstration.	
3. Explain the relationship of medication (see preceding) and diet (see further) to urinary pH.	
ROLE OF DIET IN STONE PREVENTION	
If the patient is placed on a special diet to control the incidence of future urolithiasis, provide the appropriate information. The diet will be based on the composition of the stone.	

Convalescent period

Plan for implementation	Rationale
1. Uric acid stones	
a. Reduce* intake of foods high in purine (e.g., organ meats, lean meat, whole grains, legumes).	Uric acid is a metabolite of purine.
b. Reduce* intake of foods that produce an acid urine (e.g., eggs, meat, whole grains, cheese, cranberries, plums, prunes).	Uric acid crystals are more likely to form in an acid medium.
2. Calcium stones	
a. Reduce* intake of foods high in calcium (e.g., milk, cheese, green leafy vegetables).	Decreasing the intake of calcium may decrease the amount of calcium in the urine.
3. Oxalate stones	
a. Avoid excessive intake of foods high in oxalate (e.g., rhubarb, spinach, beets, coffee, tea, chocolate).	Decreasing the intake of oxalate may decrease the amount of oxalate in the urine.
b. Avoid high doses of ascorbic acid.	Intake of ascorbic acid that exceeds 2 g per day may increase the amount of oxalate excreted in the urine. This should be mentioned to the patient because vitamin C is a popular self-prescribed drug.

*The permissible amount of these foods is decided on by the patient's physician. Some of these foods cannot be eliminated entirely without severely jeopardizing the patient's nutritional status.

Convalescent period

CHAPTER 29

Endoscopic removal of ureteral calculus (stone basketing)

Endoscopic removal of a ureteral stone is indicated when the stone is in the lower third of the ureter and the patient is either having severe pain from the stone or the stone is large and causing potentially damaging ureteral obstruction. Otherwise, the patient is generally treated conservatively (i.e., high fluid intake, analgesic administration), since the majority of these stones will eventually pass by themselves.

For the procedure the patient is placed in a lithotomy position (Fig. 29-1) and a cystoscope is inserted. A basketing instrument is passed into the ureter beyond the stone and is then slowly removed (Fig. 29-2) using a gentle, rotating motion. Care is taken not to strip any of the ureteral mucosa, since this would result in stricture formation. Once the stone is dislodged into the bladder, it is irrigated out through the cystoscope.

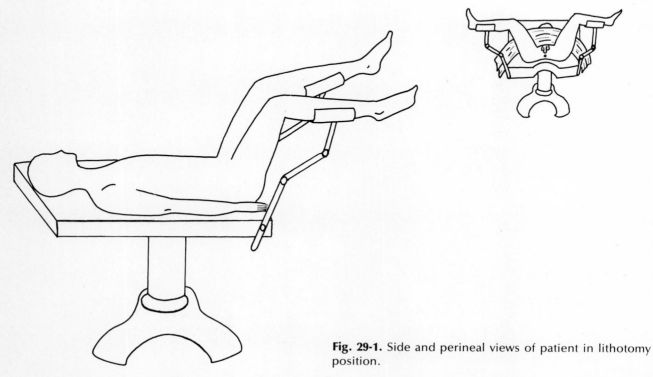

Fig. 29-1. Side and perineal views of patient in lithotomy position.

Some surgeons insert a ureteral catheter to prevent possible postoperative obstruction of the ureter because the manipulation sometimes causes edema. The catheter extends from the renal pelvis through the urethra. An indwelling urethral catheter also is inserted, and the two catheters are usually tied together with suture material.

ENDOSCOPIC REMOVAL OF URETERAL CALCULUS
Outline of Care Plan
ANTICIPATED NURSING DIAGNOSES:

Preoperative period
1. Need for preoperative teaching.
2. Need for discharge planning.

Early postoperative period
3. Potential for postoperative complications (shock, atelectasis, pneumonia, deep vein thrombosis, infection).
4. Need for management of indwelling urethral catheter.
5. Need for management of ureteral catheter.*
6. Postoperative pain.

Late postoperative period
7. Potential for urinary complications following removal of urethral (and ureteral) catheter(s).

Convalescent period
8. Need for discharge teaching.

_____

*May not apply.

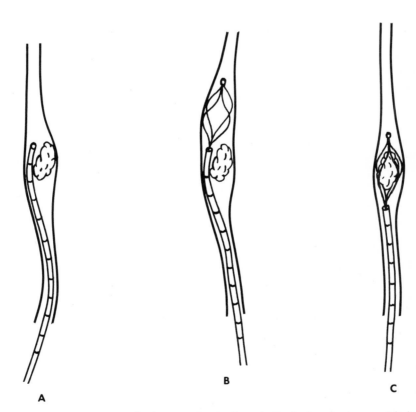

Fig. 29-2. Endoscopic removal of ureteral calculus. **A,** Basketing instrument is inserted into the ureter, compressed within the rod portion of the apparatus. **B,** Once the flexible rod is adjacent to the stone, the basket is advanced through the rod beyond the stone. The flexible wires spread out within the ureter. **C,** The stone is engaged in the wires and is removed from the ureter.

NURSING CARE PLAN FOR THE PATIENT UNDERGOING ENDOSCOPIC REMOVAL OF URETERAL CALCULUS

1. NURSING DIAGNOSIS: Need for preoperative teaching

Objectives of nursing intervention

If necessary, clarification of reason for hospitalization and type of surgery to be performed

Elimination of any negative or inaccurate notions regarding the forthcoming surgery

Explanation of preoperative tests and procedures

Psychologic preparation for general anesthesia (omit if the patient is to have spinal anesthesia)

Explanation of events expected in the early postoperative period

Explanation of body conditions expected in the early postoperative period

Identification of any known allergies

Expected outcomes

Verbal indication that explanations are understood

Verbal indication of optimistic expectations (within realistic limits) related to forthcoming surgery

Cooperation during preoperative tests and procedures

Verbal or behavioral indication of reduction of anxiety

Absence of postoperative complications

Absence of allergic reactions

Preoperative period

Plan for implementation	Rationale
See master care plan for the patient receiving preoperative teaching.	
In addition to the topics covered in the master care plan, include the following items in the preoperative teaching:	
1. Be aware that, in addition to routine preoperative tests, the following diagnostic studies may have been performed, and answer any questions the patient has regarding them.	
a. Plain x-ray film of the abdomen (KUB)	This is done to locate the stone in the ureter. It is performed when the patient is admitted to the hospital, but it must be repeated immediately before surgery so that any changes in the location of the stone can be determined.
b. Intravenous pyelogram	This is done to determine renal function and the presence of radiolucent stones in the urinary tract.
c. Cystoscopy	This is occasionally done to assess the condition of the bladder and ureteral orifice.
d. Retrograde pyelogram	This may be done to assess more precisely the location of the stone.

Plan for implementation	Rationale
2. The preoperative shave is from the umbilicus to mid-thigh.	Although the shave is sometimes omitted altogether, many surgeons will request it in case of accidental perforation of the ureter or other technical problems that may require an incision to correct. The physician usually tells the patient beforehand that it may not be possible to extract the stone endoscopically, in which case an abdominal incision will be required (see Chapter 30). The possibility of open surgery is therefore included on the informed consent document that the patient signs.
3. The patient will be permitted oral fluids shortly after returning from the recovery room, and his diet will be advanced as tolerated.	These patients can usually tolerate oral intake a few hours after the surgery. For this reason, the intravenous infusion used during surgery is frequently discontinued in the recovery room or shortly after the patient returns to the urology floor and tolerates fluids.
4. There will be an indwelling urethral catheter in place for 24 to 48 hours after surgery and possibly a ureteral catheter as well.	
5. The urine may be pink in the immediate postoperative period.	

Preoperative period

2. **NURSING DIAGNOSIS:** Need for discharge planning

Objectives of nursing intervention { Early commencement of discharge planning
Accurate estimate of time required for all discharge teaching

Expected outcome Smooth transition of care after discharge

Plan for implementation	Rationale
See master care plan for the patient requiring discharge preparations: discharge planning.	

In addition to the topics covered in the master care plan, the following items should be considered:
1. The duration of hospitalization for this type of surgery is usually 2 or 3 days.

2. Required teaching includes:
   a. General postoperative discharge teaching
   b. Possibly instructions for a stone prevention regimen

3. NURSING DIAGNOSIS: Potential for postoperative complications (shock, atelectasis, pneumonia, deep vein thrombosis, infection)

Objective of nursing intervention　　Prevention or early detection of postoperative complications

Expected outcomes
Pulse and blood pressure normal, skin dry, color normal
Respirations regular and unlabored, absence of pulmonary congestion
Early ambulation tolerated well
Absence of chills or fever

Plan for implementation	Rationale

1. Check the patient's vital signs every 4 hours and notify the physician of any indications of impending shock. These include:
  a. Increasing pulse and respiratory rates
  b. Decreasing blood pressure
  c. Diaphoresis and pallor
  d. Feelings of apprehension
	Although shock is a potential complication after any kind of surgery, it is a relatively small risk after endoscopic removal of ureteral calculus, since no blood vessels are cut and surgery is usually not prolonged.

2. Encourage coughing and abdominal breathing if the patient's lungs sound congested, and notify the physician if any of the following conditions are present:
 	
  a. The patient is unable to cough and his lungs sound congested.
  b. Sputum volume is copious.
  c. Sputum color is other than clear or white.
  d. There is a rise in the patient's temperature.
  e. Breath sounds are diminished.
	Although precautions must be taken, respiratory complications are unlikely after this type of surgery because the period of anesthesia is short. Furthermore, there is no abdominal incision to inhibit effective coughing.
	These conditions require additional treatment. The physician may order therapies such as incentive spirometry, nasotracheal suctioning, postural drainage, or intermittent positive pressure breathing, depending on the extent of respiratory embarrassment.

3. Use methods to prevent deep vein thrombosis. (See master care plan for the patient at risk for deep vein thrombosis.)	Deep vein thrombosis is a complication that must be considered after this type of surgery. Although the duration is short, the surgery is performed with the patient in the lithotomy position, which can injure the popliteal vessels.

4. Notify the physician if any indications of infection occur. These include:
  a. Chills
  b. Fever
  c. Flushed skin
	Bacteremia can occur after instrumentation of the urinary tract as a result of absorption of bacteria through the urethral and ureteral mucosa. Blood and urine specimens often are ordered to determine the type and sensitivity of the offending organism, and the patient is usually given antibiotic therapy.

Early postoperative period

4. NURSING DIAGNOSIS: Need for management of indwelling urethral catheter

Objectives of nursing intervention

Appropriate care of catheter and equipment

Prevention or early detection of infection

Care of tissue surrounding catheter

Maintenance of accurate records of urine output

Appropriate administration of hand-irrigation of catheter

Management of discomfort or pain caused by the catheter

Satisfactory collection of urine specimens from catheter

Expected outcomes

Absence of severe bladder spasms and suprapubic distention

Urine draining freely through system

Absence of fever, chills, and foul-smelling urine

Absence of urethral discharge and tissue inflammation

Minimal discomfort caused by the catheter

Urine specimens in optimum condition for all necessary tests

Plan for implementation	Rationale
See master care plan for the patient with an indwelling urethral catheter: care after insertion of the catheter.	
In addition to the topics covered in the master care plan, the following interventions are required:	
1. Notify the physician if the urine turns bright red and has a high viscosity. The urine should be blood tinged to clear within 24 to 48 hours.	There should be relatively little blood in the urine after this type of surgery. No blood vessels are cut, and the only "normal" cause of bleeding is from the rupture of capillaries during instrumentation.
2. If a ureteral catheter is used, label both collecting containers accordingly, and record output from each system separately.	The two sources of output should not be combined, or valuable information concerning the functioning of each system will be lost.

Early postoperative period

5. NURSING DIAGNOSIS: Need for management of ureteral catheter*

Objective of nursing intervention	Prevention or early detection of complications caused by the ureteral catheter

Expected outcomes { Urine draining freely through system
Absence of fever, chills, or foul-smelling urine

Plan for implementation	Rationale
1. Irrigate the catheter only if specifically ordered and only after the technique has been previously mastered.	Unless done with extreme care and skill, irrigation of a ureteral catheter could cause serious damage to the ureter and kidney. Rarely is irrigation required after this type of surgery.
2. Keep the catheter securely taped to the patient's thigh.	This helps to prevent inadvertent traction on the catheter. Often it is tied to the urethral catheter at the point where they both emerge from the urethra. Both drainage tubes then can be taped together on the patient's thigh.
3. Maintain accurate records of output. (It may vary considerably from patient to patient, depending on the diameter of the ureter in relation to the catheter.)	
4. If scanty or nonexistent output is noted: a. Milk the catheter and tubing. b. If no results, notify the physician.	The catheter may be obstructed. However, this is highly unlikely after this type of surgery, since the catheter bypasses the point where bleeding (and thus clot formation) might occur.
5. Disconnect the tubing only if absolutely necessary. Maintain sterile technique and prevent contamination of open ends of tubing.	Any break in the closed system may result in contamination of the urinary tract.
6. If the physician has ordered that the patient remain in bed while the catheter is in place: a. Explain to the patient that he must remain in bed to prevent accidental displacement of the catheter. b. The patient may not sit in a completely upright position. c. The patient may sit in a semiupright position and and turn from side to side while lying in bed. (See p. 232 for additional interventions for the patient on bed rest.)	Bed rest may be ordered because the catheter is not held in place with sutures. Understanding the reason for a specific regimen increases patient cooperation. The patient should be aware that, if he assumes an erect position, gravity may cause the ureteral catheter to become dislodged and slip into the bladder. It may then require replacement, which is a complicated procedure.

Early postoperative period

---

*May not apply; a ureteral catheter is not always used after this type of surgery.

Plan for implementation	Rationale

7. If the catheter is to be irrigated, use the following guidelines:
  a. Use a syringe with an appropriate size needle that fits snugly into the ureteral catheter.
  b. Aspirate **before** irrigating to relieve distention.
  c. With a different syringe, instill no more than 3 ml of irrigant at one time.
  d. Irrigate very gently.
  e. Maintain sterility throughout the procedure.
	Irrigation may be required if there is no drainage from the catheter **and** the patient is in pain. The absence of drainage indicates obstruction. The presence of pain, in this case, indicates ureteral distention proximal to the obstruction because urine cannot drain through the ureter. Lack of drainage **without** pain usually is not an indication for irrigation because, in this case, urine is draining around the catheter, and the obstruction is not causing structural damage to the urinary tract.

6. NURSING DIAGNOSIS: Postoperative pain

Objective of nursing intervention   Appropriate management of pain or discomfort

Expected outcome   Behavioral and/or verbal indication that pain is adequately reduced or absent

Plan for implementation	Rationale
Determine the source of the pain. It may be related to the catheter(s) or the surgical manipulation.	Pain from different sources usually requires different intervention.
1. Question and observe the patient to obtain information about the pain.	
2. Be aware that pain is a unique and individual experience. Although the different sources of pain can usually be determined by their characteristics, there are also many variations.	
3. Be alert for indications (verbal or behavioral) that the patient is experiencing discomfort other than physical pain, and attempt to resolve the problem.	Fear, loneliness, depression, and numerous other conditions may be sources of extreme discomfort for the patient, who may unconsciously translate these feelings into pain.

PERSISTENT, SEVERE, INCREASING PAIN IN SUPRAPUBIC AREA

See Chapter 11, part one, nursing objective 6.	This pain is probably caused by an obstructed indwelling urethral catheter.

SPASMODIC, INTERMITTENT PAIN IN SUPRAPUBIC AREA, OR PAIN RADIATING TO URETHRAL AREA

See Chapter 11, part one, nursing objective 6.	This pain is probably caused by the urethral catheter's irritating effect on the bladder and irritation of urethral tissue from instrumentation.

Early postoperative period

259

Plan for implementation	Rationale

SPASMODIC PAIN IN FLANK; MAY RADIATE TO SCROTUM OR LABIA

1. If the patient has a ureteral catheter:
   a. Check for obstruction. If it is not draining properly despite milking of the catheter, notify the physician and obtain an order for hand-irrigation of the catheter. (Do not irrigate a ureteral catheter without an order.)

   b. If the catheter is draining well:

      (1) Provide analgesic or antispasmodic medication as ordered.
      (2) Encourage slow abdominal breathing during spasms.

      (3) Reassure the patient that the pain is from the catheter and will disappear after the catheter is removed.

The pain may be caused by an obstructed ureteral catheter that is occluding the ureteral lumen and causing distention in the urinary tract proximal to the catheter.

The ureteral catheter sometimes causes an increase in ureteral peristaltic activity as the ureter attempts to rid itself of the foreign object (i.e., the catheter). This can occur even if the catheter is draining well.
Analgesics reduce the perception of pain; antispasmodics decrease ureteral peristaltic activity.
Deep breathing promotes general relaxation. Concentrating on breathing during spasms may also provide temporary distraction from pain.
This pain may be quite severe and upsetting to the patient, especially since he may have been in similar pain **prior to** surgery because of the ureteral stone.

2. If no ureteral catheter is present:

   a. Notify the physician.
   b. Provide analgesic or antispasmodic medication as ordered.
   c. Encourage slow abdominal breathing during spasms.
   d. Provide reassurance that the pain is temporary and will probably subside within 24 to 48 hours.

The pain may be caused by a clot in the ureter or edema from endoscopic manipulation. Both these conditions may cause temporary obstruction to the flow of urine, which in turn causes distention of the ureter and pain. However, these conditions usually resolve spontaneously.

See rationale for no. 1, b, (1).

See rationale for no. 1, b, (2).

Early postoperative period

7. NURSING DIAGNOSIS: Potential for urinary complications following removal of indwelling urethral (and ureteral) catheter(s)

Objective of nursing intervention
Prevention or early detection of complications

Expected outcomes
{ Resumption of normal voiding pattern
Absence of dysuria
Absence of flank pain, nausea, and vomiting

Plan for implementation	Rationale
See master care plan for the patient with an indwelling urethral catheter: care after removal of the catheter.	
In addition to the items covered in the master care plan, the following nursing action should be included after removal of ureteral catheter (if used).	
Be alert for flank pain, nausea, or vomiting, and notify physician if they occur.	These are symptoms of ureteral obstruction. Although it is highly unlikely that the ureter will become occluded by edema, this possibility must be considered after the removal of the ureteral catheter.

Late postoperative period

8. NURSING DIAGNOSIS: Need for discharge teaching

Objectives of nursing intervention
{ Explanation of basic information about medications to be taken at home
Explanation of information regarding follow-up care
Explanation of residual effects of the condition and/or treatment
Explanation of instructions concerning postdischarge activities
Explanation of symptoms that constitute a reason to contact the physician
Review of admitting diagnosis and mode of treatment

Expected outcomes
{ Accurate return verbalization and/or demonstration of all material learned
Smooth transition of care after discharge
Absence or early detection of complications arising after discharge
Ability to provide future health care practitioners with important data about health history

Plan for implementation	Rationale
See master care plan for the patient requiring discharge preparations: discharge teaching.	
In addition to the topics covered in the master care plan, include the following items in the discharge teaching:
1. At the follow-up office visit the physician will obtain a urine specimen for culture.	Urinary tract infection must be completely eradicated if the patient is to remain free from urinary calculi in the future.

Convalescent period

Plan for implementation	Rationale
2. The physician may prescribe periodic x-ray examinations to check for recurrence of calculi if the patient is a chronic stone former.	Detection of calculi before they become symptomatic may prevent serious renal damage.
3. The expected residual effects of this surgery are minimal. The patient is generally able to resume all usual activities 1 week after surgery.	
4. The patient should notify the physician if any of the following occur: chills, fever, hematuria, flank pain.	These would indicate the presence of a urinary tract infection.
5. Unless contraindicated by coexisting medical conditions, the patient should maintain a fluid intake of **at least** 2.5 L per day for the rest of his life. (See p. 249 for details on hydration regimen.)	A brisk flow of urine through the urinary tract discourages stone formation. Even mild dehydration should be avoided at all times, since crystallization of various constituents of the urine is more likely to occur in a concentrated solution.
6. If medication, dietary limitations, or pH monitoring has been prescribed, provide the patient with all necessary information. (See pp. 250 and 251 for a complete stone prevention regimen.)	

Convalescent period

CHAPTER 30

Ureterolithotomy

Removal of a ureteral calculus by means of an open approach is indicated in the following situations: the stone is in the upper two thirds of the ureter and is therefore impossible to remove endoscopically; it is larger than 1 cm in diameter, so it is unlikely to pass all the way through the ureter; it is obstructing the ureter and is causing renal damage; or it is causing severe symptoms.

Positioning the patient for the procedure depends on the location of the stone. When it is in the upper or middle third of the ureter, the patient is placed on his side (see Fig. 22-1), and a flank incision is made. If the stone is in the lower third of the ureter, the patient is placed in a supine position and an incision is made into the lower abdominal quadrant. The ureter is approached extraperitoneally, and the stone is identified and secured so that it does not dislodge into another portion of the ureter and become inaccessible. A longitudinal incision is made into the ureter, and the stone is removed (Fig. 30-1). This incision is then closed with fine catgut sutures, an incisional drain is inserted, and the main incision is closed. A dressing is applied, and usually an indwelling urethral catheter is inserted to ensure adequate drainage of urine.

URETEROLITHOTOMY
Outline of Care Plan
ANTICIPATED NURSING DIAGNOSES:

Preoperative period
 1. Need for preoperative teaching.
 2. Need for discharge planning.
Early postoperative period
 3. Potential for shock.
 4. Potential for wound complications.
 5. Need for management of indwelling urethral catheter.
 6. Postoperative pain.
 7. Need for management of intravenous infusion.
 8. Potential for respiratory complications related to surgical intervention.
 9. Potential for deep vein thrombosis.
 10. Alterations in gastrointestinal function.
Late postoperative period
 11. Potential for gastrointestinal complications related to resumption of oral intake.
 12. Potential for voiding complications following removal of indwelling urethral catheter.
 13. Potential for wound complications following removal of incisional drain.
Convalescent period
 14. Need for discharge teaching.

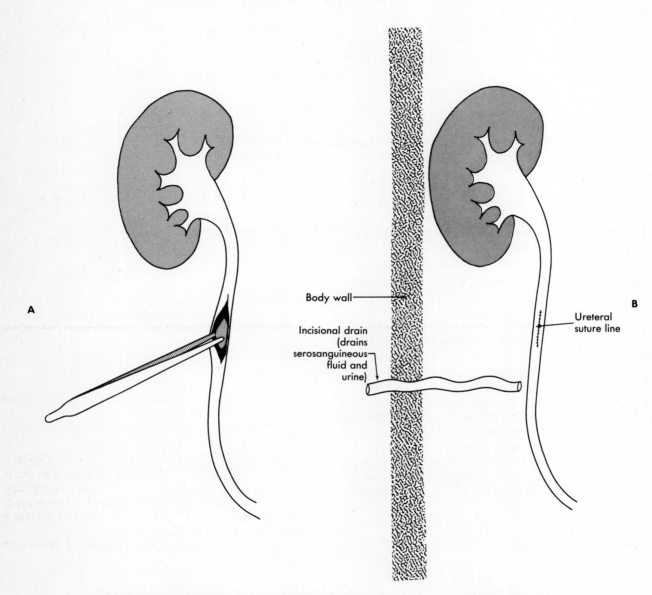

Fig. 30-1. A, Ureterolithotomy; ureteral calculus being removed via an incision in the ureter. **B,** Completed ureterolithotomy; location of drain and ureteral sutures.

NURSING CARE PLAN FOR THE PATIENT UNDERGOING URETEROLITHOTOMY

1. NURSING DIAGNOSIS: Need for preoperative teaching

Objectives of nursing intervention

- If necessary, clarification of reason for hospitalization and type of surgery to be performed
- Elimination of any negative or inaccurate notions regarding the forthcoming surgery
- Explanation of preoperative tests and procedures
- Psychologic preparation for general anesthesia (omit if the patient is to have spinal anesthesia)
- Explanation of events expected in the early postoperative period
- Explanation of body conditions expected in the early postoperative period
- Identification of any known allergies

Expected outcomes

- Verbal indication that explanations are understood
- Verbal indication of optimistic expectations (within realistic limits) related to forthcoming surgery
- Cooperation during preoperative tests and procedures
- Verbal or behavioral indication of reduction of anxiety
- Absence of postoperative complications
- Absence of allergic reactions

Plan for implementation	Rationale
See master care plan for the patient receiving preoperative teaching.	
In addition to the topics covered in the master care plan, include the following items in the preoperative teaching:	
1. Be aware that, in addition to the routine preoperative tests, the following diagnostic studies may have been performed, and answer any questions the patient has regarding them:	
a. Plain x-ray film of the abdomen (KUB)	This is done to locate the stone in the ureter. It will be performed when the patient is admitted to the hospital, but it must be repeated immediately before surgery so that any changes in the location of the stone can be determined.
b. Intravenous pyelogram	This is done to determine renal function and the presence of radiolucent stones in the urinary tract.
c. Retrograde pyelogram	This may be done to assess more precisely the location of the stone.
2. The preoperative shave will be from the nipple line to midthigh on the affected side.	
3. Oral intake will probably be withheld for 24 hours after surgery or until bowel sounds are heard and the patient passes flatus.	There is sometimes a period of intestinal atony following ureterolithotomy due to irritation of the peritoneum. Within 24 to 48 hours it generally resolves itself, but premature oral intake will cause severe abdominal discomfort, distention, and vomiting.

Preoperative period

Plan for implementation	Rationale
4. There will be an indwelling uretheral catheter in place for 1 or 2 days.	
5. The patient will have an incision either in his flank or lower abdomen (depending on the location of the stone). It will be covered with a dressing that may require frequent changing for the first few postoperative days.	

2. NURSING DIAGNOSIS: Need for discharge planning

Objectives of nursing intervention { Early commencement of discharge planning
Accurate estimate of time required for all discharge teaching

Expected outcome Smooth transition of care after discharge

Plan for implementation	Rationale
See master care plan for the patient requiring discharge preparations: discharge planning.	
In addition to the topics covered in the master care plan, the following items should be considered:	
1. The duration of hospitalization for this procedure is approximately 10 days.	
2. Required teaching includes: a. General postoperative discharge teaching b. Possibly instructions for a stone prevention regimen	

Preoperative period

3. NURSING DIAGNOSIS: Potential for shock

Objective of nursing intervention	Prevention or early detection of shock

Expected outcomes {
Vital signs normal, skin dry, color normal
Absence of bright red drainage

Plan for implementation	Rationale
1. Check the patient's vital signs every 2 to 4 hours once stable (every 15 minutes if unstable).	Shock is a potential complication, as it is with any surgery. Although relatively few blood vessels are cut, the duration of surgery may be considerable because sometimes the ureter and the stone are difficult to locate. Therefore neurogenic shock and cardiogenic shock are possibilities that must be considered.
2. Be alert for increasing pulse and respiratory rates, decreasing blood pressure, diaphoresis, pallor, and feelings of apprehension.	
3. Notify the physician at once if indications of impending shock occur.	

4. NURSING DIAGNOSIS: Potential for wound complications

Objective of nursing intervention	Prevention or early detection of complications arising from the incisional area

Expected outcome	Absence of fever, purulent exudate, erythema, edema, dehiscence, hematoma, and other abnormal wound conditions

Plan for implementation	Rationale

1. Check the dressing frequently (every 2 to 4 hours during the first 24 to 48 hours after surgery). Change it when it becomes wet, and use sterile technique for the procedure.	The dressing may become saturated rapidly with serosanguineous fluid and urine from the incision. This is because the suture line in the ureter may not become watertight for at least 48 hours after surgery. A wet dressing must be changed as soon as possible for the following reasons:
	 1. It is a source of infection.
	   a. It acts as a wick, enabling microorganisms on the skin to move toward the incision.
	   b. It provides a good medium for bacterial multiplication.
	 2. It is highly irritating to the skin because of the presence of urine in the drainage.

Early postoperative period

267

Plan for implementation	**Rationale**

2. Note the odor of the drainage. The characteristic odor of urine is not abnormal, but if it is foul smelling:
  a. Notify the physician.
  b. Obtain a wound culture specimen.
	This would indicate a wound infection.
	
	This will facilitate identification of the infecting organism so that appropriate treatment can be instituted quickly.

3. Use caution when removing soiled dressings to prevent inadvertent removal of the incisional drain.	Premature removal of a drain may result in the development of a urinoma and prolonged healing.
4. Cut and arrange gauze pads around the incisional drain, which is usually a Penrose drain.	This prevents the dressings from flattening the drain and possibly obstructing the flow of drainage from the wound.
5. If the dressing requires frequent changing, use Montgomery straps instead of adhesive tape.	This eliminates the need to remove the adhesive tape from the patient's skin each time the dressing is changed. Skin irritation and patient discomfort can be considerably reduced by this method.
6. Note the condition of the suture line. Chart its appearance and the presence of edema, erythema, hematoma, ecchymosis, or other abnormal conditions.	This provides a frame of reference for other staff members caring for the patient.
7. Notify the physician if there is any evidence of dehiscence.	
8. Check the patient's temperature every 4 hours and notify the physician if there is an elevation above 101°.	Wound infection must always be suspected when the patient runs a fever postoperatively. Other causes include respiratory complications and pharmacologic intervention.

Early postoperative period

5. NURSING DIAGNOSIS: Need for management of indwelling urethral catheter

Objectives of nursing intervention

Appropriate care of catheter and equipment
Prevention or early detection of infection
Care of tissue surrounding catheter
Maintenance of accurate records of urine output
Appropriate administration of hand-irrigation of catheter
Management of discomfort or pain caused by catheter
Satisfactory collection of urine specimens from catheter

Expected outcomes

Absence of severe bladder spasms and suprapubic distention
Urine draining freely through system
Absence of fever, chills, and foul-smelling urine
Absence of urethral discharge and tissue inflammation
Minimal discomfort caused by the catheter
Urine specimens in optimum condition for all necessary tests

Plan for implementation	Rationale
See master care plan for the patient with an indwelling urethral catheter: care after insertion of the catheter.	
In addition to the topics covered in the master care plan, the following interventions are required:	
1. Notify the physician if the urine turns bright red and has a high viscosity. The urine should be blood tinged to clear amber within 48 hours after surgery.	There should be relatively little blood in the urine after this type of surgery because the incision in the ureter is usually small and hemostasis is not a problem. The appearance of bright red urine requires investigation.
2. Be aware that the urine output through the catheter is only part of the patient's total output. Frequently a great deal of urine passes through the incisional drain into the dressing in the early postoperative period.	Until the suture line in the ureter becomes watertight, urine will leak into the abdominal cavity. It will then flow out of the body through the incisional drain.

Early postoperative period

6. NURSING DIAGNOSIS: Postoperative pain

<table>
<tr><td>**Objective of nursing intervention**</td><td>Appropriate management of pain or discomfort</td></tr>
<tr><td>**Expected outcome**</td><td>Behavioral and/or verbal indication that pain is adequately reduced or absent</td></tr>
</table>

Plan for implementation	Rationale
Determine the source of the pain. It may be related to the catheter or the surgical wound.	Pain from different sources usually requires different intervention.
1. Question and observe the patient to obtain information about the pain.	
2. Be aware that pain is a unique and individual experience. Although the different sources of pain can usually be determined by their characteristics, there are also many variations.	
3. Be alert for indications (verbal or behavioral) that the patient is experiencing discomfort other than physical pain, and attempt to resolve the problem.	Fear, loneliness, depression, and numerous other conditions may be sources of extreme discomfort for the patient, who may unconsciously translate these feelings into pain.

Early postoperative period

PERSISTENT, SEVERE, INCREASING PAIN IN SUPRAPUBIC AREA

See Chapter 11, part one, nursing objective 6.	This pain is probably caused by an obstructed catheter.

SPASMODIC, INTERMITTENT PAIN IN SUPRAPUBIC AREA, OR PAIN RADIATING TO URETHRAL AREA

See Chapter 11, part one, nursing objective 6.	This pain is probably caused by the catheter's irritating effect on the bladder.

MODERATE TO SEVERE PAIN AT SURGICAL SITE, USUALLY AGGRAVATED BY PHYSICAL ACTIVITY

1. Be certain the catheter is not obstructed. Although pain with these characteristics is usually of incisional origin and is expected, the patient may not be able to identify accurately the precise location of the pain.	Catheter obstruction must be ruled out first because it cannot remain untreated. However, after this type of surgery it is unlikely for the catheter to become obstructed because there is rarely enough blood in the drainage for clots to form, and no tissue particles are normally passed in the urine.
2. Administer analgesics as ordered.	Analgesic medication usually provides considerable relief from incisional pain.

Plan for implementation	Rationale
3. Plan the patient's activities to coincide with a time when there is a high level of pain medication in the patient's bloodstream.	The patient will cooperate better with coughing exercises, ambulating, bathing, etc. when the pain is well under control.
4. Notify the physician if the patient's requests for pain medication do not decrease within 48 to 72 hours.	Although the intensity of postoperative pain varies enormously between patients, there should be a marked decrease in the apparent severity of the pain within 2 or 3 days. If this does not occur, it may indicate the development of wound complications.

7. NURSING DIAGNOSIS: Need for management of intravenous infusion

Objectives of nursing intervention

- Appropriate administration of specific types of intravenous solutions
- Prevention or early detection of local complications
- Prevention or early detection of systemic complications
- Management of discomfort caused by the intravenous infusion
- Maintenance of proper function of intravenous equipment
- Maintenance of accurate records of the patient's hydration status

Expected outcomes

- Normal hydration status
- Normal electrolyte status
- Absence of thrombophlebitis, infiltration, infection, fluid overload, and pulmonary embolism
- Absence of discomfort caused by the intravenous infusion

Plan for implementation	Rationale
See master care plan for the patient receiving intravenous therapy.	These patients usually receive isotonic dextrose and saline solutions. Antibiotics will be given also if the urine was infected before surgery.

Early postoperative period

271

Early postoperative period

8. NURSING DIAGNOSIS: Potential for respiratory complications related to surgical intervention

Objective of nursing intervention	Prevention or early detection of atelectasis and/or pneumonia

Expected outcomes	Cooperation with therapeutic respiratory regimen
	Absence of fever or audible lung congestion
	Sputum clear or white and easily mobilized

Plan for implementation	Rationale
See master care plan for the patient at risk for respiratory complications, nursing objective 3.	

9. NURSING DIAGNOSIS: Potential for deep vein thrombosis

Objectives of nursing intervention	Explanation and maintenance of precautions against deep vein thrombosis
	Early detection of deep vein thrombosis

Expected outcomes	Cooperation with regimen to prevent deep vein thrombosis
	Absence of local pain, swelling, and redness of a lower extremity
	Absence of fever

Plan for implementation	Rationale
See master care plan for the patient at risk for deep vein thrombosis.	

10. NURSING DIAGNOSIS: Alterations in gastrointestinal function

Objectives of nursing intervention { Prohibition of oral intake as ordered
Promotion of patient comfort

Expected outcome   Return of bowel sounds and passage of flatus within 24 to 48 hours

Plan for implementation	Rationale
1. Inform the patient that he is to have no oral intake. Notify the auxiliary staff as well, so that no one inadvertently gives the patient something to eat or drink.	There is often a period of intestinal atony following this type of surgery. Within 48 hours it usually resolves itself, but premature oral intake will cause severe abdominal discomfort, distention, and vomiting. Although most patients will not feel like eating at this time, the nurse cannot rely on this alone as a deterrent to oral intake. If water is left at the patient's bedside, he may drink it.
2. Provide mouth care as needed.	Lack of salivary stimulation often causes dryness and an unpleasant taste in the patient's mouth.
3. Check periodically for bowel sounds and passage of flatus, and notify the physician when they occur.	These are indications that the intestines are regaining their function.

Early postoperative period

11. NURSING DIAGNOSIS: Potential for gastrointestinal complications related to resumption of oral intake

Objective of nursing intervention   Early detection of gastrointestinal complications

Expected outcomes { Absence of abdominal distension, tympany, nausea, or vomiting
Return to normal bowel function

Plan for implementation	Rationale
1. Permit oral intake of fluids and food only on the physician's orders.	The physician will usually wait until bowel sounds are heard and the patient passes flatus before permitting him to have anything by mouth.
2. Note the presence of distention, tympany, nausea, or vomiting. Otherwise, if ordered, advance the diet as tolerated.	
3. Inform the physician if the patient has not had a bowel movement for more than 2 days after resumption of oral intake.	A cathartic is usually indicated at this stage in the patient's recuperation if he has not moved his bowels spontaneously.

Late postoperative period

Late postoperative period

12. NURSING DIAGNOSIS: Potential for voiding complications following removal of indwelling urethral catheter

| **Objective of nursing intervention** | Prevention or early detection of complications |

| **Expected outcomes** | { Resumption of normal voiding pattern
Absence of dysuria |

Plan for implementation	**Rationale**
See master care plan for the patient with an indwelling urethral catheter: care after removal of the catheter.	

13. NURSING DIAGNOSIS: Potential for wound complications following removal of incisional drain

| **Objective of nursing intervention** | Prevention of skin irritation and breakdown at or near incisional area |

| **Expected outcomes** | { Absence of skin discoloration
Absence of disruption of skin integrity
Gradual termination of incisional drainage |

Plan for implementation	**Rationale**
1. Check the dressing frequently and change it as soon as it becomes saturated.	Urine may continue to drain from the wound for a few days after removal of the incisional drain. If wet dressings remain in contact with the skin, the urine will cause skin breakdown.
2. If copious drainage is a problem, place an ostomy bag over the incision.	This protects the surrounding skin and provides more accurate information about the volume of drainage than does a dressing.
a. Use a skin barrier such as Stomahesive before applying the bag.	This protects the surrounding skin and facilitates adherence of the bag.
b. Do not use any karaya products near the wound.	Karaya melts when it is in contact with urine, and particles may enter the wound.
c. When possible, use a bag with an antireflux valve so that there is no stasis of urine over the former drain site.	These bags are not sterile. Contamination of the wound may occur if drainage is permitted to remain in contact with any portion of the wound.

14. NURSING DIAGNOSIS: Need for discharge teaching

Objectives of nursing intervention

Explanation of basic information about medications to be taken at home
Explanation of information regarding follow-up care
Explanation of residual effects of the condition and/or treatment
Explanation of instructions concerning postdischarge activities
Explanation of symptoms that constitute a reason to contact the physician
Review of admitting diagnosis and mode of treatment

Expected outcomes

Accurate return verbalization and/or demonstration of all material learned
Smooth transition of care after discharge
Absence or early detection of complications arising after discharge
Ability to provide future health care practitioners with important data about health history

Plan for implementation	Rationale
See master care plan for the patient requiring discharge preparations: discharge teaching.	
In addition to the topics covered in the master care plan, include the following items in the discharge teaching:	
1. At the follow-up office visit the physician will obtain a urine specimen for culture and will check the incision for adequate healing.	Urinary tract infection must be completely eradicated if the patient is to remain free from urinary calculi in the future.
2. The physician may prescribe periodic x-ray examinations to check for recurrence of calculi if the patient has a history of urolithiasis.	Detection of calculi before they become symptomatic may prevent serious renal damage.
3. The expected residual effects of this surgery are incisional discomfort and fatigue during the next few weeks.	
4. The patient should notify the physician if any of the following occur: a. Chills, fever, hematuria, flank pain b. Fever, pain, and/or increasing redness at the incisional site	These may indicate a urinary tract infection. This may indicate a wound infection.
5. Unless contraindicated by coexisting medical conditions, the patient should maintain a fluid intake of **at least** 2.5 L per day for the rest of his life. (See p. 249 for details on hydration regimen.)	A brisk flow of urine through the urinary tract discourages stone formation. Even mild dehydration should be avoided at all times, since crystallization of various constituents of the urine is more likely to occur in a concentrated solution.

Convalescent period

Plan for implementation	**Rationale**

Convalescent period

6. If medication, dietary limitations, or pH monitoring has been prescribed, provide the patient with all necessary information. (See pp. 250 and 251 for complete stone prevention regimen.)

7. If the wound is still draining at time of discharge:
   a. Teach the patient and/or significant other wound care.
   b. Obtain adequate return verbalization and demonstration.
   c. Provide the patient with an adequate supply of dressings and tape.

CHAPTER 31

Ureteroneocystostomy (ureteral reimplantation)

There are numerous methods of ureteral reimplantation. The following description concerns that used for the most common conditions requiring this type of surgery—ureterovesical reflux, distal ureteral strictures, and ureteral injuries.

For the procedure the patient is placed in a supine position, and a transverse suprapubic incision is made. The bladder is opened, and the ureteral orifice is identified. An incision is made around the orifice, and the ureter is mobilized. An opening is made in the bladder wall (usually superior to the original orifice), and a tunnel is created between the bladder mucosa and the muscle. The ureter is then reinserted into the bladder through this tunnel and sutured to the bladder. This tunneling procedure results in a longer segment of ureter under the bladder mucosa, which produces a valvelike mechanism in preventing reflux (Fig. 31-1).

A ureteral catheter is left in place to prevent obstruction of the ureter from edema, and an indwelling urethral catheter is inserted and tied to the ureteral catheter to maintain the position of the ureteral catheter in the ureter. The wound is closed with an incisional drain, and a dressing is applied.*

---

*When this procedure is done for undiversion of an ileal or colon conduit, the conduit itself may be anastomozed to the bladder. This procedure involves a larger incision and a longer recovery period. However, a ureteral catheter is usually not used.

URETERONEOCYSTOSTOMY
Outline of Care Plan
ANTICIPATED NURSING DIAGNOSES:
Preoperative period
   1. Need for preoperative teaching.
   2. Need for discharge planning.
Early postoperative period
   3. Potential for shock.
   4. Potential for wound complications.
   5. Need for management of indwelling urethral catheter.
   6. Need for management of ureteral catheter.
   7. Postoperative pain.
   8. Need for management of intravenous infusion.
   9. Potential for deep vein thrombosis.
  10. Potential for respiratory complications related to surgical intervention.
Late postoperative period
  11. Potential for complications following removal of ureteral catheter.
  12. Potential for voiding complications following removal of indwelling urethral catheter.
Convalescent period
  13. Need for discharge teaching.

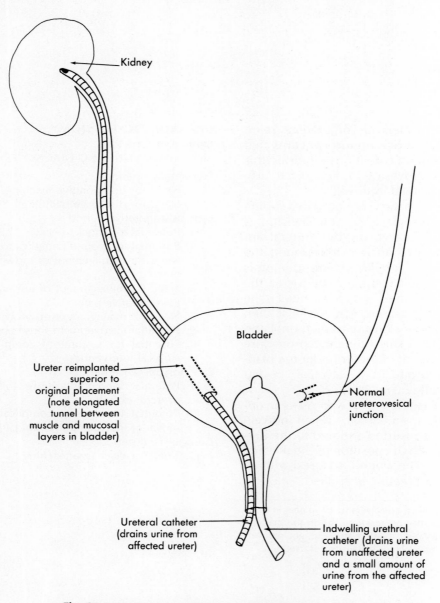

Kidney

Bladder

Ureter reimplanted
superior to
original placement
(note elongated
tunnel between
muscle and mucosal
layers in bladder)

Normal
ureterovesical
junction

Ureteral catheter
(drains urine from
affected ureter)

Indwelling urethral
catheter (drains urine
from unaffected ureter
and a small amount of
urine from the affected
ureter)

Fig. 31-1. Ureteroneocystostomy (reimplantation of ureter).

NURSING CARE PLAN FOR THE PATIENT UNDERGOING URETERONEOCYSTOSTOMY (URETERAL REIMPLANTATION)

1. NURSING DIAGNOSIS: Need for preoperative teaching

Objectives of nursing intervention

If necessary, clarification of reason for hospitalization and type of surgery to be performed

Elimination of any negative or inaccurate notions regarding the forthcoming surgery

Explanation of preoperative tests and procedures

Psychologic prepration for general anesthesia (omit if the patient is to have spinal anesthesia)

Explanation of events expected in the early postoperative period

Explanation of body conditions expected in the early postoperative period

Identification of any known allergies

Expected outcomes

Verbal indication that explanations are understood

Verbal indication of optimistic expectations (within realistic limits) related to forthcoming surgery

Cooperation during preoperative tests and procedures

Verbal or behavioral indication of reduction of anxiety

Absence of postoperative complications

Absence of allergic reactions

Plan for implementation	Rationale
See master care plan for the patient receiving preoperative teaching.	
In addition to the topics covered in the master care plan, include the following items in the preoperative teaching:	
1. Be aware that, in addition to routine preoperative tests, the following diagnostic studies may have been performed prior to this surgery, and answer any questions the patient has regarding them:	
a. Intravenous pyelogram	This is done to determine pathologic conditions in the upper urinary tract that often result from reflux.
b. Voiding cystourethrogram	This is done to visualize more accurately the presence and degree of reflux.
2. The preoperative shave will be from umbilicus to mid-thigh.	
3. The patient may be permitted a light meal in the evening after surgery.	

Preoperative period

Plan for implementation	Rationale
4. The patient will have two tubes coming out of his urethra through which urine will drain. One tube is a catheter from the bladder; the other (smaller) one is from the ureter. Depending on the physician's discretion, the patient may have to remain in bed for as long as the ureteral catheter is present (3 to 5 days) to prevent it from becoming displaced.	
5. The patient should not be alarmed if his urine is blood tinged.	
6. There will be an incision in the patient's abdomen that will be covered with a dressing. The dressing may require frequent changing in the early postoperative period.	

2. NURSING DIAGNOSIS: Need for discharge planning

Objectives of nursing intervention
- Early commencement of discharge planning
- Accurate estimate of time required for all discharge teaching

Expected outcome Smooth transition of care after discharge

Plan for implementation	Rationale
See master care plan for the patient requiring discharge preparations: discharge planning.	
In addition to the topics covered in the master care plan, the following items should be considered:	
1. The duration of hospitalization for this procedure is approximately 10 days.	
2. Required teaching consists of general postoperative discharge teaching.	

Preoperative period

3. NURSING DIAGNOSIS: Potential for shock

Objective of nursing intervention   Prevention or early detection of shock

Expected outcomes   { Vital signs normal, skin dry, color normal
Absence of bright red drainage

Plan for implementation	Rationale
1. Check the patient's vital signs every 4 hours once stable (every 15 minutes if unstable).	Shock is a potential complication after surgery requiring general anesthesia and an incision. However, blood loss from this type of surgery is generally minimal, and the incidence of shock is relatively low.
2. Be alert for increasing pulse and respiratory rates, decreasing blood pressure, diaphoresis, pallor, and feelings of apprehension.	
3. Notify the physician at once if indications of impending shock occur.	

Early postoperative period

4. NURSING DIAGNOSIS: Potential for wound complications

Objective of nursing intervention   Prevention or early detection of complications arising from the incisional area

Expected outcome   Absence of fever, purulent exudate, erythema, edema, dehiscence, hematoma, and other abnormal wound conditions

Plan for implementation	Rationale
1. Check the dressing frequently (every 2 to 4 hours during the first 24 to 48 hours after surgery.) Change it when it becomes wet and use sterile technique for the procedure.	The dressing may become saturated rapidly with serosanguineous fluid and urine from the incision. This is because the suture line in the bladder may not become watertight for at least 48 hours after surgery. A wet dressing must be changed as soon as possible for the following reasons:
	1. It is a source of infection.
	a. It acts as a wick, enabling microorganisms on the skin to move toward the incision.
	b. It provides a good medium for bacterial multiplication.
	2. It is highly irritating to the skin because of the presence of urine in the drainage.

Plan for implementation	Rationale

2. Note the odor of the drainage. The characteristic odor of urine is not abnormal, but if it is foul smelling:
  a. Notify the physician.
  b. Obtain a wound culture specimen.
	This would indicate a wound infection.
	
	This will facilitate identification of the infecting organism so that appropriate treatment can be instituted quickly.

3. Use caution when removing soiled dressings to prevent inadvertent removal of the incisional drain.	Premature removal of a drain may result in the development of a urinoma and prolonged healing.
4. Cut and arrange gauze pads around the incisional drain, which is usually a Penrose drain.	This prevents the dressings from flattening the drain and possibly obstructing the flow of drainage from the wound.
5. If the dressing requires frequent changing, use Montgomery straps instead of adhesive tape.	This eliminates the need to remove the adhesive tape from the patient's skin each time the dressing is changed. Skin irritation and patient discomfort can be considerably reduced by this method.
6. Note the condition of the suture line. Chart its appearance and the presence of edema, erythema, hematoma, ecchymosis, or other abnormal conditions.	This provides a frame of reference for other staff members caring for the patient.
7. Notify the physician if there is any evidence of dehiscence.	
8. Check the patient's temperature every 4 hours and notify the physician if there is an elevation above 101°.	Wound infection must always be suspected when the patients runs a fever postoperatively. Other causes include respiratory complications and pharmacologic intervention.

Early postoperative period

5. NURSING DIAGNOSIS: Need for management of indwelling urethral catheter

Objectives of nursing intervention

Appropriate care of catheter and equipment

Prevention or early detection of infection

Care of tissue surrounding catheter

Maintenance of accurate records of urine output

Appropriate administration of hand-irrigation of catheter

Management of discomfort or pain caused by catheter

Satisfactory collection of urine specimens from catheter

Expected outcomes

Absence of severe bladder spasms and suprapubic distention

Urine draining freely through system

Absence of fever, chills, and foul-smelling urine

Absence of urethral discharge and tissue inflammation

Minimal discomfort caused by the catheter

Urine specimens in optimum condition for all necessary tests

Plan for implementation	Rationale
See master care plan for the patient with an indwelling urethral catheter: care after insertion of catheter.	
In addition to the topics covered in the master care plan, the following interventions are required:	
1. Notify the physician if the urine turns bright red and has a high viscosity. The urine is usually blood tinged to clear within 48 hours after this type of surgery.	There should be relatively little active bleeding into the bladder after this type of surgery. The appearance of bright red blood requires investigation.
2. Label the collecting container appropriately to distinguish it from that of the ureteral catheter.	This reduces the risk of making a mistake in recording the output from the urethral catheter. Urine draining through this catheter is from the unaffected ureter and may include a small amount of urine from the affected ureter, since some urine usually drains around the ureteral catheter.
3 Keep the urethral and ureteral catheters tied together with suture material.	The catheters are usually tied in the operating room, and rarely does the suture material need replacing. The purpose of tying the catheters is to help maintain the position of the ureteral catheter in the ureter.
4. If the catheter requires irrigation, use gentle pressure on the syringe.	Excessive pressure may disrupt the suture line in the bladder.

Early postoperative period

6. NURSING DIAGNOSIS: Need for management of ureteral catheter

Objective of nursing intervention   Prevention or early detection of complications related to the ureteral catheter

Expected outcomes { Urine draining freely through system
Absence of fever, chills, or foul-smelling urine

Plan for implementation	Rationale
1. Irrigate the catheter only if specifically ordered and only after the technique has been previously mastered.	Unless done with extreme care and skill, irrigation of a ureteral catheter could cause serious damage to the ureter and kidney. Rarely is irrigation required after this type of surgery.
2. Keep the catheter securely taped to the patient's thigh.	This helps to prevent inadvertent traction on the catheter. Often it is tied to the urethral catheter at the point where they both emerge from the urethra. Both drainage tubes can then be taped together on the patient's thigh.
3. Maintain accurate records of output. It may vary considerably from patient to patient, depending on the diameter of the ureter in relation to the catheter.	

4. If scanty or nonexistent output is noted:
  a. Milk the catheter and tubing.
  b. If no results, notify the physician.
	The catheter may be obstructed. However, this is highly unlikely after this type of surgery, since the catheter bypasses the point where bleeding (and thus clot formation) might occur.

5. Disconnect the tubing only if absolutely necessary. Maintain sterile technique and prevent contamination of open ends of tubing.	Any break in the closed system may result in contamination of the urinary tract.

6. If the physician has ordered that the patient remain in bed while the catheter is in place:
  a. Explain to the patient that he must remain in bed to prevent accidental displacement of the catheter.
  b. The patient may not sit in a completely upright position.
  c. The patient may sit in a semiupright position and turn from side to side while lying in bed. (See p. 232 for additional interventions for the patient on bed rest.)
	Bed rest may be ordered because the catheter is not held in place with sutures.
	Understanding the reason for a specific regimen increases patient cooperation. The patient should be aware that, if he assumes an erect position, gravity may cause the ureteral catheter to become dislodged and slip into the bladder. It may then require replacement, which is a complicated procedure.

Early postoperative period

Plan for implementation	Rationale
7. If the catheter is to be irrigated, use the following guidelines: a. Use a syringe with an appropriate size needle that fits snugly into the ureteral catheter. b. Aspirate **before** irrigating to relieve distention. c. With a different syringe, instill no more than 3 ml of irrigant at one time. d. Irrigate very gently. e. Maintain sterility throughout the procedure.	Irrigation may be required if there is no drainage from the catheter **and** the patient is in pain. The absence of drainage indicates obstruction. The presence of pain, in this case, indicates ureteral distention proximal to the obstruction because urine cannot drain through the ureter. Lack of drainage **without** pain is usually not an indication for irrigation because, in this case, urine is draining around the catheter, and the obstruction is not causing structural damage to the urinary tract.

7. NURSING DIAGNOSIS: Postoperative pain

Objective of nursing intervention   Appropriate management of pain or discomfort

Expected outcome   Behavioral and/or verbal indication that pain is adequately reduced or absent

Plan for implementation	Rationale
Determine the source of the pain. It may be related to the catheters or the surgical wound. 1. Question and observe the patient to obtain information about the pain.	Pain from different sources usually requires different intervention.
2. Be aware that pain is a unique and individual experience. Although the different sources of pain can usually be determined by their characteristics, there are also many variations.	
3. Be alert for indications (verbal or behavioral) that the patient is experiencing discomfort other than physical pain, and attempt to resolve the problem.	Fear, loneliness, depression, and numerous other conditions may be sources of extreme discomfort for the patient, who may unconsciously translate these feelings into pain.

PERSISTENT, SEVERE, INCREASING PAIN IN SUPRAPUBIC AREA

See Chapter 11, part one, nursing objective 6.	This pain is probably caused by an obstructed indwelling urethral catheter.

SPASMODIC, INTERMITTENT PAIN IN SUPRAPUBIC AREA, OR PAIN RADIATING TO URETHRAL AREA

See Chapter 11, part one, nursing objective 6.	This pain is probably caused by the urethral catheter's irritating effect on the bladder.

Early postoperative period

Plan for implementation	Rationale

SPASMODIC PAIN IN FLANK; MAY RADIATE TO SCROTUM OR LABIA

Plan for implementation	Rationale
1. Check for obstruction of ureteral catheter. If it is not draining properly despite milking of the tubing, notify the physician and obtain an order for hand-irrigation of the catheter. (Do **not** irrigate a ureteral catheter without an order.)	The pain may be caused by an obstructed ureteral catheter that is occluding the ureteral lumen and causing distention in the upper urinary tract.
2. If the catheter is draining well:	The ureteral catheter sometimes causes an increase in ureteral peristaltic activity as the ureter attempts to rid itself of the foreign object (i.e., the catheter). This can occur even if the catheter is draining well.
a. Provide analgesic or antispasmodic medication as ordered.	Analgesics reduce the perception of pain; antispasmodics decrease ureteral peristaltic activity.
b. Encourage slow abdominal breathing during spasms.	Deep breathing promotes general relaxation. Concentrating on breathing during spasms may also provide temporary distraction from pain.
c. Reassure the patient that the pain is from the catheter and will disappear after the catheter is removed (usually 3 to 5 days).	

MODERATE TO SEVERE PAIN AT SURGICAL SITE, USUALLY AGGRAVATED BY PHYSICAL ACTIVITY

Plan for implementation	Rationale
1. Be certain the catheters are not obstructed. Although pain with these characteristics is usually of incisional origin and is expected, the patient may not be able to identify accurately the precise location or quality of the pain.	Catheter obstruction must be ruled out first because it cannot remain untreated. However, after this type of surgery it is unlikely for the catheters to become obstructed because there is rarely enough blood in the drainage for clots to form, and no tissue particles are normally passed in the urine.
2. Administer analgesics as ordered.	Analgesic medication usually provides considerable relief from incisional pain.
3. Plan the patient's activities to coincide with a time when there is a high level of pain medication in the patient's bloodstream.	The patient will cooperate better with coughing exercises, ambulating, bathing, etc. when the pain is well under control.
4. Notify the physician if the patient's requests for pain medication do not decrease within 48 to 72 hours.	Although the intensity of postoperative pain varies enormously between patients, there should be a marked decrease in the apparent severity of the pain within 2 or 3 days. If this does not occur, it may indicate the development of wound complications.

Early postoperative period

8. NURSING DIAGNOSIS: Need for management of intravenous infusion

Objectives of nursing intervention
- Appropriate administration of specific types of intravenous solutions
- Prevention or early detection of local complications
- Prevention or early detection of systemic complications
- Management of discomfort caused by the intravenous infusion
- Maintenance of proper function of intravenous equipment
- Maintenance of accurate records of the patient's hydration status

Expected outcomes
- Normal hydration status
- Normal electrolyte status
- Absence of thrombophlebitis, infiltration, infection, fluid overload, and pulmonary embolism
- Absence of discomfort caused by the intravenous infusion

Plan for implementation	Rationale
See master care plan for the patient receiving intravenous therapy.	These patients usually receive isotonic dextrose and saline solutions. Antibiotics may be ordered if the patient had infected urine prior to the surgery or for prophylactic reasons.

9. NURSING DIAGNOSIS: Potential for deep vein thrombosis

Objectives of nursing intervention
- Explanation and maintenance of precautions against deep vein thrombosis
- Early detection of deep vein thrombosis

Expected outcomes
- Cooperation with regimen to prevent deep vein thrombosis
- Absence of local pain, swelling, and redness of a lower extremity
- Absence of fever

Plan for implementation	Rationale
See master care plan for the patient at risk for deep vein thrombosis.	These patients may be at increased risk for deep vein thrombosis if they must remain in bed for a few days after surgery to maintain placement of the ureteral catheter. In this case the possibility of venous stasis is increased.

Early postoperative period

Early postoperative period

10. NURSING DIAGNOSIS: Potential for respiratory complications related to surgical intervention

Objective of nursing intervention

Prevention or early detection of atelectasis and/or pneumonia

Expected outcomes

Cooperation with therapeutic respiratory regimen

Absence of fever or audible lung congestion

Sputum clear or white and easily mobilized

Plan for implementation	Rationale
See master care plan for the patient at risk for respiratory complications, nursing objective 2.	

Late postoperative period

11. NURSING DIAGNOSIS: Potential for complications following removal of ureteral catheter

Objective of nursing intervention

Early detection of ureteral obstruction

Expected outcomes

Absence of ureteral colic

Urine output proportional in quantity to input

Plan for implementation	Rationale
1. Continue to keep accurate records of the patient's urinary output (via the indwelling urethral catheter).	The urethral catheter is usually left indwelling for 24 to 48 hours after removal of the ureteral catheter.
2. Notify the physician if any of the following conditions occur: a. The patient has colicky pain in the flank or radiating to the scrotum or labia. b. The patient experiences nausea and vomiting.	Although it is highly unlikely that the ureter will become occluded, the possibility of continued edema at the surgical site must be considered. Any indications of this must be reported so appropriate treatment (usually recatheterization) can be instituted.
3. If the patient has been on best rest while the ureteral catheter was in place, have him dangle his legs over the side of the bed for a few minutes before standing up.	This is a precaution against orthostatic hypotension. It enables the vascular bed to adjust to changes in the patient's position. This sometimes takes longer than usual after sustained bed rest.

12. NURSING DIAGNOSIS: Potential for voiding complications following removal of indwelling urethral catheter

Objective of nursing intervention	Prevention or early detection of complications

Expected outcomes	{ Resumption of normal voiding pattern Absence of dysuria

Plan for implementation	**Rationale**
See master care plan for the patient with an indwelling urethral catheter: care after removal of the catheter.	

13. NURSING DIAGNOSIS: Need for discharge teaching

Objectives of nursing intervention	{ Explanation of basic information about medications to be taken at home Explanation of information regarding follow-up care Explanation of residual effects of the condition and/or treatment Explanation of instructions concerning postdischarge activities Explanation of symptoms that constitute a reason to contact the physician Review of admitting diagnosis and mode of treatment

Expected outcomes	{ Accurate return verbalization and/or demonstration of all material learned Smooth transition of care after discharge Absence or early detection of complications arising after discharge Ability to provide future health care practitioners with important data about health history

Plan for implementation	**Rationale**
See master care plan for the patient requiring discharge preparations: discharge teaching.	
In addition to the topics covered in the master care plan, include the following items in the discharge teaching:	
1. At the follow-up office visit the physician will check the wound for adequate healing and will obtain a urine specimen for culture.	The urine culture is particularly important because many of these patients had chronic urinary tract infection before surgery.
2. During the next few weeks the expected residual effects of the surgery are incisional discomfort and fatigue.	

Plan for implementation	Rationale
3. The patient should notify the physician if any of the following occur:	
a. Chills, fever, flank pain, or hematuria	These may indicate a urinary tract infection.
b. Severe pain and/or increasing discomfort at the incisional site	These may indicate a wound infection.
4. The patient may be scheduled for periodic x-ray examinations or renal scans during the next few years to assess the condition of the ureter.	Intravenous pyelograms, cystograms, or renal scans are performed to determine the degree of postoperative ureteral dilatation and then to monitor the ureter's return to normal structure and function.

Convalescent period

References and bibliography

BIBLIOGRAPHY

Blandy, J.: Operative urology, London, England, 1975, Blackwell Scientific Publications.

Goodman, L.S., and Gilman, A.: The pharmacologic basis of therapeutics, ed. 6, New York, 1980, Macmillan Publishing Co., Inc.

Lamensdorf, H., Compere, D.E., and Begley, G.F.: Forceful endoscopic extraction of ureteral calculi, Urology **4:**301, 1973.

Lapides, J.: Fundamentals of urology, Philadelphia, 1976, W.B. Saunders Co.

Morel, A., and Wise, J.W.: Urologic endoscopic procedures, ed. 2, St. Louis, 1979, The C.V. Mosby Co.

Physician's desk reference, ed. 35, Oradell, N.J., 1981, Medical Economics Co.

Smith, D.R.: General urology, ed. 9, Los Angeles, 1978, Lange Medical Publications.

Winter, C.W., and Morel, A.: Nursing care of patients with urologic disease, ed. 4, St. Louis, 1977, The C.V. Mosby Co.

UNIT VII

PROCEDURES FOR DISORDERS
OF
THE BLADDER

CHAPTER 32

Cystolitholapaxy and cystolithotripsy

Endoscopic removal of a bladder calculus is indicated when the stone is soft enough to crush or shatter and when there is no urethral pathologic condition contraindicating instrumentation.

For the procedure the patient is placed in a lithotomy position, and a cystoscopy is performed to assess the size of the stone and to rule out other bladder disorders such as a tumor or diverticulum. If additional disease exists, an open procedure might be indicated.

If litholapaxy is to be performed, a lithotrite is inserted and the bladder is filled with saline. The stone is engaged in the jaws of the instrument and is crushed (Fig. 32-1). If a lithotripsy is to be performed, a lithotriptor is inserted and the bladder is filled with a nonconducting fluid such as glycine. An electrode is advanced into the bladder to make contact with the stone, and a few bursts of high-voltage current disintegrate the stone instantaneously.

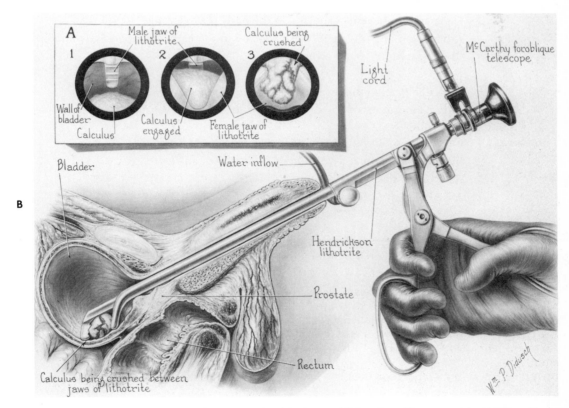

Fig. 32-1. Vesical calculus being crushed in jaws of lithotrite. (Courtesy Mr. William P. Didusch and American Cystoscope Makers, Inc., Stamford, Conn.)

After the stone is either crushed or disintegrated, the fragments are irrigated out through the cystoscope, and an indwelling urethral catheter is inserted to ensure adequate drainage.

CYSTOLITHOLAPAXY OR CYSTOLITHOTRIPSY
Outline of Care Plan
ANTICIPATED NURSING DIAGNOSES:

Preoperative period
1. Need for preoperative teaching.
2. Need for discharge planning.

Early postoperative period
3. Potential for postoperative complications (shock, atelectasis, pneumonia, deep vein thrombosis, infection).
4. Need for management of indwelling urethral catheter.
5. Postoperative pain.

Late postoperative period
6. Potential for voiding complications following removal of indwelling urethral catheter.

Convalescent period
7. Need for discharge teaching.

NURSING CARE PLAN FOR THE PATIENT UNDERGOING CYSTOLITHOLAPAXY OR CYSTOLITHOTRIPSY

1. NURSING DIAGNOSIS: Need for preoperative teaching

Objectives of nursing intervention	If necessary, clarification of reason for hospitalization and type of surgery to be performed
	Elimination of any negative or inaccurate notions regarding the forthcoming surgery
	Explanation of preoperative tests and procedures
	Psychologic preparation for general anesthesia (omit if the patient is to have spinal anesthesia)
	Explanation of events expected in the early postoperative period
	Explanation of body conditions expected in the early postoperative period
	Identification of any known allergies
Expected outcomes	Verbal indication that explanations are understood
	Verbal indications of optimistic expectations (within realistic limits) related to forthcoming surgery
	Cooperation during preoperative tests and procedures
	Verbal or behavioral indication of reduction of anxiety
	Absence of postoperative complications
	Absence of allergic reactions

Preoperative period

Plan for implementation	Rationale
See master care plan for the patient receiving preoperative teaching.	
In addition to the topics covered in the master care plan, include the following items in the preoperative teaching:	
1. Be aware that, in addition to routine preoperative tests, the following diagnostic studies may have been performed, and answer any questions the patient has regarding them:	
a. Plain x-ray examination of the abdomen (KUB)	This is done to locate the stone in the bladder and determine the presence of any other (radiopaque) stones in the upper tract. Radiolucent stones will not show up on this type of x-ray examination.

Plan for implementation	Rationale
b. Intravenous pyelogram	This is done to determine renal function and the presence of other (radiolucent) stones in the upper tract.
2. The preoperative shave is from the umbilicus to mid-thigh.	Although the shave is sometimes omitted altogether, many surgeons will request it in case of accidental perforation of the bladder, which will require an incision to correct. The physician usually tells the patient beforehand that it may not be possible to extract the stone endoscopically, in which case an abdominal incision will be required (see Chapter 33). The possibility of open surgery is therefore included on the informed consent document that the patient signs.
3. The patient will probably be permitted oral fluids a few hours after surgery, and his diet will be advanced as tolerated.	These patients can usually tolerate oral intake a few hours after surgery. For this reason the intravenous infusion used during surgery is often discontinued in the recovery room or shortly after the patient returns to the urology floor and tolerates fluids.
4. There will be an indwelling catheter in place for 24 to 48 hours after surgery.	
5. The urine may be pink in the immediate postoperative period.	

Preoperative period

2. NURSING DIAGNOSIS: Need for discharge planning

Objectives of nursing intervention { Early commencement of discharge planning
Accurate estimate of time required for all discharge teaching

Expected outcome Smooth transition of care after discharge

Plan for implementation	Rationale
See master care plan for the patient requiring discharge preparations: discharge planning.	

In addition to the topics covered in the master care plan, the following items should be considered:
1. The duration of hospitalization for this type of procedure is approximately 3 days.

2. Required teaching includes:
   a. General postoperative discharge teaching
   b. Possibly instruction for a stone prevention regimen

3. NURSING DIAGNOSIS: Potential for postoperative complications (shock, atelectasis, pneumonia, deep vein thrombosis, infection)

Objective of nursing intervention   Prevention or early detection of postoperative complications

Expected outcomes
Pulse and blood pressure normal, skin dry, color normal
Respirations regular and unlabored, absence of pulmonary congestion
Early ambulation tolerated well
Absence of chills or fever

Plan for implementation	Rationale
1. Check the patient's vital signs every 4 hours and notify the physician of any indications of impending shock. These include: a. Increasing pulse and respiratory rates b. Decreasing blood pressure c. Diaphoresis and pallor d. Feelings of apprehension	Although shock is a potential complication after any kind of surgery, it is a relatively small risk after cystilitholapaxy or cystolithotripsy because no blood vessels are cut and the duration of surgery is short.
2. Encourage coughing and abdominal breathing if the patients lungs sound congested, and notify the physician if any of the following conditions are present: a. The patient is unable to cough and his lungs sound congested. b. Sputum volume is copious. c. Sputum color is other than clear or white. d. There is a rise in the patient's temperature. e. Breath sounds are diminished.	Although precautions must be taken, respiratory complications are unlikely after this type of surgery because the period of anesthesia is very short. Furthermore, there is no abdominal incision to inhibit effective coughing. These conditions require additional treatment. The physician may order therapies such as incentive spirometry, nasotracheal suctioning, postural drainage, or intermittent positive pressure breathing, depending on the extent of respiratory embarrassment.
3. Use precautions to prevent deep vein thrombosis. (See master care plan for the patient at risk for deep vein thrombosis.)	Although deep vein thrombosis is a relatively small risk after this type of surgery, it still must be considered, and adequate precautions should be taken.
4. Notify the physician if the patient shows any indications of infection. These include: a. Chills b. Fever c. Flushed skin	Bacteremia can occur after any instrumentation of the urinary tract. This happens as a result of absorption of bacteria through the walls of the urethral mucosa. Blood and urine specimens are often ordered to determine the type and sensitivity of the offending organism, and the patient is usually given antibiotic therapy.

Early postoperative period

4. NURSING DIAGNOSIS: Need for management of indwelling urethral catheter

Objectives of nursing intervention

Appropriate care of catheter and equipment
Prevention or early detection of infection
Care of tissue surrounding catheter
Maintenance of accurate records of urine output
Appropriate administration of hand-irrigation of catheter
Management of discomfort or pain caused by catheter
Satisfactory collection of urine specimens from catheter

Expected outcomes

Absence of severe bladder spasms and suprapubic distention
Urine draining freely through system
Absence of fever, chills, and foul-smelling urine
Absence of urethral discharge and tissue inflammation
Minimal discomfort caused by the catheter
Urine specimens in optimum condition for all necessary tests

Plan for implementation	Rationale
See master care plan for the patient with an indwelling urethral catheter: care after insertion of the catheter.	
In addition to the topics covered in the master care plan, the following intervention is required:	
Notify the physician if the urine is bright red for more than a few hours after surgery. Usually it is lightly blood tinged to amber within 24 hours.	Since no tissue has been cut, prolonged hematuria requires investigation. The urine may be pink for the first day because small blood vessels might have been broken during urethral instrumentation.

Early postoperative period

5. NURSING DIAGNOSIS: Postoperative pain

Objective of nursing intervention	Appropriate management of pain or discomfort
Expected outcome	Behavioral and/or verbal indication that pain is adequately reduced or absent

Plan for implementation	Rationale
Determine the source of the pain. It may be related to the catheter or the surgical manipulation.	Pain from different sources usually requires different intervention.
1. Question and observe the patient to obtain information about the pain.	
2. Be aware that pain is a unique and individual experience. Although the different sources of pain can usually be determined by their characteristics, there are also many variations.	
3. Be alert for indications (verbal or behavioral) that the patient is experiencing discomfort other than physical pain, and attempt to resolve the problem.	Fear, loneliness, depression, and numerous other conditions may be sources of extreme discomfort for the patient, who may unconsciously translate these feelings into pain.

PERSISTENT, SEVERE, INCREASING PAIN IN SUPRAPUBIC AREA

See Chapter 11, part one, nursing objective 6.	This pain is probably caused by an obstructed catheter.

SPASMODIC, INTERMITTENT PAIN IN SUPRAPUBIC AREA, OR PAIN RADIATING TO URETHRAL AREA

See Chapter 11, part one, nursing objective 6.	This pain is probably caused by the catheter's irritating effect on the bladder and irritation of urethral tissue from instrumentation.

Early postoperative period

6. NURSING DIAGNOSIS: Potential for voiding complications following removal of indwelling urethral catheter

Objective of nursing intervention	Prevention or early detection of complications
Expected outcomes	Resumption of normal voiding pattern Absence of dysuria

Plan for implementation	Rationale
See master care plan for the patient with an indwelling urethral catheter: care after removal of the catheter.	

Late postoperative period

7. NURSING DIAGNOSIS: Need for discharge teaching

Objectives of nursing intervention

- Explanation of basic information about medications to be taken at home
- Explanation of information regarding follow-up care
- Explanation of residual effects of the condition and/or treatment
- Explanation of instructions concerning postdischarge activities
- Explanation of symptoms that constitute a reason to contact the physician
- Review of admitting diagnosis and mode of treatment

Expected outcomes

- Accurate return verbalization and/or demonstration of all material learned
- Smooth transition of care after discharge
- Absence or early detection of complications arising after discharge
- Ability to provide future health care practitioners with important data about health history

Plan for implementation	Rationale
See master care plan for the patient requiring discharge preparations: discharge teaching.	
In addition to the topics covered in the master care plan, include the following items in the discharge teaching:	
1. At the follow-up office visit the physician will obtain a urine specimen for culture.	Urinary tract infection must be completely eradicated if the patient is to remain free from urinary calculi in the future.
2. The physician may prescribe periodic x-ray examinations to check for recurrence of calculi if the patient is a chronic stone former.	Detection of calculi before they become symptomatic may prevent serious renal damage.
3. The expected residual effects of this surgery are minimal. The patient is generally able to resume most usual activities 1 week after discharge.	
4. The patient should notify the physician if any of the following occur: chills, fever, hematuria, flank pain.	These would indicate a urinary tract infection.
5. Unless contraindicated by coexisting medical conditions, the patient should maintain a fluid intake of **at least** 2.5 L per day for the rest of his life. (See p. 249 for details on a hydration regimen.)	A brisk flow of urine through the urinary tract discourages stone formation. Even mild dehydration should be avoided at all times, since crystallization of various constituents of the urine is more likely to occur in a concentrated solution.
6. If medication, dietary limitations, or pH monitoring has been prescribed, provide the patient with all necessary information. (See pp. 250 and 251 for a complete stone prevention regimen.)	

Convalescent period

CHAPTER 33

Cystolithotomy

A cystolithotomy is performed for a vesical calculus that cannot be removed endoscopically. An open approach is indicated when urethral strictures or adhesions or a very small urethra (as in a child) make endoscopic removal of a stone hazardous. Uric acid stones also are usually removed via an open procedure because they are extremely hard and therefore difficult to crush with a lithotrite or pulverize with a hydraulic lithotriptor.

For a cystolithotomy the patient is placed in a supine position and a transverse suprapubic incision is made. The bladder is distended with saline (via a urethral catheter) and is then incised. The stone is removed, and an incisional drain and urethral catheter are left in place. The incision is closed and a dressing is applied.

CYSTOLITHOTOMY
Outline of Care Plan
ANTICIPATED NURSING DIAGNOSES:

Preoperative period
   1. Need for preoperative teaching.
   2. Need for discharge planning.
Early postoperative period
   3. Potential for shock.
   4. Potential for wound complications.
   5. Need for management of indwelling urethral catheter.
   6. Need for management of intravenous infusion.
   7. Postoperative pain.
   8. Potential for respiratory complications related to surgical intervention.
   9. Potential for deep vein thrombosis.
Late postoperative period
   10. Potential for voiding complications following removal of urethral catheter.
Convalescent period
   11. Need for discharge teaching.

NURSING CARE PLAN FOR THE PATIENT UNDERGOING CYSTOLITHOTOMY

1. NURSING DIAGNOSIS: Need for preoperative teaching

Preoperative period

Objectives of nursing intervention

If necessary, clarification of reason for hospitalization and type of surgery to be performed

Elimination of any negative or inaccurate notions regarding the forthcoming surgery

Explanation of preoperative tests and procedures

Psychologic preparation for general anesthesia (omit if the patient is to have spinal anesthesia

Explanation of events expected in the early postoperative period

Explanation of body conditions expected in the early postoperative period

Identification of any known allergies

302

Cystolithotomy

Cystolithotomy

Expected outcomes {
Verbal indication that explanations are understood
Verbal indication of optimistic expectations (within realistic limits) related to forth-coming surgery
Cooperation during preoperative tests and procedures
Verbal or behavioral indication of reduction of anxiety
Absence of postoperative complications
Absence of allergic reactions
}

Plan for implementation	Rationale
See master care plan for the patient receiving preoperative teaching.	
In addition to the topics covered in the master care plan, include the following items in the preoperative teaching:	
1. Be aware that, in addition to routine preoperative tests, the following diagnostic studies may have been performed, and answer any questions the patient has regarding them:	
a. Plain x-ray examination of the abdomen (KUB)	This is done to locate the stone in the bladder and determine the presence of other (radiopaque) stones in the upper tract. Radiolucent stones will not show up on this type of x-ray examination.
b. Intravenous pyelogram	This is done to determine renal function and the presence of other (radiolucent) stones in the upper tract.
2. The preoperative shave will be from umbilicus to mid-thigh.	
3. The patient will probably be permitted a light supper in the evening after surgery and will resume his normal diet in the morning.	Because the peritoneal cavity is not entered during this surgery, the incidence of postoperative gastrointestinal disturbances is relatively low.
4. There will be an indwelling urethral catheter in place for approximately 5 days.	
5. The patient will have an incision on his lower abdomen. It will be covered by a dressing that will require frequent changing during the first 24 to 48 hours after surgery.	
6. Urine is expected to be blood tinged in the early postoperative period.	

2. NURSING DIAGNOSIS: Need for discharge planning

Objectives of nursing intervention
{ Early commencement of discharge planning
Accurate estimate of time required for all discharge teaching

Expected outcome   Smooth transition of care after discharge

Plan for implementation	Rationale
See master care plan for the patient requiring discharge preparations: discharge planning.

In addition to the topics covered in the master care plan, the following items should be considered:
1. The duration of hospitalization for this procedure is approximately 1 week.

2. Required teaching includes:
   a. General postoperative discharge teaching
   b. Possibly instruction for a stone prevention regimen | |

3. NURSING DIAGNOSIS: Potential for shock

Objective of nursing intervention   Prevention or early detection of shock

Expected outcomes
{ Vital signs normal, skin dry, color normal
Absence of bright red drainage

Plan for implementation	Rationale
1. Check the patient's vital signs every 4 hours once stable (every 15 minutes if unstable).

2. Be alert for increasing pulse and respiratory rates, decreasing blood pressure, diaphoresis, pallor, and feelings of apprehension.

3. Notify the physician at once if indications of impending shock occur. | Although shock is a potential complication after any kind of surgery, it is a relatively small risk after a cystolithotomy because few blood vessels are cut, and the duration of surgery is short. |

4. NURSING DIAGNOSIS: Potential for wound complications

Objective of nursing intervention   Prevention or early detection of complications arising from the incisional area

Expected outcome   Absence of fever, purulent exudate, erythema, edema, dehiscence, hematoma, and other abnormal wound conditions

Plan for implementation	Rationale

1. Check the dressing frequently (every 2 to 4 hours during the first 24 to 48 hours after surgery). Change it when it becomes wet and use sterile technique for the procedure.	The dressing may become saturated rapidly with serosanguineous fluid and urine from the incision. This is because the suture line in the bladder may not become watertight for at least 48 hours after surgery. A wet dressing must be changed as soon as possible for the following reasons:
	1. It is a source of infection.
	   a. It acts as a wick, enabling microorganisms on the skin to move toward the incision.
	   b. It provides a good medium for bacterial multiplication.
	2. It is highly irritating to the skin because of the presence of urine in the drainage.

2. Note the odor of the drainage. The characteristic odor of urine is not abnormal, but if it is foul smelling: a. Notify the physician. b. Obtain a wound culture specimen.	This would indicate a wound infection. This will facilitate identification of the infecting organism so that appropriate treatment can be instituted quickly.
3. Use caution when removing soiled dressings to prevent inadvertent removal of the incisional drain.	Premature removal of a drain may result in the development of a urinoma and prolonged healing.
4. Cut and arrange gauze pads around the incisional drain, which is usually a Penrose drain.	This prevents the dressings from flattening the drain and possibly obstructing the flow of drainage from the wound.
5. If the dressing requires frequent changing, use Montgomery straps instead of adhesive tape.	This eliminates the need to remove the adhesive tape from the patient's skin each time the dressing is changed. Skin irritation and patient discomfort can be considerably reduced by this method.
6. Note the condition of the suture line. Chart its appearance and the presence of edema, erythema, hematoma, ecchymosis, or other abnormal conditions.	This provides a frame of reference for other staff members caring for the patient.
7. Notify the physician if there is any evidence of dehiscence.	
8. Check the patient's temperature every 4 hours and notify the physician if there is an elevation above 101°.	Wound infection must always be suspected when the patient runs a fever postoperatively. Other causes include respiratory complications and pharmacologic intervention.

Early postoperative period

5. NURSING DIAGNOSIS: Need for management of indwelling urethral catheter

Objectives of nursing intervention
- Appropriate care of catheter and equipment
- Prevention or early detection of infection
- Care of tissue surrounding catheter
- Maintenance of accurate records of urine output
- Appropriate administration of hand-irrigation of catheter
- Management of discomfort or pain caused by catheter
- Satisfactory collection of urine specimens from catheter

Expected outcomes
- Absence of severe bladder spasms
- Urine draining freely through system
- Absence of fever, chills, and foul-smelling urine
- Absence of urethral discharge and tissue inflammation
- Minimal discomfort caused by the catheter
- Urine specimens in optimum condition for all necessary tests

Plan for implementation	Rationale
See master care plan for the patient with an indwelling urethral catheter: care after insertion of the catheter. In addition to the topics covered in the master care plan, the following interventions are required: 1. Notify the physician if the urine turns bright red and has a high viscosity. The urine should be blood tinged to clear within 24 to 48 hours after surgery.	There should be relatively little active bleeding into the bladder after this type of surgery. The appearance of bright red urine requires investigation.
2. If the catheter requires irrigation, use caution not to overdistend the bladder with irrigant.	This may result in disruption of the surgical site.

Early postoperative period

6. NURSING DIAGNOSIS: Need for management of intravenous infusion

Objectives of nursing intervention
- Appropriate administration of specific types of intravenous solutions
- Prevention or early detection of local complications
- Prevention or early detection of systemic complications
- Management of discomfort caused by intravenous infusion
- Maintenance of proper function of intravenous equipment
- Maintenance of accurate records of the patient's hydration status

Expected outcomes
- Normal hydration status
- Normal electrolyte status
- Absence of thrombophlebitis, infiltration, infection, fluid overload, and pulmonary embolism
- Absence of discomfort caused by the intravenous infusion

Plan for implementation	Rationale
See master care plan for the patient receiving intravenous therapy.	These patients usually receive isotonic dextrose and saline solutions. Antibiotics may also be given if the urine was infected before surgery.

7. NURSING DIAGNOSIS: Postoperative pain

Objective of nursing intervention   Appropriate management of pain or discomfort

Expected outcome   Behavioral and/or verbal indication that pain is adequately reduced or absent

Plan for implementation	Rationale
Determine the source of the pain. It may be related to the catheter or the surgical wound.	Pain from different sources usually requires different intervention.

1. Question and observe the patient to obtain information about the pain.

2. Be aware that pain is a unique and individual experience. Although the different sources of pain can usually be determined by their characteristics, there are also many variations.

Early postoperative period

Plan for implementation	Rationale
3. Be alert for indications (verbal or behavioral) that the patient is experiencing discomfort other than physical pain, and attempt to resolve the problem.	Fear, loneliness, depression, and numerous other conditions may be sources of extreme discomfort for the patient, who may unconsciously translate these feelings into pain.

PERSISTENT, SEVERE, INCREASING PAIN IN SUPRAPUBIC AREA

See Chapter 11, part one, nursing objective 6.	This pain is probably caused by an obstructed catheter.

SPASMODIC, INTERMITTENT PAIN IN THE SUPRAPUBIC AREA, OR PAIN RADIATING TO URETHRAL AREA

See Chapter 11, part one, nursing objective 6.	This pain is probably caused by the catheter's irritating effect on the bladder.

MODERATE TO SEVERE PAIN AT SURGICAL SITE, USUALLY AGGRAVATED BY PHYSICAL ACTIVITY

1. Be certain the catheter is not obstructed. Although pain with these characteristics is usually of incisional origin and is expected, it is very difficult to differentiate between incisional pain and the pain of an obstructed catheter after this type of surgery.	Catheter obstruction must be ruled out first because it cannot remain untreated. However, after this type of surgery it is unlikely for the catheter to become obstructed because there is rarely enough blood in the drainage for clots to form, and no tissue particles are normally passed in the urine.
2. Administer analgesics as ordered.	Analgesic medication usually provides considerable relief from incisional pain.
3. Plan the patient's activities to coincide with a time when there is a high level of pain medication in the patient's bloodstream.	The patient will cooperate better with coughing exercises, ambulating, bathing, etc. when the pain is well under control.
4. Notify the physician if the patient's requests for pain medication do not decrease within 48 to 72 hours.	Although the intensity of postoperative pain varies enormously between patients, there should be a marked decrease in the apparent severity of the pain within 2 or 3 days. It this does not occur, it may indicate the development of wound complications.

Early postoperative period

8. NURSING DIAGNOSIS: Potential for respiratory complications related to surgical intervention

Objective of nursing intervention   Prevention or early detection of atelectasis and/or pneumonia

Expected outcomes
Cooperation with therapeutic respiratory regimen
Absence of fever or audible lung congestion
Sputum clear or white and easily mobilized

Plan for implementation	Rationale
See master care plan for the patient at risk for respiratory complications, nursing objective 2.	

9. NURSING DIAGNOSIS: Potential for deep vein thrombosis

Objectives of nursing intervention
Explanation and maintenance of precautions against deep vein thrombosis
Early detection of deep vein thrombosis

Expected outcomes
Cooperation with regimen to prevent deep vein thrombosis
Absence of local pain, swelling, and redness of a lower extremity
Absence of fever

Plan for implementation	Rationale
See master care plan for the patient at risk for deep vein thrombosis.	

10. NURSING DIAGNOSIS: Potential for voiding complications following removal of indwelling urethral catheter

Objective of nursing intervention   Prevention or early detection of complications

Expected outcomes
Resumption of normal voiding pattern
Absence of dysuria

Plan for implementation	Rationale
See master care plan for the patient with an indwelling urethral catheter: care after removal of the catheter.	

Early postoperative period

Late postoperative period

309

11. NURSING DIAGNOSIS: Need for discharge teaching

Objectives of nursing intervention

{ Explanation of basic information about medications to be taken at home

Explanation of information regarding follow-up care

Explanation of residual effects of the condition and/or treatment

Explanation of instructions concerning postdischarge activities

Explanation of symptoms that constitute a reason to contact the physician

Review of admitting diagnosis and mode of treatment

Expected outcomes

{ Accurate return verbalization and/or demonstration of all material learned

Smooth transition of care after discharge

Absence or early detection of complications arising after discharge

Ability to provide future health care practitioners with important data about health history

Plan for implementation	Rationale
See master care plan for the patient requiring discharge preparations: discharge teaching.	
In addition to the topics covered in the master care plan, include the following items in the discharge teaching:	
1. At the follow-up office visit, the physician will obtain a urine specimen for culture and will check the wound for adequate healing.	Urinary tract infection must be completely eradicated if the patient is to remain free from urinary calculi in the future.
2. The physician may prescribe periodic x-ray examinations to check for recurrence of calculi if the patient is a chronic stone former.	Detection of calculi before they become symptomatic may prevent serious renal damage.
3. The expected residual effects of this surgery are incisional discomfort and fatigue during the next few weeks.	
4. The patient should notify the physician if any of the following occur: a. Chills, fever, hematuria, flank pain b. Fever, pain and/or increasing redness at the incisional site	These may indicate a urinary tract infection. These may indicate a wound infection.

Convalescent period

Plan for implementation	Rationale
5. Unless contraindicated by coexisting medical conditions, the patient should maintain a fluid intake of **at least** 2.5 L per day for the rest of his life. (See p. 249 for details on a hydration regimen.)	A brisk flow of urine through the urinary tract discourages stone formation. Even mild dehydration should be avoided at all times, since crystallization of various constituents of the urine is more likely to occur in a concentrated solution.
6. If medication, dietary limitations, or pH monitoring has been prescribed, provide the patient with all necessary information. (See pp. 250 and 251 for a complete stone prevention regimen.)	

Convalescent period

CHAPTER 34

Biopsy of bladder tumor

Biopsy of a bladder tumor is done to determine the presence of carcinoma of the bladder. The procedure is usually performed during cystoscopy with the patient under general anesthesia.

For the procedure the patient is placed in a lithotomy position, and a cystoscope is inserted into the bladder (see Chapter 7). After the bladder has been systematically visualized through the cystoscope, a cup biopsy forceps is inserted through the cystoscope, and a small tissue sample of any questionable area is removed and placed in a formalin solution. Because more than one biopsy specimen is usually obtained, special care is taken to label each specimen appropriately, usually according to the site in the bladder from which it was removed. If bleeding is encountered, the area may be lightly fulgurated. Sometimes an indwelling urethral catheter is inserted and left in place for 24 hours to ensure adequate drainage from the bladder.

BIOPSY OF BLADDER TUMOR
Outline of Care Plan
ANTICIPATED NURSING DIAGNOSES:

Preoperative period
1. Need for preoperative teaching.
2. Need for discharge planning.

Postoperative period
3. Potential for postoperative complications (shock, atelectasis, pneumonia, deep vein thrombosis, infection).
4. Need for management of indwelling urethral catheter.*
5. Potential for urinary retention (if no indwelling catheter is used).*
6. Postoperative pain.

Convalescent period
7. Potential for voiding complications following removal of indwelling urethral catheter.*
8. Need for discharge teaching.

*May not apply.

NURSING CARE PLAN FOR THE PATIENT UNDERGOING BIOPSY OF BLADDER TUMOR

Preoperative period

1. NURSING DIAGNOSIS: Need for preoperative teaching

Objectives of nursing intervention

If necessary, clarification of reason for hospitalization and type of surgery to be performed

Elimination of any negative or inaccurate notions regarding the forthcoming surgery

Explanation of preoperative tests and procedures

Psychologic preparation for general anesthesia (omit if the patient is to have spinal anesthesia)

Explanation of events expected in the early postoperative period

Explanation of body conditions expected in the early postoperative period

Identification of any known allergies

Expected outcomes	Verbal indication that explanations are understood
	Verbal indication of optimistic expectations (within realistic limits) related to forthcoming surgery
	Cooperation during preoperative tests and procedures
	Verbal or behavioral indication of reduction of anxiety
	Absence of postoperative complications
	Absence of allergic reactions

Plan for implementation	**Rationale**
See master care plan for the patient receiving preoperative teaching.	
In addition to the topics covered in the master care plan, include the following items in the preoperative teaching:	
1. Be aware that, in addition to the routine preoperative tests, an intravenous pyelogram is usually performed before this procedure, and answer any questions the patient might have regarding it.	This is done to determine the presence of any filling defects in the urinary system, which may indicate tumor growth.
2. The patient will probably be permitted oral fluids a few hours after surgery, and his diet will be advanced as tolerated.	These patients can usually tolerate oral intake a few hours after surgery. For this reason the intravenous infusion used during surgery is frequently discontinued in the recovery room or shortly after the patient returns to the urology floor and tolerates fluids.
3. The patient may have a catheter in place for approximately 1 day.	A catheter is inserted at the surgeon's discretion. Usually, if considerable bleeding is encountered, a catheter will be used to prevent obstruction of the urethra by clots.
4. The urine may be blood tinged in the early postoperative period.	

Preoperative period

2. NURSING DIAGNOSIS: Need for discharge planning

Objectives of nursing intervention
{ Early commencement of discharge planning
Accurate estimate of time required for all discharge teaching

Expected outcome   Smooth transition of care after discharge

Plan for implementation	Rationale
See master care plan for the patient requiring discharge preparations: discharge planning. In addition to the topics covered in the master care plan, the following items should be considered: 1. The duration of hospitalization for this procedure is approximately 2 or 3 days. However, it will be extended considerably if malignant tissue is found. 2. Required teaching will depend on whether additional surgery is necessary and the type of surgery performed. If the biopsy is negative, no specific teaching is required.	

Preoperative period

3. NURSING DIAGNOSIS: Potential for postoperative complications (shock, atelectasis, pneumonia, deep vein thrombosis, infection)

Objective of nursing intervention   Prevention or early detection of postoperative complications

Expected outcomes
Pulse and blood pressure normal, skin dry, color normal
Respirations regular and unlabored, absence of pulmonary congestion
Early ambulation tolerated well
Absence of chills or fever

Plan for implementation	Rationale

1. Check the patient's vital signs every 4 hours and notify the physician of any indications of impending shock. These include:
  a. Increasing pulse and respiratory rates
  b. Decreasing blood pressure
  c. Diaphoresis and pallor
  d. Feelings of apprehension
	Although shock is a potential complication after any kind of surgery, it is a relatively small risk after biopsy of a bladder tumor because usually few blood vessels are cut, and the duration of surgery is short.

2. Encourage coughing and abdominal breathing if the patient's lungs sound congested, and notify the physician if any of the following conditions are present:
 	
  a. The patient is unable to cough and his lungs sound congested.
  b. Sputum volume is copious.
  c. Sputum color is other than clear or white.
  d. There is a rise in the patient's temperature.
  e. Breath sounds are diminished.
	Although precautions must be taken, respiratory complications are unlikely after this type of surgery because the period of anesthesia is very short. Furthermore, there is no abdominal incision to inhibit effective coughing.
	These conditions require additional treatment. The physician may order therapies such as incentive spirometry, nasotracheal suctioning, postural drainage, or intermittent positive pressure breathing, depending on the extent of respiratory embarrassment.

3. Use precautions to prevent deep vein thrombosis. (See master care plan for the patient at risk for deep vein thrombosis.)	Although deep vein thrombosis is a relatively small risk after this type of surgery, it still must be considered, and adequate precautions should be taken.

4. Notify the physician if the patient shows any indications of infection. These include:
  a. Chills
  b. Fever
  c. Flushed skin
	Bacteremia can occur after any instrumentation of the urinary tract. This happens as a result of absorption of bacteria through the walls of the urethral mucosa. Blood and urine specimens are often ordered to determine the type and sensitivity of the offending organism, and the patient is usually given antibiotic therapy.

Postoperative period

4. NURSING DIAGNOSIS: Need for management of indwelling urethral catheter*

Objectives of nursing intervention

Appropriate care of catheter and equipment

Prevention or early detection of infection

Care of tissue surrounding catheter

Maintenance of accurate records of urine output

Appropriate administration of hand-irrigation of catheter

Management of discomfort or pain caused by catheter

Satisfactory collection of urine specimens from catheter

Expected outcomes

Absence of severe bladder spasms and suprapubic distention

Urine draining freely through system

Absence of fever, chills, and foul-smelling urine

Absence of urethral discharge and tissue inflammation

Minimal discomfort caused by the catheter

Urine specimens in optimum condition for all necessary tests

Plan for implementation	Rationale
See master care plan for the patient with an indwelling urethral catheter: care after insertion of the catheter.	
In addition to the topics covered in the master care plan, the following intervention is required:	
Notify the physician if the urine turns bright red at any time. Normally it is lightly blood tinged to clear within 24 hours.	Frank bleeding is abnormal after this type of procedure and should be reported.

Postoperative period

---

*May not apply; an indwelling urethral catheter is not always used after biopsy of a bladder tumor.

5. NURSING DIAGNOSIS: Potential for urinary retention*

Objectives of nursing { Maintenance of accurate records of urinary output
intervention { Early detection of retention

Expected outcome Normal voiding pattern resumed within 6 hours after surgery

Plan for implementation	Rationale
1. Instruct the patient to notify the nurse when he needs to void for the first time after surgery, and leave a urinal by the bedside.	The effects of anesthesia may cause temporary urinary retention; a blood clot or tissue particle might cause urethral obstruction. In either case early detection and correction of the problem will prevent discomfort and possible aggravation of bleeding.
2. Keep accurate records of volume, frequency, and character of each voiding for at least 24 hours after surgery.	
3. If the patient has not voided within 6 hours after surgery: a. Be certain he is receiving adequate fluids. b. Palpate the suprapubic area for distention. c. Depending on the condition of the patient, assist a male patient to a standing position with a urinal, and help a female patient to sit on a commode by the bedside. d. Provide the patient with adequate privacy. e. Notify the physician.	Occasionally dehydration may be the cause of anuria. If the patient is in severe retention, the suprapubic area will be hard and distended. Assuming the accustomed position for voiding will help the patient to void if the retention is due to psychologic factors. Catheterization may be necessary.

Postoperative period

*May not apply; some patients have an indwelling urethral catheter after biopsy of a bladder tumor.

6. NURSING DIAGNOSIS: Postoperative pain

Objective of nursing intervention	Appropriate management of pain or discomfort
Expected outcome	Behavioral and/or verbal indication that pain is adequately reduced or absent

Plan for implementation	Rationale
Determine the source of the pain. It may be related to the catheter (if used) or the surgical manipulation.	Pain from different sources usually requires different intervention.
1. Question and observe the patient to obtain information about the pain.	
2. Be aware that pain is a unique and individual experience. Although the different sources of pain can usually be determined by their characteristics, there are also many variations.	
3. Be alert for indications (verbal or behavioral) that the patient is experiencing discomfort other than physical pain, and attempt to resolve the problem.	Fear, loneliness, depression, and numerous other conditions may be sources of extreme discomfort for the patient, who may unconsciously translate these feelings into pain.

Postoperative period

PERSISTENT, SEVERE, INCREASING PAIN IN SUPRAPUBIC AREA*

See Chapter 11, part one, nursing objective 6.	This pain is probably caused by an obstructed catheter.

SPASMODIC, INTERMITTENT PAIN IN SUPRAPUBIC AREA, OR PAIN RADIATING TO URETHRAL AREA*

See Chapter 11, part one, nursing objective 6.	This pain is probably caused by the catheter's irritating effect on the bladder.

DYSURIA†

1. Provide reassurance that the discomfort is transient.	Urethral manipulation often causes mild inflammation of the urethra, which is aggravated by the presence of concentrated urine.
2. Encourage a high fluid intake.	This dilutes the urine, thus reducing its irritating effect.
3. If the patient is in considerable discomfort, suggest that an analgesic that is specific to the urinary tract (e.g., phenazopyridine [Pyridium]) be ordered.	

*Applies to the patient with an indwelling urethral catheter.
†Applies to the patient who does not have an indwelling urethral catheter.

7. NURSING DIAGNOSIS: Potential for voiding complications following removal of indwelling urethral catheter*

| Objective of nursing intervention | Prevention or early detection of complications |

Expected outcomes { Resumption of normal voiding pattern
Absence of dysuria

Plan for implementation	Rationale
See master care plan for the patient with an indwelling urethral catheter: care after removal of the catheter.	

*May not apply; many patients do not have a catheter after biopsy of a bladder tumor.

---

8. NURSING DIAGNOSIS: Need for discharge teaching*

Objectives of nursing intervention {
Explanation of basic information about medications to be taken at home
Explanation of information regarding follow-up care
Explanation of residual effects of the condition and/or treatment
Explanation of instructions concerning postdischarge activities
Explanation of symptoms that constitute a reason to contact the physician
Review of admitting diagnosis and mode of treatment

Expected outcomes {
Accurate return verbalization and/or demonstration of all material learned
Smooth transition of care after discharge
Absence or early detection of complications arising after discharge
Ability to provide future health care practitioners with important data about health history

Plan for implementation	Rationale
See master care plan for the patient requiring discharge preparations: discharge teaching. In addition to the topics covered in the master care plan, include the following items in the discharge teaching: 1. If the patient is scheduled for a follow-up office visit, the physician will probably obtain a urine specimen for culture and determine the need for further antimicrobial treatment.	Sometimes a suspicious lesion may be caused by chronic inflammation. In this case the physician will treat the patient according to the cause of the inflammation (e.g., antimicrobial medication may be prescribed if the inflammation is bacterial in origin).
2. A long-range appointment may be scheduled (6 months after discharge) if the results of the biopsy were at all uncertain.	The patient's condition will be reviewed at this time.

Convalescent period

*Only applies to the patient whose biopsy was negative. A patient with a positive biopsy will probably require additional surgery (see Chapters 35, 36, and 38).

Plan for implementation	Rationale

Convalescent period 3. The patient should notify the physician if any of the following occur:
   a. Chills, fever, flank pain
 	
   b. Hematuria
	These are symptoms of a urinary tract infection. However, if the patient showed no signs of infection within 24 to 48 hours after the procedure, it is unlikely that he will develop an infection after discharge.
	This may be caused by exacerbation of the lesion(s), and reevaluation of the patient's condition will be required.

CHAPTER 35

Transurethral resection and/or fulguration of bladder tumors

Transurethral resection and fulguration of bladder tumors are endoscopic procedures commonly performed to eradicate lesions that are localized or superficial.

For the procedures the patient is placed in a lithotomy position, and a resectoscope is inserted through the urethra. A clear, nonconducting solution is infused into the bladder to maintain visibility, and the tumors are either cut out (resected) or cauterized (fulgurated). An electric current is used for both processes. The resected tissue is examined under the microscope to grade and stage the extent of tumor invasion.

Fulguration alone is adequate to destroy tumor cells of a lesion that is very small. Large tumors usually require resection and then fulguration to destroy any remaining segments of the tumor and to close bleeding vessels.

An indwelling urethral catheter is usually inserted afterward (unless only very small lesions are involved) to ensure adequate drainage of the bladder. If hemostasis is a problem, continuous bladder irrigation or periodic hand-irrigation may be started.

TRANSURETHRAL RESECTION AND/OR FULGURATION OF BLADDER TUMORS
Outline of Care Plan
ANTICIPATED NURSING DIAGNOSES:

Preoperative period
1. Need for preoperative teaching.
2. Need for discharge planning.

Early postoperative period
3. Potential for shock.
4. Need for management of indwelling urethral catheter.
5. Need for management of continuous bladder irrigation.*
6. Postoperative pain.
7. Need for management of intravenous infusion.
8. Potential for respiratory complications related to surgical intervention.
9. Potential for infection.
10. Potential for deep vein thrombosis.

Late postoperative period
11. Potential for voiding complications following removal of indwelling urethral catheter.
12. Dysuria.*

Convalescent period
13. Need for discharge teaching.

---

*May not apply.

NURSING CARE PLAN FOR THE PATIENT UNDERGOING TRANSURETHRAL RESECTION AND/OR FULGURATION OF BLADDER TUMORS

Preoperative period

1. NURSING DIAGNOSIS: Need for preoperative teaching

Objectives of nursing intervention

If necessary, clarification of reason for hospitalization and type of surgery to be performed

Elimination of any negative or inaccurate notions regarding the forthcoming surgery

Explanation of preoperative tests and procedures

Psychologic preparation for general anesthesia (omit if the patient is to have spinal anesthesia)

Explanation of events expected in the early postoperative period

Explanation of body conditions expected in the early postoperative period

Identification of any known allergies

Expected outcomes

Verbal indication that explanations are understood

Verbal indication of optimistic expectations (within realistic limits) related to forthcoming surgery

Cooperation with preoperative tests and procedures

Verbal or behavioral indication of reduction of anxiety

Absence of postoperative complications

Absence of allergic reactions

Plan for implementation	Rationale
See master care plan for the patient receiving preoperative teaching.	
In addition to the topics covered in the master care plan, include the following items in the preoperative teaching:	
1. Be aware that, in addition to routine preoperative tests, the following diagnostic studies may have been performed, and answer any questions the patient has regarding them:	
a. Intravenous pyelogram	This is done to determine renal function and to rule out the presence of tumors elsewhere in the urinary tract.
b. Cystoscopy and biopsy	This is done to better evaluate the location and the degree of malignancy of the tumor.
c. Bone scan and radiologic survey	These are done to rule out the presence of metastatic spread of the tumor.
d. Bilateral pedal lymphangiogram	This is occasionally done to rule out involvement of pelvic lymph nodes.
e. CT scan (computerized tomography)	This is done to rule out pelvic extension of the disease.
2. The preoperative shave is from the umbilicus to mid-thigh. However, often it is omitted altogether.	A shave is sometimes ordered to keep the suprapubic area as clean as possible in the event that an incision has to be made.

Plan for implementation	Rationale
3. The patient will probably be permitted a light supper in the evening after surgery and will resume his normal diet in the morning.	
4. There will be an indwelling urethral catheter in place for 1 to 5 days depending on the size of the tumor(s) and the degree of bleeding. If a resection is to be performed, continuous bladder irrigation may be used for approximately 24 hours after surgery. If so, the patient will be required to remain in bed until the irrigation is discontinued.	
5. Urine is expected to be blood tinged in the early postoperative period.	
NOTE: Use the word "surgery" with caution. The word "scraping" or "cauterizing" should be substituted if that is how the physician has referred to the procedure when discussing it with the patient. Also, use the word "tumor" with caution. The physician may have used a less threatening term, such as "polyp."	Although transurethral resections and fulgurations of bladder tumors are considered surgical procedures, the patient's physician may have described it as a "scraping" or a "cauterizing" to allay anxiety. Furthermore, many patients think that, if there is no external incision, the procedure is not called surgery. Therefore unexpected use of the term may provoke anxiety.

Preoperative period

2. NURSING DIAGNOSIS: Need for discharge planning

Objectives of nursing   { Early commencement of discharge planning
intervention   { Accurate estimate of time required for all discharge teaching

Expected outcome   Smooth transition of care after discharge

Plan for implementation	Rationale

See master care plan for the patient requiring discharge preparations: discharge planning.

In addition to the topics covered in the master care plan, the following items should be considered:
1. The duration of hospitalization for this procedure is anywhere from 2 days to 1 week, depending on the size and number of lesions treated and the amount of postoperative bleeding.

2. Required teaching includes:
   a. General postoperative discharge teaching
   b. Discussion of the need for frequent follow-up examinations

Preoperative period

3. NURSING DIAGNOSIS: Potential for shock

Objective of nursing intervention   Prevention or early detection of shock

Expected outcomes { Vital signs normal, skin dry, color normal
Absence of bright red drainage

Plan for implementation	Rationale
1. Check the patient's vital signs every 4 hours once stable (every 15 minutes if unstable).	Hypovolemic shock is a potential complication if the tumors are highly vascular and complete hemostasis is not achieved. Severe bleeding occasionally occurs after resection of large tumors. It may also occur if the patient has had prior radiation treatments to the bladder or other pelvic organs, since this often causes a considerable decrease in the bladder's healing capacity.
2. Be alert for increasing pulse and respiratory rates, decreasing blood pressure, diaphoresis, pallor, and feelings of apprehension.	
3. Notify the physician at once if indications of impending shock occur.	

Early postoperative period

4. NURSING DIAGNOSIS: Need for management of indwelling urethral catheter

Objectives of nursing intervention

Appropriate care of catheter and equipment

Prevention or early detection of infection

Care of tissue surrounding catheter

Maintenance of accurate records of urine output

Appropriate administration of hand-irrigation of catheter

Management of discomfort or pain caused by catheter

Satisfactory collection of urine specimens from catheter

Expected outcomes

Absence of severe bladder spasms and suprapubic distention

Urine draining freely through system

Absence of fever, chills, and foul-smelling urine

Absence of urethral discharge and tissue inflammation

Minimal discomfort caused by the catheter

Urine specimens in optimum condition for all necessary tests

Plan for implementation	Rationale
See master care plan for the patient with an indwelling urethral catheter: care after insertion of the catheter.	
In addition to the topics covered in the master care plan, the following interventions are required: 1. Notify the physician if the urine remains bright red and has a high viscosity and/or clots, despite hand-irrigation. Bright red urine is unusual after this type of surgery. Normally the drainage is blood tinged and has a low viscosity.	Although in most cases bleeding is not a problem, these tumors are often highly vascular and may continue to bleed for a few days. This is most commonly seen in patients who have had radiation treatments to the bladder (or other pelvic organs), which have caused retarded healing.
2. Notify the physician if urine output becomes obstructed and cannot be corrected by hand-irrigation.	The physician will either use more powerful instruments with which to aspirate the obstruction or will change the catheter.

3. Be alert for signs and symptoms of bladder perforation. These include
  a. Suprapubic pain
  b. Abdominal rigidity
  c. Decreasing catheter drainage despite adequate hydration
  d. Fever
	Occasionally the bladder is accidentally perforated at the time of resection. A small perforation can be difficult to detect at the time of surgery.

4. If bladder perforation is suspected, notify the physician at once and do not allow oral intake until the physician sees the patient.	Immediate intervention by the physician is required. Sometimes emergency surgery may be necessary, although small perforations often heal spontaneously.

Early postoperative period

5. NURSING DIAGNOSIS: Need for management of continuous bladder irrigation*

Objectives of nursing intervention { Maintenance of patency of irrigation system
Prevention or early detection of complications

Expected outcomes { Clear or pink-tinged drainage flowing freely
Absence of suprapubic discomfort or distention

Plan for implementation	Rationale
See p. 460.	

*May not apply; continuous bladder irrigation is used only in cases of large vascular tumor(s) and considerable bleeding.

6. NURSING DIAGNOSIS: Postoperative pain

Objective of nursing intervention Appropriate management of pain or discomfort

Expected outcome Behavioral and/or verbal indication that pain is adequately reduced or absent

Plan for implementation	Rationale
Determine the source of the pain. It may be related to the catheter or the surgical manipulation.	Pain from different sources usually requires different intervention.
1. Question and observe the patient to obtain information about the pain.	
2. Be aware that pain is a unique and individual experience. Although the different sources of pain can usually be determined by their characteristics, there are also many variations.	
3. Be alert for indications (verbal or behavioral) that the patient is experiencing discomfort other than physical pain, and attempt to resolve the problem.	Fear, loneliness, depression, and numerous other conditions may be sources of extreme discomfort for the patient, who may unconsciously translate these feelings into pain.

PERSISTENT, SEVERE, INCREASING PAIN IN SUPRAPUBIC AREA

See Chapter 11, part one, nursing objective 6.	This pain is probably caused by an obstructed catheter.

SPASMODIC, INTERMITTENT PAIN IN SUPRAPUBIC AREA, OR PAIN RADIATING TO URETHRAL AREA

See Chapter 11, part one, nursing objective 6.	This pain is probably caused by the catheter's irritating effect on the bladder and inflammation at the surgical site.

Early postoperative period

7. NURSING DIAGNOSIS: Need for management of intravenous infusion

Objectives of nursing intervention
- Appropriate administration of specific types of intravenous solutions
- Prevention or early detection of local complications
- Prevention or early detection of systemic complications
- Management of discomfort caused by the intravenous infusion
- Maintenance of proper function of intravenous equipment
- Maintenance of accurate records of the patient's hydration status

Expected outcomes
- Normal hydration status
- Normal electrolyte status
- Absence of thrombophlebitis, infiltration, infection, fluid overload, and pulmonary embolism
- Absence of discomfort caused by the intravenous infusion

Plan for implementation	Rationale
See master care plan for the patient receiving intravenous therapy.	These patients usually receive isotonic dextrose and saline solutions. The infusion is frequently discontinued shortly after the patient returns to his room if there is no evidence of serious bleeding and the patient tolerates oral intake.

8. NURSING DIAGNOSIS: Potential for respiratory complications related to surgical intervention

Objective of nursing intervention
Prevention or early detection of atelectasis and/or pneumonia

Expected outcomes
- Cooperation with therapeutic respiratory regimen
- Absence of fever or audible lung congestion
- Sputum clear or white and easily mobilized

Plan for implementation	Rationale
See master care plan for the patient at risk for respiratory complications, nursing objective 1.	

Early postoperative period

9. NURSING DIAGNOSIS: Potential for infection

Objective of nursing intervention	Prevention or early detection of infection

Expected outcome	Absence of significant rise in fever

Plan for implementation	Rationale
1. See Chapter 11, care after insertion of the catheter, nursing objective 2.	The presence of a urethral catheter predisposes the patient to infection.
2. Check the patient's temperature every 4 hours routinely and within 2 hours after any difficult irrigation during which manipulation of the catheter was required.	Bacteremia can occur after any instrumentation of the urinary tract. This happens as a result of absorption of bacteria into the bloodstream through the urethral mucosa.
3. Notify the physician if the patient's temperature rises above 101°.	Although infection of the urinary tract is the most common cause of a significant rise in temperature after urethral instrumentation, other causes must also be considered. These include respiratory complications, perforation of the bladder, and pharmacologic intervention.

10. NURSING DIAGNOSIS: Potential for deep vein thrombosis

Objectives of nursing intervention	Explanation and maintenance of precautions against deep vein thrombosis Early detection of deep vein thrombosis

Expected outcomes	Cooperation with regimen to prevent deep vein thrombosis Absence of local pain, swelling, and redness of a lower extremity Absence of fever

Plan for implementation	Rationale
See master care plan for the patient at risk for deep vein thrombosis.	

Early postoperative period

11. NURSING DIAGNOSIS: Potential for voiding complications following removal of indwelling urethral catheter

Objective of nursing intervention   Prevention or early detection of complications

Expected outcomes { Resumption of normal voiding pattern
Absence of dysuria

Plan for implementation	Rationale
See master care plan for the patient with an indwelling urethral catheter: care after removal of the catheter.	

12. NURSING DIAGNOSIS: Dysuria*

Objective of nursing intervention   Reduction of discomfort

Expected outcome   Verbal and/or behavioral indication of minimal voiding discomfort

Plan for implementation	Rationale
1. Provide reassurance that the discomfort is transient.	A burning sensation while voiding occasionally occurs for the first 24 hours after the catheter is removed, especially if the catheter has been in place for more than 3 or 4 days. This happens because the catheter causes inflammation of the urethral mucosa. If the urine is concentrated, it can be very irritating to inflamed tissue. Diluting the urine by increasing the patient's fluid intake is usually sufficient to relieve the discomfort.
2. Encourage high fluid intake.	
3. If the patient has a great deal of discomfort, suggest to the physician that an analgesic specific to the urinary tract (e.g., phenazopyridine [Pyridium]) be ordered.	

Late postoperative period

*Dysuria does not always occur after removal of a catheter following transurethral bladder surgery; therefore this may not apply.

13. NURSING DIAGNOSIS: Need for discharge teaching

Objectives of nursing intervention

Explanation of basic information about medications to be taken at home
Explanation of information regarding follow-up care
Explanation of residual effects of the condition and/or treatment
Explanation of instructions concerning postdischarge activities
Explanation of symptoms that constitute a reason to contact the physician
Review of admitting diagnosis and mode of treatment

Expected outcomes

Accurate return verbalization and/or demonstration of all material learned
Smooth transition of care after discharge
Absence or early detection of complications arising after discharge
Ability to provide future health care practitioners with important data about health history

Plan for implementation	Rationale
See master care plan for the patient requiring discharge preparations: discharge teaching.	
In addition to the topics covered in the master care plan, include the following items in the discharge teaching:	
1. At the follow-up office visits the physician will obtain a urine specimen to check for hematuria and tumor cells in the urine.	
2. During the next few weeks the expected residual effect is occasional hematuria.	
3. If the patient notices blood-tinged urine, he should increase his fluid intake until this symptom subsides.	This lessens the possibility of clot formation and urethral obstruction.
4. The patient should notify the physician if any of the following occur:	
a. Chills, fever, flank pain	These may indicate the presence of a urinary tract infection.
b. Inability to void for more than 6 hours despite adequate fluid intake	This would probably indicate obstruction of the urethra by clots or tissue particles.
c. Bright red urine that is not relieved by an increase in fluid intake	This indicates hemorrhage, which may be a result of tissue sloughing and inadequate healing mechanisms.

Convalescent period

Plan for implementation	Rationale
5. The patient must continue to have follow-up examinations every 3 months for the first year, every 6 months for the next year, and then yearly. A cystoscopy will be done at each visit, and the patient will be scheduled for periodic intravenous pyelograms to detect tumor growth in the upper tract. Urine specimens for cytologic examination will be obtained as an additional precaution if there is no other evidence of tumor growth.	Tumors of the transitional epithelium have a tendency to recur. Since this tissue is present from the renal pelvis to the urethral meatus, recurrence may take place at any point in the urinary tract. Early detection and treatment of recurrence are aimed at preventing the need for more radical treatment measures, such as partial or total cystectomy.
6. Any time after the first 6 postoperative weeks, even a brief episode of hematuria should be reported to the physician.	This may indicate recurrence of the tumor(s) that was not seen on cystoscopy. An intravenous pyelogram and a urine specimen for cytologic examination will be required to determine the presence of new lesions.

Convalescent period

CHAPTER 36

Partial cystectomy

A partial cystectomy is indicated when there is a localized, solitary tumor that has penetrated into the bladder muscle and is situated at or near the bladder dome (i.e., far away from the bladder neck and ureteral orifices).

For the procedure the patient is placed in a lithotomy position, and a transverse suprapubic or a vertical midline incision is made. The bladder is mobilized, and the area around it is carefully packed to prevent contamination of the adjacent organs by cancer cells. A wide incision is then made into the bladder, and the tumor is excised with a 2-cm margin of normal tissue around it. The bladder is then closed, an incisional drain and an indwelling urethral catheter are inserted, and a dressing is applied.

PARTIAL CYSTECTOMY
Outline of Care Plan
ANTICIPATED NURSING DIAGNOSES:

Preoperative period
1. Need for preoperative teaching.
2. Psychologic distress related to the diagnosis of cancer.
3. Need for discharge planning.

Early postoperative period
4. Potential for shock.
5. Potential for wound complications.
6. Need for management of indwelling urethral catheter.
7. Postoperative pain.
8. Need for management of intravenous infusion.
9. Potential for respiratory complications related to surgical intervention.
10. Potential for deep vein thrombosis.

Late postoperative period
11. Potential for voiding complications following removal of indwelling urethral catheter.

Convalescent period
12. Need for discharge teaching.

NURSING CARE PLAN FOR THE PATIENT UNDERGOING PARTIAL CYSTECTOMY

1. NURSING DIAGNOSIS: Need for preoperative teaching

		Preoperative period
Objectives of nursing intervention	If necessary, clarification of reason for hospitalization and type of surgery to be performed	
	Elimination of any negative or inaccurate notions regarding the forthcoming surgery	
	Explanation of preoperative tests and procedures	
	Psychologic preparation for general anesthesia (omit if the patient is to have spinal anesthesia)	
	Explanation of events expected in the early postoperative period	
	Explanation of body conditions expected in the early postoperative period	
	Identification of any known allergies	

Expected outcomes
- Verbal indication that explanations are understood
- Verbal indication of optimistic expectations (within realistic limits) related to forthcoming surgery
- Cooperation during preoperative tests and procedures
- Verbal or behavioral indication of reduction of anxiety
- Absence of postoperative complications
- Absence of allergic reactions

Plan for implementation	Rationale
See master care plan for the patient receiving preoperative teaching.	
In addition to the topics covered in the master care plan, include the following items in the preoperative teaching:	
1. Be aware that, in addition to routine preoperative tests, the following diagnostic studies may have been performed, and answer any questions the patient has regarding them:	
a. Intravenous pyelogram	This is done to determine renal function and rule out the presence of tumors elsewhere in the urinary tract.
b. Cystoscopy and biopsy	This is done to better evaluate the location and the degree of malignancy of the tumor.
c. Bone scan and radiologic survey	These are done to rule out the presence of metastatic spread of the tumor.
d. Bilateral pedal lymphangiogram	This is occasionally done to rule out involvement of pelvic lymph nodes.
e. CT scan (computerized tomography)	This is done to rule out pelvic extension of the disease.
2. The preoperative shave will be from umbilicus to mid-thigh.	
3. The patient may be permitted fluids in the evening after surgery, and his diet will be advanced as tolerated.	Because the peritoneal cavity is not entered during this surgery, the incidence of postoperative gastrointestinal disturbances is relatively low.
4. There will be an indwelling urethral catheter in place for approximately 5 days.	
5. The patient will have an incision on his lower abdomen. It will be covered by a dressing that may require frequent changing during the early postoperative period.	
6. Urine is expected to be blood tinged for a few days after surgery.	

Preoperative period

2. NURSING DIAGNOSIS: Psychologic distress related to the diagnosis of cancer

Objectives of nursing intervention { Provision of an emotionally supportive environment
Achievement of effective communication between patient, family, and staff

Expected outcomes { Verbalization by the patient of feelings about the diagnosis
Realistic decision-making
Absence of severe or protracted depression

Plan for implementation	Rationale
See Chapter 20, nursing objective 1.	

3. NURSING DIAGNOSIS: Need for discharge planning

Objectives of nursing intervention { Early commencement of discharge planning
Accurate estimate of time required for all discharge teaching

Expected outcome Smooth transition of care after discharge

Plan for implementation	Rationale
See master care plan for the patient requiring discharge preparations: discharge planning.	

In addition to the topics covered in the master care plan, the following items should be considered:
1. The duration of hospitalization for this procedure is approximately 10 days.

2. Required teaching includes:
   a. General postoperative discharge teaching
   b. Discussion of the need for frequent follow-up examinations

Preoperative period

4. NURSING DIAGNOSIS: Potential for shock

<table>
<tr><td>Objectives of nursing intervention</td><td>Prevention or early detection of shock</td></tr>
<tr><td>Expected outcomes</td><td>{ Vital signs normal, skin dry, color normal
{ Absence of bright red drainage</td></tr>
</table>

Plan for implementation	Rationale
1. Check the patient's vital signs every 4 hours once stable (every 15 minutes if unstable).	Shock is a potential complication of any surgery requiring general anesthesia and an incision. However, blood loss from this type of surgery is generally minimal, and the incidence of shock is relatively low.
2. Be alert for increasing pulse and respiratory rates, decreasing blood pressure, diaphoresis, pallor, and feelings of apprehension.	
3. Notify the physician at once if indications of impending shock occur.	

Early postoperative period

5. NURSING DIAGNOSIS: Potential for wound complications

Objective of nursing intervention   Prevention or early detection of complications arising from the incisional area

Expected outcome   Absence of fever, purulent exudate, erythema, edema, dehiscence, hematoma, and other abnormal wound conditions

Plan for implementation	Rationale
1. Check the dressing every shift. Change it when it becomes wet, and use sterile technique for the procedure.	There may be a moderate amount of serosanguineous drainage for the first few days. However, even though the bladder was opened, there may be relatively little urine in the drainage following partial cystectomy because considerable effort is usually made to attain a watertight suture line at once to prevent leakage of urine and potential spread of malignant cells.
2. If there is purulent drainage: a. Notify the physician. b. Obtain a wound culture specimen.	This would indicate that the patient has a wound infection. This will facilitate identification of the infecting organism so that appropriate treatment can be instituted quickly.
3. Use caution when removing soiled dressings to prevent inadvertent removal of the incisional drain.	Premature removal of a drain may result in prolonged healing.
4. Cut and arrange gauze pads around the incisional drain, which is usually a Penrose drain.	This prevents the dressing from flattening the drain and possibly obstructing the flow of drainage.
6. Note the condition of the suture line. Chart its appearance and the presence of edema, erythema, ecchymosis, or other abnormal conditions.	This provides a frame of reference for other staff members caring for the patient.
7. Notify the physician if there is any evidence of dehiscence.	
8. Check the patient's temperature every 4 hours and notify the physician if there is an elevation above 101°.	Wound infection must always be suspected when the patient runs a fever postoperatively. Other causes include respiratory complications and pharmacologic intervention.

Early postoperative period

6. NURSING DIAGNOSIS: Need for management of indwelling urethral catheter

Objectives of nursing intervention
{
Appropriate care of catheter and equipment
Prevention or early detection of infection
Care of tissue surrounding catheter
Maintenance of accurate records of urine output
Appropriate administration of hand-irrigation of catheter
Management of discomfort or pain caused by catheter
Satisfactory collection of urine specimens from catheter
}

Expected outcomes
{
Absence of severe bladder spasms
Urine draining freely through system
Absence of fever, chills, and foul-smelling urine
Absence of urethral discharge and tissue inflammation
Minimal discomfort caused by the catheter
Urine specimens in optimum condition for all necessary tests
}

Plan for implementation	Rationale
Early postoperative period	
See master care plan for the patient with an indwelling urethral catheter: care after insertion of the catheter.	
In addition to the topics covered in the master care plan, the following interventions are required:	
1. Notify the physician if the urine turns bright red and has a high viscosity. The urine is usually blood tinged to clear within 48 hours after this type of surgery.	There should be relatively little active bleeding into the bladder after this type of surgery. The appearance of bright red urine requires investigation.
2. If the catheter requires irrigation, use caution not to overdistend the bladder with irrigant.	This may result in disruption of the surgical site, especially if a large portion of the bladder had to be resected and the bladder capacity has been considerably diminished.

7. NURSING DIAGNOSIS: Postoperative pain

Objective of nursing intervention	Appropriate management of pain or discomfort
Expected outcome	Behavioral and/or verbal indication that pain is adequately reduced or absent

Plan for implementation	Rationale
Determine the source of the pain. It may be related to the catheter or the surgical wound.	Pain from different sources usually requires different intervention.
1. Question and observe the patient to obtain information about the pain.	
2. Be aware that pain is a unique and individual experience. Although the different sources of pain can usually be determined by their characteristics, there are also many variations.	
3. Be alert for indications (verbal or behavioral) that the patient is experiencing discomfort other than physical pain, and attempt to resolve the problem.	Fear, loneliness, depression, and numerous other conditions may be sources of extreme discomfort for the patient, who may unconsciously translate these feelings into pain.

PERSISTENT, SEVERE, INCREASING PAIN IN SUPRAPUBIC AREA

See Chapter 11, part one, nursing objective 6.	This pain is probably caused by an obstructed catheter.

SPASMODIC, INTERMITTENT PAIN IN SUPRAPUBIC AREA, OR PAIN RADIATING TO URETHRAL AREA

See Chapter 11, part one, nursing objective 6.	This pain is probably caused by the catheter's irritating effect on the bladder.

MODERATE TO SEVERE PAIN AT SURGICAL SITE, USUALLY AGGRAVATED BY PHYSICAL ACTIVITY

1. Be certain the catheter is not obstructed. Although pain with these characteristics is usually of incisional origin and is expected, it is very difficult to differentiate between incisional pain and the pain of an obstructed catheter after this type of surgery.	Catheter obstruction must be ruled out first because it cannot remain untreated. However, after this type of surgery it is unlikely for the catheter to become obstructed because there is rarely enough blood in the drainage for clots to form, and no tissue particles are normally passed in the urine.

Early postoperative period

339

Plan for implementation	**Rationale**
2. Administer analgesics as ordered.	Analgesic medication usually provides considerable relief from incisional pain.
3. Plan the patient's activities to coincide with a time when there is a high level of pain medication in the patient's bloodstream.	The patient will cooperate better with coughing exercises, ambulating, bathing, etc. when the pain is well under control.
4. Notify the physician if the patient's requests for pain medication do not decrease within 48 to 72 hours.	Although the intensity of postoperative pain varies enormously between patients, there should be a marked decrease in the apparent severity of the pain within 2 or 3 days. If this does not occur, it may indicate the development of wound complications.

8. NURSING DIAGNOSIS: Need for management of intravenous infusion

Objectives of nursing intervention

Appropriate administration of specific types of intravenous solutions
Prevention or early detection of local complications
Prevention or early detection of systemic complications
Management of discomfort caused by the intravenous infusion
Maintenance of proper function of intravenous equipment
Maintenance of accurate records of the patient's hydration status

Expected outcomes

Normal hydration status
Normal electrolyte status
Absence of thrombophlebitis, infiltration, infection, fluid overload, and pulmonary embolism
Absence of discomfort caused by the intravenous infusion

Plan for implementation	**Rationale**
See master care plan for the patient receiving intravenous therapy.	These patients usually receive isotonic dextrose and saline solutions. Sometimes antibiotics are also given.

Early postoperative period

9. NURSING DIAGNOSIS: Potential for respiratory complications related to surgical intervention

Objective of nursing intervention Prevention or early detection of atelectasis and/or pneumonia

Expected outcomes { Cooperation with therapeutic respiratory regimen
Absence of fever or audible lung congestion
Sputum clear or white and easily mobilized

Plan for implementation	Rationale
See master care plan for the patient at risk for respiratory complications, nursing objective 2.	

10. NURSING DIAGNOSIS: Potential for deep vein thrombosis

Objectives of nursing intervention { Explanation and maintenance of precautions against deep vein thrombosis
Early detection of deep vein thrombosis

Expected outcomes { Cooperation with regimen to prevent deep vein thrombosis
Absence of local pain, swelling, and redness of a lower extremity
Absence of fever

Plan for implementation	Rationale
See master care plan for the patient at risk for deep vein thrombosis.	

Early postoperative period

11. NURSING DIAGNOSIS: Potential for voiding complications following removal of indwelling urethral catheter

Objective of nursing intervention   Prevention or early detection of complications

Expected outcomes { Resumption of normal voiding pattern
Absence of dysuria

Plan for implementation	Rationale
See master care plan for the patient with an indwelling urethral catheter: care after removal of the catheter.	
In addition to the items mentioned in the master care plan, include the following interventions: 1. Explain to the patient that he may need to void frequently for the first few weeks after surgery.	Depending on the size of the tumor, a considerable portion of the bladder may have been excised. Therefore the bladder capacity in the postoperative period may be limited. Bladder tissue, however, is very elastic and will soon stretch to accommodate the same amount of urine it originally could hold.
2. Reassure the patient that decreased bladder capacity is a temporary condition, and the bladder will regain its previous capacity.	

Late postoperative period

12. NURSING DIAGNOSIS: Need for discharge teaching

Objectives of nursing intervention

Explanation of basic information about medications to be taken at home
Explanation of information regarding follow-up care
Explanation of residual effects of the condition and/or treatment
Explanation of instructions concerning postdischarge activities
Explanation of symptoms that constitute a reason to contact the physician
Review of admitting diagnosis and mode of treatment

Expected outcomes

Accurate return verbalization and/or demonstration of all material learned
Smooth transition of care after discharge
Absence or early detection of complications arising after discharge
Ability to provide future health care practitioners with important data about health history

Plan for implementation	Rationale
See master care plan for the patient requiring discharge preparations: discharge teaching.	
In addition to the topics covered in the master care plan, include the following items in the discharge teaching:	
1. At the follow-up office visit the physician will check the incision for adequate healing and will obtain a urine specimen for culture.	
2. During the next few weeks the expected residual effects of the surgery are incisional discomfort and fatigue.	

3. The patient should notify the physician if any of the following occur:
  a. Chills, fever, flank pain
  b. Severe pain and/or increasing discomfort at the incisional site
  c. Blood in the urine
	These may indicate a urinary tract infection.
	These may indicate a wound infection.
	
	If this occurs shortly after the patient returns home, it is probably caused by a urinary tract infection. Later, it may indicate recurrence of the tumor.

4. The patient must continue to have follow-up examinations every 3 months for the first year, then every 6 months for the next year, and then yearly. A cystoscopy will be performed at each examination. The patient will also be scheduled for periodic intravenous pyelograms to detect tumor growth in the upper tract. Urine specimens for cytologic examination will be obtained as an additional precaution if there is no other evidence of tumor growth.	Tumors of the transitional epithelium have a tendency to recur. Since this tissue is present from the renal pelvis to the urethral meatus, recurrence may take place at any point in the urinary tract. Early detection and treatment of recurrence are aimed at preventing the need for more radical treatment measures, such as total cystectomy with conduit diversion.

Convalescent period

CHAPTER 37

Bladder diverticulectomy

Diverticulectomy is indicated when there is one or more large diverticula that do not empty (Fig. 37-1) and are a source of infection or when a diverticulum harbors calculi or tumors. Diverticula most commonly occur as a result of long-standing prostatic obstruction (see p. 449) and are frequently removed during a transvesical prostatectomy.

For the procedure the patient is placed in a supine position, and a transverse suprapubic incision is made. The bladder is partially distended with saline (instilled through a catheter) to demonstrate the diverticulum, and the affected side of the bladder is mobilized. When the diverticulectomy is being performed independent of other surgical procedures, it

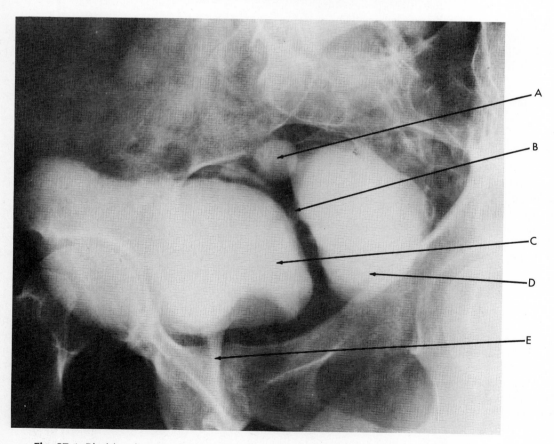

Fig. 37-1. Bladder diverticula. *A,* Small diverticulum; *B,* area of communication between large diverticulum and bladder; *C,* bladder; *D,* large diverticulum; *E,* urethra.

may be done with or without entering the bladder. The former approach is usually used when a diverticulum is low in the bladder and good visibility of the mouth of the bladder and ureteral orifices is necessary. Occasionally ureteral reimplantation may be required if the ureter is very close to the diverticulum.

Whether or not the bladder is opened, the diverticulum is excised at the level of its neck, and the defect in the bladder wall is closed. An incisional drain and an indwelling urethral catheter are inserted, and a dressing is applied.

BLADDER DIVERTICULECTOMY
Outline of Care Plan
ANTICIPATED NURSING DIAGNOSES:

Preoperative period
1. Need for preoperative teaching. (See p. 333. Initial diagnostic studies include intravenous pyelogram with postvoiding film, voiding cystourethrogram, and cystoscopy. These are done to assess the size of the bladder, the number of diverticula, and the bladder's ability to empty. Include no. 1, c, d, and e only if the diverticula are found to harbor tumors.)*
2. Need for discharge planning. (See p. 335).*

---

*Nursing care is the same as for the patient undergoing partial cystectomy.

Early postoperative period
3. Potential for shock. (See p. 336).*
4. Potential for wound complications. (See p. 337. There may be some urine in the drainage for the first 24 to 28 hours postoperatively because the suture line in the bladder may not be watertight immediately after surgery.)*
5. Need for management of indwelling urethral catheter. (See p. 338.)*
6. Postoperative pain. (See p. 339.)*
7. Need for management of intravenous infusion. (See p. 340.)*
8. Potential for respiratory complications related to surgical intervention. (See p. 341.)*
9. Potential for deep vein thrombosis. (See p. 341.)*

Late postoperative period
10. Potential for voiding complications following removal of indwelling urethral catheter. (See p. 342. These patients will have no problems with diminished bladder capacity.)*

Convalescent period
11. Need for discharge teaching. (See p. 343. Follow-up care includes periodic urine cultures to be certain that all infection has been eradicated. Include no. 4 only if the diverticulum was associated with a tumor.)*

---

*Nursing care is the same as for the patient undergoing partial cystectomy.

CHAPTER 38

Permanent supravesical diversion

In this chapter the three most commonly performed types of permanent supravesical diversion are presented, with particular emphasis on the associated complications for which the nurse must be alert.

Infection is one of the most serious long-term consequences of all these procedures. It appears that **any** interruption in the integrity of the urinary tract decreases host resistance to infection, whether it is a mechanical diversion of the urinary stream, such as an indwelling urethral catheter or a nephrostomy tube, or an anatomic change, such as the procedures to be described. Nursing care and patient teaching must always take into account the fundamental problem of infection being a constant threat to a structurally altered urinary tract.

Other complications associated with urinary diversion are more or less unique to the particular form of diversion, and all require the nurse's vigilance and conscientious teaching to prevent or reverse these serious sequelae.

Conduit diversion (ileal or colon conduit)

The surgical formation of a urinary conduit is one of the most successful means of treating serious conditions of the bladder in which normal function is (or soon will be) impossible to achieve. The procedure involves detaching the ureters from the bladder and reimplanting them into an isolated portion of the ileum or colon, the distal end of which is brought out onto the abdomen as a stoma.

The formation of an ileal conduit is indicated primarily for patients with cancer of the bladder or nonmalignant conditions such as congenital anomalies and intractable incontinence. Some surgeons perform the procedure for metastatic abdominal disease in which obstruction of the ureters is imminent.

A variation of this procedure, in which a segment of the colon is used instead of the ileum, is sometimes employed for nonmalignant conditions. A colon conduit has certain advantages over the ileal conduit. Electrolyte imbalances are minimized because the mucosa of the colon is less absorptive than the ileum, and complications associated with reflux are eliminated because a ureterocolonic anastomosis can be constructed in a nonrefluxing fashion. It is for these reasons that, whenever the life expectancy of the patient is long, the colon conduit is the treatment of choice. Thus it is most commonly seen in the pediatric age group. Elderly patients or those who have had extensive radiation to the colon area are generally not candidates for colon conduit diversion.

When urinary diversion is done for malignant conditions of the bladder, it is combined with cystectomy and possibly the removal of adjacent organs. The most common form of the procedure, total cystectomy and ileal conduit (Bricker procedure), is described next. From the floor nurse's point of view, there is little difference in terms of patient care between those who have ileal conduits and those who have colon conduits.

For the procedure the patient is placed in a Trendelenburg or modified lithotomy position. The latter is used if there are tumors in the lower bladder or urethra, necessitating a urethrectomy with the cystectomy. A midline or paramedian incision is made, and the ureters are identified and transected below the pelvic brim. Cystectomy is then performed (in the male patient the prostate is also removed), and sometimes regional lymph nodes are excised as well (radical cystectomy).

A 10- to 15-cm portion of the ileum, along with its blood supply, is separated from the rest of the small intestine, and the remaining ileum is anastomosed. The ureters are then inserted toward the proximal part of this segment of ileum (which is now completely separate from the gastrointestinal stream), and the distal end of it is brought out onto the abdomen as a stoma at a previously determined site (Fig. 38-1). Some surgeons insert ureteral catheters (stents) for temporary support of the ureterointestinal anastomosis, to prevent leakage of urine, and to prevent the possibility of edema obstructing the flow of urine. These stents are exteriorized through the stoma and drain into the ostomy pouch. One or more incisional drains (Penrose or Hemovac) are usually placed in or near the main incision.

If a urethrectomy is deemed necessary, it is done at this time, and two small Penrose drains are inserted into the groin area. If no urethrectomy is performed, an indwelling urethral catheter is inserted to drain the most dependent portion of the peritoneal cavity. Compression by the inflated balloon portion of the catheter also aids in hemostasis. When a cystectomy is not performed, an indwelling

urethral catheter is placed in the bladder to drain the small amount of mucus that tends to accumulate and promote infection.

The wound is then closed (Fig. 38-2), and retention sutures may be used. An ostomy pouch is applied, and a dressing is placed over the incision.

This operation may take 6 hours or more. Therefore the patient requires careful monitoring during the surgery and in the immediate postoperative period. An intravenous line for central venous pressure is usually started before surgery, and measurements are taken throughout the surgery and for the first 24 to 48 hours afterward. In many hospitals these patients are placed in the surgical intensive care unit for at least 48 hours so that close surveillance can be ensured.

Unfortunately the complications associated with cystectomy and ileal conduit diversion are common.

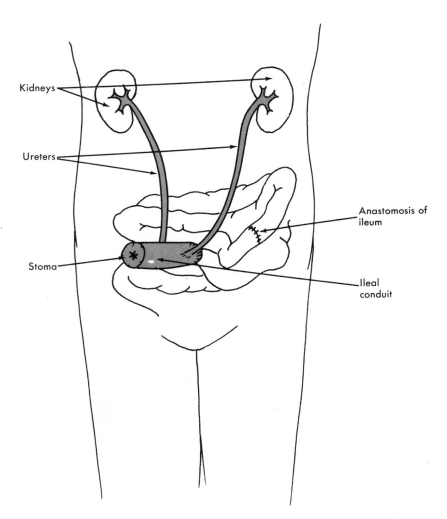

Fig. 38-1. Ileal conduit diversion. Ureters are implanted into an isolated segment of the ileum.

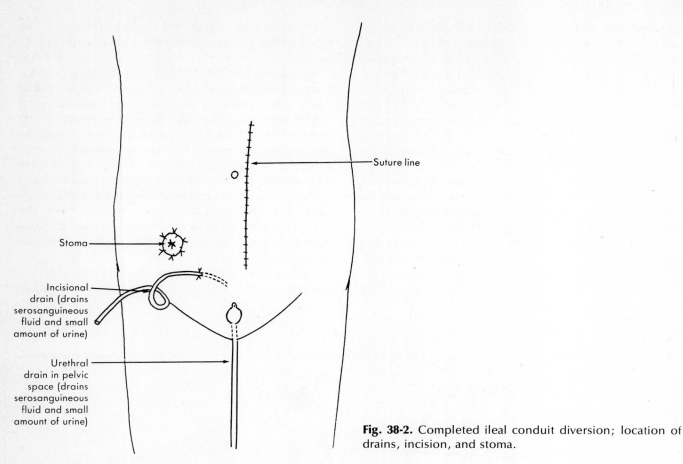

Fig. 38-2. Completed ileal conduit diversion; location of drains, incision, and stoma.

A 10-year study[7] of patients having undergone this type of surgery revealed the following incidence of early and late complications:

1. Early complications
   a. Wound infection (7.2%)
   b. Dehiscence (3.3%)
   c. Ureteral leak (2.6%)
   d. Sepsis (2.6%)
   e. Azotemia (1.3%)
2. Late complications
   a. Stomal stenosis (12.6%)
   b. Hyperchloremic acidosis (10.6%)
   c. Intestinal obstruction (10.6%)
   d. Pyelonephritis (8.6%)
   e. Ureteroileal obstruction (4.0%)
   f. Calculi (2.6%)
   g. Parastomal hernia (2.6%)
   h. Uremia (2.0%)

CONDUIT DIVERSION
Outline of Care Plan
ANTICIPATED NURSING DIAGNOSES:

Early preoperative period (2-4 days before surgery)
1. Distress related to forthcoming changes in body image.
2. Need for introductory instruction in stoma care.
3. Need for advance placement of stoma site marking.
4. Need for reduction of fecal material in the gastrointestinal tract.
5. Need for discharge planning.

Late preoperative period (24-48 hours before surgery)
6. Need for antimicrobial bowel preparation.
7. Potential for postoperative abdominal distention, pain, and vomiting.
8. Need for preoperative teaching.

Early postoperative period
9. Potential for shock.
10. Postoperative pain.
11. Potential for wound complications.
12. Need for management of urinary drainage.
13. Need for management of intravenous infusion.
14. Need for management of urethral drain or indwelling urethral catheter.*
15. Alterations in gastrointestinal function.
16. Potential for fluid and electrolyte imbalance.
17. Potential for respiratory complications related to surgical intervention.
18. Potential for deep vein thrombosis.
19. Potential for peritonitis from leakage of urine and/or intestinal contents at the surgical sites.

*May not apply.

Late postoperative period

20. Continued potential for circulatory and respiratory complications.
21. Potential for gastrointestinal complications related to resumption of oral intake.
22. Need for management of drainage from urethra following removal of urethral drain.*
23. Continued potential for complications related to urinary output.
24. Difficulty accepting changes in body image.
25. Need for stoma care.
26. Potential for complications related to stoma and peristomal skin.†

Convalescent period

27. Need for comprehensive instruction in stoma care.
28. Need for discharge teaching.

*May not apply.
†These complications are not limited to this particular period.

AUTHORS' NOTE: A segment of nursing care for the patient who is having difficulty coping with a diagnosis of cancer has not been included in this section as it has in other chapters involving procedures for treatment of cancer. It has been our experience that patients who require cystectomy are so preoccupied with changes in their body image and learning stoma care that the diagnosis of cancer does not have the psychologically devastating effect it sometimes produces. In fact, since many of these patients have been aware of their malignant tumors while receiving less radical treatment, the knowledge that cystectomy is the only chance for cure often helps the patient accept changes in his body image in preference to the alternative, succumbing to bladder cancer.

NURSING CARE PLAN FOR THE PATIENT UNDERGOING CONDUIT DIVERSION

1. NURSING DIAGNOSIS: Distress related to forthcoming changes in body image

Objectives of nursing intervention { Provision of emotional support
Provision of accurate information

Expected outcomes { Verbalization by the patient of feelings about forthcoming changes in body image
Interest in information regarding appliance care and future activities
Absence of severe or protracted depression

Plan for implementation	Rationale
1. Be aware that patients facing this type of surgery are under considerable emotional stress, regardless of how they might appear on the surface.	Understanding this enables the nurse to recognize more readily the various manifestations of psychologic conflict and deal with them in a therapeutic way.
2. When possible, include the patient's family in discussions about the surgery and the preliminary teaching of ostomy care.	One of the most frequent fears is that the patient's family (especially the spouse) will not be able to accept the stoma. The sooner the family is able to understand the changes that are to take place and begin to take an active role in helping the patient with his care, the easier the adjustment will be for all involved.
3. Encourage the patient and family to express their feelings, and convey willingness to answer all questions.	Only when the fears and worries are verbalized can they be dealt with. Often they are based on misconceptions, misinformation, or inadequate information. The nurse can frequently alleviate many of the patient's or family's concerns by providing accurate information.

Early preoperative period

Plan for implementation	Rationale
4. Be aware that irrational or inappropriate behavior often occurs as the patient works through his adjustment.	The patient's grief over his sense of loss (see further) may take the form of depression, but often it is expressed by hostility or demanding behavior, and nurses frequently get the brunt of it. By recognizing that even the most inappropriate behavior has meaning and is an expression of an emotional conflict, nurses can more easily respond to the underlying cause rather than the behavior itself. Approaching a patient's negative behavior in this way enables nurses to overcome the frustration, anger, and resentment they might initially feel in response to the behavior.
5. Recognize that grief is a normal reaction to the fantasized and real losses the patient faces. His sense of loss encompasses the following areas:	
a. Loss of normal (or socially acceptable) body image	For the rest of the patient's life he will have a stoma on his abdomen through which urine is excreted.
b. Loss of normal body function(s)	The patient will no longer void in the accustomed way. Usually male patients are unable to experience an erection.
c. Loss of autonomy	The patient will be completely dependent on the medical staff initially, and in many cases a family member may have to assume some of or all the responsibility for his care while he is convalescing at home.
d. **Feared** loss of participating in numerous recreational activities	Patients often fear that the presence of a bag of urine attached to their abdomen will keep them from taking part in sports, social events, travel, and perhaps many other activities they had previously enjoyed.
e. Threatened loss of own life from cancer	When this surgery is done for cancer, it is not certain to be curative. The patient will have to adjust to living with an element of uncertainty as to his very survival.
6. Reduce the patient's anticipation of loss by providing supportive information.	
a. Alterations in physical activity	
(1) The male patient can participate in all sports (including swimming) except for boxing, football, and other sports requiring body contact. Weight-lifting should also be avoided. Sexual activities may be altered because of the high incidence of impotence following cystectomy.	Sports requiring body contact may result in injury to the stoma. Weight-lifting may contribute to the development of a hernia.
(2) The female patient can participate in all activities except for those just listed and will not experience any physiologic change in sexual function; pregnancy is possible.	
b. Alterations in social activities	

Early preoperative period

350

Plan for implementation	Rationale

(1) There are no social limitations for either male or female patients. They should be reassured that they will not smell bad and that no one need know they have a stoma unless they choose to discuss the subject.
c. Alterations in apparel
  (1) The male patient has no clothing limitations if the stoma is well placed.
  (2) The female patient cannot wear bikinis or tight girdles. She can usually wear two-piece bathing suits (and certainly one-piece suits) if the stoma has been carefully placed and the faceplate is small.
	The pouch is odor proof; deodorants are available for use inside the pouch; medication can be taken orally to prevent odor if the patient feels particularly self-conscious (see p. 384).

7. Arrange for a visit by an ostomate.
  a. Obtain permission from the patient's physician.
  b. Discuss the plans with the patient.
  c. If the patient indicates interest, contact the United Ostomy Association.*
	The United Ostomy Association provides contact with men and women who have made a healthy adjustment to their ostomies and who are experienced at counseling potential ostomates. It can be extremely supportive and educational for the patient to talk to somebody who has gone through a similar experience. It will also give him the opportunity to obtain answers to many questions he might hesitate to ask the physician or nurse. However, it should not be arranged without prior explanation to the patient and indications of his willingness to be visited by an ostomate. The ostomate should also be briefed on the patient's condition beforehand.

8. Determine the need for psychiatric consultation.	Usually it is the patient's attending physician who makes the official request that the patient be seen by a psychiatrist during his hospitalization. However, since nurses are with the patient on a more continual basis, they may be the first to recognize the need for psychiatric assistance.

Early preoperative period

*Headquarters at 2001 West Beverly Blvd., Los Angeles, Calif. 90057. Addresses of local chapters are available through headquarters.

2. NURSING DIAGNOSIS: Need for introductory instruction in stoma care

Objectives of nursing intervention { Maintenance of an atmosphere that is conducive to optimum learning
Provision of general stoma care information

Expected outcomes { Receptive attitude toward learning stoma care
Verbal and/or behavioral indication that the information is understood

Plan for implementation	Rationale

1. Arrange for a visit by a member of the hospital's enterostomal therapy team (if such a team exists in the particular hospital).
 	
or
 	
2. Assess the patient's readiness to learn and begin introductory stoma care teaching **at his pace.**
  a. Carry out the teaching sessions in relative privacy.
  b. Provide the patient with a temporary pouch and adhesive products.
  c. Give a general explanation of the equipment.
	Nurses who are trained and certified in ostomy care are called enterostomal therapists (ETs). They usually can provide the most comprehensive teaching for ostomy patients, since they have well-developed teaching skills and current information on all varieties of appliances. However, floor nurses should be well versed in this area, even when there is an ET employed by the hospital, because continuity of care depends on knowledgeable teamwork among all the nurses who care for ostomy patients.
	Too rapid an approach may trigger anxiety and other responses that are not conducive to learning.
	
	Allowing the patient to familiarize himself with the equipment prior to surgery will facilitate learning to care for the stoma later. Some enterostomal therapists even advocate attaching the pouch to the patient's abdomen prior to surgery and filling it with some water to simulate urine. One argument in favor of extensive teaching before surgery is that the patient is not distracted by postoperative pain and weakness and will be more amenable to learning. Furthermore, the patient's tolerance of the adhesive can be assessed, the site of the stoma can be experimented with, and the patient can become accustomed to the feel of wearing the bag under his clothing. However, the equally valid argument against this method is that, if the appliance should leak or if the patient encounters difficulty in attaching the bag, he may have considerably more anxiety when he has to learn stoma care postoperatively, and he may become discouraged.

Early preoperative period

Plan for implementation	**Rationale**
3. When discussing stoma care, choose words that evoke a positive image for the patient. Use words such as "pouch" instead of "bag." The stoma can be described as "budlike." Telling the patient the original meaning of the word "stoma" (it means "mouth" in Latin) removes some of its negative association with excretion.	
4. Provide written material concerning stoma care. Diagrams may also be helpful (available from the United Ostomy Association, American Cancer Society, and some surgical manufacturers and suppliers).	Most people learn more from a combined audio-visual approach.
5. Encourage the patient to practice by himself, and leave equipment and written material at his bedside.	This allows the patient to review the material at his own pace. The strategy is particularly beneficial for the patient who appears very reluctant to learn stoma care. It provides him with an element of autonomy, giving him the opportunity to learn when **he** chooses, rather than when the nurse decides to teach.
6. Convey to the patient willingness to answer any questions whenever they come up.	This implies that the nurse expects the patient to practice on his own and that questions are welcome.

Early preoperative period

3. NURSING DIAGNOSIS: Need for advance placement of stoma site marking

Objective of nursing intervention	Determination of most advantageous site

Expected outcome	Absence of leakage, skin breakdown, and other complications related to management problems

Plan for implementation   **Rationale**

1. Assist the physician in determining the most advantageous placement of the stoma. The arbitrary rule for placement of the ileal stoma is the following: An imaginary line is drawn from the umbilicus to the anterior superior iliac spine. It is then divided into thirds, and the stoma marking is placed approximately two thirds from the umbilicus and approximately 1 cm above the line. However, there will be many patients for whom this will not apply (see further).

   Depending on hospital policy, nurses who have adequate training in enterostomal care determine the placement of the stoma (within the guidelines set by the surgeon). Proper placement of the stoma is **crucial** to the patient's well-being and to his adjustment to living with a stoma. Therefore it is necessary that the stoma site be determined in advance of the surgery. Once the patient is lying flat on the operating table, the surgeon has no way of knowing how the patient's body contours will change when he sits or stands.

2. When the aforementioned method for determining a stoma site cannot be used, an alternative site must be chosen, which should be close to the above mentioned area and have the following characteristics:

   a. The area must be accessible to the patient.
   b. The patient must be able to see the area easily when standing in front of a mirror.
   c. The area must be free from wrinkles, scars, and bony prominences. Therefore the patient must sit, stand, and move around during the process of choosing a site.
   d. The stoma site must be well away from the belt line and midline.

   There will be many patients for whom the standard rule for marking the stoma site is inappropriate. Variations in body proportions, posture, obesity, and the presence of scars from prior surgery necessitate considerable modification of this rule.

   Obesity may cause the area to be occluded when the patient is standing.
   It will be difficult to obtain a watertight seal around the stoma if the surface to which the bag must adhere is not smooth.

   Pressure from a belt may cause irritation and/or obstruction. Surgery performed at the midline generally heals more slowly and increases the risk of stomal herniation.

3. If possible, discuss with the surgeon the location of the incision and choose an area for the stoma that is at least 3 inches away from the incision, drains, and retention sutures.

   When the stoma and the incision are in close proximity, it is difficult to get a watertight seal on the pouch because of the irregularities in the surface of the abdominal skin.

4. Make a marking on the patient's abdomen by puncturing the skin with a hypodermic needle dipped in gentian violet.

   The site should be marked in such a way that it will remain visible after the surgical prep.

Early preoperative period

4. NURSING DIAGNOSIS: Need for reduction of fecal material in the gastrointestinal tract

Objectives of nursing intervention { Promotion of patient adherence to diet

Elimination of patient embarrassment and discomfort when administering enemas

Expected outcomes { Cooperation with bowel prep procedures

Absence of fecal matter in the bowel at the time of surgery

Plan for implementation	Rationale
DIETARY RESTRICTIONS	
1. Inform the patient that his diet will be limited to low-residue foods and then clear fluids starting approximately 72 hours before surgery.	The specific diet regimen is decided on by the patient's physician. The purpose of restriction of solid food is to limit the amount of fecal matter in the bowel and thus reduce the risk of contamination of the surgical site.
2. Explain to the patient why his diet is being restricted.	Understanding the reason helps the patient accept the limitations of the diet, which, for many, causes considerable frustration. Knowing the risks involved if he does not follow the diet also reduces the possibility of the patient "cheating" and eating forbidden food.
3. Whenever possible, provide the patient with choices within the limits of the prescribed diet.	This allows the patient to retain at least a small amount of autonomy and control of a situation in which he is temporarily becoming increasingly dependent and powerless.
ENEMAS	
1. Explain to the patient that he will be placed on a regimen of tap water enemas starting approximately 48 hours before surgery.	The specific regimen is decided on by the physician. The purpose is to thoroughly cleanse the bowel. Some physicians will also order laxatives.
2. Explain to the patient the reason for the enemas.	For many patients the procedure is very unpleasant, embarrassing, and often debilitating, and they need as much support as possible. An explanation of the necessity for these enemas helps to make the procedure more acceptable.
3. Provide adequate privacy for the patient.	
4. Provide petroleum jelly for external application if the rectal area becomes excoriated.	

Early preoperative period

5. NURSING DIAGNOSIS: Need for discharge planning

Objectives of nursing intervention { Early commencement of discharge planning
Accurate estimate of time required for all necessary discharge teaching

Expected outcome: Smooth transition of care after discharge

Plan for implementation	Rationale
See master care plan for discharge preparations: discharge planning.	
In addition to the topics covered in the master care plan, the following items must be considered:	
1. Evaluate the factors affecting the patient's ability to care for himself after discharge:	
a. The patient's age	Because this surgery is so extensive, elderly patients may take a long time to convalesce.
b. The patient's mental status	Unless the patient is able to understand the principles of ostomy care, he will not be able to live alone. Sometimes this is not easy to determine at this stage because the emotional distress associated with anticipation of this surgery frequently makes the patient appear unable (or unwilling) to learn. Often after the surgery, when the patient finally accepts the changes in his body image, his anxiety level is lower and he is better able to learn.
c. The patient's medical status and level of self-care	A patient who is dependent on others prior to surgery will be even more so after surgery.
d. The patient's physical dexterity	Although, initially, manipulation of ostomy equipment appears to require a highly skilled and steady hand, once the procedure becomes routine, it is very simple. So, barring any physical handicap, practically anybody can perform ostomy care.
e. The presence of a member of the patient's family or a significant other who will be able to assist the patient with his care	
2. Consult with the hospital social service department if it appears that professional care will be required after the patient's discharge.	It may be necessary for the patient to convalesce in an extended care facility. More frequently, however, the patient will only need the services of a visiting nurse. If this is the case, the necessary documents must be completed in time to be mailed and processed by the Visiting Nurse Service so that the nurse's first visit can take place on the patient's first or second day home. However, some of the information on the form cannot be completed until shortly before the patient's discharge (e.g., the level of self-care, the type of appliances used).
3. Hospitalization for this type of surgery is approximately 2 to 3 weeks.	

Early preoperative period

Plan for implementation	Rationale

4. Required teaching includes:
  a. General postoperative discharge teaching
  b. Extensive stoma care instruction
  c. Possible psychiatric counseling
  d. Discussion of the need for periodic check-ups throughout the patient's life	

5. Determine if the patient will need financial assistance to pay for ostomy supplies, and if necessary contact the hospital social service department.	In some cases government agencies or third-party payers will be able to provide financial assistance. If this is not possible, the American Cancer Society may be able to provide some of or all his equipment. (This is only done when there are no other options open to the patient.)

Early preoperative period

6. NURSING DIAGNOSIS: Need for antimicrobial bowel preparation

Objectives of nursing intervention
{ Strict adherence to medication schedule as ordered by the physician
{ Early detection of adverse effects of medication

Expected outcomes
{ Reduced bacterial content of bowel
{ Absence of postoperative infection

Plan for implementation	Rationale
1. Administer oral antibiotics at the precise time for which they were ordered.	Some surgeons order administration of antibiotics to which the bacteria in the bowel are particularly sensitive (e.g., neomycin, erythromycin, kanamycin). The purpose is to reduce the bacterial content of the bowel and thus reduce the risk of contamination of the surgical site.
2. Notify the physician if there is evidence of any side effects, allergy, and/or toxic effects of antibiotics.	See Appendix A for adverse reactions to specific medications.

3. If vomiting occurs as a reaction to the medication, the volume and the frequency should be reported to the physician, who may institute the following measures:
  a. Administration of an antiemetic
  b. Administration of intravenous infusion with additional electrolytes if needed
  c. Discontinuation of particular medication
	Some patients experience severe nausea from these medications, especially since they are often on a restricted diet and the medication schedule may require that the antibiotics be taken on a relatively empty stomach.
	
	Sodium, potassium, and water are lost in the vomitus.

4. If ordered, administer antibiotic retention enema.	Some physicians believe that this aids in the reduction of bacteria in the bowel.

Late preoperative period

7. NURSING DIAGNOSIS: Potential for postoperative abdominal distention, pain, and vomiting

Objective of nursing intervention   Assistance with satisfactory placement of nasogastric tube

Expected outcomes

Short term
  Cooperation during the procedure
  Absence of anxiety related to the procedure
Long term
  Absence of abdominal distention, pain, and vomiting postoperatively

Plan for implementation	Rationale
1. Prior to the insertion of the nasogastric tube, explain the procedure and why the tube is necessary. The purpose of the tube is to enable removal of gastric secretions proximal to the intestinal anastomosis via mild suction to reduce the incidence of abdominal pain, distention, and vomiting, which frequently occur after this type of surgery.	It will help the patient cooperate and reduce his anxiety regarding the presence of the tube if he is aware that it will make him more comfortable after surgery. Paralytic ileus commonly occurs, primarily as a result of intestinal manipulation during the formation of the conduit.
2. If a long tube (Cantor or Miller-Abbot) is used: a. Encourage the patient to lie on his right side until the tube passes out of the stomach into the intestines. This is approximately 3 feet. b. If x-ray examinations are ordered, explain their purpose. c. Tape the tube to the patient's nose and pin it to his gown once it has passed through the pylorus.	Once the tube has passed through the pylorus, peristaltic action of the small intestine will propel the tube, regardless of the patient's position. An x-ray film is often taken to confirm that the tube has advanced into the intestines. Anchoring the tube prevents it from being advanced too far into the intestinal tract (or all the way through it) by peristaltic action.

Late preoperative period

8. NURSING DIAGNOSIS: Need for preoperative teaching

Objectives of nursing intervention

If necessary, clarification of reason for hospitalization and type of surgery to be performed

Elimination of any negative or inaccurate notions regarding the forthcoming surgery

Explanation of preoperative tests and procedures

Psychologic preparation for general anesthesia

Explanation of events expected in the early postoperative period

Explanation of body conditions expected in the early postoperative period

Identification of any known allergies

Expected outcomes

Verbal indication that explanations are understood

Verbal indication of optimistic expectations (within realistic limits) related to forthcoming surgery

Cooperation during preoperative tests and procedures

Verbal or behavioral indication of reduction of anxiety

Absence of postoperative complications

Absence of allergic reactions

Plan for implementation	Rationale
See master care plan for the patient receiving preoperative teaching.	
In addition to the topics covered in the master care plan, include the following items in the preoperative teaching:	
1. Be aware that, in addition to routine preoperative tests, the following diagnostic studies may have been performed, and answer any questions the patient has regarding them*:	
a. If the surgery is being performed for carcinoma of the bladder:	
(1) Intravenous pyelogram	This is done to determine renal function and to rule out the presence of tumors elsewhere in the urinary tract.
(2) Cystoscopy and biopsy	This is done to better evaluate the tumor's location and degree of malignancy.
(3) Bone scan and radiologic survey	These are done to rule out the presence of metastatic spread of the tumor(s).
(4) Bilateral pedal lymphangiogram	This is sometimes done to rule out involvement of pelvic lymph nodes.
(5) CT scan (computerized tomography)	This is done to rule out pelvic extension of the disease.
b. If the surgery is being performed for benign conditions (e.g., incontinence):	
(1) Intravenous pyelogram	This is done to determine the effect of bladder disease on the upper tract.
(2) Cystoscopy	This is done to determine the presence of structural causes of incontinence.
(3) Urodynamic studies	These are done to rule out causes of incontinence that are correctable by less radical means.

*These studies are done well in advance of the surgery and often prior to the patient's present hospital admission. They are mentioned here, however, to conform with the format of the other chapters in which the description of diagnostic procedures is included in the section on preoperative teaching.

Late preoperative period

Plan for implementation	Rationale
2. Enemas will be continued until the morning of surgery.	Usually the physician will order the patient to have tap water enemas "until clear" in the evening and the morning just prior to surgery.
3. The preoperative shave will be from the nipple line to midthigh.	
4. After the surgery the patient will usually be in the surgical intensive care unit for approximately 48 hours.	In many hospitals, patients undergoing such extensive surgery as this will automatically be placed in the SICU so that they can be under continuous close surveillance in the immediate postoperative period.
5. Oral intake will be prohibited for at least 24 to 48 hours after surgery. During this time the nasogastric tube will be connected to a suction machine by the patient's bedside.	Oral intake, as well as gastric secretions and gas, would cause severe discomfort during the period of intestinal atony that almost always occurs after this type of surgery.
6. Once the patient passes flatus and bowel sounds are heard, he will be started on a clear fluid diet. If this is tolerated, the diet will slowly be advanced to the patient's normal diet.	
7. The patient will have a vertical incision on his abdomen that will be covered with a dressing. There is usually drainage from the incision, so the dressing will require frequent changing during the first few days after surgery.	
8. There may be a tube coming from the patient's urethra to drain fluid from the surgical area. This tube will be left in place for approximately 3 to 6 days or until the drainage is minimal.	When the urethra is not removed, some surgeons will insert an indwelling urethral catheter to prevent serous fluid from accumulating in the space that had been occupied by the bladder. If the bladder was left intact, an indwelling catheter will be in place to drain any mucus that tends to accumulate in the nonfunctioning bladder.
9. The ostomy pouch will be in place and will be attached to a bedside collecting container until the patient gets out of bed.	
10. The patient will probably be assisted out of bed to sit in a chair for a few minutes in the morning after surgery.	Despite the extensive nature of this surgery (and the typical patient's unwillingness to get out of bed the following morning), the period of immobility must be minimized to prevent postoperative complications.

Late preoperative period

9. NURSING DIAGNOSIS: Potential for shock

Objective of nursing intervention   Prevention or early detection of shock

Expected outcomes   { Vital signs normal, skin dry, color normal
Absence of bright red drainage

Plan for implementation	Rationale
1. Check the patient's vital signs every 2 to 4 hours once stable (every 15 minutes if unstable).	Hypovolemic shock is a potential complication in the early postoperative period following this type of surgery because of the removal of large amounts of tissue and loss of blood and plasma. Furthermore, the prolonged period of anesthesia contributes to the possibility of neurogenic shock, and the highly stressful nature of the surgery predisposes the patient to cardiogenic shock.
2. Be alert for increasing pulse and respiratory rates, decreasing blood pressure, diaphoresis, pallor, and feelings of apprehension.	
3. Notify the physician at once if indications of impending shock occur.	

Early postoperative period

10. NURSING DIAGNOSIS: Postoperative pain

Objective of nursing intervention	Appropriate management of pain or discomfort
Expected outcome	Behavioral and/or verbal indication that pain is adequately reduced or absent

Plan for implementation	Rationale
Determine the source of the pain. It may be related to the surgical wound, musculoskeletal manipulation, or pharyngeal irritation.	Pain from different sources usually requires different intervention.
1. Question and observe the patient to obtain information about the pain.	
2. Be aware that pain is a unique and individual experience. Although the different sources of pain can usually be determined by their characteristics, there are also many variations.	
3. Be alert for indications (verbal or behavioral) that the patient is experiencing discomfort other than physical pain, and attempt to resolve the problem.	Fear, loneliness, depression, and numerous other conditions, may be sources of extreme discomfort for the patient, who may unconsciously translate these feelings into pain.

MODERATE TO SEVERE PAIN AT SURGICAL SITE, USUALLY AGGRAVATED BY PHYSICAL ACTIVITY

Plan for implementation	Rationale
1. Administer analgesic as ordered.	Pain with these characteristics is usually incisional in origin, which is expected and often quite severe after this type of surgery.
2. Plan the patient's activities to coincide with a time when there is a high level of pain medication in the patient's bloodstream.	The patient will cooperate better with coughing exercises, ambulating, bathing, etc. when the pain is well under control.
3. Notify the physician if the patient's requests for pain medication do not begin to decrease within 48 to 72 hours.	Although the intensity of postoperative pain varies enormously between patients, there should be some decrease in the apparent severity of the pain within 2 or 3 days. If this does not occur, the possibility of wound complications should be considered. However, this surgery is extremely painful, physically as well as **emotionally,** and these patients often require analgesia considerably longer than the "average" surgical patient.

Early postoperative period

Plan for implementation	Rationale
MUSCULAR DISCOMFORT IN NECK, SHOULDERS, EXTREMITIES, ETC.	
1. Provide the patient with an explanation for the pain and reassurance that it is transient.	Because of the long duration of this surgery, the patient may feel stiffness or soreness in various parts of his body. For the first few days after surgery the administration of narcotic analgesics and the presence of severe incisional pain may mask this discomfort. Generally, reassurance that it does not indicate complications is sufficient to take the patient's mind off it.
2. Apply warm compresses to the affected area.	
3. Provide back rubs as needed.	
SORE THROAT	
1. Explain the reason for the discomfort.	The nasogastric tube, and also possible trauma caused by the endotracheal tube, may cause this discomfort. Explanation and reassurance reduce patient anxiety and therefore may provide some relief.
2. Provide reassurance that after the removal of the nasogastric tube the discomfort will be considerably reduced and should disappear within a day or two.	
3. Suggest that 2% lidocaine mouthwash (Xylocaine 2% Viscous) be ordered for gargling, as needed.	This topical anesthetic may provide some temporary relief from the discomfort.

Early postoperative period

11. NURSING DIAGNOSIS: Potential for wound complications

Objective of nursing intervention	Prevention or early detection of complications arising from the incisional area
Expected outcome	Absence of fever, purulent exudate, erythema, edema, dehiscence, hematoma, and other abnormal wound conditions

Plan for implementation	Rationale
1. Check the dressing every 4 hours during the first 24 to 48 hours and then every shift. Change it when it becomes wet and use sterile technique for the procedure.	These dressings may require changing at least once a shift in the early postoperative period, since there are usually one or two drains present. The drainage is serosanguineous fluid with a relatively large proportion of lymph.
2. Report the presence of purulent drainage or the presence of urine or stool draining from the suture line.	See nursing diagnosis 19, p. 373.
3. Use caution when removing soiled dressings to prevent the inadvertent removal of the incisional drains and ostomy bag. The drains may be Penrose drains or Hemovacs. (See p. 634 for nursing management of Hemovacs.)	Premature removal of a drain may result in prolonged wound healing.
4. If the edge of the ostomy pouch and the incision are in close proximity, trim the adhesive of the pouch as much as possible (without compromising adherence) and attach the bag **first.** Then apply the dressing. (Sometimes applying the pouch sideways helps.)	Although the temptation is first to protect the incision with a dressing **before** applying the bag, this is impractical. If the bag is applied over the dressing, it will not have a watertight seal, and the protection will not last. Therefore it is essential that the bag be attached directly to the patient's skin uniformly around the stoma. Then the dressing can be applied.
5. Cut and arrange gauze pads around the drains when applying new dressings.	This prevents the dressings from flattening the drains and possibly obstructing the flow of drainage.
6. Note the condition of the suture line. Chart its appearance and the presence of edema, erythema, ecchymosis, or other abnormal conditions.	This provides a frame of reference for other staff members caring for the patient.
7. Notify the physician if there is any evidence of dehiscence.	
8. Check the patient's temperature every 4 hours, and notify the physician if there is an elevation above 101°.	Wound infection must always be suspected when the patient runs a fever postoperatively. Other causes include respiratory complications and pharmacologic intervention.

Early postoperative period

12. NURSING DIAGNOSIS: Need for management of urinary drainage

Objectives of nursing intervention
{ Prevention or early detection of complications related to urinary output
  Precautions against mechanical failure of drainage equipment

Expected outcomes
{ Stoma red or dark pink, without change in shape
  Urine clear amber or light blood tinged in color, mucus shreds present
  Drainage equipment patent, ostomy pouch intact

Plan for implementation	Rationale
STOMA	
1. Check the size, shape, and color of the stoma every 2 hours for the first 24 hours and then twice a shift for the next 2 or 3 days. (The disposable ostomy pouch is transparent and therefore should not be removed for this.)	Sudden changes in the appearance of the stoma may indicate prolapse, inversion, ischemia, or potentially obstructive edema.
2. Notify the physician if the color of the stoma is not red or dark pink or if the shape of the stoma appears to be changing.	The color of the stoma should be similar to that of the mucous lining of the mouth (i.e., rose pink). A cyanotic appearance indicates ischemia.
3. Check for bleeding from skin adjacent to the stoma. If anything more than scanty bleeding is observed, notify the physician.	A small amount of blood may occasionally ooze from the stoma area. This is especially common if the bag requires changing within the first 72 hours and the area has not had ample time to heal. Any **continuous** bleeding indicates open blood vessels at the stoma edge, which may require surgical correction.
4. Note presence of stents (ureteral catheters) extending from the stoma into the bag.	Many surgeons insert these small plastic ureteral catheters to preserve the patency of the newly implanted ureters and ileal segment. It is a precaution against edema, which could impede the flow of urine, resulting in increased intrarenal pressure and damage to the kidneys.
URINE CHARACTERISTICS	
1. Check and record urine output hourly for the first 24 hours and then twice a shift.	A sudden decrease in output may indicate dehydration, shock, or, if no stents are present, obstruction from edema.
2. Report output of less than 30 ml per hour or **any** sudden change in output that is not proportional to the intravenous infusion rate.	
3. Note color of urine, which should be pink to amber within 48 hours.	

Early postoperative period

Plan for implementation	Rationale
4. Report the presence of bright red urine.	
5. Do not confuse mucus shreds in the urine (which is normal) with pus (which is definitely abnormal and must be reported). The latter will cause a uniformly cloudy urine. Mucus generally appears as yellowish shreds in clear amber urine.	The ileum is lined with mucus-producing cells. Since the conduit and stoma have been constructed from a segment of the ileum, mucus will continue to be produced, although the amount will vary from person to person.

CARE OF EQUIPMENT

Plan for implementation	Rationale
1. Keep the ostomy bag connected to a bedside collecting container unless the patient is out of bed.	This prevents a large volume of urine from accumulating in the bag. Excess urine in the bag would greatly increase the risk of the bag detaching from the patient's skin because of the extra weight. Keeping the pouch from filling with urine also keeps stagnant urine away from the stoma, thus reducing the risk of ascending infection.
2. Check the ostomy pouch periodically for leakage and change it at once if necessary.	A transparent, disposable pouch will have been applied in the operating room. Usually this pouch remains intact for a few days because the ureteral stents help to keep urine from seeping under the adhesive portion of the pouch.
3. Be certain that mucus is not clogging the outlet of the pouch where it is attached to bedside drainage equipment.	If urine is permitted to accumulate in the pouch, the risk of its leaking or breaking is increased.
4. Be certain that the patient is positioned in bed so that the flow of urine in the pouch and tubing is unimpeded.	The ostomy pouch is not sterile. Stasis of urine over the stoma should be avoided because it may be highly contaminated and thus contribute to the development of an infection.

CHANGING THE OSTOMY POUCH*

Plan for implementation	Rationale
1. Assemble all materials. They include a basin of water, 4 × 4-inch sponges, mild soap, pencil, scissors, Stomahesive wafer (or other skin barrier), urostomy pouch of suitable size, adhesive remover, and paper tape (optional).	
2. Remove the used pouch by gently peeling it (with the Stomahesive) away from the patient's skin, starting at the most superior point. Use adhesive remover for any areas that do not readily detach.	Removing the bag from its most superior edge first minimizes spillage of urine.

Early postoperative period

*In the early postoperative period the pouch should be changed only if it is leaking or if the stoma appears abnormal and requires closer observation.

Plan for implementation	Rationale
3. Measure stoma with stencil (provided in box of Stomahesive and also in box of disposable pouches).	
a. Choose the size that is no more than $\frac{1}{16}$ inch larger than the stoma.	Peristomal skin should be exposed to as little urine as possible to prevent skin breakdown.
b. Record the measurement of the stoma.	This will save time for the next pouch change. However, shrinkage will occur, and frequent remeasuring will be required.
c. Trace the appropriate size circle from the stencil onto the Stomahesive wafer.	
4. Cut the circle out of the Stomahesive wafer and put the wafer aside.	
5. Wash stoma and peristomal area thoroughly with soap and water; rinse thoroughly.	The area must be clean and free from soap to preserve skin integrity.
6. Dry the area **thoroughly.** If no stents are present, a 4 × 4-inch gauze pad must be placed over the stomal meatus to keep urine from draining onto the dried area. This usually requires three hands and is an excellent way to introduce the patient to caring for his stoma; ask him to hold the pad in place. If stents are used, this is usually not necessary because most of the urine can be directed away from the peristomal area by proper placement of the distal ends of the stents.	Any moisture under the adhesive portion of the Stomahesive wafer and ostomy pouch will prevent the appliances from adhering.
7. Apply Stomahesive to stoma area and gently press it against the skin. (This requires removal of the gauze pad; see no. 6). To prevent urine from wetting the field, have the patient cough **before** removing the gauze pad.	Coughing increases intraabdominal pressure and causes urine to be expressed out of the distal portion of the conduit. Usually this is followed by a brief pause in the drainage, allowing enough time for application of Stomahesive. The maneuver can be repeated before placing the pouch.
8. Apply the pouch and press it onto the Stomahesive and abdominal skin.	
9. Apply paper tape around edges to anchor it more securely.	
10. Connect the pouch to the bedside drainage system.	

Early postoperative period

13. NURSING DIAGNOSIS: Need for management of intravenous infusion

Objectives of nursing intervention

Appropriate administration of specific types of intravenous solutions

Prevention or early detection of local complications

Prevention or early detection of systemic complications

Management of discomfort caused by the intravenous infusion

Maintenance of proper function of intravenous equipment

Maintenance of accurate records of the patient's hydration status

Expected outcomes

Normal hydration status

Normal electrolyte status

Absence of thrombophlebitis, infiltration, infection, fluid overload, and pulmonary embolism

Absence of discomfort caused by the intravenous infusion

Plan for implementation	Rationale
See master care plan for the patient receiving intravenous therapy.	
In addition to the topics covered in the master care plan, the following items may be included:	
1. If the patient is receiving fluids through a central line, additional precautions are required. These include:	Sometimes the surgeon will want periodic readings of the patient's central venous pressure. Therefore a central line will be inserted. This may be used for fluid replacement considerably longer than for CVP measurements.
a. Keep the dressing on the central line meticulously clean and use sterile technique if it requires changing.	This line goes directly to the right atrium, so the risk of serious infection is an important consideration.
b. Keep the tubing anchored securely to the patient's skin.	Dislodgement of the tube should be prevented. Replacing a central line is not a simple procedure.
c. Do not permit any air to enter the line.	This could result in a pulmonary embolism.
d. Be certain all connections of the tubing are tight.	If the tubing becomes disconnected, the negative pressure in the line will cause blood to flow out of the line, and dangerous blood loss might occur.
2. If the patient is placed on a regimen in which the volume of fluid output (urine and nasogastric drainage) determines the amount and type of electrolyte solution to be infused, keep precise records of urine and nasogastric output.	

14. NURSING DIAGNOSIS: Need for management of urethral drain or indwelling urethral catheter*

Objective of nursing intervention

Prevention or early detection of complications related to drainage from the pelvic space or from the nonfunctioning bladder

*This may not apply. If the urethra was removed, small incisional drains will be in or near the perineal suture line instead.

Expected outcomes
If cystectomy: gradually decreasing amounts of blood-tinged or straw-colored fluid draining through urethral drain

If bladder left in situ: whitish or clear mucus draining through indwelling urethral catheter

Plan for implementation	Rationale
FOR CYSTECTOMY (i.e., if catheter is for drainage of serosanguineous fluid in pelvic cavity)	
1. **Do not** irrigate this catheter. As an extra precaution, refer to it as a **urethral drain** on the Kardex so it is not mistaken for a catheter to the bladder and inadvertently irrigated.	This catheter is used to facilitate drainage from the pelvic space and to provide early detection of any active abdominal bleeding if it occurs. The proximal end of the catheter is in the space from which the bladder (and often other pelvic organs) have been removed. Instillation of fluid into this catheter could result in peritonitis.
2. Record the volume of drainage each shift and notify the physician if there is a sudden increase in the amount of drainage.	Excessive drainage may indicate continuous leakage of urine into the pelvic space from the surgical site. A small amount of leakage, however, is not unusual and generally corrects itself within a few days.
3. Note color and consistency of drainage.	The drainage is composed of plasma and normally only very small amounts of urine, if any. There should be minimal blood in the drainage by the third postoperative day.
4. Report **sudden** cessation of drainage. It should subside gradually over a week or more.	This may indicate internal obstruction of the catheter, causing it to function as a plug rather than a conduit.
5. Prevent external obstruction of the drain and tubing. Prevent kinking of the tubing, and position the patient so that he is not lying on it.	Fluid collecting in the pelvic space must be permitted to drain out of the body. If it is trapped in the body, it may lead to abscess formation because it is potentially contaminated by communication (via the urethra) with the external environment.
FOR BLADDER LEFT IN SITU	
1. Record the volume of drainage through the catheter each shift.	Whitish mucus tends to accumulate in the nonfunctioning bladder. A catheter may be left in place for a few days postoperatively to encourage drainage of this mucus.
2. Prevent external obstruction of the catheter and tubing. Prevent kinking of the tubing, and position the patient so that he is not lying on it.	
3. Provide hand-irrigation of the catheter as ordered.	If pyocystis occurs, antibiotic irrigation of the catheter is often ordered on a specific time schedule.
4. See master care plan for the patient with an indwelling urethral catheter for more detailed nursing actions.	

Early postoperative period

369

15. NURSING DIAGNOSIS: Alterations in gastrointestinal function

Objectives of nursing intervention
{ Appropriate management of nasogastric suction
Prevention or early detection of complications heralded by changes in nasogastric drainage

Expected outcomes
{ Moderate amount of greenish brown drainage through suction apparatus
Absence of pain, abdominal distention, nausea, and vomiting

Plan for implementation	Rationale
1. Keep nasogastric tube securely taped to the patient's nose and pinned to the patient's gown.	This prevents inadvertent traction on the tube, which would cause the patient discomfort.
2. Maintain suction through the tube as ordered, and irrigate it with normal saline at regular intervals (usually every 2 hours).	
3. Record volume and characteristics of drainage each shift. (Drainage is usually greenish.)	Records of the volume of drainage are extremely important. Frequently the physician will order intravenous replacement of fluid and electrolytes to compensate for what was lost in the gastrointestinal secretions.
4. Be alert for sudden changes in color or volume of drainage. a. If drainage ceases, irrigate with normal saline; if no results, check suction device and replace it if necessary. b. If there appears to be blood in the drainage: (1) Notify the physician at once. (2) Obtain a specimen for a test for occult blood.	Sudden reduction of output may indicate obstruction of tubing or faulty suction equipment. Drainage that is bright red or has brownish particles in it indicates bleeding somewhere in the gastrointestinal tract.
5. Do not allow oral intake, as ordered.	
6. Provide mouth care as needed.	The mouth often becomes uncomfortably dry with nasogastric suction.
7. Lubricate nares with petroleum jelly as needed.	This reduces some of the irritation caused by the nasogastric tube.
8. Check periodically for bowel sounds and passage of flatus.	These are indicators that the intestines are regaining function.

Early postoperative period

16. NURSING DIAGNOSIS: Potential for fluid and electrolyte imbalance

Objective of nursing interventiion
Prevention or early detection of fluid and electrolyte imbalance

Expected outcomes
{ Normal laboratory values for serum electrolytes
Absence of signs and symptoms of fluid and electrolyte imbalance

Plan for implementation	Rationale
1. Check laboratory values for abnormalities in blood chemistry, and report if present.	The patient is losing sodium, potassium, and hydrochloric acid in gastric suction and is losing potassium in the wound drainage. Careful observation of the patient and his laboratory values is extremely important during the early postoperative period. Low potassium is particularly dangerous if the patient is receiving a digitalis preparation because it predisposes him to cardiac arrhythmias.
2. Notify the physician if symptoms of fluid and electrolyte imbalance occur. In general, these include: a. Changes in level of consciousness (from somnolence to agitation) b. Changes in respiratory rate and depth c. Abnormalities in muscle tone (from flaccidity to convulsions) d. Cardiac irregularities	
3. Keep accurate records of all fluid input. (Remember: nasogastric irrigation fluid that is not immediately aspirated is counted as input.)	This provides continuity of fluid replacement guidelines for subsequent nursing shifts and allows the physician to assess rapidly the patient's hydration status.
4. If, for any reason, intravenous fluids have not been infusing as ordered, this must be reported.	The physician may choose to compensate for deficits or overloads by temporarily changing intravenous orders.
5. In general, normal saline should be used for irrigation of the nasogastric tube.	Frequent irrigation with anything other than an isotonic solution may cause a hypoosmolar condition due to the absorption of hypotonic fluid from the gastrointestinal tract. However, the patient's condition must be evaluated; patients on sodium restriction may require irrigations with water to prevent a sodium overload. If there is any uncertainty, consult the physician before irrigating.

Early postoperative period

17. NURSING DIAGNOSIS: Potential for respiratory complications related to surgical intervention

Objective of nursing intervention   Prevention or early detection of atelectasis and/or pneumonia

Expected outcomes
Cooperation with therapeutic respiratory regimen
Absence of fever or audible lung congestion
Sputum clear or white and easily mobilized

Plan for implementation	Rationale
See master care plan for the patient at risk for respiratory complications, nursing objective 3.	These patients are especially prone to respiratory complications because of the long period under anesthesia and the severe postoperative pain, which inhibits coughing.

18. NURSING DIAGNOSIS: Potential for deep vein thrombosis

Objectives of nursing intervention
Explanation and maintenance of precautions against deep vein thrombosis
Early detection of deep vein thrombosis

Expected outcomes
Cooperation with regimen to prevent deep vein thrombosis
Absence of local pain, swelling, and redness of a lower extremity
Absence of fever

Plan for implementation	Rationale
See master care plan for the patient at risk for deep vein thrombosis.	

Early postoperative period

19. NURSING DIAGNOSIS: Potential for peritonitis from leakage of urine and/or intestinal contents at the surgical sites

Objective of nursing intervention

Early detection of peritonitis

Expected outcomes

Absence of abdominal distention

Return of bowel sounds within 72 hours

Nonpurulent serosanguineous or serous drainage from wound and urethra

Cooperation with diagnostic regimen if peritonitis is suspected

Plan for implementation	Rationale

1. Be alert for the following signs of peritonitis:
  a. Abnormal drainage from wound or urethra (e.g., large quantities of cloudy, purulent fluid; stool in the drainage)
  b. Prolonged abdominal distention with rebound tenderness
  c. Prolonged absence of bowel sounds
  d. A sudden rise in temperature accompanied by any of the signs just listed
	Although it is a rare complication, inadequate anastomosis of the ureteral conduit junction or the intestinal tract may result in leakage of urine or intestinal contents into the peritoneal cavity.

2. Notify the physician if any of these signs occur.	
3. If a methylene blue test is performed, explain to the patient that his urine might appear bluish temporarily because of the dye.	To detect the presence of urine in the drainage, the physician will inject the patient with methylene blue dye. This dye will be excreted in the urine in approximately 15 minutes. If the drainage also turns blue, it indicates that the urine is leaking into the peritoneal cavity. Leakage of urine may resolve itself if the volume is small. But peritonitis requires immediate medical intervention, including aggressive antibiotic therapy. Stool in the drainage is pathognomonic of a faulty intestinal anastomosis and requires prompt surgical correction.

Early postoperative period

20. NURSING DIAGNOSIS: Continued potential for circulatory and respiratory complications

Objective of nursing intervention Prevention or early detection of deep vein thrombosis, atelectasis, and pneumonia

Expected outcomes
Cooperation with regimen to increase activity tolerance and promote adequate circulation

Absence of lung congestion

or

Cooperation with regimen to improve respiratory function

Plan for implementation	Rationale
1. Encourage the patient to sit in a chair at least twice daily and to ambulate (with assistance if necessary) increasing distances as tolerated.	This increases the patient's tolerance for activity and promotes adequate circulation and lung expansion.
2. Do not permanently remove antiembolic stockings or Ace bandages until the patient is ambulating well (usually at least 10 days after surgery).	Until the patient is out of bed most of the day, elastic support of the legs is considered useful in preventing venous stasis.
3. Auscultate for lung congestion and continue turning, coughing, and deep breathing exercises as needed.	
4. Note changes in characteristics of cough, and notify the physician if the sputum becomes yellow, green, or brown, and/or is foul smelling.	Any indications of pneumonia must be reported to the physician so appropriate treatment can be started as soon as possible.

Late postoperative period

21. NURSING DIAGNOSIS: Potential for gastrointestinal complications related to resumption of oral intake

Objective of nursing intervention	Early detection of gastrointestinal complications

Expected outcomes { Absence of abdominal distention, tympany, nausea, and vomiting
Return to normal bowel function

Plan for implementation	Rationale
1. Disconnect the nasogastric tube as ordered.	Once bowel sounds are heard and the patient passes flatus, nasogastric suction is no longer required. The patient will usually be permitted sips of water, with the nasogastric tube clamped. If this is tolerated, the tube will be removed.
2. If a long (intestinal) tube is used, assist the physician with its removal.	A tube that extends into the intestines must be removed gradually over a period of a few hours to avoid damage to the gastrointestinal tract.
3. Notify the physician if nausea and vomiting occur.	
4. Note the patient's response to the diet, which usually begins with clear fluids and is then advanced as tolerated. The development of distention, tympany, nausea, or vomiting indicates that the patient is not yet able to tolerate oral intake.	
5. Be aware that diarrhea often occurs as the bowel regains normal function. If it should occur: a. Reassure the patient that this is a common occurrence and, although uncomfortable, is not serious. b. Estimate the amount of liquid stool and record it as output. c. If diarrhea persists (more than three episodes) notify the physician, who may order medication to control it.	The oral antibiotics given in the bowel preparation before surgery, the disruption of bowel continuity during surgery, and the absence of solid food may cause this temporary condition.
6. Be certain the patient is eating adequately, once he is back on his regular diet, to ensure adequate wound healing.	Nutritional deficiencies are a potential complication of this type of surgery because of the diet limitations before surgery and the period of fasting afterward.

Late postoperative period

22. NURSING DIAGNOSIS: Need for management of drainage from urethra following removal of urethral drain*

| Objectives of nursing intervention | Promotion of patient comfort
Early detection of complications |

Expected outcome   Gradual reduction and eventual absence of urethral drainage

Plan for implementation	Rationale
1. Note presence of drainage, its color, and approximate volume.	Usually the drain is not removed until the drainage becomes scanty. Therefore it is unlikely that the drainage will be more than a few milliliters, and an estimate can be made from the amount of staining that occurs.
2. Reassure the patient that it is normal for some drainage to continue for a few weeks, especially after the patient has been lying down for a while and then stands up.	Fluid will accumulate in the pelvic space when the patient is supine and drain with gravity when the patient is in a vertical position.
3. For the male patient, suggest the use of a combine wrapped **loosely** around the penis. However, it should be made clear to him that this should be used **only** when ambulating and never left in place for long periods.	Under no circumstances should the combine be wrapped tightly around the penis or left in place for any length of time. The fluid must be permitted to drain out of the body for adequate healing to take place.
4. For the female patient, suggest the use of a perineal pad. If used, be certain it is changed frequently to prevent skin breakdown.	
5. Notify the physician if there is a sudden increase in drainage or change in color.	Although it is unlikely at this point, there is a possibility that urine will leak from the internal surgical site, or a late postoperative hemorrhage may occur as tissue is sloughed.

Late postoperative period

---

*May not apply. Some patients will have an indwelling urethral catheter for a nonfunctioning bladder or perineal drains instead.

23. NURSING DIAGNOSIS: Continued potential for complications related to urinary output

Objective of nursing intervention Prevention or early detection of complications heralded by changes in characteristics of urine

Expected outcome Clear amber urine with occasional mucus shreds, draining approximately 100 ml/hour

Plan for implementation	Rationale
1. Check and record output each shift.	
2. Pay particular attention to the urine output during the 24-hour period following removal of ureteral stents (if used).	The possibility of edema occluding the ureters or conduit is small but must be considered nonetheless.
3. Note characteristics of the urine and report any abnormalities. It should no longer be blood tinged; mucus particles will be present.	
4. Provide maximum amount of fluid intake permitted by the physician (usually 2500 to 3000 ml per day).	Unless contraindicated by a coexisting medical condition, these patients should maintain a high fluid intake for the rest of their lives to discourage stasis of urine in the conduit and ascending infection.

24. NURSING DIAGNOSIS: Difficulty accepting changes in body image

Objectives of nursing intervention { Promotion of the patient's acceptance of his stoma
If married, promotion of the spouse's acceptance of the stoma

Expected outcomes { Willingness to look at and touch the stoma
Interest in learning stoma care
Willingness to participate in stoma care

Plan for implementation	Rationale
PROMOTING POSITIVE PATIENT ATTITUDE TOWARD STOMA	
1. Do not wear gloves when changing the patient's pouch.	If the nurse wears gloves, it gives the patient the impression that the stoma is either dirty or very delicate and easily contaminated. Actually the urine should be sterile (unless the patient has a urinary tract infection), and the stoma is like any other body orifice—it need only be kept reasonably clean.

Late postoperative period

Plan for implementation	Rationale
2. Express approval when looking at the stoma for the first time. This can be done verbally or with a smile and nod.	Nurses are usually the first people the patient will observe looking at his stoma. Their reaction will inevitably influence his reaction to the appearance of it.
3. Have the patient touch the stoma.	The sense of touch aids in the patient's acceptance of the stoma. Any fear of pain or sensitivity will be diminished once he realizes there is no feeling in the stoma and it will not fall off.
4. Have the patient participate in changing the pouch as soon as possible.	Early participation leads to early independence.

PROMOTING POSITIVE ATTITUDE OF PATIENT'S SPOUSE TOWARD STOMA

1. Continue to include the spouse in all teaching and discussion.	
2. If the spouse has not been present during the preoperative teaching, explain the following beforehand:	This prepares the spouse for the appearance of a stoma. It is especially important for somebody who has never seen an ostomy before and does not know what to expect. The redness of the stoma often gives the mistaken impression that it is delicate, inflamed, and painful to touch.
a. The stoma should be red or dark pink.	
b. The stoma has no pain receptors, so there is no pain associated with it.	
c. The cells of the stoma secrete a yellowish mucus.	
3. If circumstances permit, speak to the spouse about his or her facial reaction to the sight of the stoma. Any negative feelings should not be allowed to show on the spouse's face, which is probably what the patient will be watching the first time the spouse views the stoma.	Although open communication of feelings between the spouse and the patient is to be encouraged, the spouse's initial reaction to the stoma will leave its imprint in the patient's mind. If any negative reaction is visible, it may be remembered by the patient unconsciously, even if the spouse eventually makes a very positive adjustment to the stoma.
4. Convey to the spouse willingness to discuss any concerns, feelings, or questions about the surgery.	

Late postoperative period

25. NURSING DIAGNOSIS: Need for stoma care

Objectives of nursing intervention
{
Promotion of optimum healing of stoma site

Prevention or early detection of complications arising in peristomal area

Comprehensive teaching of stoma care to patient and/or family member
}

Expected outcomes
{
Stoma red or deep pink

Absence of skin breakdown or signs of inflammation in peristomal area

Understanding and application of stoma care information
}

Plan for implementation	Rationale
OBSERVATIONS TO BE MADE AND TAUGHT TO PATIENT	
1. The stoma should be red or deep pink.	These (nos. 1 to 5) are normal conditions. (See pp. 381 to 384 for abnormal conditions requiring intervention.)
2. The stoma should be free from encrustations.	
3. The peristomal skin should be the same color and texture as the rest of the abdominal skin.	
4. There should be no prolonged bleeding from the stoma opening or its stem. Occasional bleeding may occur when the stoma is cleansed because of the many capillaries near its surface.	
5. There should be no unusual odor from the stoma.	
CHANGING THE POUCH	

1. Change the pouch for the following reasons:
  a. Leakage
  b. Teaching purposes
  c. Every 4 or 5 days
	Even if the pouch remains intact for this length of time (and it should, if it is properly fitted), the peristomal skin should be evaluated no less frequently than every 5 days and considerably more frequently if there are any skin problems.

2. Lay out all necessary materials beforehand.	Stopping the procedure to locate missing equipment interrupts the teaching session and creates a disorganized atmosphere.
3. Maintain a confident attitude throughout the procedure.	The more calm the nurse is throughout the procedure, the easier it will appear to the patient.

Late postoperative period

Plan for implementation	**Rationale**
4. Be certain the patient is positioned to allow good visibility of the stoma.	
5. Provide reasons for each step of the procedure. (See p. 366 for step-by-step procedure for changing a urostomy pouch.)	It is easier to remember sequence and details when one understands why they are necessary.
6. Ask the patient simple questions throughout the procedure.	This enables the nurse to acertain the patient's degree of understanding, it enhances the learning process, and it provides a good review.
7. Encourage the patient to get involved in the procedure by initially giving him simple tasks to do (e.g., holding the gauze over the stoma, trimming or cutting the equipment to the required shape, and emptying the bag between changes).	
8. When possible, change the pouch in the early morning, when urine output is minimal.	Because there is no sphincter control, urine will continually flow out of the stoma. This hinders application of the pouch, which will adhere only to a completely dry surface. Therefore changing the pouch in the morning is easiest, since the patient has had relatively little fluid intake in the preceding 6 to 8 hours.
9. If urine flow from the stoma is heavy enough to interfere with the application of the pouch, have the patient cough a few times immediately before applying the pouch.	The increase in intraabdominal pressure that occurs during coughing usually expresses enough urine through the distal ureters and conduit to temporarily halt the flow of urine long enough to apply the pouch to a dry surface.
10. If retention sutures are used and are very close to the area where the pouch must be applied, reassure the patient that, once they are removed, there will be more of a uniform surface on the abdomen and the pouch will be easier to apply.	These large sutures cause temporary indentations in the abdomen, which may be in the area onto which the pouch must adhere. This causes a channel through which urine can leak. Extra care must be taken in applying the pouch to press the skin flat so that there is a good foundation to which the adhesive portion of the pouch can adhere.

Late postoperative period

26. NURSING DIAGNOSIS: Potential for complications related to the stoma and peristomal area

Objective of nursing intervention

Prevention, early detection, or early correction of stomal and peristomal problems

Expected outcomes

Stoma that is free from encrustations
Peristomal skin that is indistinguishable in appearance from other abdominal skin
Absence of odor

Although this section has been placed in the late postoperative period of the nursing care plan, it is not limited to this period. Preventative measures against stomal and peristomal complications begin in the preoperative period (choosing the optimum stomal site) and in the operative period (constructing a conduit that is as short as possible with a stoma that protrudes at least 1 cm beyond the surface of the abdomen). Prevention of complications then extends throughout the patient's life and depends on adequate patient teaching, appropriate appliances, and patient motivation. The following problems are those most commonly seen after urinary conduit surgery. However, inexperienced urology nurses should, if possible, consult with an enterostomal therapist before carrying out extensive nursing care of a patient with a urinary stoma so that they may provide truly comprehensive care. Prevention and early correction of stomal and peristomal problems fall primarily in the domain of the nurses, and their importance cannot be stressed enough. To say that the patient's life depends on optimum stomal care is not an exaggeration. If he does not disinfect his bag properly or if he does not have adequate fit of his appliance, his bag will leak and he will smell of urine; all psychosocial aspects of his life will be affected.[2] Furthermore, he may develop an infection that will ascend to his kidneys, resulting in potentially fatal renal damage from pyelonephritis; or constant stomal irritation may cause strictures, urinary retention, electrolyte imbalances, and structural damage necessitating more surgery.

Maintaining an acid urine appears to be a key factor in preventing some of the stomal and peristomal complications (e.g., alkaline encrustations, pseudoepitheliomatous hyperplasia, and odor).[1] However, controversy exists regarding how this should be accomplished. Acidification by high doses of vitamin C has been a popular method. However, some studies have indicated the acidification is very limited[5] or only occurs when there is no urinary tract infection.[6] Cranberry juice, a traditional nursing remedy, does not appear to adequately lower the urine pH even in very high quantities.[3] Furthermore, indiscriminate use of acidifying agents may be hazardous for any urinary conduit patient unless hyperchloremic acidosis (a common complication) has been ruled out. Otherwise, further lowering of the serum pH may compound the imbalance. For this reason the nurse should consult the physician about this aspect of patient management.

Plan for implementation	Rationale
WHITE ENCRUSTATIONS FORMING ON STOMA	

1. If the pouch does not have an antireflux valve:
  a. Instill 100 ml of white vinegar into the pouch. It can be full strength or diluted with water up to 1 : 4.
  b. Have the patient lie down, and allow the vinegar to slosh over the stoma for 30 minutes.
  c. Repeat the above procedure three or four times a day until crystals are gone.
	Alkaline crystals sometimes form on the stoma when the urine pH is elevated. They can be very irritating and may eventually obstruct the meatus if not removed. The irritation may also be a forerunner of stricture formation. The crystals can be dissolved by soaking in an acid solution such as vinegar.

Late postoperative period

Plan for implementation	Rationale

Late postoperative period

2. If the pouch has an antireflux valve:
   a. Remove the pouch and apply a gauze pad soaked in vinegar to the stoma for 30 minutes. Use a fresh pad every 5 minutes.
   b. Dry the stomal area thoroughly before reapplying the pouch.

IRREGULAR AREA OF RED IRRITATED SKIN AROUND STOMA, COVERED WITH WHITISH SLOUGH; MAY HAVE A WARTLIKE APPEARANCE

1. If this is accompanied by frequent leakage (i.e., the bag requires changing more than once every 4 or 5 days), evaluate and correct unsatisfactory parts of the equipment or application technique.

or

2. Check the relationship of the opening of the bag and the skin barrier to the stoma size. There should be no more than $1/16$ to $1/8$ inch of exposed skin around the stoma.

| | This condition is caused by continuous seepage of urine onto the skin and subsequent skin overgrowth. The technical name for the condition is pseudoepitheliomatous hyperplasia. |

3. Check the pH of the urine.
   a. Use fresh urine for the test.
   b. Apply Nitrazine paper to urine that has rolled off the stoma onto the skin.

   c. Notify the physician if the pH is above 6.5.

| | Urine from the bag will give an inaccurate reading. Nitrazine paper, placed directly on the stoma, may give a falsely high pH because of the alkalinity of the intestinal (stomal) mucosa. This skin condition is less likely to occur if the urine pH is relatively low. The physician may therefore choose to administer a systemic acidifying agent if infection or hyperchloremic acidosis is absent. |

4. Expose the skin to the air for 30 minutes twice a day and dry it thoroughly with a hair dryer (on "cool" setting).

5. Use a skin barrier such as Stomahesive or Colly-Seel to protect macerated skin. Do not use a karaya product for this purpose.

| | Karaya should never be used around a urinary stoma because it melts in urine. Leakage and skin breakdown will occur, and the spout on the bag may become clogged by pieces of karaya. |

PRURITIC, REDDENED RASH THAT SPREADS RAPIDLY AROUND STOMA

1. Report this to the physician. It is probably caused by a yeast infection, which will require an antifungal powder.

Plan for implementation	Rationale
2. Apply prescribed medication to clean, dry skin. A steroid spray* is often ordered, to be follow by an antifungal medication.	
3. Remove excess medication and apply equipment as usual.	An excessive amount of powder will prevent adequate adherence of the appliance.
4. If there is no improvement in 24 hours, the condition requires further evaluation.	

RED AREA AROUND STOMA THAT DOES NOT SPREAD AND HAS DEFINITE BORDERS; EDEMA OR SMALL
MULTIPLE VESICLES MAY BE PRESENT

1. Determine which part of the equipment is in direct contact with the affected skin.	Hypersensitivity to any of the ostomy products is a frequent occurrence, and alternative equipment must be substituted.
2. Change the particular piece of equipment to a related product made by a different ostomy supply company.	
3. If there is no improvement in 24 hours, the condition requires further evaluation.	

ODOR

1. Determine the cause. a. If infection is the suspected cause: (1) Obtain a urine specimen for culture and sensitivity tests (see Appendix C for catheterization of a urinary stoma). (2) If the urine is infected, notify the physician.	Infected urine must be investigated and treated at once to avoid pyelonephritis.
b. If poor hygiene is the suspected cause: (1) Emphasize the importance of meticulous cleanssing of the peristomal area. (2) If the patient is using a reusable pouch, he should wash it with dishwashing detergent, soak it in white vinegar or Uri-Kleen for 10 minutes, and allow it to dry thoroughly between wearings. If this regimen cannot be followed, the patient should switch to a disposable pouch. (3) The patient should remember to dry the spout on the pouch after each emptying.	This prevents urine sediment from building up on the outside of the pouch.

Late postoperative period

*Topical steroids should not be applied indiscriminately. Prolonged use may cause weakening and thinning of the epidermis.

Plan for implementation	**Rationale**

2. In general:
   a. Avoid asparagus.
   b. Add ostomy deodorant to the pouch each time it is emptied.
 	
   c. If further steps are desired, an oral medication, methionine (Pedameth), is available.
	Asparagus causes the urine to have a pungent odor.
	A few deodorants are made especially for this purpose. They are sold by the companies that make other ostomy products.
	This medication reduces the ammonia odor of urine.

INFLAMMATION OF HAIR FOLLICLES AROUND STOMA

1. Shave hair on peristomal area with an electric razor or cut it with small scissors.	Folliculitis can result from frequent pulling of hair when removing the adhesive portion of the appliance. Furthermore, the presence of hair reduces the watertight seal necessary to keep the pouch intact.
2. Use adhesive remover when removing any adhesive-backed portions of the equipment.	Removing slowly with remover is preferable to ripping off the adhesive seal (and the skin to which it is attached).

Late postoperative period

27. NURSING DIAGNOSIS: Need for comprehensive instruction in stoma care

Objective of nursing intervention   Adaptation of teaching regimen to suit the individual patient's needs

Expected outcomes   { Short term: Patient independence in stoma care
Long term: Absence of complications related to stoma management

Plan for implementation	Rationale
1. Measure the patient for a reusable appliance, and order equipment the patient will take home with him. The patient should be aware that the stoma may continue to shrink slightly during the next few months, and he may need to be refitted one or more times during this period.	The size of the stoma will decrease during the first week after surgery as postoperative edema resolves. Therefore measurements for a reusable appliance cannot be made until the second week after surgery. In some hospitals the patient is sent home with a single-use pouch and is not fitted for a reusable one until 2 months after surgery. This is because slight shrinkage may continue for as long as 1 year after surgery, and it is easier to adjust the size of the orifice of a disposable pouch than of a reusable one. Others recommend that the stoma be recalibrated every 3 weeks for 6 months and the appliance orifice be reduced as needed.[1]
2. Teach application of the reusable appliance to the patient and/or family member. Plan at least three teaching sessions.	
3. Emphasize the importance of thorough cleaning and **drying** of the pouch between wearings. (This means the patient should have at least 2 reusable pouches).	This is one of the most important measures in reducing urinary tract infection and odor.
4. Suggest the use of a pouch cover, particularly for the patient who perspires heavily and for use in a warm climate.	Cloth covers made to fit around the pouch reduce the irritation and chafing that often occur as the plastic pouch presses against the bare skin of the abdomen.
5. Encourage the patient to connect the bag to a bedside collecting container at night for the following reasons: a. This eliminates the need for the patient to awaken every few hours to empty his pouch. b. It reduces the possibility of the pouch being pulled off by the weight of the urine during the night. c. It reduces the risk of ascending infection because stagnant urine flows into the collecting container rather than remaining near the stoma.	
6. Explain the potential complications and how to observe for them at home (see pp. 381 to 384).	

Convalescent period

28. NURSING DIAGNOSIS: Need for discharge teaching

Objectives of nursing intervention
- Explanation of basic information about medications to be taken at home
- Explanation of information regarding follow-up care
- Explanation of residual effects of the condition and/or treatment
- Explanation of instructions concerning postdischarge activities
- Explanation of symptoms that constitute a reason to contact the physician
- Review of admitting diagnosis and mode of treatment

Expected outcomes
- Accurate return verbalization and/or demonstration of all material learned
- Smooth transition of care after discharge
- Absence or early detection of complications arising after discharge
- Ability to provide future health care practitioners with important data about health history

Plan for implementation	Rationale
See master care plan for the patient requiring discharge preparations: discharge teaching.	
In addition to the topics covered in the master care plan, include the following items in the discharge teaching:	
1. Information regarding follow-up medical care	
a. The initial follow-up appointments with the physician are usually scheduled for approximately 1 week and then 1 month after discharge. Other appointments are usually scheduled every 3 months for the first year and then every 6 months or yearly thereafter.	
b. At each visit a urine specimen will be obtained (for culture and pH) and the stoma will be examined. Therefore the patient should always bring extra equipment for a pouch change.	Urinary tract infection is a constant threat to these patients. The physician will also check for the development of stenosis, which is a serious and often silent complication.
c. The patient will be scheduled for periodic intravenous pyelograms and have periodic cytology studies done on his urine (if he had bladder carcinoma).	The intravenous pyelogram is to detect structural changes, such as stenosis of the ureteroileal anastomosis or hydronephrosis. The cytologic examination is to detect malignant cells in the urinary tract.
d. The patient's blood chemistry will be checked periodically.	These patients are prone to electrolyte imbalances. Hyperchloremic acidosis is a problem if stomal stenosis occurs because drainage from the conduit is impeded.
2. Information regarding follow-up nursing or enterostomal therapist care	
a. Explain to the patient that arrangements have been made with the Visiting Nurse Service (or whichever service has been contacted).	Reassuring the patient about arrangements with other support systems outside the hospital reduces the feeling that he has been left totally on his own to cope with what might be the biggest change in his entire life.
b. Provide the patient with a telephone number with which to reach the enterostomal therapist or nurse who was caring for him.	Few patients take undue advantage of this reassuring courtesy, and many small problems can be solved by telephone instead of through an office or clinic consultation.

Convalescent period

Plan for implementation	Rationale
3. Encourage the patient to contact ostomy associations and attend meetings at local chapters. The United Ostomy Association and the American Cancer Society have local chapters throughout the country. (See p. 147 for addresses of headquarters.)	These organizations are an ideal source of information about new ostomy appliances, equipment, and techniques. They also provide the patient with contact with other ostomates and are therefore the best form of emotional support.
4. During the next few weeks the expected residual effects of the surgery include incisional discomfort and especially fatigue.	The patient will tire more rapidly than most postoperative patients because of the extensive nature of this surgery, the period of fasting, possible blood loss, and tremendous emotional adjustments. Many patients worry that their inability to "bounce back" quickly is due to residual disease. They need to be reassured that slow progress is considered normal.
5. Fluid intake should be 2 to 3 L per day (unless contraindicated by a coexisting medical condition). The patient should learn to observe the color of his urine and increase his fluid intake if it becomes concentrated.	These patients are prone to ascending urinary tract infections. A rapid flow of urine through the urinary tract discourages bacterial multiplication by reducing urinary stasis.
6. The patient should notify the physician if any of the following occur:	
a. Chills, fever, hematuria, cloudy or foul-smelling urine, flank pain	These are signs and symptoms of a urinary tract infection.
b. Sudden decrease in urinary output despite adequate intake	The patient may be developing stenosis and obstruction.
c. Changes in stoma color or shape	Stomal ischemia, retraction, or hernia may be occurring.
d. Abdominal pain	This may indicate obstruction of the gastrointestinal tract from adhesions.
e. Persistent dry mouth, thirst, nausea, vomiting, paresthesia, lethargy	These are symptoms of hyperchloremic acidosis, a complication that may occur if electrolytes are absorbed through the walls of the conduit.
f. Suprapubic tenderness, palpable mass in bladder area, and fever	If cystectomy was **not** performed, the bladder sometimes becomes infected (pyocystis). This may occur at any time throughout the patient's life, since there is continuous mucus secretion within the bladder, which sometimes becomes a medium for bacterial growth.
7. Provide the patient with a list of supplies he will need, where they can be purchased, and the catalogue number of each item.	
8. If deemed appropriate, provide the patient with information concerning sexual counseling organizations.	When the prostate gland and bladder are removed, this surgery usually causes the male patient to become impotent because of interruptions in the parasympathetic nerve pathways. Therefore sexual counseling for a man and his wife may be extremely helpful. Furthermore, surgical techniques have been developed to provide the man with a silicone implant in his penis to enable vaginal penetration (see Chapter 50).

Convalescent period

Ureterosigmoidostomy

The indications for ureterosigmoidostomy are the same as those for conduit diversion. Both procedures are methods of urinary diversion for patients with bladder carcinoma, congenital anomalies, intractable incontinence, and certain other conditions. Although there may be more physiologic complications associated with this procedure than with intestinal conduits, the psychologic problems associated with a stoma are avoided. Therefore this method is often used in children for whom the formation of a stoma may be too psychologically traumatic or for adults who refuse to have a stoma. Even this procedure, however, requires considerable psychologic adjustment, since the patient will have to become accustomed to evacuating stool and urine through the same orifice.

For the procedure the patient is placed in a supine position. A vertical midline or paramedian incision is made (occasionally a very wide, transverse lower abdominal incision is used instead), and the peritoneal cavity is entered. The ureters are located, clamped, and transected, and, if the surgery is being performed for carcinoma of the bladder, a radical cystectomy and prostatectomy are done. The sigmoid colon is then incised in two adjacent areas, and the ureters are inserted through a sub-mucosal tunnel, which reduces the possibility of reflux (Fig. 38-3). Ureteral stents are usually inserted to support the anastomosis and to ensure adequate drainage until edema subsides. They generally extend from the renal pelvis through the anal sphincter. An incisional drain is then inserted, and the abdominal wound is closed. A rectal tube (or balloon-type indwelling catheter) is placed in the rectum to provide a continuous flow of urine, thereby preventing reabsorption of urinary electrolytes.

If a cystectomy is not performed, an indwelling urethral catheter is inserted into the nonfunctioning bladder to drain the mucus that accumulates in the bladder and increases the risk of infection in the early postoperative period (Fig. 38-4). If a cystec-

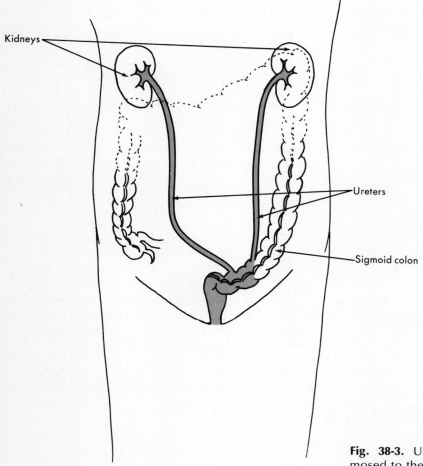

Fig. 38-3. Ureterosigmoidostomy; ureters are anastomosed to the sigmoid colon.

tomy is performed but the urethra is left intact, the same type of catheter is inserted through the urethra into the pelvic space where the bladder had been to allow for drainage of serosanguineous fluid, which accumulates in this area. A cystectomy **and** urethrectomy require only an incisional drain at the perineal suture line.

Complications following this type of surgery are associated with the colon's high bacterial content, its absorptive characteristics, and its relatively high pressure. Pyelonephritis may occur as a result of fecal reflux and ascending organisms. Hyperchloremic acidosis may occur, accompanied by severe hypokalemia, because a selective exchange of ions takes place in the colonic mucosa when urine is present; urinary chloride and hydrogen ions are absorbed back into the bloodstream, and potassium and bicarbonate ions are taken from the bloodstream and excreted in the feces. An additional late complication has recently been reported in patients

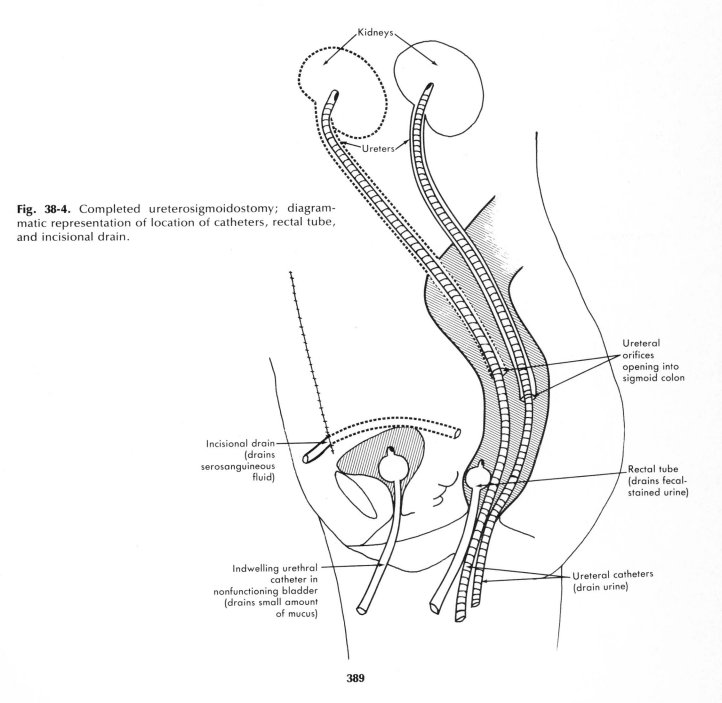

Fig. 38-4. Completed ureterosigmoidostomy; diagrammatic representation of location of catheters, rectal tube, and incisional drain.

undergoing this surgery for carcinoma of the bladder. An unusually high proportion of these patients develop carcinoma of the colon.[4] Other problems associated with this procedure are uremia, azotemia, and the development of structural abnormalities such as hydronephrosis, hydroureter, and strictures at the site of the anastomoses.

In spite of all these complications, this surgery is often chosen above other forms of diversion because the numerous problems (physical and psychologic) associated with a stoma are absent. Of course, this surgery is contraindicated if the patient has an incompetent anal sphincter, since he will be completely reliant on his rectum for remaining continent of urine as well as stool. Many surgeons also consider severely dilated ureters to be a contraindication, since all the problems associated with reflux will be more pronounced with this condition.

URETEROSIGMOIDOSTOMY
Outline of Care Plan
ANTICIPATED NURSING DIAGNOSES:

Early preoperative period (2 to 4 days before surgery)
1. Need for evaluation of anal sphincter competence. (See p. 391.)†
2. Need for reduction of fecal matter in the gastrointestinal tract. (See p. 355.)*
3. Need for discharge planning. (See p. 392.)†

Late preoperative period (24 to 48 hours before surgery)
4. Need for antimicrobial bowel preparation. (See p. 357.)*

---

*Nursing care is the same as for the patient undergoing conduit diversion.

†Nursing care is described on the following pages.

5. Potential for postoperative abdominal distention, pain, and vomiting. (See p. 358).*
6. Need for preoperative teaching. (See p. 392.)†

Early postoperative period
7. Potential for shock. (See p. 361.)*
8. Postoperative pain. (See p. 362.)*
9. Potential for wound complications. (See p. 364. Omit No. 4; these patients do not have a stoma.)*
10. Need for management of urinary drainage. (See p. 394.)†
11. Need for management of intravenous infusion. (See p. 368.)*
12. Need for management of urethral drain or indwelling urethral catheter. (See p. 368.)*
13. Alterations in gastrointestinal function. (See p. 370.)*
14. Potential for respiratory complications related to surgical intervention. (See p. 372.)*
15. Potential for deep vein thrombosis. (See p. 372.)*
16. Potential for peritonitis. (See p. 373. If leakage occurs, it will be at the ureterosigmoid anastomosis.)*

Late postoperative period
17. Continued potential for circulatory and respiratory complications. (See p. 374).*
18. Potential for gastrointestinal complications related to resumption of oral intake. (See p. 396.)†
19. Need for management of drainage from urethra following removal of urethral drain. (See p. 376.* May not apply.)
20. Continued potential for complications related to urinary output. (See p. 397.)†

Convalescent period
21. Need for discharge teaching. (See p. 398.)†

---

*Nursing care is the same as for patients undergoing conduit diversion.

†Nursing care is described on the following pages.

PARTIAL NURSING CARE PLAN FOR THE PATIENT UNDERGOING URETEROSIGMOIDOSTOMY

1. NURSING DIAGNOSIS: Need for evaluation of anal sphincter competence

Objective of nursing intrevention	Explanation and administration of saline enema
Expected outcome	Retention of enema for a minimum of 1 hour

Plan for implementation	Rationale
1. Explain to the patient the purpose of the enema. It is a test to ascertain the ability of the anal sphincter to retain fluid.	Most patients associate enemas with catharsis only. It should be made quite clear that the purpose is to simulate the presence of urine in the rectum.
2. Instill approximately 300 ml normal saline into the patient's rectum.	Normal saline is used (as opposed to tap water) because it is isotonic and therefore will not cause electrolyte problems if it is absorbed through the colon.
3. For the next hour have the patient get up, ambulate, and participate in normal activities while retaining the enema.	
4. Check for leakage of saline and report findings to the physician.	
5. Have the patient expel the enema.	

Early preoperative period

3. NURSING DIAGNOSIS: Need for discharge planning

Objectives of nursing intervention { Early commencement of discharge planning
Accurate estimate of time required for all discharge teaching

Expected outcome Smooth transition of care after discharge

Plan for implementation	Rationale

See master care plan for the patient requiring discharge preparations: discharge planning.
 	
In addition to the topics covered in the master care plan, the following items should be considered:
1. Hospitalization for this procedure is approximately 10 days to 2 weeks.
 	
2. Required teaching includes:
  a. General postoperative discharge teaching
  b. Instructions on the need for frequent voiding and the use of nighttime rectal drainage
  c. Discussion of the need for periodic check-ups throughout the patient's life	

Early preoperative period

6. NURSING DIAGNOSIS: Need for preoperative teaching

Objectives of nursing intervention {
If necessary, clarification of reason for hospitalization and type of surgery to be performed
Elimination of any negative or inaccurate notions regarding the forthcoming surgery
Explanation of preoperative tests and procedures
Psychologic preparation for general anesthesia
Explanation of events expected in the early postoperative period
Explanation of body conditions expected in the early postoperative period
Identification of any known allergies

Expected outcomes {
Verbal indication that explanations are understood
Verbal indication of optimistic expectations (within realistic limits) related to forthcoming surgery
Cooperation during preoperative tests and procedures
Verbal or behavioral indication of reduction of anxiety
Absence of postoperative complications
Absence of allergic reactions

Late preoperative period

Plan for implementation	**Rationale**
See master care plan for the patient receiving preoperative teaching.	
In addition to the topics covered in the master care plan, include the following items in the preoperative teaching:	
1. Be aware that, in addition to routine preoperative procedures, the diagnostic procedures for ureterosigmoidostomy are the same as for conduit diversion (see p. 359), and answer any questions the patient may have regarding them.	
2. Enemas will be continued until the evening before or the morning of surgery.	Usually the physician will order the patient to have tap water enemas "until clear" in the evening and sometimes also in the morning before surgery.
3. The preoperative shave will be from the nipple line to midthigh.	
4. Oral intake will be prohibited for at least 24 to 48 hours after surgery. During this time the nasogastric tube will be connected to a suction machine by the patient's bedside.	Oral intake, as well as gastric secretions and gas, would cause severe discomfort during the period of intestinal atony, which almost always occurs after any manipulation of the intestinal tract.
5. Once the patient passes flatus and bowel sounds are heard, he will be started on a clear liquid diet. This will be advanced to a low-residue diet on which the patient will remain for approximately 1 week.	A low-residue diet limits the amount of formed stool in the colon while the ureteral anastomosis is healing.
6. The patient will have drainage tubes coming from his rectum for about 1 week. Two of these tubes extend up to his kidneys and facilitate the drainage of urine. The third is a larger tube that ends in the rectum. This tube will be removed as needed for the patient to defecate.	The rectal tube prevents urine from accumulating in the colon. If this were to occur, it would cause distention at the surgical site.
7. There may be a tube coming from the patient's urethra to drain fluid from the surgical area (or from the bladder if cystectomy was not performed). This tube will be left in place for approximately 1 week or until the drainage is minimal.	When a cystectomy is performed without a urethrectomy, some surgeons insert an indwelling urethral catheter to prevent serous fluid from accumulating in the space that was occupied by the bladder. In instances where the bladder has been left intact, the catheter will drain the small amount of mucus that tends to accumulate in the bladder. Unless permitted to drain from the body, any accumulation of fluid will contribute to the development of infection.
8. The patient will have an incision on his abdomen that will be covered with a dressing. There is usually drainage from the incision, so the dressing will require frequent changing during the first few days after surgery.	

Late preoperative period

10. NURSING DIAGNOSIS: Need for management of urinary drainage

| Objective of nursing intervention | Prevention or early detection of complications associated with urinary output |

Objective of nursing intervention   Prevention or early detection of complications associated with urinary output

Expected outcome   Clear amber urine draining through ureteral catheters at approximately 100 ml/ hour

Plan for implementation	Rationale
1. Keep ureteral catheters and rectal tube (or balloon-type indwelling catheter) securely taped to the patient's thigh. Some surgeons will suture the ureteral catheters to the perineum.	This prevents inadvertent traction and possible displacement of the tubes. The ureteral catheters are in place to support the anastomosis and prevent obstruction from edema. The rectal tube prevents any additional urine (that which flows around the catheters rather than through them) from accumulating in the area. This prevents distention near the surgical site and eliminates the possibility of reabsorption of urinary electrolytes through the colon wall.
2. Label each collecting container accordingly: rectal tube, right ureteral catheter, left ureteral catheter. (Unless the surgeon marked the ureteral catheters in the operating room, the floor nurse will not be able to distinguish right from left.)	This enables rapid evaluation of each kidney's urine output.
3. Keep accurate records of volume and character of urine from each source. Urine from the ureteral catheters should be clear amber. Urine from the rectal tube may be blood tinged and/or fecal stained.	Urine from the catheters is flowing directly from the kidneys and does not communicate with the anastomosis or fecal content of the colon. Urine through the rectal tube has passed through the anastomosis and the rectum. Therefore it may have some blood and/or fecal matter in it.
4. Notify the physician if any of the following occur: a. The appearance of bright red urine b. Significant decrease or absence of urine from any of the three tubes	

Early postoperative period

Plan for implementation	Rationale

5. Irrigate the tubes only if specifically ordered, using the following guidelines:
  a. Irrigation fluid must be an isotonic solution.
  b. Irrigation must be done gently to prevent trauma to the kidneys (via the ureteral catheters) and to the suture lines (via the rectal tube).	

6. If the rectal tube (or balloon-type indwelling catheter) requires replacement (i.e., it falls out or requires removal so the patient can defecate), use the following guidelines: a. If this occurs within the first 4 days after surgery, notify the physician. Usually he will replace it himself.	In the early postoperative period there is a risk of perforation at the surgical site if the tube is replaced by somebody who lacks precise knowledge of the location of the anastomosis.
b. Use a no. 30 French tube or catheter.	This size provides adequate drainage of urine mixed with feces.
c. Use a water-soluble local anesthetic on the tip of the tube.	This eliminates discomfort while the tube is being inserted.
d. Do not insert the tube more than 3 or 4 inches into the rectum.	This prevents trauma to the anastomosis, which is usually 6 to 8 inches above the anus.
e. If a balloon-type indwelling catheter is used, do not instill more than 5 to 10 ml of fluid into the balloon.	Distending the balloon more than this amount is unnecessary and may be uncomfortable for the patient.

Early postoperative period

18. NURSING DIAGNOSIS: Potential for gastrointestinal complications related to resumption of oral intake

Objective of nursing intervention   Early detection of gastrointestinal complications

Expected outcomes { Absence of abdominal distention, tympany, nausea, or vomiting
Reestablishment of intestinal peristalsis

Plan for implementation	Rationale
1. Disconnect the nasogastric tube as ordered.	Once bowel sounds are heard and the patient passes flatus, nasogastric suction is no longer required. The patient will usually be permitted sips of water with the tube clamped. If this is tolerated, the tube will be removed.
2. If a long (intestinal) tube is used, assist the physician with its removal.	A tube that extends into the intestines must be removed gradually over a period of a few hours to prevent damage to the gastrointestinal tract.
3. Notify the physician if nausea and vomiting occur.	
4. Note the patient's response to the diet, which usually begins with clear fluids and is then advanced to low residue. The patient will usually remain on this diet for as long as the ureteral catheters are in place.	This limits the amount of formed stool in the colon during the period when the anastomoses are the most delicate.
5. Remove the rectal tube so the patient can defecate.	
6. Reinsert the tube after the patient defecates.	
7. Inform the patient that his stool will be diarrhea-like when the ureteral catheters are removed.	The low-residue diet and the diluting effect of the urine in the colon will make the stool softer than what the patient is accustomed to.
8. Explain to the patient that he will learn to distinguish the difference between the need to urinate and the need to defecate even though his stool will remain relatively loose.	

Late postoperative period

20. NURSING DIAGNOSIS: Continued potential for complications related to urinary output

Objective of nursing intervention	Prevention or early detection of urinary and/or electrolyte abnormalities

Expected outcomes { Cooperation with regimen for emptying colon
Absence of indications of electrolyte imbalances

Plan for implementation	Rationale
1. Following removal of rectal tube and ureteral catheters, encourage the patient to empty his rectum every 3 to 4 hours during the day.	If urine is permitted to accumulate in the rectum, electrolytes will be reabsorbed through the wall of the colon. Severe electrolyte imbalance (hyperchloremic acidosis and hypokalemia) is one of the most serious hazards of this type of surgery.
2. Check and record the output each shift.	
3. Note characteristics of the urine and report any abnormalities such as the presence of blood.	
4. Pay particular attention to the urine output during the first 24 hours after the removal of the ureteral catheters.	The possibility of edema occluding the ureters is very small but must be considered nonetheless.
5. Provide the maximum amount of fluid intake permitted by the patient's physician (usually 2500 ml per day).	Unless contraindicated by a coexisting medical condition, these patients should remain on a relatively high fluid intake for life to discourage the incidence of ascending infection.
6. Insert a rectal tube for nighttime drainage, and teach the patient the procedure. (See p. 399.)	Many surgeons recommend that the patient use a nighttime drainage system even after discharge so urine does not accumulate in the rectum, where electrolytes may be reabsorbed. This also eliminates the need for the patient to awaken several times at night to empty his rectum.

7. Notify the physician of any evidence of electrolyte imbalance.
 a. Check laboratory values for serum chemistry (especially chloride, potassium, sodium, bicarbonate, BUN [blood urea nitrogen], and creatinine).
 b. Be alert for symptoms of hypokalemia.
  (1) Arrhythmias
  (2) Anorexia
  (3) Lethargy
  (4) Confusion
  (5) Flaccid paralysis
 c. Be alert for symptoms of metabolic acidosis.
  (1) Apathy
  (2) Disorientation
  (3) Weakness
  (4) Kussmaul respirations

Late postoperative period

21. NURSING DIAGNOSIS: Need for discharge teaching

Objectives of nursing intervention

Explanation of basic information about medications to be taken at home

Explanation of information regarding follow-up care

Explanation of residual effects of the condition and/or treatment

Explanation of instructions concerning postdischarge activities

Explanation of symptoms that constitute a reason to contact the physician

Review of admitting diagnosis and mode of treatment

Expected outcomes

Accurate return verbalization and/or demonstration of all material learned

Smooth transition of care after discharge

Absence or early detection of complications arising after discharge

Ability to provide future health care practitioners with important data about health history

Plan for implementation	Rationale
See master care plan for the patient requiring discharge preparations: discharge teaching.	
In addition to the topics covered in the master care plan, include the following items in the discharge teaching:	
1. At the initial follow-up visit the physician will check the abdominal wound for adequate healing and will obtain a blood specimen for electrolyte determination.	
2. The patient will be scheduled for additional office visits at intervals of approximately 3 months for the first year, every 6 months for the next year, and then annually. Serum electrolytes wll be checked, and the patient will have periodic intravenous pyelograms.	Any changes in the patient's electrolyte status must be corrected. Intravenous pyelograms are done at the physician's discretion to detect any structural changes in the urinary tract.
3. When this surgery is done for bladder cancer, additional precautions are required. a. The stool is checked for blood every 3 months. b. Intravenous pyelograms are obtained on a yearly basis (usually beginning 5 years postoperatively). c. Periodic sigmoidoscopies, colonoscopies, and/or barium enemas are performed.	There is a high incidence of recurrence of cancer elsewhere in the urinary tract and in the colon after this type of surgery. Although the exact pathogenesis is uncertain, it is thought that carcinogenic factors in the urine itself may be the cause.[4]
4. During the next few weeks expected residual effects of the surgery include incisional discomfort and fatigue.	

Convalescent period

Plan for implementation	Rationale
5. The patient must continue to empty his rectum every 3 or 4 hours while awake and at least once a night if a rectal tube has not been prescribed.	Urine must not be permitted to accumulate in the rectum for more than a few hours or serious electrolyte abnormalities will occur as a result or reabsorption of urinary electrolytes back into the bloodstream.

6. If a rectal tube has been prescribed, give the patient a list of equipment he will need, names of places to buy the equipment, and the following written instructions:
a. Assemble all materials before hand.
  (1) Plastic tubing and collecting container
  (2) No. 28 rectal tube
  (3) Adhesive tape (four 6-inch strips)
  (4) Water-soluble lubricant
  (5) Plastic sheet and/or incontinence pads
  (6) Tincture of benzoin (optional)
  (7) Benzalkonium solution (1:750)	

b. Apply plastic bed shields as needed.	Some patients will have occasional leakage during the night.
c. Connect rectal tube, tubing, and collecting container. d. Apply two strips of tape under whichever buttock will be facing the collecting container.	These tapes give a good foundation for the tubing and remaining tape. If the patient has sensitive skin, tincture of benzoin should be applied first to protect the skin.
e. Lubricate the tube and insert it 4 inches into the rectum. f. Place the other two pieces of tape over the rectal tube and the first pieces of tape, and press firmly to secure the tape to the skin.	The anastomosis is usually 6 to 8 inches above the anus, and the tube must be distal to this point.

g. When removing the tube in the morning, wrap it in tissue to avoid soiling the bedding.
h. Clean equipment daily.
  (1) Wash collecting container, rectal tube, and plastic tubing thoroughly with soap and water.
  (2) Soak rectal tube and plastic tubing in benzalkonium solution for 15 minutes.
  (3) Rinse rectal tube and tubing in cold water.
  (4) Boil the rectal tube for 10 minutes.
	Thorough cleaning of equipment is essential to control odor and ensure adequate hygiene.

7. The patient should not receive enemas or take laxatives at any time for the rest of his life.	These treatments are not only unnecessary (the patient's stool will remain soft because of the presence of urine in the colon) but also may exacerbate electrolyte irregularities.
8. The patient should notify the physician if any of the following occur: a. Chills, fever, flank pain, or hematuria	These may be indications of a urinary tract infection. Hematuria may be also caused by a colonic or renal lesion.
b. Sudden decrease in urinary output despite adequate intake	This may be an indication of ureteral obstruction.

Convalescent period

Convalescent period

Plan for implementation	Rationale
c. Persistent dry mouth, thirst, anorexia, nausea, vomiting, paresthesia	These are symptoms of hyperchloremic acidosis.
d. Lethargy, confusion, abnormal behavior	These are symptoms of hypokalemia. Changes in mental status are also symptoms of low magnesium, another electrolyte that may be excreted in abnormally large quantities.
9. If deemed appropriate, provide the patient with information concerning sexual counseling organizations.	When the bladder and prostate are removed, this surgery usually causes the male patient to become impotent because of interruptions in the parasympathetic nerve pathways. Therefore sexual counseling for a man and his wife may be extremely helpful. Furthermore, surgical techniques have been developed to provide the man with a silicone implant in his penis to enable vaginal penetration (see Chapter 50).

Cutaneous ureterostomy

Cutaneous ureterostomy is most commonly employed in adults as a palliative treatment for advanced malignancies of the bladder or other pelvic organs for which supravesical diversion is necessary. It is also performed for certain types of urinary incontinence or irreversible damage to the urinary tract.

There are various forms of cutaneous ureterostomy. When only one ureter is suitable for externalization, the other one is anastomosed to it, proximal to the stoma, and urine from both kidneys drains through the single ureteral stoma (ureteroureterostomy). Other forms involve externalization of both ureters into adjacent stomas (double-barreled cutaneous ureterostomy), or both ureters are externalized on either side of the abdomen (bilateral cutaneous ureterostomy).

For the procedure the patient is placed in a supine position, and a midline or paramedian incision is made. The ureters are identified, transected, and brought out anteriorly through the skin. In some cases the stoma site is determined preoperatively. However, the condition of the ureters is a major consideration in the choice of stoma placement, and often there are not many options.

Any additional surgery (e.g., cystectomy) may be performed at this time. If ureteroureterostomy is being done, an incisional drain is inserted near the anastomosis. The incision is then closed and the ostomy appliance(s) and dressings are applied. In most cases the bladder is left intact, and an indwelling urethral catheter is inserted to drain the mucus that accumulates in the bladder and contributes to the development of infection.

Advantages of this form of diversion over the more commonly performed procedures are that the surgery is short, it eliminates the intestinal complications associated with procedures involving an intestinal conduit, and it is less complicated surgery (it can often be done extraperitoneally), so it may be used for patients who would be unable to tolerate extensive surgery.

However, there are numerous complications associated with cutaneous ureterostomy, including stenosis of the stoma and pyelonephritis. Because stomal stenosis is such a common complication, the procedure is usually only performed as a temporary measure or for a patient whose life expectancy is relatively short. When it is used as a permanent form of diversion in a patient with an otherwise normal life expectancy, it is usually done only if at least one of the ureters is chronically hypertrophied and dilated, making stomal stenosis less likely.

CUTANEOUS URETEROSTOMY
Outline of Care Plan

Nursing care plans for patients undergoing a cutaneous ureterostomy will vary considerably, depending on the general condition of the patient and the extent of any additional surgery. Since this procedure is most commonly done for the patient with a relatively short life expectancy (except for the pediatric patient for whom the procedure may be done with the intent of undiversion later on), many of the psychosocial considerations relating to changes in body image may not apply. In these patients, declining health and poor long-term prognosis will be the major focus of the nurse's attention with regard to the patient's psychosocial needs. However, assessment of patients in otherwise relatively good health will include all the psychosocial considerations discussed in the care plan for the patient undergoing conduit diversion.

ANTICIPATED NURSING DIAGNOSES:

Preoperative period

1. Need for preoperative teaching. (See p. 401.)†
2. Need for discharge planning. (See p. 403.)†
3. Dependence on assistance in coping with changes in life-style imposed by advanced cancer. (May not apply. See Chapter 20, nursing objective 2.)

Early postoperative period

4. Potential for shock. (See p. 404.)†
5. Postoperative pain. (See p. 362. Omit material concerning muscle and throat pain. This pain is usually less severe than the pain after conduit diversion because the surgery is not as extensive.)*
6. Potential for wound complications. (See p. 364.) Drainage may not be heavy, depending on the type of ureterostomy performed and the presence of incisional drains.)*
7. Need for management of urinary drainage. (See p. 365. The urine does not contain mucus particles.)*
8. Need for management of intravenous infusion. (See p. 368. Type and duration of infusion will depend on the patient's general condition.)*

---

*Nursing care is the same as for the patient undergoing conduit diversion.
†Nursing care is described on the following pages.

9. Need for management of indwelling urethral catheter. (See p. 405.)†
10. Potential for respiratory complications related to surgical intervention. (See p. 372. Respiratory complications do not occur as frequently after cutaneous ureterostomy because the duration of this surgery is relatively short.)*
11. Potential for deep vein thrombosis. (See p. 372.)*

Late postoperative period

12. Continued potential for complications related to urinary output. (See p. 377. The urine does not contain mucus particles.)*
13. Need for stoma care. (See p. 379.)*
14. Potential complications involving stoma and peristomal skin. (See p. 381.* Add information on stomal stenosis discussed in discharge teaching section.)

Convalescent period

15. Need for discharge teaching. (See p. 406.)†

---

*Nursing care is the same as for patients undergoing conduit diversion.
†Nursing care is described on the following pages.

PARTIAL NURSING CARE PLAN FOR THE PATIENT UNDERGOING CUTANEOUS URETEROSTOMY

1. NURSING DIAGNOSIS: Need for preoperative teaching

Objectives of nursing intervention

- If necessary, clarification of reason for hospitalization and type of surgery to be performed
- Elimination of any negative or inaccurate notions regarding the forthcoming surgery
- Explanation of preoperative tests and procedures
- Psychologic preparation for general anesthesia
- Explanation of events expected in the early postoperative period
- Explanation of body conditions expected in the early postoperative period
- Identification of any known allergies

Expected outcomes

- Verbal indication that explanations are understood
- Verbal indication of optimistic expectations (within realistic limits) related to forthcoming surgery
- Cooperation during preoperative tests and procedures
- Verbal or behavioral indication of reduction of anxiety
- Absence of postoperative complications
- Absence of allergic reactions

Preoperative period

Plan for implementation	Rationale

See master care plan for the patient receiving preoperative teaching.

In addition to the topics covered in the master care plan, include the following items in the preoperative teaching:
1. Be aware that, in addition to routine preoperative procedures, the diagnostic tests preceding cutaneous ureterostomy may be the same as for conduit diversion (see p. 359), depending on the primary problem for which the patient is being treated. Answer any questions the patient may have regarding these procedures.

2. The preoperative shave will be from nipple line to mid-thigh.

3. The patient will probably be permitted clear fluids in the evening after surgery, and his diet will be advanced as tolerated.

Because the peritoneal cavity is not entered during this surgery, the incidence of postoperative gastrointestinal disturbances is relatively low.

4. There will be a vertical incision on the patient's abdomen, which will be covered by a dressing.

5. Urine will flow from the stoma(s) and will be contained in a pouch attached to the abdomen.

NOTE: Depending on the patient's condition, detailed preoperative discussion and teaching regarding the stoma should be done at least a few days before surgery. (See care plan for the patient undergoing conduit diversion.) In many cases, however, this is inappropriate. The patient's mental condition is often deteriorated, or the surgery is done as an emergency to correct obstruction, and there is no time for lengthy psychologic preparation.

Preoperative period

2. NURSING DIAGNOSIS: Need for discharge planning

Objectives of nursing intervention { Early commencement of discharge planning

Accurate estimate of time required for all discharge teaching

Expected outcome Smooth transition of care after discharge

Plan for implementation	Rationale
See master care plan for the patient receiving discharge preparations: discharge planning.	
In addition to the topics covered in the master care plan, the following items should be considered:	
1. The duration of hospitalization for this procedure will vary considerably, depending on the patient's general condition and/or the duration of hospitalization for the primary problem.	
2. Discharge teaching may include general postoperative discharge teaching as well as comprehensive teaching of stoma care.	
3. Refer the patient to the hospital's social service department if it appears that professional care will be required after discharge.	It may be necessary for the patient to be discharged to an extended care facility, depending on his general condition. These plans should be made well in advance so that necessary forms can be completed by the time the patient is ready to leave the hospital.

Preoperative period

4. NURSING DIAGNOSIS: Potential for shock

Objective of nursing intervention   Prevention or early detection of shock

Expected outcomes   { Vital signs normal, skin dry, color normal
Absence of bright red drainage

Plan for implementation	Rationale
1. Check the patient's vital signs every 4 hours once stable (every 15 minutes if unstable).	The risk of shock after this type of surgery is generally small because few blood vessels are cut, and the surgery itself is not highly complex. However, often these patients are already in a compromised physical condition, and the added stress of surgery makes shock a potential complication that must be considered.
2. Be alert for increasing pulse and respiratory rates, decreasing blood pressure, diaphoresis, pallor, and feelings of apprehension.	
3. Notify the physician at once if indications of impending shock occur.	

Early postoperative period

9. NURSING DIAGNOSIS: Need for management of indwelling urethral catheter

Objective of nursing intervention Prevention or early detection of complications related to nonfunctioning bladder

Expected outcome Whitish, clear, or blood-tinged mucus draining through indwelling urethral catheter

Plan for implementation	Rationale
1. Record volume and characteristics of drainage each shift.	A catheter is usually left in the nonfunctioning bladder for the following reasons: 1. Mucus tends to accumulate in the bladder. A catheter will facilitate drainage, especially in a patient confined to bed, as many of these patients are. Stasis of this mucus predisposes the patient to infection of the bladder (pyocystis). 2. Many of these patients have cancer of the bladder, which is inoperable. These lesions frequently bleed, and the catheter facilitates drainage from the area.
2. Prevent external obstruction of the catheter and tubing. Prevent kinking of the tubing, and position the patient so that he is not lying on it.	
3. Provide hand-irrigation of the catheter only if ordered.	If pyocystis occurs, antibiotic irrigation of the catheter is often ordered on a specific time schedule.
4. See master care plan for the patient with an indwelling urethral catheter for more detailed nursing actions.	

Early postoperative period

15. NURSING DIAGNOSIS: Need for discharge teaching

Objectives of nursing intervention

Explanation of basic information about medications to be taken at home

Explanation of information regarding follow-up care

Explanation of residual effects of the condition and/or treatment

Explanation of instructions concerning postdischarge activities

Explanation of symptoms that constitute a reason to contact the physician

Review of admitting diagnosis and mode of treatment

Expected outcomes

Accurate return verbalization and/or demonstration of all material learned

Smooth transition of care after discharge

Absence or early detection of complications arising after discharge

Ability to provide future health care practitioners with important data about health history

Convalescent period

Plan for implementation	Rationale
See master care plan for the patient requiring discharge preparations: discharge teaching.	
The extent and depth of discharge teaching will vary considerably depending on the patient's general condition and who will be providing his care.	Many of these patients will not be discharged home because of their primary medical problems, which require continued professional care.
1. Follow discharge teaching guidelines on pp. 386 and 387. Eliminate or modify information as necessary.	Discharge care after cutaneous ureterostomy is similar to that following conduit diversion. However, since some of these patients may not be going home, much of this information may instead be transcribed onto a document from another institution or hospital department to which the patient will be transferred. Instead of providing discharge teaching, the nurse will write the information as a recommendation for follow-up nursing care.
2. Emphasize the importance of observing the stoma for signs of stenosis. The physician must be notified if any occur. They include: a. Reduced urine output despite adequate fluid intake b. Retraction or dimpling of the stoma	Stomal stenosis is the most common complication when a portion of the ureter is reconstructed into a stoma. Stenosis causes reduction in the diameter of the ureteral lumen and eventual obstruction. Although decreased output may also be due to other causes, such as dehydration or renal failure, stomal stenosis must be investigated and corrected at once to prevent structural damage to the urinary tract.

CHAPTER 39

Surgery for stress incontinence

Stress incontinence is a condition that primarily affects older and multiparous women. It is defined as the involuntary loss of urine through the urethra associated with sudden increases in intraabdominal pressure in an otherwise normal individual. Thorough urodynamic and radiologic studies are necessary to rule out other causes of incontinence, such as neurogenic bladder, vesicovaginal fistula, and urinary retention with overflow.

There are a variety of surgical procedures to correct the condition, which use a vaginal approach, a suprapubic approach, or a combination of the two. The vaginal correction (anterior vaginal colporrhaphy) is usually done by gynecologists and is therefore rarely seen on a urology floor. For this reason only the other types of procedures are discussed.

SUPRAPUBIC SUSPENSION PROCEDURES

The three most common procedures in this category are the Marshall-Marchetti-Krantz procedure, the Lapides anterior vesicopexy, and the Burch colposuspension. All involve elevating the bladder into the abdominal cavity, which results in lengthening the urethra and thus producing better resistance in the urethral lumen (Fig. 39-1). In the Marshall-Marchetti-Krantz procedure the urethra is sutured to the posterior surface of the pubic bone with three sutures on each side. In some cases additional sutures may be placed between the anterior surface of the bladder and the rectus muscle to provide further elevation. In the Lapides procedure the neck of the bladder is sutured to the pubic bone at the midline, and one suture is made on each side, connecting the vaginal fornices to the Cooper ligament. In the Burch procedure the same effect is created without placing any sutures into the urethra. It is done by suturing the lateral vaginal fornices to the Cooper ligament.

For all of these procedures the patient is in a modified lithotomy position. A transverse suprapubic incision is made, the rectus muscles are separated, the retropubic space is defined, and the bladder neck and urethra are mobilized. The sutures are then placed according to the procedure of choice. At the end of the surgery an incisional drain and indwelling urethral catheter or suprapubic tube are inserted.

PEREYRA PROCEDURE

This procedure produces the same effect on the bladder and urethra as do the three just described but uses a combination of the vaginal and suprapubic approaches. It involves the least amount of surgical manipulation and takes the least amount of time to complete. For the surgery the patient is placed in a modified lithotomy position. An anterior vaginal and a small suprapubic incision are made. By means of special needles, sutures are placed into the anterior aspect of the vagina on either side of the bladder neck. These sutures are then pulled up through the suprapubic incision and tied to the rectus sheath, elevating the bladder neck. The result can be visualized by imagining the anterior vaginal wall as a hammock lifting the bladder neck. A cystoscopy is performed to ascertain that the sutures have not penetrated the bladder wall or urethra. Both incisions are then closed, and a small dressing is applied. No incisional drains are used. An indwelling urethral catheter is inserted to maintain adequate drainage of the bladder, and vaginal packing is applied.

The nursing care following all of these procedures is essentially the same. Some patients will have indwelling urethral catheters and others will have a suprapubic tube. However, this depends on the surgeon's preference and not on the particular procedure used (except for the Pereyra procedure, which always requires an indwelling urethral catheter).

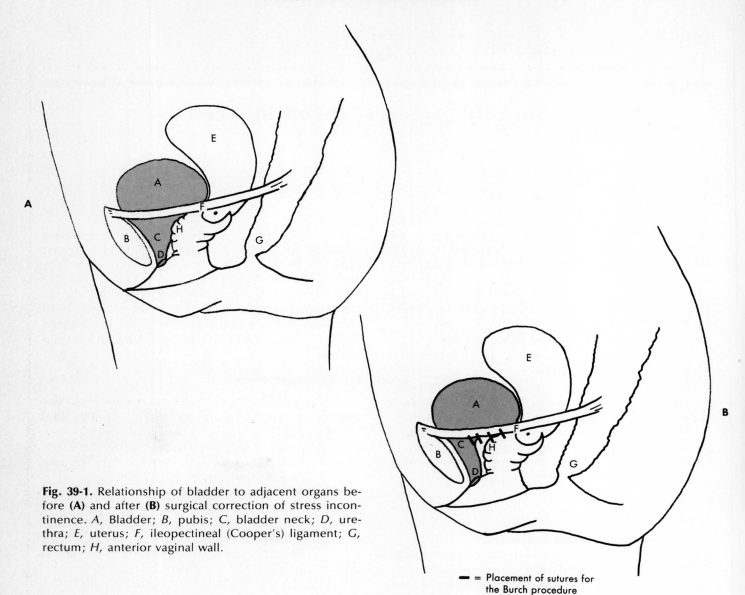

Fig. 39-1. Relationship of bladder to adjacent organs before **(A)** and after **(B)** surgical correction of stress incontinence. *A,* Bladder; *B,* pubis; *C,* bladder neck; *D,* urethra; *E,* uterus; *F,* ileopectineal (Cooper's) ligament; *G,* rectum; *H,* anterior vaginal wall.

— = Placement of sutures for the Burch procedure

SURGICAL CORRECTION OF STRESS INCONTINENCE
Outline of Care Plan
ANTICIPATED NURSING DIAGNOSES:

Preoperative period
1. Discomfort related to urinary incontinence.
2. Need for preoperative teaching.
3. Need for discharge planning.

Early postoperative period
4. Potential for shock.
5. Potential for wound complications.
6. Need for management of indwelling urethral catheter.*
   or
7. Need for management of suprapubic tube.*
8. Postoperative pain.
9. Need for management of intravenous infusion.
10. Potential for respiratory complications related to surgical intervention.
11. Potential for deep vein thrombosis.

Late postoperative period
12. Potential for voiding complications following removal of indwelling urethral catheter or clamping of suprapubic tube.
13. Need for intermittent, clean self-catheterization.*

Convalescent period
14. Need for discharge teaching.

*May not apply.

*May not apply.

NURSING CARE PLAN FOR THE PATIENT UNDERGOING SURGERY FOR STRESS INCONTINENCE

1. NURSING DIAGNOSIS: Discomfort related to urinary incontinence

Objective of nursing intervention   Promotion of patient comfort

Expected outcomes { Absence of skin irritation in perineal area
Absence of embarrassment related to incontinence

Plan for implementation	Rationale
1. Determine the integrity of the patient's skin where it is exposed to urine (buttocks, thighs, sacral area, etc.).	Prolonged contact with urine will result in skin irritation and breakdown.
2. Notify the physician if topical medications (e.g., zinc oxide powders or ointments) are required, and apply as ordered.	
3. Check the patient frequently for wetness. In most cases the patient can be relied on to notify the nurse when she is wet.	Urine should not be permitted to remain in contact with the skin for any prolonged period of time (see preceding rationale).
4. Provide adequate amounts of perineal pads or large combines, and change them frequently. In most cases the patient can be relied on to do this herself.	
5. Provide privacy whenever possible.	The patient may be embarrassed by her incontinence. Being in a multibed room may increase her psychologic discomfort.

Preoperative period

409

2. NURSING DIAGNOSIS: Need for preoperative teaching

Objectives of nursing intervention

If necessary, clarification of reason for hospitalization and type of surgery to be performed

Elimination of any negative or inaccurate notions regarding the forthcoming surgery

Explanation of preoperative tests and procedures

Psychologic preparation for general anesthesia (omit if the patient is to have spinal anesthesia)

Explanation of events expected in the early postoperative period

Explanation of body conditions expected in the early postoperative period

Identification of any known allergies

Expected outcomes

Verbal indication that explanations are understood

Verbal indication of optimistic expectations (within realistic limits) related to forthcoming surgery

Cooperation during preoperative tests and procedures

Verbal or behavioral indication of reduction of anxiety

Absence of postoperative complications

Absence of allergic reactions

Preoperative period

Plan for implementation	Rationale
See master care plan for the patient receiving preoperative teaching.	
In addition to the topics covered in the master care plan, include the following items in the preoperative teaching: 1. Be aware that, in addition to routine preoperative tests, the following diagnostic studies may have been performed, and answer any questions the patient has regarding them: a. Urodynamic studies	These are done to establish that the condition is true stress incontinence. Otherwise the surgical procedure will not be successful.
b. Voiding cystourethrogram c. Cystoscopy	These are sometimes done to rule out other types of bladder disease.
2. The preoperative shave is from the umbilicus to mid-thigh.	
3. The patient will probably be permitted a light supper in the evening after surgery and will resume her normal diet the next morning.	Because the peritoneal cavity is not entered during this surgery, the incidence of postoperative gastrointestinal disturbances is relatively low.

Plan for implementation	Rationale
4. There will be an indwelling urethral catheter or a suprapubic tube in place for approximately 4 to 6 days (except after Pereyra procedure, in which case the catheter will be removed after 2 days).	
5. The patient will have a dressing on her lower abdomen that may require changing periodically.	
6. Urine is expected to be pink in the early postoperative period.	

3. NURSING DIAGNOSIS: Need for discharge planning

Objectives of nursing intervention { Early commencement of discharge planning
Accurate estimate of time required for all discharge teaching

Expected outcome Smooth transition of care after discharge

Plan for implementation	Rationale
See master care plan for the patient requiring discharge preparations: discharge planning.	
In addition to the topics covered in the master care plan, the following items should be considered: 1. The duration of hospitalization for this type of procedure is approximately 7 to 10 days.	

2. Required teaching includes:
  a. General postoperative discharge teaching
  b. Possibly intermittent clean self-catheterization	

Preoperative period

4. NURSING DIAGNOSIS: Potential for shock

Objective of nursing intervention   Prevention or early detection of shock

Expected outcomes   { Vital signs normal, skin dry, color normal
Absence of bright red drainage

Plan for implementation	Rationale
1. Check the patient's vital signs every 4 hours once stable (every 15 minutes if unstable).	Although shock is a potential complication after any kind of surgery, it is a relatively small risk after surgery for stress incontinence because few blood vessels are cut and the duration of surgery is usually short.
2. Be alert for increasing pulse and respiratory rates, decreasing blood pressure, diaphoresis, pallor, and feelings of apprehension.	
3. Notify the physician at once if indications of impending shock occur.	

Early postoperative period

5. NURSING DIAGNOSIS: Potential for wound complications

Objective of nursing intervention	Prevention or early detection of complications arising from the incisional area
Expected outcome	Absence of fever, purulent exudate, erythema, edema, dehiscence, hematoma, and other abnormal wound conditions

Plan for implementation	Rationale
1. Check the dressing every 4 hours for the first 24 hours and then once a shift. Change it if it becomes wet, and use sterile technique for the procedure.	Incisional drainage is usually not heavy. Small amounts of serosanguineous fluid are expected to drain after all these types of surgery except the Pereyra procedure, for which no incisional drain is used.
2. If there is purulent drainage: a. Notify the physician. b. Obtain a wound culture specimen.	This would indicate a wound infection. This will facilitate identification of the infecting organism so that appropriate treatment can be instituted quickly.
3. Use caution when removing soiled dressings to prevent inadvertent removal of the incisional drain or suprapubic tube (if used).	Premature removal of a drain may result in prolonged wound healing.
4. Cut and arrange gauze pads around the incisional drain and suprapubic tube (if used).	This prevents the dressings from flattening the drainage mechanisms and possibly obstructing the flow of drainage from the wound.
5. Note the condition of the suture line. Chart its appearance and the presence of edema, erythema, ecchymosis, or other abnormal conditions.	This provides a frame of reference for other staff members caring for the patient.
6. Notify the physician if there is any evidence of dehiscence.	
7. Check the patient's temperature every 4 hours and notify the physician if there is an elevation above 101°.	Wound infection must always be suspected when the patients runs a fever postoperatively. Other causes include respiratory complications and pharmacologic intervention.
8. If the Pereyra procedure was performed, remove vaginal packing as ordered by the physician and: a. Notify the physician if drainage has a purulent odor. b. Check for vaginal bleeding during the next 24 hours. c. Notify the physician if vaginal bleeding requires more than one change of Peri-Pad per shift.	Vaginal bleeding should be scanty or nonexistent after packing is removed.

Early postoperative period

6. NURSING DIAGNOSIS: Need for management of indwelling urethral catheter*

Objectives of nursing intervention

{
Appropriate care of catheter and equipment

Prevention or early detection of infection

Care of tissue surrounding catheter

Maintenance of accurate records of urine output

Appropriate administration of hand-irrigation of catheter

Management of discomfort or pain caused by catheter

Satisfactory collection of urine specimens from catheter
}

Expected outcomes

{
Absence of severe bladder spasms

Urine draining freely through system

Absence of fever, chills, and foul-smelling urine

Absence of urethral discharge and tissue inflammation

Minimal discomfort caused by the catheter

Urine specimens in optimum condition for all necessary tests
}

Plan for implementation	Rationale
See master care plan for the patient with an indwelling urethral catheter: care after insertion of the catheter. In addition to the topics covered in the master care plan, the following intervention is required: Notify the physician if the urine turns bright red and has a high viscosity. The urine should be blood tinged to clear within 24 to 48 hours after surgery.	There should be relatively little bleeding into the bladder after this type of surgery. The appearance of bright red urine requires investigation.

Early postoperative period

*This may not apply. The patient may have a suprapubic tube or trocar cystostomy instead.

7. NURSING DIAGNOSIS: Need for management of suprapubic tube*

Objective of nursing intervention   Prevention or early detection of complications related to the suprapubic tube

Expected outcome   Pink to amber urine draining freely through suprapubic tube

Plan for implementation	Rationale
1. Keep collecting container below the level of the patient's bladder.	Urine flows through the tubing via gravity. Elevation of the collecting container will result in urine flowing back into the bladder from the distal portion of the system, which has the greatest potential for being contaminated.
2. Keep the tubing free from kinks and external pressure.	Flattening or sharply bending the tubing will decrease its patency.
3. Anchor the tubing securely to the patient's abdomen with tape.	This prevents inadvertent traction on the tube and possible displacement of it.
4. Hand-irrigate the tube only if it is obstructed, and use sterile technique for the procedure.	Unnecessary disconnection of the tubing increases the risk of contamination of the drainage system.
5. Keep the area around the suprapubic tube clean and dry.	
6. Maintain accurate records of volume and character of suprapubic tube drainage.	

Early postoperative period

*This may not apply; the patient may have an indwelling urethral catheter. If the patient has a trocar cystostomy, see p. 538.

8. NURSING DIAGNOSIS: Postoperative pain

Objective of nursing intervention	Appropriate management of pain or discomfort
Expected outcome	Behavioral and/or verbal indication that pain is adequately reduced or absent

Plan for implementation	Rationale
Determine the source of the pain. It might be related to the catheter (if used) or the surgical wound. 1. Question and observe the patient to obtain information about the pain.	Pain from different sources usually requires different intervention.
2. Be aware that pain is a unique and individual experience. Although the different sources of pain can usually be determined by their characteristics, there are also many variations.	
3. Be alert for indications (verbal or behavioral) that the patient is experiencing discomfort other than physical pain, and attempt to resolve the problem.	Fear, loneliness, depression, and numerous other conditions may be sources of extreme discomfort for the patient, who may unconsciously translate these feelings into pain.

PERSISTENT, SEVERE, INCREASING PAIN IN SUPRAPUBIC AREA*

See Chapter 11, part one, nursing objective 6.	This pain is probably caused by an obstructed catheter.

SPASMODIC, INTERMITTENT PAIN IN SUPRAPUBIC AREA, OR PAIN RADIATING TO URETHRAL AREA*

See Chapter 11, part one, nursing objective 6.	This pain is probably caused by the catheter's irritating effect on the bladder.

MODERATE TO SEVERE PAIN AT SURGICAL SITE, USUALLY AGGRAVATED BY PHYSICAL ACTIVITY

1. If the patient has a catheter, be certain it is not obstructed. Although pain with these characteristics is usually of incisional origin and is expected, it is very difficult to differentiate between incisional pain and pain from an obstructed catheter after this type of surgery.	Catheter obstruction must be ruled out first because it cannot remain untreated. However, after this type of surgery it is unlikely for the catheter to become obstructed because there is rarely enough blood in the drainage for clots to form, and no tissue particles are normally passed in the urine.
2. If the patient does not have a catheter, administer analgesics as ordered.	Analgesic medication usually provides considerable relief from incisional pain.

*Applies only to the patient with an indwelling urethral catheter.

Plan for implementation	Rationale
3. Plan the patient's activities to coincide with a time when there is a high level of pain medication in the patient's bloodstream.	The patient will cooperate better with coughing exercises, ambulating, bathing, etc. when the pain is well under control.
4. Notify the physician if the patient's requests for pain medication do not decrease within 48 to 72 hours.	Although the intensity of postoperative pain varies enormously between patients, there should be a marked decrease in the apparent severity of the pain within 2 or 3 days. If this does not occur, it may indicate the development of wound complications.

9. NURSING DIAGNOSIS: Need for management of intravenous infusion

Objectives of nursing intervention
- Appropriate administration of specific types of intravenous solutions
- Prevention or early detection of local complications
- Prevention or early detection of systemic complications
- Management of discomfort caused by the intravenous infusion
- Maintenance of proper function of intravenous equipment
- Maintenance of accurate records of the patient's hydration status

Expected outcomes
- Normal hydration status
- Normal electrolyte status
- Absence of thrombophlebitis, infiltration, infection, fluid overload, and pulmonary embolism
- Absence of discomfort caused by the intravenous infusion

Plan for implementation	Rationale
See master care plan for the patient receiving intravenous therapy.	These patients usually receive isotonic dextrose and saline solutions.

Early postoperative period

417

10. NURSING DIAGNOSIS: Potential for respiratory complications related to surgical intervention

Objective of nursing intervention   Prevention or early detection of atelectasis and/or pneumonia

Expected outcomes
Cooperation with therapeutic respiratory regimen
Absence of fever or audible lung congestion
Sputum clear or white and easily mobilized

Plan for implementation	Rationale
See master care plan for the patient at risk for respiratory complications, nursing objective 2.	

11. NURSING DIAGNOSIS: Potential for deep vein thrombosis

Objectives of nursing intervention
Explanation and maintenance of precautions against deep vein thrombosis
Early detection of deep vein thrombosis

Expected outcomes
Cooperation with regimen to prevent deep vein thrombosis
Absence of local pain, swelling, and redness of a lower extremity
Absence of fever

Plan for implementation	Rationale
See master care plan for the patient at risk for deep vein thrombosis.	

12. NURSING DIAGNOSIS: Potential for voiding complications following removal of indwelling urethral catheter or clamping of suprapubic tube

Objective of nursing intervention   Prevention or early detection of complications

Expected outcomes
Adequate volume of clear amber or slightly pink urine
Absence of urgency, frequency, dysuria, and suprapubic distention
Resumption of normal voiding pattern

Plan for implementation	Rationale
IF INDWELLING URETHRAL CATHETER WAS USED FOR URINARY DRAINAGE	
See master care plan for the patient with an indwelling urethral catheter: care after removal of the catheter.	

Early postoperative period

Late postoperative period

Plan for implementation	**Rationale**

IF SUPRAPUBIC TUBE OR TROCAR CYSTOSTOMY TUBE WAS USED FOR URINARY DRAINAGE

1. Clamp the tube as ordered. Usually the patient will start voiding spontaneously within a few hours.

2. Provide the following instructions:
   a. The patient should drink 8 to 12 glasses of fluid during the day (but avoid drinking within 3 hours of her bedtime).
   b. Voiding may be frequent, and the patient may experience some urgency.

The fluid intake should remain high to assess rapidly the patient's voiding ability. However, it should be limited to daytime to allow the patient uninterrupted sleep.
The patient should know that this is a common complication and easily handled. It may be transient or may be caused by urinary retention (see further).

3. Maintain accurate records of the volume, frequency, and character of each voiding for 48 to 72 hours.

This facilitates rapid assessment of the patient's voiding ability and hydration status.

IF THE PATIENT IS UNABLE TO VOID NORMALLY

1. If the patient has not voided for more than 6 hours after removal of the indwelling urethral catheter or clamping of the suprapubic tube, notify the physician. **One** of the following actions will probably be ordered:
   a. Begin intermittent catheterization (see further).
   b. Replace indwelling urethral catheter.
   c. Unclamp suprapubic tube or trocar cystostomy tube (if used).

The patient may be in urinary retention as a result of postoperative edema or for psychologic reasons (i.e., the patient may be so fearful of having pain when she voids that she is unable to void).

2. If the patient is voiding unusually small amounts with frequency (i.e., more than once an hour), notify the physician. **One** of the following actions will be ordered:
   a. Begin postvoiding intermittent catheterization and record volume of residual urine.
   b. If suprapubic tube is still in place, keep it clamped until after the patient voids, and then unclamp it to measure the volume of residual urine.

This may indicate that the patient is not completely emptying her bladder.

This enables the physician to assess the degree of urinary retention due to incomplete voiding.
Same as preceding rationale.

Late postoperative period

13. NURSING DIAGNOSIS: Need for intermittent, clean self-catheterization*

Objectives of nursing intervention

{ Performance and teaching of intermittent catheterization as ordered

Maintenance of an atmosphere conducive to optimum learning

Explanation of all necessary information related to intermittent self-catheterization

Expected outcome   Accurate return demonstration and explanation of self-catheterization procedure

Plan for implementation	Rationale

1. Reduce any anxiety the patient may be feeling by the following actions:
  a. Explain that the temporary need for intermittent catheterization is not unusual after this type of surgery and does not indicate a long-term condition.
  b. Inform the patient that she will be taught to do the procedure herself in case she is discharged before her normal voiding pattern has been reestablished.
 	
  c. Maintain a calm, confident attitude while performing the procedure.
 	
  d. Do not wear gloves for the procedure.
	If the patient's physician has not discussed the possibility, the patient may be extremely upset by being unable to void normally.
	If the patient is unable to void normally, intermittent, clean self-catheterization is generally the method of choice for draining the bladder during the late postoperative and convalescent periods until complete healing has taken place and edema subsides.
	Any anxiety or uncertainty on the part of the nurse may be transmitted easily to the patient, who is often apprehensive about learning the procedure.
	The use of gloves conveys to the patient that her urine is "unclean." This notion may hamper her ability to catheterize herself without gloves.

2. Provide privacy and adequate visibility of the perineum for the patient during the teaching sessions. Adequate light and mirror placement are essential. (See Appendix C for step-by-step procedure.)	
3. If available, use a clear plastic, no. 14 French, regular length Robinson catheter.	This type of catheter provides the following advantages: 1. The transparency gives immediate indication of when the catheter is in the bladder. 2. Its length makes disposal of urine more convenient than with a short catheter. 3. Its flexibility minimizes urethral trauma. 4. It can be easily stored and transported.

Late postoperative period

*This only applies if the patient is unable to completely empty her bladder after removal of indwelling urinary drainage equipment.

Plan for implementation	**Rationale**
4. If ordered, catheterize the patient immediately after each voiding to determine residual volume.	
or	
5. If ordered, catheterize the patient according to the prescribed time schedule, and adhere to the schedule precisely. Usually the schedule is every 3 hours during the day and once at night or every 4 to 6 hours around the clock.	Strict adherence to the prescribed schedule is essential so that the bladder is not permitted to become distended. If this were to happen, the circulation to the mucosal lining would become impaired, and host resistance to bacterial infection might be compromised.[2,4]
6. Emphasize to the patient that this procedure does not pose a risk of infection, provided that the bladder is never allowed to become distended with urine. The catheter need only be clean; washing her hands and catheter tip prior to insertion is adequate.	The primary emphasis of patient teaching should be on **regularity of catheterization** rather than cleanliness. In fact, if the patient has no access to washing facilities, it is preferable for her to catheterize herself without washing rather than to allow distention to occur, which would impair her defenses against pathogens.[1,3]

Late postoperative period

421

14. NURSING DIAGNOSIS: Need for discharge teaching

Objectives of nursing intervention

Explanation of basic information about medications to be taken at home

Explanation of information regarding follow-up care

Explanation of residual effects of the condition and/or treatment

Explanation of instructions concerning postdischarge activities

Explanation of symptoms that constitute a reason to contact the physician

Review of admitting diagnosis and mode of treatment

Expected outcomes

Accurate return verbalization and/or demonstration of all material learned

Smooth transition of care after discharge

Absence or early detection of complications arising after discharge

Ability to provide future health care practitioners with important data about health history

Plan for implementation	Rationale
See master care plan for the patient requiring discharge preparations: discharge teaching.	
In addition to the topics covered in the master care plan, include the following items in the discharge teaching:	
1. At the follow-up office visit the physician will check the wound for adequate healing, obtain a urine specimen for culture, and assess the patient's voiding ability.	
2. During the next few weeks the expected residual effects are some fatigue and incisional discomfort.	
3. The patient should notify the physician if any of the following occur: a. Chills, fever, flank pain, hematuria b. Severe pain and/or increasing redness at the incisional site	This may indicate a urinary tract infection. This may indicate a wound infection.
4. If intermittent self-catheterization is still required at the time of discharge, provide written instructions of the procedure and review the key points (i.e., never allow the bladder to become distended; always carry an extra catheter whenever away from home).	Regularity of catheterization is the single most important element in the self-catheterization regimen.
5. Provide the patient with a telephone number with which to reach the nurse or enterostomal therapist who provided the self-catheterization teaching, in case any questions arise.	

Convalescent period

CHAPTER 40

Neurogenic bladder

Neurogenic bladder is a condition of dysfunction caused by interference with the normal conduction of nerve fibers associated with urination. It usually results in some form of urinary incontinence and is often associated with damage to the upper urinary tract, a high incidence of urinary tract infection, and urolithiasis.

There are numerous causes of this condition, and its manifestations vary considerably depending on the etiology. The bladder, urogenital diaphragm (external sphincter), and bladder neck (internal sphincter) may all be directly affected by neurologic disease, or only one or two of these structures may be involved. However, abnormalities in the emptying of the bladder will occur if there is any neurologic dysfunction associated with these parts of the system. Urodynamic studies are essential for proper identification and evaluation of the condition.

The behavior of a neurogenic bladder will fall into either of two broad categories—**hyperreflexive** (or uninhibited) activity and **hypotonic** (or atonic) behavior. A hyperreflexive neurogenic bladder is caused by interruptions in the innervation of the bladder that occur at a level superior to the sacral nerves, such as cerebral vascular accident, Parkinson's disease, and most forms of spinal cord injuries. It is manifested by small bladder capacity and uncontrolled frequent voiding (see Fig. 6-3, A). The opposite condition occurs with the hypotonic bladder (see Fig. 6-3, B). In this case the capacity is extremely large (it may reach as much as 2000 ml) because contraction of the bladder does not readily occur. This condition is the result of interruption in the bladder innervation at the level of the sacral nerves. It occurs with lesions of the cauda equina (the collection of nerve roots in the vertebral canal below the spinal cord) and congenital deformities, injuries, or tumors of the sacral part of the spinal cord. Incontinence occurs only when the bladder becomes so full that small amounts of urine are forced out (overflow incontinence).

Atonic behavior may be subdivided into additional categories according to the cause. A **sensory paralytic** bladder may occur as a result of syphilis, diabetes, and certain types of surgery on the spinal cord. This condition is manifested by an atonic bladder caused by overdistention. The distention occurs because the patient lacks the desire to void. A **motor-paralytic** bladder results in the same overfilling and eventual loss of tone. In this case the patient feels the desire to void, but he is unable to do so because the impulse triggering bladder contraction is lost. This condition sometimes occurs as a result of poliomyelitis.

The two basic voiding patterns (hyperreflexive and hypotonic) are often further compounded by disease involving the external or internal sphincters. Normal voiding can occur only if bladder contraction is simultaneous with the relaxation of the sphincters. If either the internal or external sphincter is in a state of contraction while the other is relaxed (i.e., dyssynergic sphincters), the resulting condition and treatment thereof become more complicated.

The various forms of neurogenic bladder can often be controlled by medication. Anticholinergics such as propantheline bromide (Pro-Banthine) and oxybutynin chloride (Ditropan) may be used to treat hyperreflexive neurogenic conditions by suppressing unwanted contractions (i.e., those which occur when the bladder has only a small volume of urine in it). Parasympathomimetics such as bethanechol chloride (Urecholine) may be used for hypotonic bladders to stimulate contractions at a normal bladder volume. Alpha-adrenergic blockers such as phenoxybenzamine (Dibenzyline) and phentolamine (Regitine) may be used to relax spastic bladder necks. Sympathomimetics such as ephedrine may be used to increase deficient bladder neck and urethral tone, which occurs in certain cases of stress incontinence. Striated muscle relaxers such as dantrolene sodium (Dantrium) and diazepam (Valium) may be used to relax spastic external sphincters.

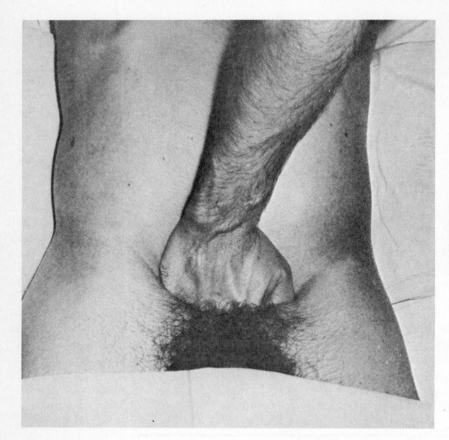

Fig. 40-1. Credé maneuver. (From Pearman, J.W., and England, E.J.: The urological management of the patient following spinal cord injury, ed. 1, Springfield, Ill., 1973. Courtesy Charles C Thomas, Publisher.)

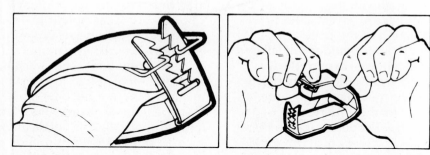

Fig. 40-2. Cunningham clamp. (Courtesy Bard Home Health Division, Berkeley Heights, N.J.)

There are numerous other methods of management, depending on the bladder disease and the general condition of the patient. Those who are unable to empty their bladders completely (hypotonic bladders) and who have adequate manual dexterity may be taught intermittent, clean self-catheterization. The Credé maneuver (sustained manual suprapubic pressure) (Fig. 40-1) and the Valsalva maneuver are other possible options for these patients. However, these maneuvers must **not** be used if there is unusually strong sphincter resistance because this will result in extremely high intravesical pressure during the procedure and possibly cause ureteral reflux and thus infection.

Patients suffering from incontinence caused by deficient sphincter tone may be helped by perineal exercises, provided that only the external sphincter is affected and the bladder neck is intact. Male patients with more extensive sphincter damage may be managed successfully with a Cunningham clamp (Fig. 40-2). However, this may not be sufficient in cases where bladder contractions are excessive, so an external catheter may be required.

Appropriate management of incontinence pre-

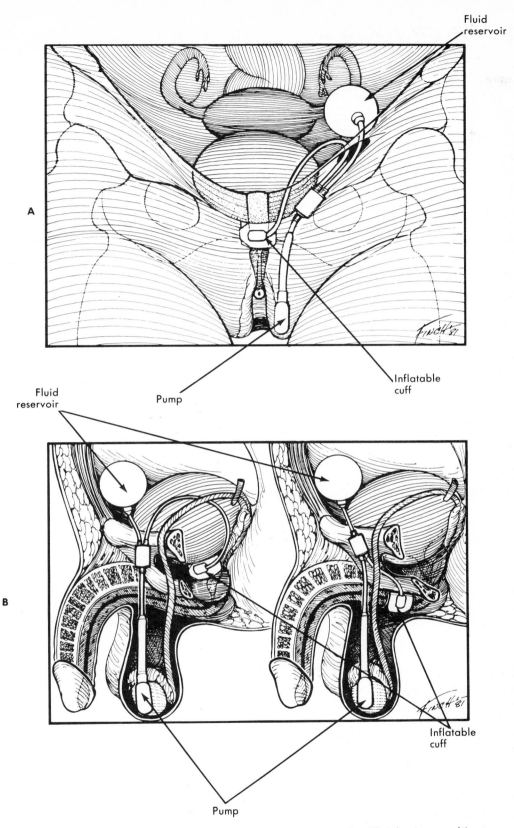

Fig. 40-3. Artificial inflatable urinary sphincter. **A,** Location of artificial urinary sphincter in the female. **B,** Location of artificial urinary sphincter in the male; note that position of cuff may be around either the bladder neck or the bulbous urethra. (Courtesy American Medical Systems, Inc., Minneapolis, Minn.)

sents a more complex problem in the female patient, many of whom must use indwelling urethral catheters, despite the numerous hazards associated with this type of drainage. However, recent surgical advances have made the implantation of an artificial inflatable sphincter a potential option for certain patients. It may also be used for males, although it is of far greater significance for the incontinent female who has relatively few other satisfactory options available. Although this procedure is being done in only a few major medical centers to date, all nurses should be aware of the mechanics of these devices in the event that they are required to care for a patient with such an implant, who has been hospitalized for a condition that renders her unable to communicate (such as a coma or severe mental confusion). Special nursing care will be required, such as the necessity of valve deflation every 4 to 6 hours to empty the bladder and deflation prior to catheterization (Fig. 40-3). It is also important to place a note concerning the artificial sphincter on a conspicuous part of the patient's chart so that, if the patient requires abdominal surgery, the surgeon knows beforehand to use caution. This prevents inadvertent severing of part of the device. These patients should (and usually do) wear a Medic-Alert tag to notify any caregiver of their condition.

Other devices that sometimes provide a degree of relief from incontinence in the female are the pessary, the Edward occlusive device, the Vincent balloon binder device, and the Crowley suction device (for immobilized patients only). Some types of incontinence must be managed surgically via permanent urinary diversion, and, in cases where surgery is not an option, various forms of absorbent pads and briefs may be used.

Nursing care of the incontinent patient is extremely challenging, mentally as well as physically. The importance of meticulous skin care cannot be emphasized enough, and the psychologic aspects of incontinence are always an important consideration, even for a patient who appears to be adjusted to the condition. In all patients, to some degree, it symbolizes the return to the helpless condition of early childhood when even the most fundamental control over one's body was not possible. Every attempt must be made to help the patient maintain as normal a life-style as possible because the psychologic consequences of incontinence can be devastating.

NEUROGENIC BLADDER
Outline of Care Plan
POSSIBLE NURSING DIAGNOSES*:

1. Potential for life-threatening systemic manifestations of hyperreflexive bladder conditions.
2. Potential for disruption of skin integrity from prolonged exposure to urine.
3. Potential for social isolation due to urinary incontinence.
4. Need for instruction on Valsalva or Credé maneuvers.
5. Need for instruction and assistance in intermittent, clean (self)-catheterization.
6. Need for instruction and assistance in the use of an external catheter.
7. Need for instruction and assistance in the use of a Cunningham clamp.
8. Need for management of an indwelling urethral catheter.
9. Need for sexual counseling.

---

*No single patient will have all these nursing diagnoses; they apply to different types of neurogenic bladder conditions and varying degrees of incontinence and activity limitations.

NURSING CARE PLAN FOR THE PATIENT WITH NEUROGENIC BLADDER

1. NURSING DIAGNOSIS: Potential for life-threatening systemic manifestations of hyperreflexive bladder conditions*

Objective of nursing intervention	Prevention of dangerous effects of autonomic hyperreflexia by means of education and close observation of the patient
Expected outcomes	Patient ability to identify and verbalize the presence of autonomic hyperreflexive syndrome Absence of severe headache, bradycardia, paroxysmal hypertension, diaphoresis, and piloerection (gooseflesh)

---

*This only applies to certain patients with a hyperreflexive bladder caused by a spinal cord lesion at or above the seventh thoracic vertebra.

Plan for implementation	**Rationale**

1. Be aware that patients with spinal cord injuries at or above the seventh thoracic vertebra may experience life-threatening symptoms when their bladders (and/or rectums) are distended. The syndrome includes:
  a. Bradycardia
  b. Paroxysmal hypertension
  c. Diaphoresis (particularly on the forehead)
  d. Severe headache
  e. Piloerection
	Afferent impulses from a full bladder travel up the spinal cord to higher centers, setting off certain sympathetic reflexes involving vasoconstriction and therefore a rise in blood pressure. In a normal individual these are mitigated by compensatory mechanisms inducing bradycardia and vasodilation. However, in some patients with high spinal cord lesions, impulses triggering the compensatory vasodilation cannot travel beyond the lesion, and only the slowing of the heart rate occurs to compensate for the hypertension. This may result in extreme bradycardia as well as continued hypertension and the additional associated symptoms.

2. Instruct the patient to notify the nurse if he develops a headache.	A headache usually indicates the onset of the syndrome.

3. If the patient complains of a headache:
  a. Encourage him to void or empty his rectum (if possible).
  b. Monitor his pulse and blood pressure.
  c. Do not give aspirin or other pain medication if his vital signs are abnormal.
  d. Palpate for bladder distention.
  e. If an indwelling catheter is in place:
    (1) Check the catheter for patency.
    (2) Terminate any continuous bladder irrigation.
 	
    (3) Do not hand-irrigate the catheter. However, if the catheter is obstructed, attempt to aspirate the obstruction from the catheter with a bulb syringe.
  f. If ordered, administer alpha-adrenergic blockers such as phenoxybenzamine (Dibenzyline).
  g. Notify the physician if any of the following conditions are present:
    (1) The symptoms do not subside after the bladder (or rectum) is emptied.
    (2) The bladder (and/or rectum) is full and cannot be emptied.
    (3) The medication does not relieve the symptoms within 10 to 30 minutes (depending on route of administration).
	Irrigation of a catheter will increase bladder pressure and thus exacerbate the syndrome.
	
	This medication inhibits vasoconstriction and thus lowers the patient's blood pressure.

4. Prevent recurrence of autonomic hyperreflexia by the following measures:
  a. If an indwelling catheter is to be clamped, take extra precautions to prevent its being forgotten and left clamped for longer than required.
  b. Encourage adequate bowel function.
 	
  c. Avoid stimulation of other trigger zones besides the bladder and rectum.
	
	A full rectum may also trigger or contribute to the severity of the syndrome.
	In some patients, stimulation of certain areas on the thighs may cause the syndrome. It may also be the result of severe decubitus ulcers.

2. NURSING DIAGNOSIS: Potential for disruption of skin integrity from prolonged exposure to urine

Objective of nursing intervention Maintenance of appropriate hygienic measures to prevent skin breakdown

Expected outcome Normal appearance of skin on perineum, buttocks, and thighs

Plan for implementation	Rationale
1. Inspect the patient's skin for redness and areas of excoriation.	Prolonged contact with urine will result in skin irritation and breakdown.
2. Notify the physician if topical medications (e.g., zinc oxide ointments or powders) are required, and apply as ordered.	Once the skin is broken, medication should be used to prevent infection and additional skin damage.
3. Check the patient frequently for wetness.	
4. Maintain dry, clean linen and absorbent materials (e.g., large combines, incontinence underpads, briefs).	The skin must be permitted to dry thoroughly between episodes of incontinence, or breakdown will be accelerated.
5. Clean the affected area with mild soap and water as often as necessary, and rinse and dry thoroughly.	
6. Keep plastic bed shields out of direct contact with the patient's skin at all times (i.e., keep absorbent material between the skin and the plastic).	Plastic material directly against the skin prevents evaporation of moisture and therefore contributes to skin breakdown.

3. NURSING DIAGNOSIS: Potential for social isolation due to urinary incontinence

Objective of nursing intervention   Promotion of a management regimen that eliminates patient embarrassment

Expected outcomes   Verbal or behavioral indication that the regimen is psychologically acceptable

Ability to socialize without embarrassment

Plan for implementation	Rationale
1. Suggest methods for the patient to control odor.	Real or **imagined** urinary odor is one of the strongest inhibitors to socialization in an incontinent individual.
a. He should maintain good hygiene. This means a thorough washing and drying of the perineal area a minimum of once a day.	
b. He should avoid asparagus.	This food tends to cause the urine to have a particularly strong odor.
c. He should launder his clothes frequently and change his underwear a minimum of once a day.	
d. He should notify his physician if his urine develops a strong odor despite the preceding measures.	Urinary tract infection is the primary cause of strong urinary odor. It requires medical intervention as soon as possible for the sake of the patient's physical health as well as his psychosocial well-being.
2. Suggest guidelines for the patient to follow regarding choice of clothing.	
a. The material should be washable and quick-drying.	
b. There should be adequate zippers and flaps so that changes of incontinence pads or briefs are relatively easy.	
c. The patient may want to avoid wearing very light colors.	Staining shows more with light colors. Deeper shades are also a better camouflage of various undergarments, which may be bulky.
d. The patient's clothing should be of relatively absorbent materials, such as cotton or wool jersey.	These types of materials do not show wetness as much as thinner, flatter weaves. Natural fibers also provide better ventilation for the skin.
3. Suggest that the patient restrict his fluid intake for 2 or 3 hours before a long car ride or other situation in which he cannot easily get to a bathroom.	
He should, however, be certain to compensate for any fluid restrictions afterward, so that his total intake is approximately 2 to 3 L per 24-hour period.	A liberal fluid intake is an important measure in preventing urinary tract infection.
4. Provide emotional support and encouragement.	

4. NURSING DIAGNOSIS: Need for instruction on Valsalva or Credé maneuvers*

Objective of nursing intervention	Provision of instruction on emptying the bladder via Valsalva or Credé maneuvers
Expected outcome	Ability to empty bladder completely via one or both procedures

Plan for implementation	Rationale
1. Maintain a regular schedule for emptying the bladder via Valsalva or Credé maneuvers. Usually it is done every 4 to 6 hours when the patient's fluid intake is 2 to 3 L per 24-hour period.	The bladder should not be permitted to become over-distended. However, an adequate amount of urine should be present before either procedure is attempted.
2. Teach the Valsalva maneuver. a. Place the patient in a comfortable position to void. This should be as close as possible to his accustomed voiding position. b. Have the patient perform the Valsalva maneuver by describing it in relation to straining to defecate.	Valsalva maneuver (forced exhalation against a closed glottis) results in an increase in intrathoracic and intra-abdominal pressure. This is sometimes adequate to express sufficient quantities of urine through the urethra and completely empty the bladder.
3. If the Valsalva maneuver is inadequate, teach the Credé maneuver. a. Place the patient in a comfortable position to void. This should be as close as possible to his accustomed voiding position. b. Apply sustained manual pressure over the suprapubic area in the direction of the perineum (see Fig. 40-1). c. Repeat the maneuver until urine is no longer expressed.	
4. With either procedure, make every effort to empty the bladder completely.	Residual urine predisposes the patient to urinary tract infection.
5. Monitor fluid intake and output, and maintain accurate records.	This provides general information about the effectiveness of these methods of emptying the bladder.

*Only applies to the patient with an atonic bladder **whose sphincters are also relatively relaxed.**

5. NURSING DIAGNOSIS: Need for instruction and assistance in intermittent, clean (self)-catheterization*

Objectives of nursing intervention
{
Provision of intermittent, clean catheterization

Provision of instructions on intermittent, clean, self-catheterization (if the patient is a candidate for self-catheterization)

Expected outcomes
{
Complete emptying of the bladder with each catheterization

Absence of urinary tract infection

Patient is able to perform catheterization without anxiety or awkwardness (if the patient is a candidate for self-catheterization)

Plan for implementation	Rationale
1. Maintain a strict schedule of catheterization. It is usually ordered for every 4 or every 6 hours around the clock.	Strict adherence to the prescribed schedule is essential so that the bladder is not permitted to become distended. If this were to happen, the circulation to the mucosal lining would become impaired, and host resistance to bacterial infection might be compromised.[2,4]
2. If the patient is to be taught the procedure, provide privacy and adequate visibility of the urinary meatus during teaching sessions. Adequate light and mirror placement are essential for the female patient. (See Appendix C for step-by-step procedure.)	
3. Wash the catheter thoroughly with soap and water before each catheterization.	Sterilization of a catheter is not necessary for intermittent catheterization, provided it is done regularly and the bladder is not permitted to become distended.[1,3]
4. Maintain a calm, confident attitude while performing or teaching the procedure.	Any anxiety or uncertainty on the part of the nurse may be transmitted easily to the patient.
5. Do not wear gloves for the procedure.	The use of gloves conveys to the patient that his urine is "unclean." If he is a candidate for self-catheterization, this notion may impair his ability to perform it comfortably without gloves.
6. If available, use a clear plastic, no. 14 French, regular length, Robinson catheter.	This type of catheter provides the following advantages: 1. The transparency gives immediate indication of when the catheter is in the bladder. 2. Its length makes disposal of urine more convenient than with a short catheter. 3. Its flexibility minimizes urethral trauma. 4. It can be stored easily and transported.
7. Administer antibiotics as ordered.	Some physicians order antibiotics for a limited period of time after commencement of intermittent catheterization as a prophylactic measure. Once regular emptying of the bladder by this method has been established, antibiotics are usually unnecessary because the urine remains sterile.

*Applies to patients whose bladders cannot be emptied by voiding, Valsalva maneuver, or Credé maneuver. This includes patients with cord injuries and those with sphincter dyssynergia.

Plan for implementation	**Rationale**
8. Maintain the prescribed schedule for regular monitoring of urine composition. Usually this involves monthly urine cultures for the first 3 months and then, if no infection is present, urinalyses every 2 months.	This provides the physician with information regarding changes in the constituents of the urine. It is especially important in the detection of asymptomatic urinary tract infection.
9. If the patient will be doing self-catheterization after discharge, emphasize to him that it does not pose a risk of infection, provided that the bladder is never allowed to become distended with urine. The catheter need only be clean; washing his hands and catheter prior to insertion is adequate.	The primary emphasis of patient teaching should be on **regularity of catheterization** rather than cleanliness. In fact, if the patient has no access to washing facilities, it is preferable for him to catheterize himself **without** washing rather than to allow distention to occur, since this would impair his defenses against pathogens.[1,3]

6. NURSING DIAGNOSIS: Need for instruction or assistance in the use of an external catheter

Objective of nursing intervention Promotion of effective, safe use of external catheter drainage equipment

Expected outcomes { Absence of skin breakdown or edema on the penis
Urine draining freely through catheter and tubing

Plan for implementation	**Rationale**
1. Demonstrate the application of a condom catheter in the following way: 　a. Cut any pubic hair that might come in contact with skin bond cement or adhesive. 　b. Clean and dry the penis thoroughly. If the patient is uncircumcised, this includes cleaning under the prepuce as well.	This eliminates the discomfort of pulling hairs when the catheter is removed. Thorough cleaning is especially important for these patients because they are highly prone to urinary tract infections. Any pooled urine in the distal portion of the condom may be forced back up the urethra, bringing with it contaminants from the skin.
c. Apply skin bond cement to the penis shaft and allow it to dry. (Cement may not be necessary for certain patients; its use is determined by the size of the penis and the degree of patient activity.) 　d. Place the **rolled** condom onto the tip of the penis and then unroll the condom onto the shaft of the penis. 　e. Be certain to leave approximately 1 inch of space at the tip of the condom. 　f. Wrap an elasticized adhesive strip (usually enclosed in the catheter package) around the proximal end of the catheter. It should be snug but not so tight that it impedes circulation to or from the penis.	This prevents pressure buildup of voided urine.

Plan for implementation	**Rationale**
2. Minimize stasis of urine at the distal end of the catheter. a. Prevent twisting of the condom at the point where it is connected to drainage tubing. b. Prevent loops or kinks in the tubing. c. Keep collecting container below hip level at all times.	Pooled urine near the tip of the penis may be forced back up the urethra and is therefore a potential source of urinary tract contamination. Among patients with neurogenic bladders there is a considerably higher incidence of urinary tract infections in patients wearing external catheters than in those wearing no appliance.[6] Stasis of contaminated urine near the distal part of the urethra may be a contributing factor.
3. Obtain a satisfactory return demonstration before permitting the patient to apply the catheter without supervision.	
4. Encourage the patient not to use the catheter for 24 hours a day. The skin should have an opportunity to dry thoroughly a few times during the day.	This helps to preserve skin integrity. Prolonged contact with urine predisposes the skin to breakdown.

7. NURSING DIAGNOSIS: Need for instruction and assistance in the use of a Cunningham clamp

Objective of nursing intervention   Promotion of safe, effective use of Cunningham clamp

Expected outcomes { Accurate return verbalization and demonstration of use of clamp
Absence of skin breakdown or edema on penis

Plan for implementation	Rationale
If the physician has ordered that the patient be fitted for a penile clamp, give the following instructions, show the patient how it works, and obtain a return verbalization and demonstration on the use of the device.	
1. Wash, dry, and apply powder to the penis.	This prevents moisture from being trapped under the rubber part of the clamp and irritating the skin.
2. Apply the clamp after voiding. It should be placed in a horizontal fashion behind the glans (see Fig. 40-2).	
3. Remove the clamp approximately every 4 hours to void.	Urine should not be permitted to remain in the bladder for more than 4 hours, since stasis of urine can contribute to the development of a urinary tract infection.
4. Periodically, check the skin under the area where the clamp presses.	Skin breakdown should be detected at once to prevent further complications. The clamp may have to be refitted or not used at all until the skin heals.
5. Check the glans for swelling. If it occurs, use the clamp on a looser notch.	Swelling of the glans occasionally occurs from excessive compression, which results in decreased venous return and thus edema.
6. Alternate the clamp with a condom catheter.	This reduces the amount of skin irritation sometimes caused by the clamp.

8. NURSING DIAGNOSIS: Need for management of indwelling urethral catheter

Objectives of nursing intervention
- Appropriate care of catheter and equipment
- Prevention or early detection of infection
- Care of tissue surrounding catheter
- Maintenance of accurate records of urine output
- Appropriate administration of hand-irrigation of catheter
- Management of discomfort or pain caused by catheter
- Satisfactory collection of urine specimens from catheter

Expected outcomes
- Absence of severe bladder spasms and suprapubic distention
- Urine draining freely through system
- Absence of fever, chills, and foul-smelling urine
- Absence of urethral discharge and tissue inflammation
- Minimal discomfort caused by the catheter
- Urine specimens in optimum condition for all necessary tests

Plan for implementation	Rationale
See master care plan for the patient with an indwelling urethral catheter: care after insertion of the catheter.	
In addition to the topics covered in the master care plan, the following interventions are required: 1. Do not use an indwelling catheter unless all other methods to control incontinence have failed.	The long-term use of an indwelling urethral catheter results in urinary tract infection and contributes to the formation of urinary calculi and urethral strictures.
2. Use a catheter made of an inert material (e.g., silicone or latex).	Inert materials are less likely to cause an inflammatory reaction than are catheters made of rubber.
3. Use a small-caliber catheter (no. 14 French).	A small caliber permits urethral secretions to drain freely. A tight-fitting catheter causes these secretions to accumulate and contribute to inflammation.
4. If ordered, irrigate the catheter with 10% Renacidin solution daily according to the prescribed regimen. Usually the catheter is clamped briefly after Renacidin is instilled and then irrigated with normal saline.	Renacidin irrigations reduce the amount of phosphate precipitation in the catheter lumen. A buildup of phosphate crystals will eventually cause obstruction of the lumen.
5. If ordered, administer prophylactic antibiotics.	The long-term presence of an indwelling urethral catheter almost inevitably causes some degree of urinary tract infection.

Plan for implementation	Rationale
6. Change the catheter every 2 weeks and the tubing and collecting container weekly. This should be done more often if the catheter or tubing feel gritty when rolled between the thumb and forefinger.	The longer the particular elements of the drainage system remain in place, the more likely they are to become contaminated. A gritty feeling in the tubing indicates a build-up of phosphate crystals and will eventually cause obstruction.
7. If the patient is a male and suffers from paralysis of the perineal area, tape the catheter to his abdomen instead of his thigh.	When paralysis involves the perineal area, the penis may lie in such a way that the urethra, at the penoscrotal junction, forms a sharp angle. This causes the catheter to create pressure against the urethra, which contributes to stricture and fistula formation. Taping the catheter to the patient's abdomen reduces the pressure on the urethra and thus hazardous sequelae.

9. NURSING DIAGNOSIS: Need for sexual counseling

Objective of nursing intervention Provision of suggestions to help the patient establish a satisfactory level of sexual expression

Expected outcomes { Absence of patient anxiety regarding discussion of sexual needs
Development of appropriate methods of sexual satisfaction

Plan for implementation	Rationale
1. When possible, make provisions for the patient to have contact with a professional sex counselor. If this is not possible, the nurse who has had the most contact with the patient may be in an appropriate position to discuss the subject.	Somebody who specializes in this field of therapy is usually able to provide more help than individuals who have not received training in this area. The problems that arise are highly individual and require a considerable amount of experience on the part of the counselor to assist with the development of a suitable means of sexual expression. If direct communication is not possible between the patient and a sex counselor, staff contact with such an individual may indirectly help the patient.
2. Be aware of one's own attitude toward frank discussion of sexual matters and various forms of sexual expression other than vaginal-penile intercourse. a. If uncomfortable with the subject, suggest that another nurse assume the responsibility for this aspect of patient rehabilitation. b. Avoid moral judgments. c. Avoid forming concepts of what is sexually "normal."	Embarrassment on the part of the nurse is usually transmitted to the patient and will lessen the likelihood of frank, constructive communication.

Plan for implementation	Rationale
3. Encourage discussion of concerns the patient might have regarding sexual function. This may be done by beginning the discussion with less threatening topics, such as personal concerns, habits, and previous sexual experiences.	Usually the patient will not initiate this discussion, although it may be foremost on his mind.
4. Provide basic information regarding the physiologic aspects of sexual function, and distinguish between sex for procreation and sex as a means of intimate human communication.	Many patients simply lack basic knowledge about the physiology of sexual function. The "permission-giving" aspect inherent in discussions of sex as an important element in human relationships often enables the patient to approach his own needs more realistically.
5. Avoid making any predictions about the effect of neurologic damage on sexual function. Erection and the sensory experience of orgasm depend on the level and extent of neurologic damage, and no two patients are completely alike in their responses to the impairment. The **fear** of impotence may, in some cases, inhibit erection more than the actual disease process.	Patients with lesions above the sacrum usually have adequate erections (which may be achieved by stimulation of trigger zones), and intercourse can be carried out. Patients with lesions at the sacral part of the cord or the cauda equina may not be able to achieve erections. In these cases surgical implantation of a penile prosthesis may be a viable option (see Chapter 50). Some of these patients may experience orgasm; some may have retrograde ejaculation.
6. If the patient has a sexual partner, encourage open communication between both parties, and include the partner in any discussions relating to sexual matters.	
7. Encourage the patient to explore methods of sexual expression other than penile/vaginal intercourse (if genital intercourse appears to be impossible).	Although religious upbringing may have a considerable influence on the patient's ability to accept alternative modes of sexual expression, the "permission-giving" aspect of frank discussion of the subject may be helpful.

8. Provide useful suggestions of methods for making the sexual experiences more satisfactory within the limitations of the patient's condition. Although every patient will have individual needs and problems, the following may be helpful:
a. The patient should empty his bladder before sexual activity.
or
b. The patient should tape his suprapubic tube securely to his abdomen.
or
c. The patient should leave an indwelling urethral catheter in place.
  (1) A male patient should bend it close to the meatus, tape it to the penis, and cover it with a condom.
  (2) A female patient should push the catheter higher up into the bladder and tape it securely to her thigh or abdomen.
	This prevents distention and the possibility of incontinence during sexual activity.
	
	This reduces the possibility of the tube becoming dislodged.
	
	Not only does this solve the problem of incontinence, it also sometimes helps the patient with erectile problems because of the splinting effect of the catheter.
	This prevents traction on the tube and pressure on the neck of the bladder from the balloon portion of the catheter.

Plan for implementation	Rationale
9. Explain to the patient that in most cases fertility is not impaired.	If it is the male partner who is affected, semen can sometimes be retrieved after retrograde ejaculation by separating it from the urine if the bladder is emptied immediately after intercourse. Artificial insemination may then be employed. If it is the female partner who is affected, pregnancy is usually not contraindicated, although careful urologic management will be required during the pregnancy. Labor is under hormonal (not neurologic) control and therefore is not affected, regardless of the level of the spinal lesion. However, the patient may not be able to feel the contractions or be able to bear down, so forceps are frequently required.[5]
10. Inform the couple who does not want to have children that contraception may be necessary (depending on the particular patient's condition). If the patient is a female, she should consult with a gynecologist about a suitable contraceptive method.	Careful evaluation of the type of contraception must be made. Oral contraceptives may not be advisable because of the increased risk of thrombophlebitis.[5]

References and bibliography

REFERENCES
Chapter 38

1. Jeter, K.F., and Lattimer, J.K.: Common stomal problems following ileal conduit urinary diversion, Urology **3:**399-403, 1974.
2. Jones, M.A., Breckman, B., and Hendry, W.F.: Life with an ileal conduit: results of questionnaire surveys of patients and urological surgeons, Br. J. Urol. **52:**21, 1980.
3. Kahn, H.D., et al.: Effect of cranberry juice on urine, J. Am. Dietet. Assoc. **51:**251, 1967.
4. Leadbetter, G.W., Jr., Zickerman, P., and Pierce, E.: Ureterosigmoidostomy and cancer of the colon, J. Urol. **121:**732, 1979.
5. McLeod, D.C., and Nahata, M.C.: Inefficacy of ascorbic acid as a urinary acidifier, N. Engl. J. Med. **296:**1413, 1977.
6. Murphy, F.J., Zelman, S., and Mau, W.: Ascorbic acid as a urinary acidifying agent. 2. Its adjunctive role in chronic urinary infection, J. Urol. **94:**300, 1965.
7. Remigailo, R.V., et al.: Ileal conduit urinary diversion—ten year review, Urology **3:**343, 1976.

Chapter 39

1. Champion, V.L.: Clean technique for intermittent self-catheterization, Nurs. Res. **25:**13, 1976.
2. Lapides, J.: Tips on self-catheterization, Urology Digest, July 1977, p. 11.
3. Lapides, J., et al.: Further observations on self-catheterization, J. Urol. **116:**169, 1976.
4. Lowe, B.S.: The how-to of self-catheterization, ET J., Winter 1975-1976, p. 6.

Chapter 40

1. Champion, V.L.: Clean technique for intermittent self-catheterization, Nurs. Res. **25:**13, 1976.
2. Lapides, J.: Tips on self-catheterization, Urology Digest, July 1977, p. 11.
3. Lapides, J., et al.: Further observations on self-catheterization, J. Urol. **116:**169, 1976.
4. Lowe, B.S.: The how-to of self-catheterization, ET J. Winter 1975-1976, p. 6.
5. McCluer, S.: Pregnancy and fertility in women with spinal cord injury, Paper presented at Symposium on Long-term Genito-urinary Tract Management: Neurogenic Bladder, Spinal Cord Lesion, Sexuality, Minneapolis, April 1981.
6. Newman, E., and Price, M.: Urinary tract infection and sources of infection with different modes of urinary drainage, Paper presented at Symposium on Long-term Genito-urinary Tract Management: Neurogenic Bladder, Spinal Cord Lesion, Sexuality, Minneapolis, April 1981.

BIBLIOGRAPHY

Beland, G.: Present status of supravesical external urinary diversion, Urology **12**(3):261, 1978.
Boyarsky, S., et al.: Care of the patient with neurogenic bladder, Boston, 1979, Little, Brown & Co.
Broadwell, D., and Jackson, B.: Principles of ostomy care, St. Louis, 1981, The C.V. Mosby Co.
Castro, J.E., and Ram, M.D.: Electrolyte imbalance following ileal conduit diversion, Br. J. Urol. **42:**29, 1970.
Cockett, A.T.K., and Koshiba, K.: Manual of urologic surgery, New York, 1979, Springer-Verlag.
Dericks, V.C., and Donoval, C.T.: The ostomy patient really needs you, Nursing **6:**30, Sept. 1976.
Gault, P.L.: Six patients with bladder cancer . . . and how they fared after surgery, Nursing **7:**48, Nov. 1977.
Giaquinta, B.: Helping families face the crisis of cancer, Am. J. Nurs. Oct. 1977, p. 1585.
Glen, J.F., and Boyce, W.H., editors: Urologic surgery, ed. 2, New York, 1975, Harper & Row, Publishers.
Hock, W.H., Shanser, J.D., and Burns, R.A.: Ureterosigmoidostomy: a 59 year followup and review of long-term urinary diversion, J. Urol. **122:**407, Sept. 1979.
Lennenberg, E.S., and Sohn, N.: Modern concepts in the management of patients with intestinal stomas, New York, 1972, Harper & Row, Publishers.
Lerner, J., Harsh, J., and Eisenstat, T.E.: Why pre-op stoma planning is a must . . . and how you can make sure it's done right, RN **43:**48, Aug. 1980.
Mahoney, J.M.: Guide to ostomy nursing care, Boston, 1976, Little, Brown & Co.

Milroy, M.D., et al.: Permanent cutaneous ureterostomy: 18 years of experience, J. Urol. **120:**682, Dec. 1978.

Morel, A., and Wise, J.W.: Urologic endoscopic procedures, ed. 2, St. Louis, 1979, The C.V. Mosby Co.

Smith, R.B., and Skinner, D.G., editors: Complications of urologic surgery—prevention and management, Philadelphia, 1976, W.B. Saunders Co.

Sullivan, R.A., and Rago, M.: Specialized care of the spinal cord injured patient, J. Pract. Nurs. **26:**36, July 1976.

Wear, J.B., and Barquin, O.P.: Ureterosigmoidostomy—long-term results, Urology **1:**192, March 1973.

Wilson, M.F.: Bladder training for the chronically ill, RN **38:**36, June 1975.

Winter, C.W., and Morel, A.: Nursing care of patients with urologic disease, ed. 4, St. Louis, 1977, The C.V. Mosby Co.

Yeaworth, R.C.: Symposium on gerontological nursing. Foreword, Nurs. Clin. North Am. **11**(1):115, 1976.

UNIT VIII

PROCEDURES FOR DISORDERS
OF
THE PROSTATE

CHAPTER 41

Management of the patient in acute urinary retention

Acute urinary retention is one of the most common reasons for emergency admissions onto a urology unit. It has a variety of causes, but benign prostatic hyperplasia is by far the most common, especially in men over 50 years of age.

When a patient is admitted in acute urinary retention, he has been in considerable discomfort for many hours and is often apprehensive about the unexpected hospitalization. He is usually catheterized in the emergency room, where the volume of urine is carefully monitored. He is then admitted as an inpatient with the catheter in place. X-ray examinations (intravenous pyelogram and voiding cystourethrogram) and urodynamic studies are performed,* and, if an obstructive prostate is found to be the cause of the retention, the patient is scheduled for a prostatectomy (see Chapters 42 and 44).

If the tests indicate that the cause of retention is not a result of prostatic obstruction, other factors are often implicated, such as prior intake of anti-

*The less common conditions resulting in urinary retention (e.g., hemorrhagic cystitis and neurologic disorders) are characterized by distinctive signs and symptoms that indicate the type of diagnostic investigation required.

cholinergics (found in many nonprescription "cold" medications) or an unusually high alcohol intake. In these cases the time usually required to complete the diagnostic tests (48 hours) is generally sufficient for vesical tone to be reestablished. The catheter is then removed, and, if there are no voiding difficulties, the patient is usually discharged 24 hours later.

ACUTE URINARY RETENTION
Outline of Care Plan
ANTICIPATED NURSING DIAGNOSES:

Period of acute symptoms
1. Anxiety and physical discomfort related to hospitalization.
2. Need for management of indwelling urethral catheter.
3. Need for management of intravenous infusion.
4. Need for psychologic and physical preparation for diagnostic procedures.

Convalescent period
5. Potential for voiding complications following removal of indwelling urethral catheter.*
6. Need for discharge teaching.*

*May not apply.

NURSING CARE PLAN FOR THE PATIENT HOSPITALIZED FOR ACUTE URINARY RETENTION

1. NURSING DIAGNOSIS: Anxiety and physical discomfort related to hospitalization

Objective of nursing intervention	Appropriate management of anxiety and physical discomfort
Expected outcome	Behavioral and/or verbal indication of adequate reduction of anxiety and physical discomfort

Plan for implementation	Rationale

1. Be aware that the patient admitted with a diagnosis of acute urinary retention probably will have experienced the following:
  a. Extreme bladder discomfort for the last 24 hours or more
  b. Severe anxiety about being unable to void
  c. The discomfort of an indwelling urethral catheter
 	
  d. The psychologic stress of sudden hospitalization
  e. The psychologic stress of **possible** impending surgery
	Acute urinary retention is usually painful and frightening for the patient.
	
	Although this relieves the discomfort of urinary retention, the catheter may cause bladder spasms and provoke anxiety.
	
	Uncertainty about forthcoming events sometimes provokes more anxiety than the certainty of a potentially unpleasant event.

2. Provide analgesia and/or sedative as ordered.	
3. Explain all procedures beforehand.	
4. Allow the patient to express feelings.	
5. Convey willingness to listen, and answer all questions.	
6. Provide encouragement and reassurance.	

7. If the patient appears anxious about the presence of hematuria:
  a. Explain the reason for its occurrence.
 	
  b. Provide reassurance that the condition is transient.
 	
  c. Explain that only a few spoonfuls of blood will turn the urine red.
	If the bladder was greatly distended during the period of acute retention, decompression often causes the capillaries in the mucosa to rupture, causing the urine to turn deep pink.
	In most cases the bleeding stops spontaneously within 24 hours.

Period of acute symptoms

2. NURSING DIAGNOSIS: Need for management of indwelling urethral catheter

Objectives of nursing intervention

Appropriate care of catheter and equipment
Prevention or early detection of infection
Care of tissue surrounding catheter
Maintenance of accurate records of urine output
Appropriate administration of hand-irrigation of catheter
Management of discomfort or pain caused by catheter
Satisfactory collection of urine specimens from catheter

Expected outcomes

Absence of severe bladder spasms and suprapubic distention
Urine draining freely through system
Absence of fever, chills, and foul-smelling urine
Absence of urethral discharge and tissue inflammation
Minimal discomfort caused by the catheter
Urine specimens in optimum condition for all necessary tests

Plan for implementation	Rationale
See master care plan for the patient with an indwelling urethral catheter: care after insertion of catheter.	
In addition to the topics covered in the master care plan, the following interventions are required: 1. If there is a great deal of blood in the urine, maintain the patient's fluid intake at 3 L or more per day (unless contraindicated by a coexisting medical condition).	There is less risk of obstruction from clots if the urine is dilute.
2. In the initial phase of decompression, follow the physician's orders **precisely** regarding intermittent clamping or partial continuous clamping of the catheter.	Slow decompression (keeping the tube partially clamped or intermittently clamped) is sometimes employed to reduce the degree of postobstructive hematuria.
3. If the urine turns bright red and has a moderate viscosity and/or clots, notify the physician.	Hemorrhage is a potential complication following decompression.
4. If urine output exceeds 200 ml/hour (after the initial decompression in the emergency room), notify the physician and make preparations to carry out the following orders: a. Start intravenous infusion (if not already present).	Postobstructive diuresis may occur, resulting in the kidney's production of abnormally large amounts of dilute urine. Excessive amounts of water and sodium are lost, so dehydration and electrolyte imbalance must be prevented. Usually the condition resolves within 12 hours.
b. Obtain urine specimen for electrolyte analysis and osmolarity. c. Obtain blood specimen for electrolytes.	

Period of acute symptoms

Plan for implementation	Rationale
5. If the aforementioned condition occurs, check the patient's vital signs carefully and be alert for irregularities in the patient's pulse. If any abnormalities are noted, inform the physician.	Potassium may also be lost in abnormal quantities, predisposing the patient to cardiac arrhythmias.

3. NURSING DIAGNOSIS: Need for management of intravenous infusion

Objectives of nursing intervention

- Appropriate administration of specific types of intravenous solutions
- Prevention or early detection of local complications
- Prevention or early detection of systemic complications
- Management of discomfort caused by the intravenous infusion
- Maintenance of proper function of intravenous equipment
- Maintenance of accurate records of the patient's hydration status

Expected outcomes

- Normal hydration status
- Normal electrolyte status
- Absence of thrombophlebitis, infiltration, infection, fluid overload, and pulmonary embolism
- Absence of discomfort caused by the intravenous infusion

Plan for implementation	Rationale
See master care plan for the patient receiving intravenous therapy.	These patients are often given intravenous therapy to prevent the dehydration and electrolyte imbalance that sometimes occurs from postobstructive diuresis. They may be given isotonic saline solutions and placed on a regimen in which the volume of urine output determines the amount of intravenous fluid to be infused. Various electrolytes may be added to the solutions, depending on the electrolyte loss in the urine.

Period of acute symptoms

4. NURSING DIAGNOSIS: Need for psychologic and physical preparation for diagnostic procedures

Objectives of nursing intervention
Reduction of patient anxiety
Provision of description and explanation of purpose for the procedures
Provision of physical preparation for the procedures

Expected outcomes
Absence of anxiety about diagnostic procedures
Cooperation during procedures
Specimens and x-ray films in satisfactory condition for diagnosis

Plan for implementation	Rationale
1. Provide information and physical preparation for whichever of the following tests are ordered: a. Urinalysis b. Intravenous pyelogram c. Cystoscopy d. Urodynamic studies	Some of or all these tests may be required to determine the underlying cause of the retention. The patient may need considerable support and reassurance, since some of these tests may cause discomfort.
2. If the tests indicate that the urinary retention is caused by prostatic enlargement proceed with the following actions after the physician has discussed the surgery with the patient: a. Determine the type of surgery the patient is to have. b. Begin preoperative teaching.	If the patient is to have surgery, the care plan for the patient in acute urinary retention terminates here. (See Chapter 42 or 44 for the next steps in the nursing care plan for this patient.)

5. NURSING DIAGNOSIS: Potential for voiding complications following removal of indwelling urethral catheter*

Objective of nursing intervention
Prevention or early detection of complications

Expected outcomes
Resumption of normal voiding pattern
Absence of dysuria

Plan for implementation	Rationale
See master care plan for the patient with an indwelling urethral catheter: care after removal of the catheter.	

*This only applies to the patient for whom the diagnostic procedures have established that the obstruction is **not** related to prostatic enlargement. Otherwise, the catheter will remain in place, and the patient will be scheduled for surgery.

Period of acute symptoms

Convalescent period

6. NURSING DIAGNOSIS: Need for discharge teaching*

Objectives of nursing intervention

{ Explanation of basic information about medications to be taken at home

Explanation of information regarding follow-up care

Explanation of residual effects of the condition and/or treatment

Explanation of instructions concerning postdischarge activities

Explanation of symptoms that constitute a reason to contact the physician

Review of admitting diagnosis and mode of treatment }

Expected outcomes

{ Accurate return verbalization and/or demonstration of all material learned

Smooth transition of care after discharge

Absence or early detection of complications arising after discharge

Ability to provide future health care practitioners with important data about health history }

Plan for implementation	Rationale
See master care plan for the patient requiring discharge preparations: discharge teaching.	
In addition to the topics covered in the master care plan, include the following items in the discharge teaching:	
1. The patient will probably be given a prescription for antibiotics to take at home.	This is usually done prophylactically because the catheter has predisposed him to urinary tract infection.
2. The patient should drink at least 2 L of fluid daily.	This also reduces the possibility of a urinary tract infection resulting from the indwelling urethral catheter.
3. He will be given a follow-up office appointment for his physician to check his voiding pattern.	
4. If the retention was caused by excessive anticholinergic intake, the patient should avoid the use of over-the-counter cold and allergy preparations unless he checks with his physician beforehand to determine the type and amount of medication he should use.	Nasal decongestants and cold preparations often contain anticholinergic medications. These may cause urinary retention if consumed in large enough quantities because they inhibit parasympathetic activity and thus bladder contractions.

*The patient may be scheduled for a prostatectomy; therefore this may not apply.

Convalescent period

CHAPTER 42

Simple prostatectomies

Simple prostatectomy is the type of surgery performed for patients with prostatic enlargement caused by benign prostatic hyperplasia.* Descriptions of the three different forms of this surgery follow. However, a few words should be said about the implications of benign prostatic hyperplasia, since it is such a common affliction of men over 50 years of age.

In the early stages of the condition the bladder undergoes hypertrophy to compensate for the increased resistance in the prostatic urethra. The muscle bundles of the bladder wall begin to lift up the bladder mucosa, forming a honeycomb appearance (trabeculation), and, as the process continues, portions of the mucosa (diverticula) balloon out between the muscle bundles into the perivesical fat. Finally the bladder muscles can no longer exert enough force to completely expel urine through the narrowing urethral lumen. Decompensation occurs, and urine is retained in the bladder, predisposing the patient to infection and calculus formation. Meanwhile, the increased voiding pressure in the bladder may have resulted in progressive ureterohydronephrosis, impairment of renal function, and finally uremia.

Therefore the hazard of benign prostatic hyperplasia is not so much the enlarged prostate itself, but the effects of its obstruction on other organs of the urinary tract. In its most extreme form the obstruction may have fatal consequences, although rarely is it allowed to progress this far.

Symptoms usually begin with hesitancy and decreased force of the urinary stream. The patient may develop frequency (due to bladder instability) and nocturia. Hematuria might also occur if dilated veins

in the bladder neck rupture. When the prostatic obstruction develops to the degree that voiding becomes impossible, the patient is said to be in acute urinary retention. Surgery is essential when the condition progresses to this point, but it is often performed before such an acute condition occurs because of the patient's discomfort with urinary frequency and the progressive damage to the urinary tract, which begins well in advance of complete obstruction.

• • •

There are three different types of simple prostatectomies, all of which involve removal of the enlarged portion of the prostate gland while leaving the prostatic capsule in place. The term "adenectomy" is often used to differentiate these procedures from radical prostatectomy, which involves removal of the entire gland, including the capsule, and is done for malignant conditions (see Chapter 44).

A simple prostatectomy may be performed via the urethra (transurethral prostatectomy) or by means of an abdominal incision. When an open procedure is used, the prostate may be approached through an incision in the bladder (transvesical prostatectomy) or by cutting into the prostatic capsule (retropubic prostatectomy).

Either form of open procedure has frequently been described by comparing the prostate gland and its capsule to a walnut within a shell. The shell is entered, and only the meat of the nut (the adenoma) is removed. For this reason the term "enucleation" of the prostate is often used. As with the transurethral approach, these open prostatectomies do no involve removal of the entire gland; therefore the possibility of future enlargement exists.

Occasionally a vasectomy is performed with transvesical or retropubic operations as prophylaxis

---

*The terms "hyperplasia" and "hypertrophy" have sometimes been used interchangeably when referring to benign prostatic enlargement. Technically, however, hyperplasia is the correct term, since the condition involves **new** cellular growth within the gland, as opposed to enlargement of existing cells.

against epididimoorchitis. If this procedure is to be done, it should be indicated on the surgical consent form the patient signs.

TRANSURETHRAL PROSTATECTOMY

The purpose of a transurethral prostatectomy is to correct the urethral obstruction resulting from benign prostatic hyperplasia, without an abdominal incision. It is the treatment of choice when the prostate gland is only moderately enlarged.

The surgery is performed with the patient in a lithotomy position. A resectoscope is inserted through the urethra, and the enlarged portion of the prostate gland is sliced out (resected) in small pieces (Fig. 42-1). Visualization of the surgical field is maintained by constant infusion of a clear solution into the bladder and urethra. Hemostasis is achieved with coagulation current. All prostatic chips are irrigated out through the resectoscope, and an indwelling catheter is inserted to ensure adequate drainage of the bladder.

If venous bleeding is encountered, some surgeons will apply traction to the catheter by taping it to the patient's thigh in such a way that the catheter remains very taut, and the balloon portion creates pressure against the prostatic fossa (Fig. 42-2). Traction may also be achieved by tying a strip of gauze around the catheter at the penile meatus to keep it from ascending to its natural position with the balloon in the bladder.

Also, at the surgeon's discretion, continuous bladder irrigation (Fig. 42-3) or periodic hand-irrigation may be instituted to prevent clot retention within the bladder.

TRANSURETHRAL PROSTATECTOMY
Outline of Care Plan
ANTICIPATED NURSING DIAGNOSES:

Preoperative period
1. Need for preoperative teaching.
2. Need for discharge planning.

Early postoperative period
3. Potential for shock.
4. Potential for hyponatremia.
5. Potential for respiratory complications related to surgical intervention.
6. Need for management of indwelling urethral catheter.
7. Need for management of traction on catheter.*
8. Need for management of continuous bladder irrigation.*
9. Postoperative pain.
10. Need for management of intravenous infusion.
11. Potential for infection.
12. Potential for deep vein thrombosis.
13. Potential for injury to surgical site from rectal trauma.
14. Anxiety about visible hematuria.†
15. Bleeding from penile meatus.†

Late postoperative period
16. Potential for voiding complications following removal of indwelling urethral catheter.
17. Dysuria.†
18. Disturbance in urinary control.†

Convalescent period
19. Need for discharge teaching.
20. Continued disturbance in urinary control at time of discharge.†
21. Knowledge deficit—minor alterations in sexual function.

---

*Used at the discretion of the surgeon; may not apply.
†May not apply.

450

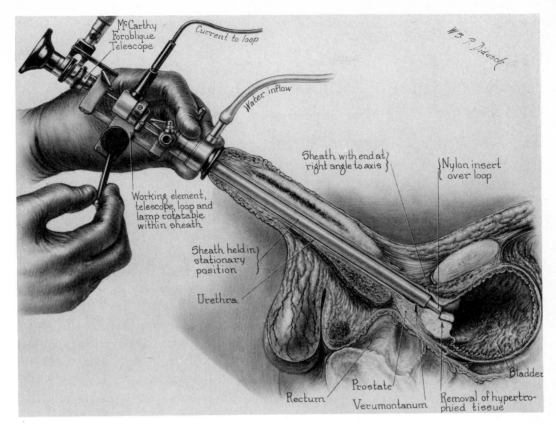

Fig. 42-1. Stern-McCarthy resectoscope in prostatic urethra removing prostatic tissue. (Courtesy William P. Didusch and American Cystoscope Makers, Inc., Stamford, Conn.)

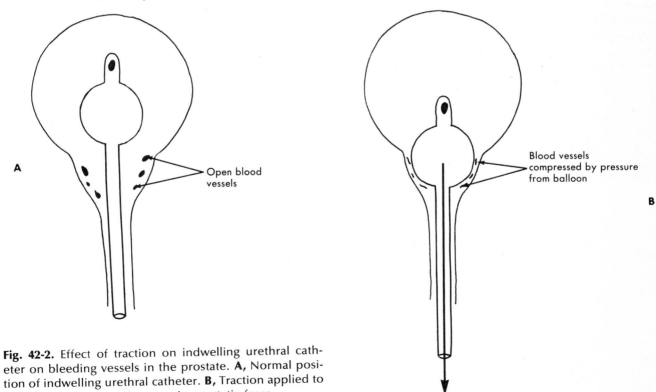

Fig. 42-2. Effect of traction on indwelling urethral catheter on bleeding vessels in the prostate. **A,** Normal position of indwelling urethral catheter. **B,** Traction applied to catheter; balloon portion now in prostatic fossa.

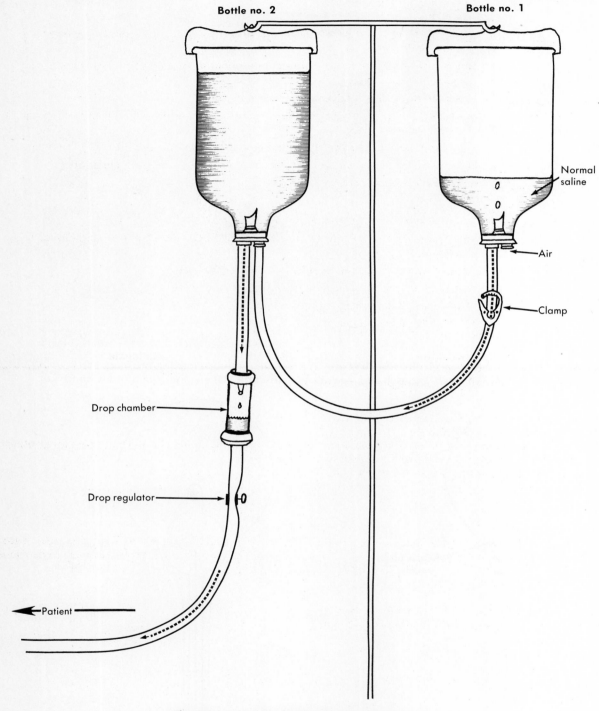

Fig. 42-3. Continuous bladder irrigation set-up.

NURSING CARE PLAN FOR THE PATIENT UNDERGOING TRANSURETHRAL PROSTATECTOMY

1. NURSING DIAGNOSIS: Need for preoperative teaching

Objectives of nursing intervention

If necessary, clarification of reason for hospitalization and type of surgery to be performed

Elimination of any negative or inaccurate notions regarding the forthcoming surgery

Explanation of preoperative tests and procedures

Psychologic preparation for general anesthesia (omit if the patient is to have spinal anesthesia)

Explanation of events expected in the early postoperative period

Explanation of body conditions expected in the early postoperative period

Identification of any known allergies

Expected outcomes

Verbal indication that explanations are understood

Verbal indication of optimistic expectations (within realistic limits) related to forthcoming surgery

Cooperation during preoperative tests and procedures

Verbal or behavioral indication of reduction of anxiety

Absence of postoperative complications

Absence of allergic reactions

Plan for implementation	Rationale
See master care plan for the patient receiving preoperative teaching.	
In addition to the topics covered in the master care plan, include the following items in the preoperative teaching: 1. Be aware that, in addition to the routine preoperative tests, an intravenous pyelogram is usually performed, and answer any questions the patient may have regarding the procedure.	This is done to detect any associated anatomic abnormalities.
2. The preoperative shave is from the umbilicus to mid-thigh. Occasionally it is omitted altogether.	A shave is usually ordered to keep the area as clean as possible in the event that an incision has to be made.
3. The patient will probably be permitted a light supper in the evening after surgery and will resume his normal diet in the morning.	

Preoperative period

Plan for implementation	Rationale
4. There will be an indwelling urethral catheter in place for several days. It may be connected to continuous bladder irrigation for approximately 24 hours after surgery. If so, the patient will be required to remain in bed until the irrigation is discontinued.	
5. Urine is expected to be blood tinged in the early postoperative period. NOTE: Use the word "surgery" with caution. The word "scraping" can be substituted if necessary.	Although technically a transurethral prostatectomy is considered a surgical procedure, the patient's physician may have described it as a "scraping" rather than a "cutting," to allay anxiety. Furthermore, many patients think that, if there is no external incision, the procedure is not called surgery. Therefore the unexpected use of the term may provoke anxiety.

2. NURSING DIAGNOSIS: Need for discharge planning

Objectives of nursing intervention
- Early commencement of discharge planning
- Accurate estimate of time required for all discharge teaching

Expected outcome Smooth transition of care after discharge

Plan for implementation	Rationale

See master care plan for the patient requiring discharge preparations: discharge planning.
 	
In addition to the topics covered in the master care plan, the following items should be considered:
1. The duration of hospitalization for this procedure is approximately 1 week.
 	
2. Required teaching includes:
  a. General postoperative discharge teaching
  b. Perineal exercises (occasionally required)
  c. Mention of minor changes in sexual function	

Preoperative period

3. NURSING DIAGNOSIS: Potential for shock

Objective of nursing intervention Prevention or early detection of shock

Expected outcomes { Vital signs normal, skin dry, color normal
Absence of bright red drainage from the catheter

Plan for implementation	Rationale
1. Check the patient's vital signs every 4 hours once stable (every 15 minutes if unstable).	Hemorrhagic shock is a potential complication after this type of surgery because the prostate gland is highly vascular. During a transurethral prostatectomy the most common bleeding is of venous origin. The source is sometimes difficult to locate at the time of surgery because the pressure of irrigating fluid is greater than the pressure of blood in the open vein, and the bleeding stops temporarily. For this reason the open vein is not identified and treated with coagulation current. Once the irrigation stops, the bleeding begins again. Considerable loss of blood occasionally occurs, and vital signs must be carefully monitored because the severity of bleeding may be difficult to determine if the patient is on continuous bladder irrigation.
2. Be alert for increasing pulse and respiratory rates, decreasing blood pressure, diaphoresis, pallor, and feelings of apprehension.	
3. Notify the physician at once if indications of impending shock occur.	

Early postoperative period

4. NURSING DIAGNOSIS: Potential for hyponatremia*

| **Objective of nursing intervention** | Early detection and management of hyponatremia |

Expected outcomes
{ Consciousness regained without delay after anesthesia
Absence of confusion, muscular twitching, convulsions

Early postoperative period

Plan for implementation	Rationale
1. Check the patient's mental status throughout the immediate postoperative period and notify the physician if the patient is confused.	This is usually the first indication of hyponatremia that the floor nurse will encounter. In many cases patients suffering from hyponatremia will also take an abnormally long time to recover from the effects of anesthesia in the recovery room.
2. Notify the physician at once if the patient develops muscular twitching and/or convulsions.	These are late symptoms of hyponatremia that may, if the imbalance is great enough, progress to unconsciousness and death unless they are rapidly treated.
3. If any of these conditions occur, notify the physician and take the following actions. a. Keep siderails on the patient's bed elevated. b. Make preparations for a blood specimen to be obtained for electrolyte determination (specifically sodium). c. Have hypertonic saline solution on hand for intravenous infusion.	This is a protective measure for the confused patient. This is necessary to confirm that the patient is indeed suffering from hyponatremia. Sodium replacement should be initiated as soon as possible.

*Hyponatremia is a potential complication of a transurethral prostatectomy because of the nature of the irrigating fluid that is used. Normal saline cannot be used during any surgery that uses electric current for cutting or hemostasis because it is ionized. The irrigant of choice is a glycine solution, since it will not conduct electric current and has good optical properties. However, because it is moderately hypotonic, its absorption through open veins in the prostate during surgery will cause an increase in the volume of circulating blood and a decrease in the sodium concentration. This fluid and electrolyte imbalance may be transient and relatively asymptomatic. However, in some cases, the hyponatremia may be severe enough to cause cerebral edema, which, if not corrected, may lead to convulsions, unconsciousness, and death. (See nursing diagnosis 5 for complications associated with hypervolemia.) The condition can, however, be rapidly reversed by intravenous infusion of hypertonic sodium solutions.

5. NURSING DIAGNOSIS: Potential for respiratory complications related to surgical intervention

Objective of nursing intervention

Prevention or early detection of pulmonary edema, atelectasis, and/or pneumonia

Expected outcomes

Absence of rales, dyspnea, and neck venous distention
Cooperation with therapeutic respiratory regimen
Absence of fever or audible lung congestion
Sputum clear or white and easily mobilized

Plan for implementation	Rationale
See master care plan for the patient at risk for respiratory complications, nursing objective 1.	
In addition to the items mentioned in the master care plan, the following interventions are required:	

1. Be alert for the following indications of fluid overload:
  a. Pulmonary congestion (rales, dyspnea)
  b. Elevation of central venous pressure, which may be manifested by prominent jugular veins when the patient is in a semi-Fowler or upright position
	During surgery excessive absorption of irrigating fluid occasionally occurs through the open veins in the prostate. If the patient is unable to eliminate this fluid quickly enough, he will develop fluid overload and pulmonary edema. Patients with a history of congestive heart failure are particularly at risk, especially if the surgery is prolonged.

2. If any of these signs occur: a. Place the patient in an upright position.	This facilitates breathing by reducing the pressure of the abdomen against the diaphragm. Furthermore, it causes excess fluid in the lungs to gravitate to the base of the lungs, making the upper portion available for exchange of gases.
b. Slow the IV to a minimal rate.	Intravenous fluid will only compound the problem.
c. Notify the physician at once.	Depending on the degree of fluid overload and the patient's homeostatic mechanisms to deal with it, the condition may be life threatening.

d. Keep the patient calm.
  e. Have a fast-acting diuretic (e.g., furosemide) on hand so that it can be administered at once if the physician should request it.
  f. Have oxygen readily available.	

Early postoperative period

6. NURSING DIAGNOSIS: Need for management of indwelling urethral catheter

Objectives of nursing intervention

Appropriate care of catheter and equipment
Prevention or early detection of infection
Care of tissue surrounding catheter
Maintenance of accurate records of urine output
Appropriate administration of hand-irrigation of catheter
Management of discomfort or pain caused by catheter
Satisfactory collection of urine specimens from catheter

Expected outcomes

Absence of severe bladder spasms and suprapubic distention
Urine draining freely through system
Absence of fever, chills, and foul-smelling urine
Absence of urethral discharge and tissue inflammation
Minimal discomfort caused by the catheter
Urine specimens in optimum condition for all necessary tests

Plan for implementation	Rationale
See master care plan for the patient with an indwelling urethral catheter: care after insertion of the catheter.	
In addition to the topics covered in the master care plan, the following interventions are required: 1. Notify the physician if the urine remains bright red and has a high viscosity and/or clots, despite hand-irrigation. Deep pink urine that lightens after irrigation is not abnormal after prostatic surgery.	If the bleeding is of venous origin, the physician might put traction on the catheter (see p. 459). If it is arterial bleeding, it may require correction in the operating room.
2. Notify the physician if the urine output or drainage from continuous bladder irrigation becomes obstructed and cannot be corrected by hand-irrigation.	The physician will either use more powerful instruments with which to aspirate the obstruction or will change the catheter.
3. Be alert for psychologic dependence on hand-irrigation of the catheter, manifested by patient requests that the catheter be irrigated, despite obvious patency.	This sometimes happens if the patient incorrectly associates hand-irrigation with the reduction of **all** bladder pain. Such a patient assumes that irrigation will reduce the discomfort of "normal" bladder spasms (which periodically occur simply from the catheter's irritating effect on the wall of the bladder), and the patient may become extremely insistent that he be irrigated with frequency.

4. If conditions in no. 3 occur:
  a. Check catheter for patency.
  b. If the catheter is patent, do not irrigate; instead, explain to the patient the hazards of unnecessary irrigation (i.e., infection) and that irrigation has no beneficial effect on limiting "normal" bladder spasms.
	If the catheter is obstructed, of course it must be irrigated.

Early postoperative period

458

Plan for implementation	Rationale
c. Provide an appropriate analgesic. (See Chapter 11, part one, nursing objective 6, spasmodic, intermittent pain in suprapubic area, or pain radiating to urethral area.)	

7. **NURSING DIAGNOSIS:** Need for management of traction on catheter*

Objectives of nursing intervention { Maintenance of traction
Prevention of complications associated with prolonged traction

Expected outcomes { Short term: Venous bleeding reduced
Long term: Absence of necrotic tissue sloughing

Plan for implementation	Rationale
1. Do not remove tape (or strip of gauze) maintaining traction on the catheter, unless there is an order to do so.	The catheter may be taped to the patient's thigh, or a strip of gauze bandage may be tied around the catheter to act as a wedge, keeping the balloon portion of the catheter from ascending into the bladder where it is normally positioned. Either method of traction causes the inflated balloon to exert pressure on the prostatic fossa to decrease venous bleeding from the surgical site (see Fig. 42-2). However, traction is controversial. Some surgeons believe that the pressure of the balloon causes the veins to distend, and thus the normal process of hemostasis, which involves venous constriction, is retarded.
2. Follow precisely the orders indicating the time the traction is to be released.	The pressure of the balloon will cause ischemia and consequent necrosis if it is not released within 3 to 6 hours.
3. If no order has been written concerning the time the traction is to be released, contact the physician.	

*Traction is not always applied to a catheter after a transurethral prostatectomy; therefore this may not apply.

Early postoperative period

8. NURSING DIAGNOSIS: Need for management of continuous bladder irrigation*

Objectives of nursing intervention

- Maintenance of patency of irrigation system
- Prevention or early detection of obstruction and other complications associated with system

Expected outcomes

- Clear or light blood-tinged drainage, flowing freely
- Absence of suprapubic distention or discomfort

Plan for implementation	Rationale
1. Use only normal saline for irrigation fluid.	It is possible for some of the irrigating fluid to be absorbed systemically through blood vessels that were not treated with coagulation current. Therefore it is essential that the fluid be isotonic to the blood to prevent massive hemolysis and other potentially fatal consequences that would occur if water were used.
2. Check the color of the drainage frequently and adjust the flow rate accordingly.	
a. If the drainage is very bloody, increase the rate.	Dilution of the blood aids in the prevention of clot formation.
b. If drainage is pale pink or clear, reduce the rate, but do not stop it altogether.	Saline, like other hospital supplies, should not be wasted, and irrigation is unnecessary unless bleeding is present. However, hemostasis may be very erratic during the immediate postoperative period, and obstructive clot formation could occur without much warning.
3. Keep the patient in bed while irrigation is in progress, unless ordered otherwise.	An accident could easily occur with irrigating fluid and drainage bottles if the patient were to ambulate. Bed rest also favors hemostasis.
4. Avoid external obstruction of tubing (e.g., kinks, patient lying on tubing).	If the bladder becomes distended with fluid, it will cause severe discomfort and potential damage to the surgical site.
5. Be alert for indications of internal obstruction (e.g., decreased drainage, bladder spasms of increasing intensity, suprapubic distention).	Clots and tissue particles may prevent irrigating fluid from draining out of the bladder, resulting in pain, distention, and potential damage to the surgical site.
6. If necessary, hand-irrigate the catheter with a 60-ml bulb syringe.	Hand-irrigation provides the negative pressure necessary to aspirate obstructive particles.
7. Be certain the fluid input regulator of the continuous bladder irrigation is turned off while hand-irrigation is in progress (and turned back on afterward).	If fluid from the continuous irrigation system is permitted to flow into the bladder during hand-irrigation, it is difficult to estimate the amount of fluid to instill with the hand-irrigation equipment, and overdistention can easily occur.
8. Notify the physician if the obstruction cannot be aspirated.	

Early postoperative period

*Continuous bladder irrigation is not always used after a transurethral prostatectomy; therefore this may not apply.

9. NURSING DIAGNOSIS: Postoperative pain

<table>
<tr><td>**Objective of nursing intervention**</td><td>Appropriate management of pain or discomfort</td></tr>
<tr><td>**Expected outcome**</td><td>Behavioral and/or verbal indication that pain is adequately reduced or absent</td></tr>
</table>

Plan for implementation	Rationale
Determine the source of the pain. It may be related to the catheter or surgical intervention.	Pain from different sources usually requires different intervention.
1. Question and observe the patient to obtain information about the pain.	
2. Be aware that pain is a unique and individual experience. Although the different sources of pain can usually be determined by their characteristics, there are also many variations.	
3. Be alert for indications (verbal or behavioral) that the patient is experiencing discomfort other than physical pain, and attempt to resolve the problem.	Fear, loneliness, depression, and numerous other conditions may be sources of extreme discomfort for the patient, who may unconsciously translate these feelings into pain.

PERSISTENT, SEVERE, INCREASING PAIN IN SUPRAPUBIC AREA

See Chapter 11, part one, nursing objective 6.	This pain is probably caused by an obstructed catheter.

SPASMODIC, INTERMITTENT PAIN IN SUPRAPUBIC AREA, OR PAIN RADIATING TO URETHRAL AREA

See Chapter 11, part one, nursing objective 6.	This pain is probably caused by the catheter's irritating effect on the bladder and inflammation at the surgical site.

Early postoperative period

10. NURSING DIAGNOSIS: Need for management of intravenous infusion

Objectives of nursing intervention

Appropriate administration of specific types of intravenous solutions
Prevention or early detection of local complications
Prevention or early detection of systemic complications
Management of discomfort caused by the intravenous infusion
Maintenance of proper function of intravenous equipment
Maintenance of accurate records of the patient's hydration status

Expected outcomes

Normal hydration status
Normal electrolyte status
Absence of thrombophlebitis, infiltration, infection, fluid overload, and pulmonary embolism
Absence of discomfort caused by the intravenous infusion

Plan for implementation	Rationale
See master care plan for the patient receiving intravenous therapy.	Prostatectomy patients usually receive isotonic dextrose and saline solutions. Many physicians also order prophylactic antibiotic administration.

11. NURSING DIAGNOSIS: Potential for infection

Objective of nursing intervention

Prevention or early detection of infection

Expected outcome

Absence of significant rise in fever

Plan for implementation	Rationale
1. See Chapter 11, care after insertion of the catheter, nursing objective 2.	The urethral catheter predisposes the patient to infection.
2. Check the patient's temperature every 4 hours routinely and within 2 hours after any difficult irrigation during which manipulation of the catheter was required.	Bacteremia can occur after any instrumentation of the urinary tract. This happens as a result of absorption of bacteria into the bloodstream through the urethral mucosa.
3. Notify the physician if the patient's temperature rises above 101°.	

Early postoperative period

12. NURSING DIAGNOSIS: Potential for deep vein thrombosis

Objectives of nursing intervention
{ Explanation and maintenance of precautions against deep vein thrombosis
Early detection of deep vein thrombosis

Expected outcomes
{ Cooperation with regimen to prevent deep vein thrombosis
Absence of local pain, swelling, and redness of a lower extremity
Absence of fever

Plan for implementation	Rationale
See master care plan for the patient at risk for deep vein thrombosis.	

13. NURSING DIAGNOSIS: Potential for injury to surgical site from rectal trauma

Objective of nursing intervention
Prevention of rectal trauma

Expected outcomes
{ Absence of perforated tissues
Uninterrupted healing process

Plan for implementation	Rationale
1. Do not insert any foreign object into the patient's rectum for 48 to 72 hours after surgery. This includes enemas, suppositories, and thermometers.	The proximity of the prostate to the rectum makes the introduction of a foreign object into the rectum potentially harmful to healing prostatic tissue.
2. If the patient requires rectal temperature readings, use **extreme caution** when inserting the thermometer. Do not delegate this job to an auxiliary staff member.	This job should not be assigned to nurses' aides or orderlies because, in most cases, they are not aware of the abovementioned information.

Early postoperative period

14. NURSING DIAGNOSIS: Anxiety about visible hematuria*

Objective of nursing intervention	Patient education regarding postoperative hematuria

Expected outcome	Verbal and/or behavioral indication of reduced anxiety

Plan for implementation	Rationale
Explain the following:	
1. Blood-tinged urine is expected after a prostatectomy.	
2. Only a few spoonfuls of blood will turn the urine red.	
3. Increased blood in the urine is not uncommon after a bowel movement.	Increased intraabdominal pressure, as well as contraction of the colon, may cause a transient increase in bleeding from the surgical site.

*May not apply.

15. NURSING DIAGNOSIS: Bleeding from penile meatus (around catheter)*

Objectives of nursing intervention	Maintenance of patient hygiene
	Prevention of skin irritation

Expected outcome	Absence of discomfort and/or meatal tissue irritation

Plan for implementation	Rationale
1. Check the catheter for obstruction (indicated by scanty drainage and suprapubic distention) and irrigate if necessary. (See Chapter 11, nursing objective 5.)	When the catheter is obstructed, the "bleeding" is really blood-tinged urine being expelled around the catheter.
2. If the catheter is patent:	In this case the bleeding is simply a result of the surgery and should not be considered abnormal unless it is severe.
a. Wrap a combine loosely around the penis to avoid soiling the patient's gown.	
b. Increase the frequency of catheter care.	Dried blood is an ideal medium for bacterial growth and is also extremely irritating to the urethral mucosa.

*May not apply.

Early postoperative period

16. NURSING DIAGNOSIS: Potential for voiding complications following removal of indwelling urethral catheter

Objective of nursing intervention   Prevention or early detection of complications

Expected outcomes { Resumption of normal voiding pattern
Absence of dysuria

Plan for implementation	Rationale
See master care plan for the patient with an indwelling urethral catheter: care after removal of the catheter.	

17. NURSING DIAGNOSIS: Dysuria*

Objective of nursing intervention   Reduction of discomfort

Expected outcome   Verbal and/or behavioral indication of minimal voiding discomfort

Plan for implementation	Rationale
1. Provide reassurance that the discomfort is transient.	A burning sensation while voiding is very common for the first 24 hours after the catheter is removed. Urine, particularly if it is concentrated, may have an irritating effect on healing tissue.
2. Encourage high fluid intake.	This dilutes the urine and thus reduces the discomfort.
3. If the patient is in a great deal of discomfort, suggest to the physician that an analgesic that is specific to the urinary tract (e.g., phenazopyridine HCl [Pyridium]) be ordered.	

Late postoperative period

*Dysuria does not always occur after removal of a catheter following a prostatectomy; this may not apply.

465

18. NURSING DIAGNOSIS: Disturbance in urinary control*

Objectives of nursing intervention { Reduction of anxiety

Instruction on perineal exercises and types of fluid restrictions

Expected outcomes { Short term

Verbal and/or behavioral indication of decreased anxiety

Accurate return verbalization of instructions on perineal exercises

Long term: Resumption of normal voiding pattern

Plan for implementation	Rationale
1. Provide reassurance by explaining that dribbling and urgency incontinence are not uncommon after a prostatectomy, but it is a **temporary** condition.	Temporary lack of complete urinary control sometimes occurs after simple prostatectomies because the surgery involves removal of portions of the bladder neck and prostatic urethra. Complete return to a normal voiding pattern may take up to 6 months, although relatively adequate control usually returns within a few days or weeks.
2. Explain perineal exercises and obtain an accurate return verbalization. a. While standing, the patient should tighten and relax his buttocks five or more times each hour.	When gluteal muscles are voluntarily contracted, all the perineal muscles contract, including the sphincter muscles. Since the urinary sphincters are under voluntary and involuntary control, some physicians feel that these exercises facilitate the return of adequate sphincter control.
b. While voiding, the patient should voluntarily stop and restart the urinary stream using sphincter muscles. c. The patient should attempt to lengthen the period of time between each voiding by consciously holding in the urine.	
3. Suggest that the patient avoid drinking tea, coffee, and cola beverages.	These drinks contain caffeine, which is a mild diuretic and might make urinary control more difficult.

*Limited urinary control does not always occur after a transurethral prostatectomy; this may not apply.

Late postoperative period

19. NURSING DIAGNOSIS: Need for discharge teaching

Objectives of nursing intervention

Explanation of basic information about medications to be taken at home

Explanation of information regarding follow-up care

Explanation of residual effects of the condition and/or treatment

Explanation of instructions concerning postdischarge activities

Explanation of symptoms that constitute a reason to contact the physician

Review of admitting diagnosis and mode of treatment

Expected outcomes

Accurate return verbalization and/or demonstration of all material learned

Smooth transition of care after discharge

Absence or early detection of complications arising after discharge

Ability to provide future health care practitioners with important data about health history

Plan for implementation	Rationale
See master care plan for the patient requiring discharge preparations: discharge teaching.	
In addition to the topics covered in the master care plan, include the following items in the discharge teaching:	
1. At the follow-up office visit the physician will check how the patient is voiding and whether there is any discomfort, and he will obtain a urine specimen.	
2. During the next few weeks the expected residual effects of the surgery include frequency, urgency, and occasional episodes of hematuria and passage of tissue particles.	
3. If blood-tinged urine occurs, the patient should increase his fluid intake until it subsides.	This lessens the possibility of clot formation and potential urethral obstruction.
4. The patient should avoid straining during a bowel movement for 4 to 6 weeks and should relieve constipation with a laxative or stool softener.	Straining causes increased venous congestion, which might result in a secondary hemorrhage.
5. The patient should notify the physician if any of the following symptoms occur: a. Chills, fever, flank pain b. Inability to void for more than 6 hours despite adequate fluid intake c. Bright red urine that is not relieved by an increase in fluid intake	This would indicate a urinary tract infection. This probably would indicate obstruction of the urethra by clots or tissue particles. This indicates a late postoperative hemorrhage, which is not uncommon around the tenth postoperative day, when normal tissue sloughing occurs.

Convalescent period

Convalescent period

20. NURSING DIAGNOSIS: Continued disturbance in urinary control at time of discharge*

Objectives of nursing intervention
- Reduction of anxiety
- Review of information on perineal exercises and fluid restrictions

Expected outcomes
- Short term
  - Expression of confidence that the condition is temporary
  - Return verbalization of regimen to reduce incontinence
- Long term: Resumption of normal voiding pattern

Plan for implementation	Rationale
1. Provide reassurance that, as the surgical site heals, good urinary control will return. The patient can expect to see considerable improvement in the next few weeks, although it may take up to 6 months for full control to be attained.	The focus of the nurse's attention should be on the mental attitude of the patient rather than on the incontinence itself. The condition is often viewed by the patient as childishness, helplessness, and "being dirty" and can be a major source of depression, even if the incontinence is not severe.
2. Encourage continued practice of the perineal exercises (see nursing diagnosis 18).	
3. **Do not** encourage the use of a condom catheter.	The patient will become dependent on the catheter and may lack the incentive to regain urinary control.
4. Suggest that the patient refrain from fluid intake for 2 or more hours before long trips.	
5. Suggest that the patient avoid drinking tea, coffee, or cola beverages until control is achieved.	These drinks contain caffeine, which is a mild diuretic and might make urinary control more difficult.

*This condition is not common and therefore may not apply. However, it does occasionally occur, especially in very elderly patients. The nurse should ascertain from the physician that it is temporary before proceeding with the following plan of care.

21. NURSING DIAGNOSIS: Knowledge deficit—minor alterations in sexual function

Objective of nursing intervention   Patient education concerning effect of a transurethral prostatectomy on sexual function

Expected outcome   Verbal indication of understanding of information

Plan for implementation	Rationale
Provide the following information.	It is usually left to the nurse's judgment whether this information should be provided if the patient does not request it. The nurse should be aware, however, that there are many questions the patient is afraid or embarrassed to ask, and he may benefit from the knowledge whether he has requested it or not.
1. Potency (the ability to sustain an erection) is unaltered.	
2. "Dry" ejaculation will occur in the majority of patients. This may terminate after a few months, and normal emission will be restored. Most men are not aware of this during intercourse. However, they should be told that the condition is normal and that the feelings associated with orgasm are unaltered.	This condition occurs because the bladder neck has been opened and semen takes the path of least resistance, flowing into the bladder rather than through the urethra. It is then excreted during voiding. The technical term is **retrograde ejaculation.**
3. The possibility of conception occurring after a simple prostatectomy is decreased as long as the retrograde ejaculation is present. Otherwise, fertility is unaffected.	The portion of the prostate gland left intact is sufficient to enable conception.

Convalescent period

469

TRANSVESICAL PROSTATECTOMY (SUPRAPUBIC PROSTATECTOMY)

The decision to perform a transvesical prostatectomy may be based on a variety of factors, including the particular physician's preference and the size of the prostate. It is indicated when there is coexisting bladder disease (e.g., diverticula or calculi) that is to be treated simultaneously.

For the procedure the patient is placed in a supine position, and a horizontal incision is made just above the symphysis pubis. The bladder is distended with fluid (instilled via a catheter), and a small incision is made in the bladder wall. The prostate gland is then enucleated through the bladder cavity (Fig. 42-4). Hemostasis is achieved by ligation or fulguration of bleeding points. Additional bladder disease is corrected at this time.

Depending on the surgeon's preference, a suprapubic tube may be inserted through the bladder wall, or the incision may be sutured with the tube extending through it. Otherwise, the bladder is completely closed without a suprapubic tube.

A Penrose drain is positioned outside the bladder for drainage of blood and urine, which may seep through the suture line during the first few postoperative days (before the suture line becomes watertight). An indwelling urethral catheter is then inserted, the abdominal muscles and skin are closed, and a dressing is applied (Fig. 42-5).

If venous bleeding is encountered, some surgeons will apply traction to the catheter (see Fig. 42-2). Also at the surgeon's discretion, continuous bladder irrigation (see Fig. 42-3) or periodic hand-irrigation to prevent clot retention within the bladder may be started.

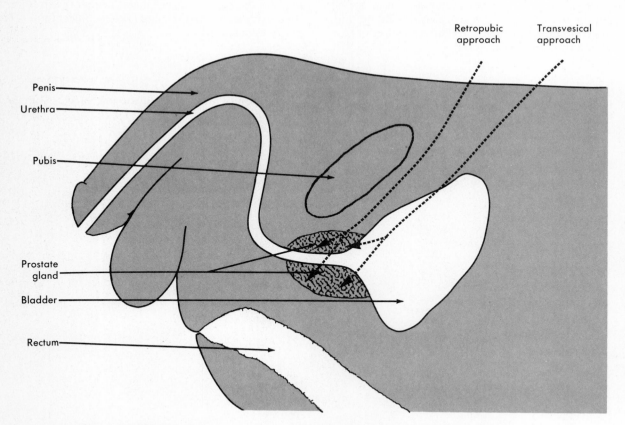

Fig. 42-4. Comparison of surgical approaches in transvesical and retropubic prostatectomies.

TRANSVESICAL PROSTATECTOMY
Outline of Care Plan
ANTICIPATED NURSING DIAGNOSES:

Preoperative period
1. Need for preoperative teaching.
2. Need for discharge planning.

Early postoperative period
3. Potential for shock.
4. Need for management of indwelling urethral catheter.
5. Need for management of continuous bladder irrigation.*
6. Need for management of suprapubic tube.*
7. Potential for wound complications.
8. Postoperative pain.
9. Need for management of intravenous infusion.
10. Potential for respiratory complications related to surgical intervention.
11. Potential for deep vein thrombosis.

12. Potential for injury to surgical site from rectal trauma.
13. Anxiety about visible hematuria.†
14. Bleeding from penile meatus.†

Late postoperative period
15. Potential for voiding complications following removal of indwelling urethral catheter (when no suprapubic tube is present).†
16. Dysuria.†
17. Disturbance in urinary control.†
18. Potential for voiding complications following removal of indwelling urethral catheter and subsequent clamping and removal of suprapubic tube.†

Convalescent period
19. Need for discharge teaching.
20. Continued disturbance in urinary control at time of discharge.†
21. Knowledge deficit—minor alterations in sexual function.

---

*Used at the discretion of the surgeon; may not apply.

†May not apply.

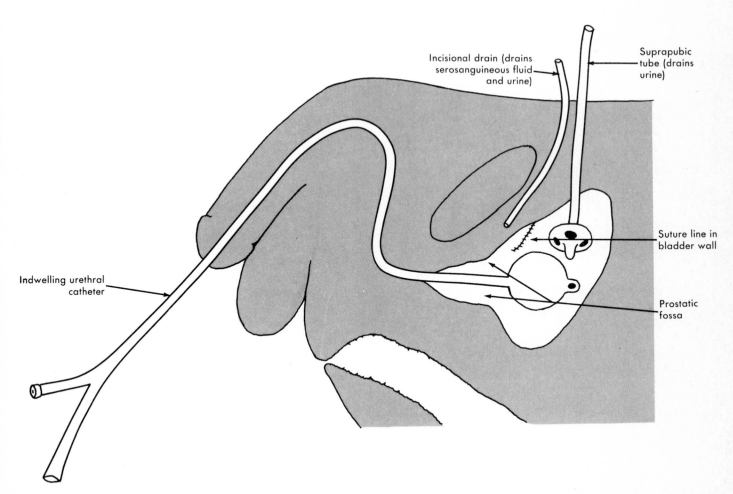

Fig. 42-5. Location of drainage mechanisms and incision after transvesical prostatectomy.

NURSING CARE PLAN FOR THE PATIENT UNDERGOING TRANSVESICAL PROSTATECTOMY

Preoperative period

1. NURSING DIAGNOSIS: Need for preoperative teaching

Objectives of nursing intervention

If necessary, clarification of reason for hospitalization and type of surgery to be performed

Elimination of any negative or inaccurate notions regarding the forthcoming surgery

Explanation of preoperative tests and procedures

Psychologic preparation for general anesthesia (omit if the patient is to have spinal anesthesia)

Explanation of events expected in the early postoperative period

Explanation of body conditions expected in the early postoperative period

Identification of any known allergies

Expected outcomes

Verbal indication that explanations are understood

Verbal indication of optimistic expectations (within realistic limits) related to forthcoming surgery

Cooperation during preoperative tests and procedures

Verbal or behavioral indication of reduction of anxiety

Absence of postoperative complications

Absence of allergic reactions

Plan for implementation	Rationale
See master care plan for the patient receiving preoperative teaching.	
In addition to the topics covered in the master care plan, include the following items in the preoperative teaching:	
1. Be aware that, in addition to the routine preoperative tests, an intravenous pyelogram is usually performed, and answer any questions the patient may have regarding the procedure.	This is done to detect any associated anatomic abnormalities.
2. The preoperative shave is from the umbilicus to mid-thigh.	
3. The patient will probably be permitted a light supper in the evening after surgery and will resume his normal diet in the morning.	Because the peritoneal cavity is not entered during this surgery, the incidence of postoperative gastrointestinal disturbances is relatively low.
4. There will be an indwelling urethral catheter in place for 5 or 6 days. It may be connected to continuous bladder irrigation for approximately 24 hours after surgery. If so, the patient will be required to remain in bed until the irrigation is discontinued.	

Plan for implementation	Rationale
5. The patient will have an incision on his lower abdomen. It will be covered by a dressing that may require frequent changing during the first 24 to 48 hours after surgery.	
6. There may be a tube coming from the patient's bladder, through the incision, to drain urine for a few days.	The use of a suprapubic tube is at the surgeon's discretion. Some believe that the additional source of drainage enhances the healing process.
7. Urine is expected to be blood tinged in the early postoperative period.	

2. NURSING DIAGNOSIS: Need for discharge planning

Objectives of nursing intervention
{ Early commencement of discharge planning
{ Accurate estimate of time required for all discharge teaching

Expected outcome   Smooth transition of care after discharge

Plan for implementation	Rationale
See master care plan for the patient requiring discharge preparations: discharge planning.	

In addition to the topics covered in the master care plan, the following items should be considered:
1. The duration of hospitalization for this procedure is usually 7 to 10 days if the patient does not have a suprapubic tube postoperatively, and possibly 2 weeks or more if a suprapubic tube is used, depending on how soon it is removed.

2. Required teaching includes:
   a. General postoperative discharge teaching
   b. Perineal exercises (occasionally required)
   c. Mention of minor changes in sexual function
   d. Wound care if there is still drainage from the incision at the time of discharge

Preoperative period

3. NURSING DIAGNOSIS: Potential for shock

Objective of nursing intervention Prevention or early detection of shock

Expected outcomes
{ Vital signs normal, skin dry, color normal
{ Absence of bright red drainage from the catheter or suprapubic tube (if used)

Plan for implementation	Rationale
1. Check the patient's vital signs every 4 hours once stable (every 15 minutes if unstable).	Hemorrhagic shock is a potential complication after this type of surgery. The prostate gland is highly vascular, and often numerous blood vessels need to be incised. Unless adequate hemostasis is achieved, considerable loss of blood occasionally occurs. Vital signs must be carefully monitored because the severity of the bleeding is sometimes difficult to determine if the patient is on continuous bladder irrigation.
2. Be alert for increasing pulse and respiratory rates, decreasing blood pressure, diaphoresis, pallor, and feelings of apprehension.	
3. Notify the physician at once if indications of impending shock occur.	

Early postoperative period

4. NURSING DIAGNOSIS: Need for management of indwelling urethral catheter

Objectives of nursing intervention
{ Appropriate care of catheter and equipment
{ Prevention or early detection of infection
{ Care of tissue surrounding catheter
{ Maintenance of accurate records of urine output
{ Appropriate administration of hand-irrigation of catheter
{ Management of discomfort or pain caused by catheter
{ Satisfactory collection of urine specimens from catheter

Expected outcomes
{ Absence of severe bladder spasms
{ Urine draining freely through system
{ Absence of fever, chills, and foul-smelling urine
{ Absence of urethral discharge and tissue inflammation
{ Minimal discomfort caused by the catheter
{ Urine specimens in optimum condition for all necessary tests

Plan for implementation	**Rationale**
See master care plan for the patient with an indwelling urethral catheter: care after insertion of the catheter.	
In addition to the topics covered in the master care plan, the following interventions are required: 1. Notify the physician if the urine remains bright red and has a high viscosity and/or clots despite hand-irrigation. Deep pink urine that lightens after irrigation is not abnormal after prostatic surgery.	If the bleeding is of venous origin, the physician might put traction on the catheter (see p. 459). If it is arterial bleeding, it may require correction in the operating room.
2. Notify the physician if the urine output (or drainage from continuous bladder irrigation) becomes obstructed and cannot be corrected by hand irrigation.	The physician will either use more powerful instruments with which to aspirate the obstruction or will change the catheter.
3. Be alert for psychologic dependence on hand-irrigation of the catheter, manifested by patient requests that the catheter be irrigated despite obvious patency.	This situation occasionally occurs if the patient incorrectly associates hand-irrigation with the reduction of **all** bladder pain. Such a patient assumes that irrigation will reduce the discomfort of "normal" bladder spasms (which periodically occur simply from the catheter's irritating effect on the wall of the bladder), and the patient may become extremely insistent that he be irrigated with frequency.
4. If the situation in no. 3 occurs: a. Check catheter for patency.	If the catheter is obstructed, of course it must be irrigated.
b. If the catheter is patent, do not irrigate; instead, explain to the patient the hazards of unnecessary irrigation (i.e., infection) and that irrigation has no beneficial effect on limiting "normal" bladder spasms. c. Provide appropriate analgesic (see Chapter 11, part one, nursing objective 6, spasmodic, intermittent pain in suprapubic area, or pain radiating to urethral area).	

Early postoperative period

5. NURSING DIAGNOSIS: Need for management of continuous bladder irrigation*

Objectives of nursing intervention { Maintenance of patency of irrigation system
Prevention or early detection of complications

Expected outcomes { Clear or light blood-tinged drainage, flowing freely
Absence of suprapubic discomfort

Plan for implementation	Rationale
1. Use only normal saline for irrigation fluid.	It is possible for some of the irrigating fluid to be absorbed systemically through blood vessels that were not treated with coagulation current. Therefore it is essential that the fluid be isotonic to the blood to prevent massive hemolysis and other potentially fatal consequences that would occur if water were used.
2. Check the color of the drainage frequently and adjust the flow rate accordingly. a. If the drainage is very bloody, increase the rate. b. If drainage is pale pink or clear, reduce the rate, but do not stop it altogether.	Dilution of the blood aids in the prevention of clot formation. Saline, like other hospital supplies, should not be wasted, and irrigation is unnecessary unless bleeding is present. However, hemostasis may be very erratic during the immediate postoperative period, and obstructive clot formation could occur without much warning.
3. Keep the patient in bed while irrigation is in progress, unless ordered otherwise.	An accident could easily occur with irrigating fluid and drainage bottles if the patient were to ambulate. Bed rest also favors hemostasis.

Early postoperative period

*Continuous bladder irrigation is not always used; this may not apply.

Plan for implementation	**Rationale**
4. Avoid external obstruction of tubing (e.g., kinks, patient lying on tubing).	If the bladder becomes distended with fluid, it will cause severe discomfort and potential damage to the surgical site.
5. Be alert for indications of internal obstruction such as decreased drainage and bladder spasms of increasing intensity. Suprapubic distention may also be present but is not palpable when there is an incision.	Clots and tissue particles may prevent irrigating fluid from draining out of the bladder, resulting in pain, distention, and potential damage.
6. If necessary, hand-irrigate the catheter with a 60-ml bulb syringe.	Hand-irrigation provides the negative pressure necessary to aspirate obstructive particles.
7. Be certain the fluid input regulator of the continuous bladder irrigation is turned off while hand-irrigation is in progress (and turned back on afterward).	If fluid from the continuous irrigation system is permitted to flow into the bladder during hand-irrigation, it is difficult to estimate the amount of fluid to instill with the hand-irrigation equipment, and overdistention can easily occur.
8. Notify the physician if the obstruction cannot be aspirated.	

NOTE: When continuous bladder irrigation is used with a suprapubic tube and indwelling urethral catheter, it is set up so that irrigation fluid is instilled through the catheter and drains out through the suprapubic tube.

Early postoperative period

6. NURSING DIAGNOSIS: Need for management of suprapubic tube*

| Objective of nursing intervention | Prevention or early detection of complications related to the suprapubic drainage system |

| Expected outcome | Amber or light blood-tinged drainage flowing through suprapubic tube |

Plan for implementation	Rationale
1. Keep collecting container below the level of the patient's bladder.	Urine flows through the tubing via gravity. Elevation of the collecting container will result in urine flowing back into the bladder from the distal portion of the system, which has the greatest potential for being contaminated.
2. Keep the tubing free from kinks and external pressure.	Flattening or sharply bending the tubing will decrease its patency.
3. Anchor the tubing securely to the patient's abdomen with tape.	This prevents inadvertent traction on the tube and possible displacement of it.
4. Hand-irrigate the tube only if it is obstructed, and use sterile technique for the procedure.	Unnecessary disconnection of the tubing increases the risk of contamination of the drainage system. Although obstruction of a suprapubic tube is less likely than obstruction of a balloon-type indwelling urethral catheter (which has a narrower lumen), these tubes do occasionally require irrigation.
5. Keep the area around the suprapubic tube clean and dry. Remove exudate with hydrogen peroxide.	
6. Maintain accurate records of volume and character of suprapubic tube drainage.	
7. Indicate on the collecting container that the drainage is from the suprapubic tube.	This is a precaution against mistakes in recording sources of output when urine is draining from more than one tube. The drainage from the urethral catheter and this tube should be charted separately to acertain whether both tubes are draining adequately.

Early postoperative period

*A suprapubic tube is not always used after this type of surgery; this may not apply.

7. NURSING DIAGNOSIS: Potential for wound complications

Objective of nursing intervention	Prevention or early detection of complications arising from the incisional area
Expected outcome	Absence of fever, purulent exudate, erythema, edema, dehiscence, hematoma, and other abnormal wound conditions

Plan for implementation	Rationale

1. Check the dressing frequently (every 2 to 4 hours during the first 24 to 48 hours after surgery). Change it when it becomes wet, and use sterile technique for the procedure.	The dressing may become saturated rapidly with serosanguineous fluid and urine from the incision. This is because the suture line in the bladder may not become watertight for at least 48 hours after surgery. If continuous bladder irrigation is used, there will also be saline in the drainage, and the dressing will become saturated even more quickly. A wet dressing must be changed as soon as possible for the following reasons:
	1. It is a source of infection.
	   a. It acts as a wick, enabling microorganisms on the skin to move toward the incision
	   b. It provides a good medium for bacterial multiplication.
	2. It is highly irritating to the skin because of the presence of urine in the drainage.

2. Note the odor of the drainage. The characteristic odor of urine is not abnormal, but if it is foul smelling:
  a. Notify the physician.
  b. Obtain a wound culture specimen.
	This would indicate that the patient has a wound infection.
	
	This will facilitate identification of the infecting organism so that appropriate treatment can be instituted quickly.

3. Use caution when removing soiled dressings to prevent inadvertent removal of the incisional drain.	Premature removal of a drain may result in the development of a urinoma and prolonged healing.
4. Cut and arrange gauze pads around the suprapubic tube (if used) and incisional drain. Usually it is a Penrose drain, but occasionally a tube drain is used. (See p. 492 for nursing management of a tube drain.)	This prevents the dressings from flattening the drainage mechanisms and possibly obstructing the flow of drainage from the wound.
5. If the dressing requires frequent changing, use Montgomery straps instead of adhesive tape.	This eliminates the need to remove the adhesive tape from the patient's skin each time the dressing is changed. Skin irritation and patient discomfort can be considerably reduced by this method.
6. Note the condition of the suture line. Chart its appearance and the presence of edema, erythema, hematoma, ecchymosis, or other abnormal conditions.	This provides a frame of reference for other staff members caring for the patient.

Early postoperative period

Plan for implementation	Rationale
7. Notify the physician if there is any evidence of dehiscence.	
8. Check the patient's temperature every 4 hours and notify the physician if there is an elevation above 101°.	Wound infection must always be suspected when the patient runs a fever postoperatively. Other causes include respiratory complications and pharmacologic intervention.

8. NURSING DIAGNOSIS: Postoperative pain

Objective of nursing intervention	Appropriate management of pain or discomfort
Expected outcome	Behavioral and/or verbal indication that pain is adequately reduced or absent

Plan for implementation	Rationale
Determine the source of the pain. It may be related to the catheter or the surgical wound.	Pain from different sources usually requires different intervention.
1. Question and observe the patient to obtain information about the pain.	
2. Be aware that pain is a unique and individual experience. Although the different sources of pain can usually be determined by their characteristics, there are also many variations.	
3. Be alert for indications (verbal or behavioral) that the patient is experiencing discomfort other than physical pain, and attempt to resolve the problem.	Fear, loneliness, depression, and numerous other conditions may be sources of extreme discomfort for the patient, who may unconsciously translate these feelings into pain.

PERSISTENT, SEVERE, INCREASING PAIN IN SUPRAPUBIC AREA

See Chapter 11, part one, nursing objective 6.	This pain is probably caused by an obstructed catheter.

SPASMODIC, INTERMITTENT, INCREASING PAIN IN SUPRAPUBIC AREA, OR PAIN RADIATING TO URETHRAL AREA

See Chapter 11, part one, nursing objective 6.	This pain is probably caused by the catheter's irritating effect on the bladder.

Early postoperative period

480

Plan for implementation	Rationale
MODERATE TO SEVERE PAIN AT SURGICAL SITE, USUALLY AGGRAVATED BY PHYSICAL ACTIVITY	
1. Be certain the catheter is not obstructed. Although pain with these characteristics is usually of incisional origin and is expected, it is very difficult to differentiate between incisional pain and pain from an obstructed catheter after this type of surgery.	Catheter obstruction must be ruled out first because it cannot remain untreated. It is also a likely cause of suprapubic pain after a prostatectomy because bleeding is common, and clots can easily obstruct the catheter lumen. An obstructed catheter is hazardous to the patient, and the pain it causes will not be relieved by analgesics.
2. Administer analgesics as ordered.	Analgesic medication usually provides considerable relief from incisional pain.
3. Plan the patient's activities to coincide with a time when there is a high level of pain medication in the patient's bloodstream.	The patient will cooperate better with coughing exercises, ambulating, bathing, etc. when the pain is well under control.
4. Notify the physician if the patient's requests for pain medication do not decrease within 48 to 72 hours.	Although the intensity of postoperative pain varies enormously between patients, there should be a marked decrease in the apparent severity of the pain within 2 or 3 days. If this does not occur, it may indicate the development of wound complications.

9. NURSING DIAGNOSIS: Need for management of intravenous infusion

Objectives of nursing intervention
- Appropriate administration of specific types of intravenous solutions
- Prevention or early detection of local complications
- Prevention or early detection of systemic complications
- Management of discomfort caused by the intravenous infusion
- Maintenance of proper function of intravenous equipment
- Maintenance of accurate records of the patient's hydration status

Expected outcomes
- Normal hydration status
- Normal electrolyte status
- Absence of thrombophlebitis, infiltration, infection, fluid overload, and pulmonary embolism
- Absence of discomfort caused by the intravenous infusion

Plan for implementation	Rationale
See master care plan for the patient receiving intravenous therapy.	Prostatectomy patients usually receive isotonic dextrose and saline solutions. Many physicians also order prophylactic administration of antibiotics.

Early postoperative period

10. NURSING DIAGNOSIS: Potential for respiratory complications related to surgical intervention

Objective of nursing intervention   Prevention or early detection of atelectasis and/or pneumonia

Expected outcomes
- Cooperation with therapeutic respiratory regimen
- Absence of fever or audible lung congestion
- Sputum clear or white and easily mobilized

Plan for implementation	Rationale
See master care plan for the patient at risk for respiratory complications, nursing objective 2.	

11. NURSING DIAGNOSIS: Potential for deep vein thrombosis

Objectives of nursing intervention
- Explanation and maintenance of precautions against deep vein thrombosis
- Early detection of deep vein thrombosis

Expected outcomes
- Cooperation with regimen to prevent deep vein thrombosis
- Absence of local pain, swelling, and redness of a lower extremity
- Absence of fever

Plan for implementation	Rationale
See master care plan for the patient at risk for deep vein thrombosis.	

Early postoperative period

12. NURSING DIAGNOSIS: Potential for injury to surgical site from rectal trauma

Objective of nursing intervention Prevention of rectal trauma

Expected outcomes { Absence of perforated tissues
Uninterrupted healing process

Plan for implementation	Rationale
1. Do not insert any foreign object into the patient's rectum for 48 to 72 hours after surgery. This includes enemas, suppositories, and thermometers.	The proximity of the prostate to the rectum makes the introduction of a foreign object into the rectum potentially harmful to healing tissue.
2. If the patient requires rectal temperature readings, use extreme caution when inserting the thermometer. Do not delegate this job to an auxiliary staff member.	This job should not be assigned to nurses' aides or orderlies because, in most cases, they are not aware of the abovementioned information.

13. NURSING DIAGNOSIS: Anxiety about visible hematuria*

Objective of nursing intervention Patient education regarding postoperative hematuria

Expected outcome Verbal and/or behavioral indication of reduced anxiety

Plan for implementation	Rationale
Explain the following:	
1. Blood-tinged urine is expected after a prostatectomy.	
2. Only a few spoonfuls of blood will turn the urine red.	
3. Increased blood in the urine is not uncommon after a bowel movement.	Increased intraabdominal pressure, as well as contraction of the colon, may cause a transient increase in bleeding from the surgical site.

*May not apply.

Early postoperative period

14. NURSING DIAGNOSIS: Bleeding from penile meatus (around catheter)*

Objectives of nursing
intervention { Maintenance of patient hygiene
Prevention of skin irritation

Expected outcome Absence of discomfort and/or meatal tissue irritation

Plan for implementation	Rationale
1. Check the catheter for obstruction (scanty drainage, suprapubic pain, etc.) and irrigate if necessary. (See Chapter 11, nursing objective 5.)	When the catheter is obstructed, the "bleeding" is really blood-tinged urine being expelled around the catheter.
2. If the catheter is patent:	In this case the bleeding is simply a result of the surgery and should not be considered abnormal unless it is severe.
a. Wrap a combine loosely around the penis to avoid soiling the patient's gown.	
b. Increase the frequency of catheter care.	Dried blood is an ideal medium for bacterial growth and is also extremely irritating to the urethral mucosa.

*May not apply.

15. NURSING DIAGNOSIS: Potential for voiding complications following removal of indwelling urethral catheter
(when no suprapubic tube is present)*

Objective of nursing
intervention Prevention or early detection of complications

Expected outcomes { Resumption of normal voiding pattern
Absence of dysuria

Plan for implementation	Rationale
See master care plan for the patient with an indwelling urethral catheter: care after removal of the catheter.	

*If the physician has left the suprapubic tube in place after removal of the catheter, see nursing diagnosis no. 18.

Early postoperative period

Late postoperative period

16. NURSING DIAGNOSIS: Dysuria*

Objective of nursing intervention	Reduction of discomfort
Expected outcome	Verbal and/or behavioral indication of minimal voiding discomfort

Plan for implementation	Rationale
1. Provide reassurance that the discomfort is transient.	The catheter often causes urethritis. Urine, particularly if it is concentrated, may cause a burning sensation on inflamed tissue.
2. Encourage high fluid intake.	This dilutes the urine, thus reducing its irritating effect.
3. If the patient is in a great deal of discomfort, suggest to the physician that an analgesic that is specific to the urinary tract (e.g., phenazopyridine HCl [Pyridium]) be ordered.	

Late postoperative period

*Dysuria does not always occur after removal of a catheter following a prostatectomy; this may not apply.

17. NURSING DIAGNOSIS: Disturbance in urinary control*

Objectives of nursing intervention { Reduction of anxiety
Instruction on perineal exercises and types of fluid restrictions

Expected outcomes { Short term
    Verbal and/or behavioral indication of decreased anxiety
    Accurate return verbalization of instructions on perineal exercises
Long term: Resumption of normal voiding pattern

Plan for implementation	Rationale
1. Provide reassurance by explaining that dribbling and urgency incontinence are not uncommon after a prostatectomy, but it is a **temporary** condition.	Temporary lack of complete urinary control sometimes occurs after simple prostatectomies because the surgery involves removal of portions of the bladder neck and prostatic urethra. Complete return to a normal voiding pattern may take up to 6 months, although relatively adequate control usually returns within a few days or weeks.
2. Explain perineal exercises and obtain an accurate return verbalization. a. While standing, the patient should tighten and relax his buttocks five or more times each hour.	When gluteal muscles are voluntarily contracted, all the perineal muscles contract, including the sphincter muscles. Since the urinary sphincters are under voluntary and involuntary control, some physicians feel that these exercises facilitate the return of adequate sphincter control.
b. While voiding, the patient should voluntarily stop and restart the urinary stream using sphincter muscles. c. The patient should attempt to lengthen the period of time between each voiding by consciously holding in the urine.	
3. Suggest that the patient avoid drinking tea, coffee, and cola beverages.	These drinks contain caffeine, which is a mild diuretic and might make urinary control more difficult.

Late postoperative period

*Limited urinary control does not always occur after a simple prostatectomy; this may not apply.

18. NURSING DIAGNOSIS: Potential for voiding complications following removal of indwelling urethral catheter and subsequent clamping and removal of suprapubic tube*

Objective of nursing intervention   Prevention or early detection of complications arising during termination of urinary drainage systems

Expected outcomes   { Resumption of normal voiding pattern
Rapid closure of suprapubic wound

Plan for implementation	Rationale
1. After removal of indwelling catheter: a. Maintain records of suprapubic tube drainage. b. If the patient voids, maintain records of the amount and character of voided urine. However, it is unlikely that the patient will void as long as the suprapubic tube is patent. c. Check the suprapubic tube for patency, and irrigate if necessary. d. Maintain a fluid intake of 2 to 3 L per day.	Urine usually will drain only from the suprapubic tube because it takes the path of least resistance. The incidence of urinary tract infection and obstruction of the suprapubic tube is reduced if there is a relatively rapid flow of urine through the urinary tract.
2. After clamping of the suprapubic tube: a. Record the time and volume of each voiding and determine whether the patient is voiding with an adequate stream. b. Be alert for suprapubic pain. c. Notify the physician if the patient has not voided for 6 hours despite adequate fluid intake.	The physician will usually keep the suprapubic tube clamped for 1 or 2 days before its removal to assess the patient's voiding ability. This may indicate urinary retention. Occasionally voiding does not occur spontaneously. Various conditions may be implicated, such as a hypotonic bladder associated with chronic urinary retention and severe urethritis associated with prolonged catheter drainage before surgery.
3. After the removal of the suprapubic tube: a. Continue to record the time and volume of each voiding for an additional 24 hours. b. Check the suprapubic dressing frequently, and change it when it becomes wet.	Although obstruction is unlikely at this point, the extra precaution facilitates rapid assessment if it occurs. Urine may continue to drain from the opening created by the suprapubic tube for a few more days. A dressing wet with urine will impede adequate healing and may cause skin breakdown if permitted to remain in contact with the patient's skin for a prolonged time.

Late postoperative period

*Only applies in cases where the physician removes the catheter **before** the suprapubic tube. Many physicians remove the suprapubic tube 24 to 48 hours after surgery and leave the indwelling urethral catheter in place for a few days more.

19. NURSING DIAGNOSIS: Need for discharge teaching

Objectives of nursing intervention

Explanation of basic information about medications to be taken at home

Explanation of information regarding follow-up care

Explanation of residual effects of the condition and/or treatment

Explanation of instructions concerning postdischarge activities

Explanation of symptoms that constitute a reason to contact the physician

Review of admitting diagnosis and mode of treatment

Expected outcomes

Accurate return verbalization and/or demonstration of all material learned

Smooth transition of care after discharge

Absence or early detection of complications arising after discharge

Ability to provide future health care practitioners with important data about health history

Plan for implementation	Rationale
See master care plan for the patient requiring discharge preparations: discharge teaching.	
In addition to the topics covered in the master care plan, include the following items in the discharge teaching: 1. At the follow-up visit the physician will check the wound for adequate healing, assess how the patient is voiding, and obtain a urine specimen for culture.	

2. During the next few weeks the expected residual effects of the surgery include frequency, urgency, and occasional episodes of hematuria. A small amount of suprapubic drainage may continue for a few more days if the patient had a suprapubic tube. If drainage is present when the patient is discharged:
  a. Be certain he has an adequate supply of dressings and tape.
  b. Demonstrate dressing change and obtain a satisfactory return demonstration from the patient or significant other.
  c. Encourage the patient to keep the area clean, but sterility for dressing changes is unnecessary.
  d. Explain to the patient that showers are permitted; a clean dressing should be applied afterward.	

3. If blood-tinged urine occurs, the patient should increase his fluid intake until it subsides.	This lessens the possibility of clot formation and potential urethral obstruction.

Convalescent period

Plan for implementation	Rationale
4. The patient should avoid straining during a bowel movement for 4 to 6 weeks and should relieve constipation with a laxative or stool softener.	Straining causes increased venous congestion, which might result in a secondary hemorrhage.
5. The patient should notify the physician if any of the following symptoms occur:	
a. Chills, fever, flank pain	This would indicate a urinary tract infection.
b. Inability to void for more than 6 hours despite adequate fluid intake	This probably would indicate obstruction of the urethra by clots.
c. Bright red urine that is not relieved by an increase in fluid intake	This indicates a late postoperative hemorrhage, which is not uncommon around the tenth postoperative day, when normal tissue sloughing occurs.
d. Severe pain and/or increasing redness at the incisional site	This may indicate a wound infection.

20. NURSING DIAGNOSIS: Continued disturbance in urinary control at time of discharge*

Objectives of nursing intervention
- Reduction of anxiety
- Review of information on perineal exercises and fluid restrictions

Expected outcomes
- Short term
  - Expression of confidence that the condition is temporary
  - Return verbalization of regimen to reduce incontinence
- Long term: Resumption of normal voiding pattern

Plan for implementation	Rationale
1. Provide reassurance that, as the surgical site heals, good urinary control will return. The patient can expect to see considerable improvement in the next few weeks, although it may take up to 6 months for full control to be attained.	The focus of the nurse's attention should be on the mental attitude of the patient rather than on the incontinence itself. The condition is often viewed by the patient as childishness, helplessness, and "being dirty" and can be a major source of depression even if the incontinence is not severe.
2. Encourage continued practice of the perineal exercises (see nursing diagnosis 17).	
3. **Do not** encourage the use of a condom catheter.	The patient will become dependent on the catheter and may lack the incentive to regain urinary control.

*This condition is not common, and therefore this may not apply. However, it does occasionally occur, especially in very elderly patients. The nurse should ascertain from the physician that it is temporary before proceeding with the following plan of care.

Convalescent period

Plan for implementation	Rationale
4. Suggest that the patient refrain from fluid intake for 2 or more hours before long trips.	
5. Suggest that the patient avoid drinking, tea, coffee, or cola beverages until control is achieved.	These drinks contain caffeine, which is a mild diuretic and might make urinary control more difficult.

21. NURSING DIAGNOSIS: Knowledge deficit—minor alterations in sexual function

Objective of nursing intervention   Patient education concerning effect of a simple prostatectomy on sexual function

Expected outcome   Verbal indication of understanding of information

Plan for implementation	Rationale
Provide the following information.	It is usually left to the nurse's judgment whether this information should be provided if the patient does not request it. The nurse should be aware, however, that there are many questions that the patient is afraid or embarrassed to ask, and he may benefit from the knowledge whether he has requested it or not.
1. Potency (the ability to sustain an erection) is unaltered.	
2. "Dry" ejaculation will occur in the majority of patients. This may terminate after a few months, and normal emission will be restored. Most men are not aware of this during intercourse. However, they should be told that the condition is normal and that the feelings associated with orgasm are unaltered.	This condition occurs because the bladder neck has been opened and semen takes the path of least resistance, flowing into the bladder rather than through the urethra. It is then excreted during voiding. The technical term is **retrograde ejaculation.**
3. The possibility of conception occurring after a simple prostatectomy is decreased as long as the retrograde ejaculation is present. Otherwise, fertility is unaffected (unless a vasectomy was performed).	The portion of the gland left intact is sufficient to enable conception.

Convalescent period

RETROPUBIC PROSTATECTOMY

The decision to perform a retropubic prostatectomy, as with a transvesical prostatectomy, is based on a variety of factors. These include the particular physician's preference and the size of the prostate. However, it is **not** done when there is coexisting bladder disease, since a transvesical approach is more suitable if the bladder must be entered.

For the procedure the patient is placed in a supine position, and a horizontal incision is made just above the symphysis pubis. A retractor is positioned to spread the muscles and expose the prostate gland, the prostatic capsule is incised, and the adenoma is removed (see Fig. 42-4). An indwelling urethral catheter is then inserted, and the capsule of the prostate is closed. One or more tube drains or Penrose drains are inserted to prevent postoperative collection of blood and urine in the retropubic space (Fig. 42-6).

The abdominal muscles and skin are then closed, and a dressing is applied. Continuous bladder irrigation (see Fig. 42-3) or periodic hand-irrigation to prevent clot retention may be started.

RETROPUBIC PROSTATECTOMY
Outline of Care Plan
ANTICIPATED NURSING DIAGNOSES:

Preoperative period
1. Need for preoperative teaching. (See p. 472. Omit references to suprapubic tube.)*
2. Need for discharge planning. (See p. 473.)*

Early postoperative period
3. Potential for shock. (See p. 474.)*
4. Need for management of indwelling urethral catheter. (See p. 474.)*
5. Need for management of continuous bladder irrigation. (See p. 476.)*
6. Potential for wound complications. (If the patient has a Penrose drain, see p. 479. Change rationale no 1: There may be urine in the drainage because the suture line in the prostatic capsule may not be watertight for at least 48 hours after surgery.)*
   or
7. Potential for wound complications. (If the patient has a tube drain, see p. 492.)†

---

*Nursing care is the same as for the patient undergoing transvesical prostatectomy.
†Nursing care is described on following pages.

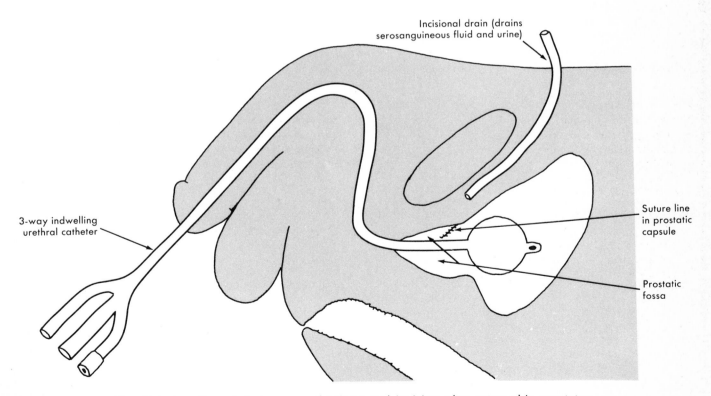

Fig. 42-6. Location of drainage mechanisms and incision after retropubic prostatectomy.

8. Postoperative pain. (See p. 480.)*
9. Need for management of intravenous infusion. (See p. 481.)*
10. Potential for respiratory complications. (See p. 482.)*
11. Potential for deep vein thrombosis. (See p. 482.)*
12. Potential for injury to surgical site from rectal trauma. (See p. 483.)*
13. Anxiety about visible hematuria. (See p. 483.)*
14. Bleeding from penile meatus. (See p. 484.)*

Late postoperative period
15. Potential for voiding complications following removal of indwelling urethral catheter. (See p. 484.)*
16. Dysuria. (See p. 485.)*
17. Disturbance in urinary control. (See p. 486.)*
Convalescent period
18. Need for discharge teaching. (See p. 488.)*
19. Continued disturbance in urinary control at time of discharge. (See p. 489.)*
20. Knowledge deficit—minor alterations in sexual function. (See p. 490.)*

*Nursing care is the same as for the patient undergoing transvesical prostatectomy.

*Nursing care is the same as for the patient undergoing transvesical prostatectomy.

---

7. NURSING DIAGNOSIS: Potential for wound complications (when tube drain is present)*

Objective of nursing intervention	Prevention or early detection of complications arising from the incisional area
Expected outcome	Absence of fever, purulent exudate, erythema, edema, dehiscence, hematoma, and other abnormal wound conditions

Plan for implementation	Rationale
1. Check the dressing every 4 hours for the first 24 hours and then every shift.	When a tube drain is present, there will be relatively little drainage on the dressing. Excess fluid accumulating in the area will drain through the tube into the attached leg bag.
2. Empty the leg bag each shift (or as needed) and record volume and character of output.	The drainage consists of serosanguineous fluid. There may also be urine in the drainage because the suture line in the prostatic capsule may not be watertight for at least 48 hours after surgery.
3. Avoid contamination of the opening on the leg bag when emptying it. a. Place cap on a sterile surface. b. Wipe rim of spout with alcohol after emptying it.	Microorganisms introduced into the system through the opening in the leg bag are a potential source of wound infection.
4. Tape the tubing of the drain securely to the patient's thigh.	This prevents inadvertent traction on the drain, which could cause it to become dislodged. The drain usually remains in place for 2 or 3 days or until drainage stops.

Early postoperative period

*A tube drain is used at the surgeon's discretion; it is not always present following this type of surgery.

Plan for implementation	**Rationale**
5. If the dressing requires changing:	
a. Use caution when removing it to prevent inadvertent displacement of the drain.	Premature removal of a drain may result in the development of a urinoma and prolonged healing.
b. Note the odor of the drainage. The characteristic odor of urine is not abnormal, but if it is foul smelling:	This would indicate a wound infection.
(1) Notify the physician.	
(2) Obtain a wound culture specimen.	This will facilitate identification of the infecting organism so that appropriate treatment can be instituted quickly.
c. Note the condition of the suture line. Charts its appearance and the presence of edema, erythema, ecchymosis, or other abnormal conditions.	
d. Notify the physician if there is any evidence of dehiscence.	
6. Check the patient's temperature every 4 hours and notify the physician if there is an elevation above 101°.	Wound infection must always be suspected when the patient runs a fever postoperatively. Other causes include respiratory complications and pharmacologic intervention.

Early postoperative period

493

CHAPTER 43

Prostatic needle biopsy

Biopsy of the prostate is done to determine the presence of cancer. The procedure is usually performed after cystourethroscopy with the patient under general anesthesia. (Occasionally it is done transrectally with the patient under local anesthesia.) After the bladder and prostatic urethra have been visualized cystoscopically (see Chapter 7), a finger is inserted into the patient's rectum, and the area to be biopsied is identified. A biopsy needle is inserted through the perineal skin and directed to the particular area in question. A small specimen is removed and placed in formalin solution. Usually more than one area is biopsied to ensure accurate representation of the tissue. Special care is taken to label each specimen appropriately.

After the procedure is completed, no dressing is applied. If bleeding from the bladder is anticipated, an indwelling urethral catheter may be inserted to remain in place for approximately 24 hours.

PROSTATIC NEEDLE BIOPSY
Outline of Care Plan
ANTICIPATED NURSING DIAGNOSES:
Preoperative period
1. Need for preoperative teaching.
2. Need for discharge planning.
Postoperative period
3. Potential for postoperative complications (shock, atelectasis, pneumonia, urinary retention, deep vein thrombosis).
4. Potential for infection.
5. Postoperative pain.
Convalescent period
6. Need for discharge teaching.

NURSING CARE PLAN FOR THE PATIENT UNDERGOING PROSTATIC NEEDLE BIOPSY

1. NURSING DIAGNOSIS: Need for preoperative teaching

Objectives of nursing intervention

If necessary, clarification of reason for hospitalization and type of surgery to be performed

Elimination of any negative or inaccurate notions regarding the forthcoming surgery

Explanation of preoperative tests and procedures

Psychologic preparation for general anesthesia (omit if the patient is to have spinal anesthesia)

Explanation of events expected in the early postoperative period

Explanation of body conditions expected in the early postoperative period

Identification of any known allergies

Expected outcomes

Verbal indication that explanations are understood

Verbal indication of optimistic expectations (within realistic limits) related to forthcoming surgery

Cooperation during preoperative tests and procedures

Verbal or behavioral indication of reduction of anxiety

Absence of postoperative complications

Absence of allergic reactions

Plan for implementation	Rationale
See master care plan for the patient receiving preoperative teaching.	
In addition to the topics covered in the master care plan, include the following items in the preoperative teaching:	
1. Be aware that, in addition to routine preoperative tests, the following diagnostic studies may have been performed, and answer any questions the patient has regarding them:	
a. Serum acid phosphatase (prostatic fraction)	This may be done if metastatic disease is suspected.
b. Intravenous pyelogram	This is done to detect any associated structural abnormalities such as obstructive conditions.
2. The patient will be allowed a light meal in the evening after surgery.	
3. The patient may have blood-tinged urine for a short time after surgery.	
4. The patient will have a tiny puncture point on his perineum that will not be covered by a dressing. He should therefore use caution after a bowel movement to avoid contamination of the area with stool.	

Preoperative period

2. NURSING DIAGNOSIS: Need for discharge planning*

Objectives of nursing intervention { Early commencement of discharge planning
Accurate estimate of time required for all necessary discharge teaching

Expected outcome Smooth transition of care after discharge

Plan for implementation	Rationale

See master care plan for discharge preparations: discharge planning.

In addition to the topics covered in the master care plan, the following items should be considered:
1. The duration of hospitalization for this procedure is approximately 2 or 3 days. However, it will be extended considerably if malignant tissue is found or if the enlarged prostate is not due to cancer but is causing serious urinary tract obstruction and urinary retention. In either case, further surgery may be required.

2. Required teaching will depend on whether additional treatment is necessary and the type of treatment. If the biopsy is negative, no specific teaching is required.

Preoperative period

*Discharge planning is often deferred until the results of the biopsy are known.

3. NURSING DIAGNOSIS: Potential for postoperative complications (shock, atelectasis, pneumonia, urinary retention, deep vein thrombosis)

Objective of nursing intervention

Prevention or early detection of postoperative complications

Expected outcomes

Pulse and blood pressure normal, skin dry, color normal
Respirations regular and unlabored, absence of pulmonary congestion
Normal voiding pattern established within 6 hours after surgery
Early ambulation tolerated well

Plan for implementation	Rationale
1. Check the patient's vital signs every 4 hours and notify the physician of any indications of impending shock. These include: a. Increasing pulse and respiratory rates b. Decreasing blood pressure c. Diaphoresis and pallor d. Feelings of apprehension	Although shock is a potential complication after any kind of surgery, it is a relatively small risk after prostatic biopsy because few blood vessels are cut and the duration of the procedure is short.
2. Encourage coughing and abdominal breathing if the patient's lungs sound congested, and notify the physician if any of the following conditions are present: a. The patient is unable to cough and his lungs sound congested. b. Sputum volume is copious. c. Sputum color is other than clear or white. d. There is a rise in the patient's temperature. e. Breath sounds are diminished.	Although precautions must be taken, respiratory complications are unlikely after this type of surgery because the period of anesthesia is very short. Furthermore, there is no abdominal incision to inhibit effective coughing. These conditions require additional treatment. The physician may order therapies such as incentive spirometry, nasotracheal suctioning, postural drainage, or intermittent positive pressure breathing, depending on the extent of respiratory embarrassment.

3. Promote resumption of normal voiding pattern by the following actions:
a. Be certain the patient is well hydrated.
b. Leave urinal at the bedside within reach of the patient.
c. Ask the patient to notify the nurse the first time he voids.
d. If the patient has not voided within 6 hours after surgery:
   (1) Assist the patient to a standing position to void.
 	
   (2) If the patient is still unable to void, notify the physician.
	Temporary urinary retention occasionally occurs as a result of anesthesia and edema from urethral manipulation during cystoscopy.
	
	Assuming the accustomed position for voiding will help the patient to void if the retention is caused by psychologic factors.
	Catheterization may be required.

4. Use precautions against deep vein thrombosis. (See master care plan for the patient at risk for deep vein thrombosis.) The patient is usually permitted out of bed in the evening after surgery.	Although deep vein thrombosis is a relatively small risk after this type of surgery, it still must be considered, and adequate precautions should be taken.

Postoperative period

4. NURSING DIAGNOSIS: Potential for infection

Objective of nursing intervention   Prevention or early detection of infection at the surgical site or originating in the urinary tract

Expected outcomes   Absence of purulent drainage, erythema, and edema at the site of the perineal wound

Absence of fever

Plan for implementation	Rationale
1. Check perineal puncture point every shift for the first 24 hours after surgery.	This type of wound rarely becomes infected. However, since the possibility exists, precautions must be taken.
2. Check the patient's temperature every 4 hours. If there is an elevation above 101°: a. Notify the physician. b. Be prepared to obtain blood and urine specimens for culture if ordered.	Bacteremia can occur after any instrumentation of the urinary tract. This happens as a result of absorption of bacteria into the bloodstream through the urethral mucosa. Blood and urine cultures often are ordered to determine the type and sensitivity of the infecting organism, and the patient is often given antibiotic therapy.

5. NURSING DIAGNOSIS: Postoperative pain

Objective of nursing intervention   Appropriate management of pain or discomfort

Expected outcome   Behavioral and/or verbal indication that pain is adequately reduced or absent

Plan for implementation	Rationale
1. Question and observe the patient to obtain information about the pain.	
2. Be alert for indications (verbal or behavioral) that the patient is experiencing discomfort other than physical pain, and attempt to resolve the problem.	Anxiety about the outcome of the biopsy, loneliness, and numerous other conditions may be sources of extreme discomfort for the patient who may unconsciously translate these feelings into pain.
3. Determine whether the patient has voided recently. If not, encourage him to do so, and note its effect on the pain.	
4. Administer analgesic as ordered.	Mild perineal pain is occasionally experienced after this procedure. It is usually well controlled by analgesic medication.

Postoperative period

6. NURSING DIAGNOSIS: Need for discharge teaching*

Objectives of nursing intervention

Explanation of basic information about medications to be taken at home
Explanation of information regarding follow-up care
Explanation of residual effects of the condition and/or treatment
Explanation of instructions concerning postdischarge activities
Explanation of symptoms that constitute a reason to contact the physician
Review of admitting diagnosis and mode of treatment

Expected outcomes

Accurate return verbalization and/or demonstration of all information
Smooth transition of care after discharge
Absence or early detection of complications arising after discharge
Ability to provide future health care practitioners with important data about health history

Plan for implementation	Rationale
See master care plan for discharge preparations: discharge teaching.	
In addition to the topics covered in the master care plan, include the following items in the discharge teaching:	
1. The patient should be certain to maintain the follow-up appointment schedule the physician makes for him. Usually patients are checked approximately 6 months after the biopsy. If the questionable area feels larger, it may be necessary to have a repeat biopsy.	Approximately 20% of clinically occult prostatic carcinomas will yield a negative biopsy. Therefore careful follow-up is important.
2. The patient should experience no residual effects from this procedure.	
3. The patient should notify the physician if he has chills, fever, hematuria, or flank pain.	These are symptoms of urinary tract infection. However, if the patient showed no signs of infection within 24 to 48 hours after the procedure, it is unlikely that he will develop an infection after he is discharged.

*Only applies if the biopsy was negative and no obstructive uropathy was found.

Convalescent period

Radical prostatectomies

For many years radical prostatectomy was considered the only curative treatment for localized carcinoma of the prostate. Although radioactive seed implantation and lymphadenectomy has been gaining popularity among surgeons because it appears to offer similar long-term results without the adverse effects of radical prostatectomy, there is still insufficient evidence to prove that this newer treatment is as good or superior. Therefore radical prostatectomy remains the most commonly performed surgery in most institutions for early stage prostatic cancer.

The decision about whether to use a perineal or a retropubic approach is usually based on the patient's general health and the surgeon's preference. Both types of procedures have the disadvantage of rendering the patient sexually impotent (nerve pathways are interrupted) and sterile (semen is no longer produced). They also pose a higher risk of urinary incontinence than do other types of prostatectomies. The physician must discuss these adverse effects with the patient before surgery, and the nurse should make certain that the patient understands what he has been told.

The retropubic approach usually includes iliac lymphadenectomy as part of the procedure. Although the removal of regional nodes has not been shown to improve survival rates, it does allow for more precise staging of the disease and thus provides important information regarding further management of the patient. Therefore this approach is more commonly used. However, the relative ease with which the perineal approach can be performed makes it a useful option for the patient whose general condition precludes abdominal surgery.

Perineal prostatectomy

For a perineal prostatectomy the patient is placed in the perineal position. This is an exaggerated lithotomy position in which the knees are against the chest, and the buttocks are elevated on a pad so that the perineal area is completely elongated and parallel to the table (Fig. 44-1). An inverted U-shaped incision is made between the ischial tuberosities, the scrotum, and the rectum. The prostate gland is then separated from the wall of the rectum, and the urethra is incised at the apex of the prostate. The bladder neck is then incised, and the entire prostate gland (including its capsule), prostatic urethra, and seminal vesicles are removed. The urethra is then anastomosed to the bladder neck around an indwelling urethral catheter. The wound is closed with a small incisional drain (Fig. 44-2), and a scrotal dressing is applied.

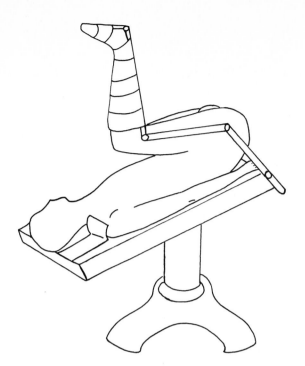
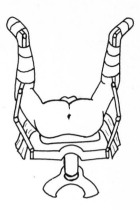

Fig. 44-1. Exaggerated lithotomy (perineal) position used for perineal prostatectomy; side view and perineal view.

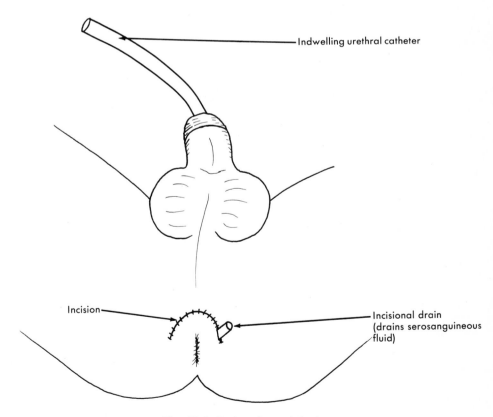

Indwelling urethral catheter

Incision

Incisional drain (drains serosanguineous fluid)

Fig. 44-2. Perineal prostatectomy.

501

PERINEAL PROSTATECTOMY
Outline of Care Plan
ANTICIPATED NURSING DIAGNOSES:

Preoperative period
1. Need for preoperative teaching.
2. Psychologic distress related to the diagnosis of cancer.
3. Potential for depression regarding effects of forthcoming surgery: impotence and sterility.
4. Need for discharge planning.

Early postoperative period
5. Potential for shock.
6. Need for management of indwelling urethral catheter.
7. Potential for wound complications.
8. Postoperative pain.

9. Potential for injury to surgical site from rectal trauma or premature bowel movement.
10. Need for management of intravenous infusion.
11. Potential for deep vein thrombosis.
12. Potential for respiratory complications related to surgical intervention.

Late postoperative period
13. Potential for wound complications following removal of incisional drain.
14. Need for management of returning bowel function.
15. Potential for voiding complications following removal of indwelling urethral catheter.

Convalescent period
16. Dysuria.*
17. Urinary incontinence.*
18. Need for discharge teaching.

*May not apply.

NURSING CARE PLAN FOR THE PATIENT UNDERGOING PERINEAL PROSTATECTOMY

1. NURSING DIAGNOSIS: Need for preoperative teaching

Preoperative period

Objectives of nursing intervention

- If necessary, clarification of reason for hospitalization and type of surgery to be performed
- Elimination of any negative or inaccurate notions regarding the forthcoming surgery
- Explanation of preoperative tests and procedures
- Psychologic preparation for general anesthesia (omit if the patient is to have spinal anesthesia)
- Explanation of events expected in the early postoperative period
- Explanation of body conditions expected in the early postoperative period
- Identification of any known allergies

Expected outcomes

- Verbal indications that explanations are understood
- Verbal indication of optimistic expectations (within realistic limits) related to forthcoming surgery
- Cooperation during preoperative tests and procedures
- Verbal or behavioral indication of reduction of anxiety
- Absence of postoperative complications
- Absence of allergic reactions

Plan for implementation	Rationale
See master care plan for the patient receiving preoperative teaching.	
In addition to the topics covered in the master care plan, include the following items in the preoperative teaching:	
1. Be aware that, in addition to routine preoperative tests, the following diagnostic studies may have been performed, and answer any questions the patient has regarding them.	
a. Needle biopsy of the prostate	In most cases the definitive diagnosis of carcinoma of the prostate is not made until cytologic examination of the prostatic tissue is performed.
b. Intravenous pyelogram	This is done to detect any associated anatomic abnormalities such as metastases or obstructive disease.

c. Serum acid phosphatase (prostatic fraction)
   d. Bone and liver scans
   e. CT scan of the pelvis for lymph node enlargement
   f. Lymphangiogram (occasionally done)
	These are done to determine the presence of metastatic spread of the disease. If any of the tests are positive, other treatment modalities are usually employed (e.g., radiotherapy or chemotherapy).

2. The preoperative shave is from the umbilicus to mid-thigh, including the perineum and scrotum.	
3. The patient will be placed on a low-residue diet for approximately 24 to 48 hours preoperatively, and the diet will be continued for 5 to 7 days postoperatively. The patient will probably be permitted to have a light meal in the evening after surgery.	The purpose of the diet is to reduce the amount of fecal matter in the bowel before surgery and then to delay defecation in the early postoperative period. This is done as a precaution because the prostatic capsule lies directly against the anterior wall of the rectum, and any inadvertent trauma to the rectum during surgery will be greatly compounded by a large amount of stool. A bowel movement in the early postoperative period may disrupt the surgical site because of the proximity of the rectum to the vesicourethral anastomosis.
4. The patient will be placed on a regimen of tap water enemas during the 24 hours before surgery. In addition, a cathartic may be ordered.	The purpose is to clean the rectum thoroughly before surgery and have the bowel as empty as possible for the above stated reasons. Some physicians will also order neomycin enemas to reduce the bacterial content of the bowel.
5. The patient will have an indwelling urethral catheter for 10 to 14 days after the surgery.	
6. There will be an incision on the perineal area. It will be covered by a dressing that may require frequent changing during the first 24 to 48 hours after surgery.	

Preoperative period

2. NURSING DIAGNOSIS: Psychologic distress related to the diagnosis of cancer

Objectives of nursing intervention
{ Provision of an emotionally supportive environment
Achievement of effective communication between patient, family, and staff

Expected outcomes
{ Verbalization by the patient of feelings about the diagnosis
Realistic decision-making
Absence of severe or protracted depression

Plan for implementation	Rationale
See Chapter 20, nursing diagnosis 1.	

3. NURSING DIAGNOSIS: Potential for depression regarding the effects of forthcoming surgery (impotence and sterility)

Objective of nursing intervention
Provision of emotional support

Expected outcomes
{ Patient expresses feelings about loss of sexual function
Absence of severe or protracted depression

Plan for implementation	Rationale
1. Be aware that the loss of sexual function is usually difficult for a man to accept, no matter what his age nor how well adjusted he appears to be regarding the effects of the forthcoming surgery.	Many patients on whom this surgery is performed are still sexually active or at least interested in sex. The loss of sexual function is so intimately connected to a man's self-esteem that his feelings of loss of manhood can be devastating.
2. Recognize that inappropriate behavior (e.g., hostility, demanding behavior, withdrawal) may be reactions to the patient's feelings of powerlessness based on his sense of loss of manhood.	
3. Encourage the patient to verbalize his feelings.	
4. Provide emotional support.	
5. If the patient is married, encourage his wife to verbalize her feelings. Sometimes this is better done, at least initially, in private (i.e., without the spouse).	

Preoperative period

504

Plan for implementation	Rationale
6. Suggest psychiatric or sexual counseling if the patient (or his wife) appears to be unable to cope adequately with the situation.	

4. NURSING DIAGNOSIS: Need for discharge planning

Objectives of nursing intervention { Early commencement of discharge planning
Accurate estimate of time required for all discharge teaching

Expected outcome Smooth transition of care after discharge

Plan for implementation	Rationale

See master care plan for the patient requiring discharge preparations: discharge planning.
 	
In addition to the topics covered in the master care plan, the following items should be considered:
1. The duration of hospitalization for this type of surgery is approximately 2 to 3 weeks.
 	
2. Required teaching includes:
  a. General postoperative discharge teaching
  b. Perineal exercises
  c. Possibly instructions on the use of a urinary collecting device or penile clamp if severe incontinence occurs.	

Preoperative period

505

5. NURSING DIAGNOSIS: Potential for shock

Objective of nursing intervention	Prevention or early detection of shock

Expected outcomes { Vital signs normal, skin dry, color normal
Absence of bright red drainage from catheter

Plan for implementation	Rationale
1. Check the patient's vital signs every 4 hours once stable (every 15 minutes if unstable).	Although shock is a potential complication after any type of surgery, it is relatively unlikely after a perineal prostatectomy because few blood vessels are cut, and the duration of surgery is short.
2. Be alert for increasing pulse and respiratory rates, decreasing blood pressure, diaphoresis, pallor, and feelings of apprehension.	
3. Notify the physician at once if indications of impending shock occur.	

Early postoperative period

6. NURSING DIAGNOSIS: Need for management of indwelling urethral catheter

Objectives of nursing intervention

Appropriate care of catheter and equipment

Prevention or early detection of infection

Care of tissue surrounding catheter

Maintenance of accurate records of urine output

Appropriate administration of hand-irrigation of catheter

Management of discomfort or pain caused by catheter

Satisfactory collection of urine specimens from catheter

Expected outcomes

Absence of severe bladder spasms and suprapubic distention

Urine draining freely through system

Absence of fever, chills, and foul-smelling urine

Absence of urethral discharge and tissue inflammation

Minimal discomfort caused by the catheter

Urine specimens in optimum condition for all necessary tests

Plan for implementation	Rationale
See master care plan for the patient with an indwelling urethral catheter: care after insertion of the catheter. In addition to the topics covered in the master care plan, the following interventions are required: 1. Use **strict** precautions to prevent accidental ejection of the catheter.	The catheter is essential for adequate healing of the vesicourethral anastomosis because it maintains decompression of the bladder and splints the suture line. Premature removal could necessitate additional surgery.

a. Keep the catheter taped **securely** to the patient's thigh or abdomen at all times. Some surgeons suture the catheter to the glans as an additional precaution.
  b. Do not allow inexperienced staff members to remove urine from the catheter without providing them with thorough instructions (see Fig. 11-2).
  c. If the patient is confused, obtain an order for arm restraints, and use them if the patient cannot be adequately supervised.
	A confused patient might pull the catheter out, balloon and all.

2. If the catheter is accidentally removed:
  a. Notify the physician **at once.**
 	
  b. Do not attempt to replace the catheter.
	Immediate recatheterization is essential to maintain proper healing of the anastomosis.
	The site of the anastomosis is extremely delicate and easily disrupted in the early postoperative period. The nurse should not attempt to recatheterize the patient because of the considerable risk of trauma to healing tissue. Often even the surgeon is unable to replace it.

3. Notify the physician if the urine is bright red and has a high viscosity and/or clots.	Although the urine may be lightly blood tinged in the early postoperative period, the amount of bleeding is usually considerably less than that after procedures leaving the prostatic capsule intact (e.g., transurethral prostatectomy or transvesical prostatectomy).

Early postoperative period

7. NURSING DIAGNOSIS: Potential for wound complications

Objective of nursing intervention	Prevention or early detection of complications arising from the incisional area
Expected outcome	Absence of fever, purulent exudate, erythema, edema, dehiscence, hematoma, and other abnormal wound conditions

Plan for implementation   Rationale

1. Check the dressing frequently (every 2 to 4 hours during the first 24 to 48 hours after surgery). Change it when it becomes wet and use sterile technique for the procedure.

   There may be a moderate amount of drainage on the dressing for the first few days after surgery. It contains serosanguineous fluid and usually a small amount of urine. The amount of drainage should decrease considerably after the first few days because the vesicourethral anastomosis becomes watertight after this period. Until then the dressing requires frequent changing for the following reasons:
   1. It is a source of infection.
      a. It acts as a wick, enabling microorganisms on the skin to move toward the incision.
      b. It provides a good medium for bacterial multiplication.
   2. It is highly irritating to the skin because of the presence of urine in the drainage.

2. When changing the dressing:
   a. Use sterile technique for the procedure.
   b. Use caution when removing the soiled dressing to prevent inadvertent removal of the incisional drain.
   c. Note the condition of the suture line. Chart its appearance and the presence of edema, erythema, or other abnormal wound conditions.
   d. Notify the physician if there is any **purulent** drainage. It is not abnormal, however, for the dressing to have an odor, since there is urine in the drainage and the apocrine glands in the groin are close to the wound.
   e. Secure the fresh dressing with a split T-binder.

   Premature removal of a drain may result in the development of a urinoma and prolonged healing.
   This provides a frame of reference for other staff members caring for the patient.

3. Check the patient's temperature every 4 hours, and notify the physician if there is an elevation above 101°.

   Wound infection must always be suspected when the patient runs a fever postoperatively. Other causes include respiratory complications and pharmacologic intervention.

Early postoperative period

8. NURSING DIAGNOSIS: Postoperative pain

Objective of nursing intervention	Appropriate management of pain or discomfort
Expected outcome	Behavioral and/or verbal indication that pain is adequately reduced or absent

Plan for implementation	Rationale
Determine the source of the pain. It may be related to the catheter, the surgical wound, or musculoskeletal manipulation.	Pain from different sources usually requires different intervention.
1. Question and observe the patient to obtain information about the pain.	
2. Be aware that pain is a unique and individual experience. Although the different sources of pain can usually be determined by their characteristics, there are also many variations.	
3. Be alert for indications (verbal or behavioral) that the patient is experiencing discomfort other than physical pain, and attempt to resolve the problem.	Fear, loneliness, depression, and numerous other conditions may be sources of extreme discomfort for the patient, who may unconsciously translate these feelings into pain.

PERSISTENT, SEVERE, INCREASING PAIN IN SUPRAPUBIC AREA

See Chapter 11, part one, nursing objective 6.	This pain is probably caused by an obstructed catheter.

SPASMODIC, INTERMITTENT PAIN IN SUPRAPUBIC AREA, OR PAIN RADIATING TO URETHRAL AREA

See Chapter 11, part one, nursing objective 6.	This pain is probably caused by the catheter's irritating effect on the bladder.

MODERATE PAIN AT SURGICAL SITE, USUALLY AGGRAVATED BY PHYSICAL ACTIVITY

1. Be certain the catheter is not obstructed. Although pain with these characteristics is usually of incisional origin and is expected, it is often difficult to differentiate between incisional pain and pain from an obstructed catheter after this type of surgery.	Catheter obstruction must be ruled out first because it cannot remain untreated. However, after this type of surgery it is unlikely for the catheter to become obstructed because there is rarely enough blood in the drainage for clots to form, and no tissue particles are normally passed in the urine.
2. Administer analgesics as ordered.	Analgesic medication usually provides considerable relief from incisional pain.

Early postoperative period

Plan for implementation	Rationale
3. Plan the patient's activities to coincide with a time when there is a high level of pain medication in the patient's bloodstream.	The patient will cooperate better with coughing exercises, ambulating, bathing, etc. when the pain is well under control.
4. Notify the physician if the patient's requests for pain medication do not decrease within 48 to 72 hours.	Although the intensity of postoperative pain varies enormously between patients, there should be a marked decrease in the apparent severity of the pain within 2 or 3 days. If this does not occur, it may indicate the development of wound complications.

MUSCULAR DISCOMFORT IN NECK, SHOULDERS, EXTREMITIES, ETC.

1. Provide the patient with an explanation for the pain and reassurance that it is transient.	Because of the unusual positioning of the patient during surgery (see Fig. 44-1), many of these patients have some stiffness or soreness in various parts of their bodies. Generally, reassurance that it does not indicate complications is sufficient to take the patient's mind off it.
2. Apply warm compresses to the affected area.	
3. If pain persists, notify the physician.	
4. If the patient complains of numbness, tingling, or paralysis of his arm, notify the physician.	Brachial palsy is a rare complication that occurs as a result of the pressure from the braces placed against the patient's shoulder during surgery. In some cases the patient may be unable to move his arm at all. Fortunately this is usually a self-limiting condition, but a neurologic evaluation is required.

Early postoperative period

9. NURSING DIAGNOSIS: Potential injury to surgical site from rectal trauma or premature bowel movement

Objectives of nursing intervention — Prevention of rectal trauma from any foreign material
Reduction of colonic activity

Expected outcomes — Absence of disruption of vesicourethral anastomosis
Absence of bowel movements for 5 days after surgery

Plan for implementation	Rationale
1. Do not insert any foreign object into the patient's rectum for at least 5 days after surgery. This includes enemas, suppositories, and thermometers.	Because of the proximity of the anterior rectal wall to the surgical site, the introduction of a foreign object into the rectum is potentially harmful to healing tissue.
2. If the patient **requires** rectal temperature readings (i.e., there is a written order that the patient is to have his temperature taken by this route because other routes are for some reason inappropriate): a. Use extreme caution when inserting the thermometer. b. Do not delegate this job to an auxiliary staff member.	This job should not be assigned to nurses' aides or orderlies because in most cases they are not aware of the abovementioned information.
3. Reduce the need for the patient to have a bowel movement by the following measures: a. Maintain the patient on a low-residue diet as ordered. b. Administer medication as ordered. Frequently codeine or diphenoxylate HCl with atropine sulfate (Lomotil) is given.	Distention of the rectum by fecal matter may cause disruption of the vesicourethral anastomosis. This will reduce the amount of solid matter in the colon. This will reduce the motility of the colon.

Early postoperative period

Early postoperative period

10. NURSING DIAGNOSIS: Need for management of intravenous infusion

Objectives of nursing intervention
- Appropriate administration of specific types of intravenous solutions
- Prevention or early detection of local complications
- Prevention or early detection of systemic complications
- Management of discomfort caused by the intravenous infusion
- Maintenance of proper function of intravenous equipment
- Maintenance of accurate records of the patient's hydration status

Expected outcomes
- Normal hydration status
- Normal electrolyte status
- Absence of thrombophlebitis, infiltration, infection, fluid overload, and pulmonary embolism
- Absence of discomfort caused by the intravenous infusion

Plan for implementation	Rationale
See master care plan for the patient receiving intravenous therapy.	These patients usually receive isotonic dextrose and saline solutions.

11. NURSING DIAGNOSIS: Potential for deep vein thrombosis

Objectives of nursing intervention
- Explanation and maintenance of precautions against deep vein thrombosis
- Early detection of deep vein thrombosis

Expected outcomes
- Cooperation with regimen to prevent deep vein thrombosis
- Absence of local pain, swelling, and redness of a lower extremity
- Absence of fever

Plan for implementation	Rationale
See master care plan for the patient at risk for deep vein thrombosis.	The risk of deep vein thrombosis is relatively high postoperatively because the unusual positioning during the surgery may impair circulation to the lower extremities (see Fig. 44-1).

12. NURSING DIAGNOSIS: Potential for respiratory complications related to surgical intervention

Objective of nursing intervention Prevention or early detection of atelectasis and/or pneumonia

Expected outcomes
{ Cooperation with therapeutic respiratory regimen
Absence of fever or audible lung congestion
Sputum clear or white and easily mobilized

Plan for implementation	Rationale
See master care plan for the patient at risk for respiratory complications, nursing objective 1.	

Early postoperative period

13. NURSING DIAGNOSIS: Potential wound complications following removal of incisional drain

Objectives of nursing intervention
{ Management of regimen to promote wound healing
Prevention and/or early detection of complications

Expected outcomes
{ Gradual disappearance of drainage from surgical site
Absence of fever, edema, erythema, or other abnormal wound conditions

Plan for implementation	Rationale
1. Observe the wound, and chart the volume and characteristics of drainage on the soiled dressing.	This provides a frame of reference for other staff members caring for the patient and provides a record of the patient's progress.
2. Assist the patient with sitz baths as ordered (usually two or three times a day for 15 to 30 minutes).	This helps keep the wound clean and promotes healing.
3. Provide the patient with a heat lamp directed at the perineal area as ordered (usually two or three times a day for 30 to 40 minutes).	This promotes healing and drying of the wound.
a. Keep the lamp close enough to the perineum to **warm** the skin, but be certain it is not so close that it will burn the skin.	
b. Provide the patient with adequate privacy during treatments.	
4. Loosely apply a sterile dressing (secured with a split T-binder) after these procedures.	

Late postoperative period

Plan for implementation	Rationale
5. Notify the physician when the drainage stops completely.	The heat lamp and sitz bath are no longer required once the wound is dry.

Late postoperative period

14. NURSING DIAGNOSIS: Need for management of returning bowel function

Objective of nursing intervention	Maintenance of diet, medication and exercise regimen

Expected outcome	Resumption of normal bowel movements within 5 to 7 days after surgery

Plan for implementation	Rationale
1. Have the patient resume his regular diet as ordered (usually 5 to 7 days postoperatively).	
2. If the patient has not had a bowel movement for 1 week following surgery: a. Administer stool softeners and/or cathartics as ordered. b. Encourage high fluid intake, especially fruit juices. c. Keep an accurate record of the patient's bowel movements.	
3. Give the patient the following perineal exercise instructions and obtain an accurate return verbalization: a. The patient should assume a standing position. b. He should tighten and relax his buttocks five or more times per hour. c. He should repeat this every hour.	This exercise will cause contraction of all the perineal muscles, including the anal sphincter. Although these exercises are mainly to correct **urinary** incontinence once the catheter is removed, they serve an additional purpose by being started within the first week after surgery because occasionally some patients are temporarily incontinent of stool following perineal surgery. This is because the surgery causes relaxation of the perineal muscles. Fecal incontinence can be psychologically upsetting for the patient, and if possible such an incidence should be avoided.
4. If fecal incontinence occurs, reassure the patient that this is not uncommon after this type of surgery and it is **temporary.**	

15. NURSING DIAGNOSIS: Potential for voiding complications following removal of indwelling urethral catheter

Objective of nursing intervention Prevention or early detection of complications

Expected outcomes { Resumption of normal voiding pattern

Absence of dysuria

Plan for implementation	Rationale
See master care plan for the patient with an indwelling urethral catheter: care after removal of the catheter.	
In addition to the items covered in the master care plan, the following intervention is often helpful:	
Explain to the patient that he might have some degree of urinary incontinence shortly after removal of the catheter, but this is usually temporary.	Before surgery the physician discussed with the patient the possibility of permanent incontinence as a result of the surgery. The patient should be told, however, that incontinence during the first few days after removal of the catheter is very common and does not necessarily mean permanent urinary incontinence.

16. NURSING DIAGNOSIS: Dysuria*

Objective of nursing intervention Promotion of regimen to reduce discomfort

Expected outcome Verbal and/or behavioral indication of minimal voiding discomfort

Plan for implementation	Rationale
1. Provide reassurance that the discomfort is transient.	The catheter often causes urethritis. Urine, particularly if it is concentrated, may cause a burning sensation on inflamed tissue.
2. Encourage a high fluid intake.	This dilutes the urine, thus reducing its irritating effect.
3. If the patient is in considerable discomfort, suggest that an analgesic specific to the urinary tract (e.g., phenazopyridine [Pyridium]) be ordered.	

Late postoperative period

Convalescent period

*This may not apply. Dysuria does not always occur after removal of a catheter following a radical prostatectomy.

17. NURSING DIAGNOSIS: Urinary incontinence*

Objectives of nursing intervention
{ Reduction of psychologic discomfort about incontinence
Instruction on perineal exercises and the use of incontinence device(s)

Expected outcomes
{ Expression of optimism regarding reduction of incontinence
Absence of protracted depression if incontinence continues
Accurate return verbalization of perineal exercises and use of incontinence device(s)
Performance of perineal exercises at least six to eight times daily
Absence of skin breakdown from use of incontinence device(s)

Plan for implementation	Rationale
1. Provide reassurance that the condition can be improved.	During the next 6 months, as healing is completed, there will be some reduction in the degree of incontinence. Although the nurse cannot say with certainty that the patient will regain complete continence, every effort must be made to help the patient maintain an optimistic attitude. In this way he will be more willing to comply with the perineal exercise regimen and not simply give in to a condition that may be correctable.
2. If the incontinence persists, maintain an attitude of acceptance. Caring for an incontinent patient can be very frustrating for the nurse, who has to keep him clean and dry. Take extra precautions not to convey any negative feelings toward the patient.	Incontinence has many symbolic meanings to a patient, all of which are sources of emotional discomfort for him. He may view it as an indication of helplessness, childishness, and "being dirty." The nurse's attitude can either reinforce these feelings of poor self-worth or keep the patient interested in continuing perineal exercises and learning to use a urinary collecting device or clamp if necessary.
3. Explain perineal exercises and obtain an accurate return verbalization. a. While standing, the patient should tighten and relax his buttocks five or more times each hour. b. While voiding, the patient should voluntarily stop and restart the urinary stream using his sphincter muscles. c. The patient should attempt to lengthen the period of time between each voiding by consciously holding in the urine.	When gluteal muscles are voluntarily contracted, all the perineal muscles contract, including the urinary sphincters. Since the urinary sphincters are under voluntary and involuntary control, some physicians feel that these exercises facilitate the return of sphincter control.
4. Suggest that the patient avoid drinking tea, coffee, and cola beverages.	These drinks contain caffeine, which is a mild diuretic and might make urinary control more difficult.
5. If the patient is unable to ambulate without leaking urine, place his penis in a rubber glove and secure the glove to his abdomen with a piece of tape when he is walking around.	This will enable the patient to socialize without embarrassment yet still preserve some motivation to correct the incontinence, since this is clearly a temporary measure.

Convalescent period

*This may not apply. Only a small percentage of patients are totally incontinent after a radical prostatectomy. Many, however, will have varying degrees of stress incontinence, especially in the early convalescent period.

Plan for implementation	**Rationale**

6. If the incontinence is severe and the physician has ascertained that it may be permanent:
   a. Demonstrate the application of a condom catheter in the following way:
      (1) Cut any pubic hair that might come in contact with the skin bond cement or adhesive.
      (2) Clean and dry the penis thoroughly. If the patient is uncircumcised, this includes cleaning under the prepuce as well.
      (3) Apply skin bond cement to penile shaft and allow it to dry. (Cement may not be necessary for certain patients, depending on the size of the penis and the degree of activity.)
      (4) Place the **rolled** condom onto the tip of the penis and then unroll the condom onto the shaft of the penis. Be certain to leave approximately 1 inch of space at the tip of the condom to prevent pressure buildup of voided urine.
      (5) Wrap an elasticized adhesive (a strip is enclosed in the catheter package) around the proximal end of the catheter. It should be snug but not so tight that it impedes circulation to the penis.
   b. Obtain a satisfactory return demonstration before permitting the patient to apply the catheter without supervision.
   c. Encourage the patient not to use the catheter all the time for the following reasons:
      (1) The skin should be permitted to air dry thoroughly a few times during the day.
      (2) The patient is more likely to remember to do perineal exercises and make an effort to regain continence if he is not wearing the catheter all the time.

Rationale (item 6): If the patient is unable to remain relatively dry, even with makeshift devices like a rubber glove or perineal pads, the psychosocial and physiologic hazards of social withdrawal and immobility must be weighed against the possible premature development of psychologic dependence on a condom catheter. The use of an incontinence device is discouraged after simple prostatectomies because the patient is expected to regain full urinary control. However, after a radical prostatectomy continence is not assured, and the patient should not be deprived of some relief from discomfort if the incontinence is incapacitating and if it appears that the incontinence will not improve.

Rationale (item 6c(1)): This helps prevent skin breakdown from the constant contact with urine.

7. If the physician has ordered that the patient be fitted for a penile clamp, give the following instructions, show the patient how it works, and obtain a return verbalization and demonstration on the use of the device.
   a. Wash, dry, and apply powder to the penis.

   b. Apply the clamp after voiding. It should be placed horizontally behind the glans (see Fig. 40-2).
   c. Remove the clamp approximately every 4 hours to void.

   d. Periodically check the skin under the area where the clamp presses.

   e. Check the glans for swelling. If it occurs, use the clamp on a looser notch.

   f. Alternate the clamp with a condom catheter.

Rationale (item 7a): This prevents moisture from being trapped under the rubber part of the clamp and irritating the skin.

Rationale (item 7c): Urine should not be permitted to remain in the bladder for more than 4 hours, since this can contribute to the development of a urinary tract infection.

Rationale (item 7d): Skin breakdown should be detected at once to prevent further complications. The clamp may have to be refitted or not used at all until the skin heals.

Rationale (item 7e): Swelling of the glans occasionally occurs from excessive compression, which results in decreased venous return and edema.

Rationale (item 7f): This reduces the amount of skin irritation sometimes caused by the clamp.

Convalescent period (margin note, right side)

18. NURSING DIAGNOSIS: Need for discharge teaching

Objectives of nursing
intervention

Explanation of basic information about medications to be taken at home
Explanation of information regarding follow-up care
Explanation of residual effects of the condition and/or treatment
Explanation of instructions concerning postdischarge activities
Explanation of symptoms that constitute a reason to contact the physician
Review of admitting diagnosis and mode of treatment

Expected outcomes

Accurate return verbalization and/or demonstration of all material learned
Smooth transition of care after discharge
Absence or early detection of complications arising after discharge
Ability to provide future health care practitioners with important data about health history

Plan for implementation	Rationale
See master care plan for the patient requiring discharge preparations: discharge teaching.	
In addition to the topics covered in the master care plan, include the following items in the discharge teaching: 1. At the follow-up office visit the physician will check how the wound is healing and assess the patient's voiding control.	
2. The patient will be scheduled for periodic examinations during which blood tests and x-ray and rectal examinations will be done.	Levels of serum acid phosphatase will be monitored, and chest and pelvic x-ray films will be taken to determine the presence of metastatic spread of the disease. Rectal examinations will be done to detect local recurrence.
3. The possible residual effects of this surgery include varying degrees of incontinence that may improve during the next 3 to 6 months and a small amount of drainage from the perineal wound, which should terminate within a few weeks.	
4. The patient should notify the physician if any of the following occur: a. Inability to urinate or a marked decrease in the size and force of the stream	This may indicate the development of strictures at the site of the anastomosis.
b. Chills and/or fever	This may indicate an infection or leakage from the anastomosis.
c. An **increase** in the amount of perineal drainage	This may indicate leakage from the anastomosis.
d. Hematuria	This may be caused by incomplete healing of ligated vessels.

Convalescent period

Radical retropubic prostatectomy

For a radical retropubic prostatectomy the patient is placed in a supine position, and a vertical midline incision is made from the umbilicus to the pubis. The muscles are separated, and the iliac lymph nodes are dissected on both sides. A frozen section is obtained to determine the presence of previously unidentified metastasis; if the lymph node test is negative, the surgeon proceeds with the actual prostatectomy. The entire prostate gland (including its capsule), prostatic urethra, and seminal vesicles are removed. As a general rule, a direct anastomosis is made between the bladder neck and the urethra. An indwelling urethral catheter is inserted, and sometimes a suprapubic tube is used as well. A Penrose drain or Hemovac is placed in the wound, the incision is closed, and a dressing is applied.

RADICAL RETROPUBIC PROSTATECTOMY
Outline of Care Plan
ANTICIPATED NURSING DIAGNOSES:

Preoperative period
1. Need for preoperative teaching. (See p. 522. The patient will have an indwelling urethral catheter and possibly a suprapubic tube for approximately 2 weeks.)*
2. Psychologic distress related to diagnosis of cancer. (See Chapter 20, nursing diagnosis 1.)

3. Potential for depression regarding the effects of forthcoming surgery. (See p. 504.)†
4. Need for discharge planning. (See p. 505.)†

Early postoperative period
5. Potential for shock. (See p. 525.)*
6. Need for management of indwelling urethral catheter. (See p. 507.)†
7. Need for management of suprapubic tube (if present). (See p. 478.)‡
8. Potential for wound complications. (See p. 525.)*
9. Postoperative pain. (See p. 528.)*
10. Potential injury to surgical site from rectal trauma. (See p. 511. Omit section concerning regulation of bowel movements.)†
11. Need for management of intravenous infusion. (See p. 527.)*
12. Potential for respiratory complications related to surgical intervention. (See p. 530.)*
13. Potential for deep vein thrombosis. (See p. 530.)*

Late postoperative period
14. Potential for voiding complications after removal of indwelling urethral catheter. (See p. 515.)†

Convalescent period
15. Dysuria. (See p. 515.)†
16. Need for management of urinary incontinence. (See p. 516.)†
17. Need for discharge teaching. (See p. 518. Omit mention of perineal drainage. Add to no. 4: The patient should notify the physician if there is severe pain or increasing redness at the surgical site.)†

---

*Nursing care is the same as for the patient undergoing radioactive iodine seed implantation and lymphadenectomy.
†Nursing care is the same as for the patient undergoing perineal prostatectomy.
‡Nursing care is the same as for the patient undergoing transvesical prostatectomy.

CHAPTER 45

Radioactive iodine seed implantation and iliac lymphadenectomy

Radioactive iodine (¹²⁵I) seed* implantation into the prostate gland, accompanied by iliac lymphadenectomy, is gaining popularity as the treatment of choice for prostatic cancer when there is no evidence of metastatic extension beyond the prostatic capsule.

The procedure is performed with the patient in a modified lithotomy position. A midline incision is made from the umbilicus to the pubis, the muscles are separated, and the iliac lymph nodes are dissected on both sides (Fig. 45-1). A frozen section is obtained to determine the presence of previously unidentified metastases.

The prostate gland is then defined, and radioactive iodine seeds are inserted into the gland. The number of seeds is proportional to the size of the gland. These seeds are a source of interstitial radiation and remain in the prostate permanently (Fig. 45-2). The radioactivity will gradually disappear (the half-life of ¹²⁵I seeds is 60 days). An indwelling urethral catheter is then inserted to ensure adequate drainage of the bladder. Incisional drains are usually placed on both sides of the surgical site to drain the considerable amount of lymph that tends to accumulate in the area as a consequence of the lymphadenectomy. The main incision is then closed and a dressing is applied.

---

*Some institutions use radioactive gold seeds instead of iodine. Nursing care is the same, regardless of the material used.

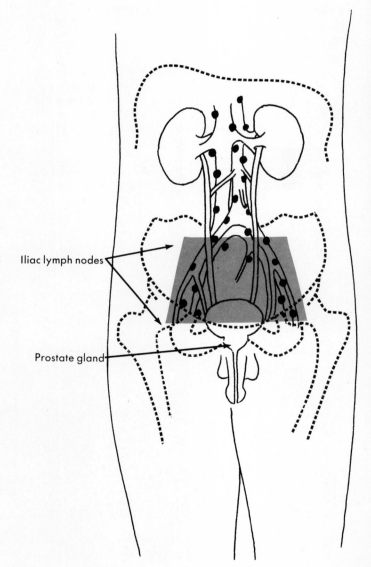

Fig. 45-1. Organs involved in surgical implantation of radioactive iodine seeds into the prostate gland and iliac lymphadenectomy.

RADIOACTIVE IODINE SEED IMPLANTATION AND LYMPHADENECTOMY
Outline of Care Plan
ANTICIPATED NURSING DIAGNOSES:

Preoperative period
1. Need for preoperative teaching.
2. Psychologic distress related to diagnosis of cancer.
3. Anxiety about radiation emitted from radioactive seeds.
4. Need for discharge planning.

Early postoperative period
5. Potential for shock.
6. Potential for wound complications.
7. Need for management of indwelling urethral catheter.
8. Need for management of intravenous infusion.
9. Postoperative pain.
10. Potential for displacement of radioactive seeds.
11. Potential for respiratory complications related to surgical intervention.
12. Potential for deep vein thrombosis.

Late postoperative period
13. Potential for voiding complications following removal of indwelling urethral catheter.

Convalescent period
14. Need for discharge teaching.

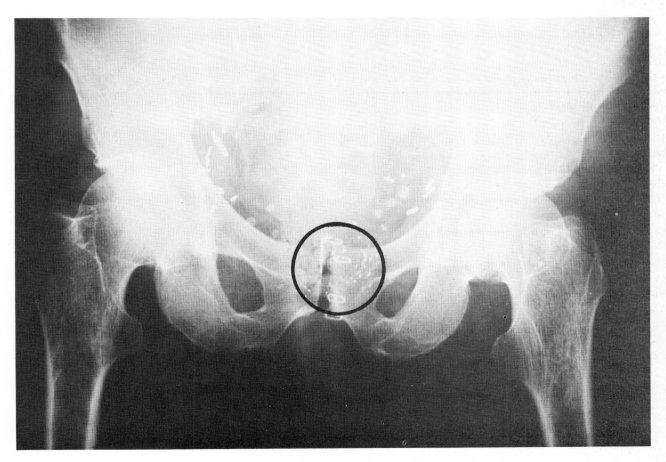

Fig. 45-2. X-ray film of pelvis after radioactive iodine seed implantation. Seeds appear as small white dots within the circle. Surgical clips and staples are also visualized.

521

NURSING CARE PLAN FOR THE PATIENT UNDERGOING RADIOACTIVE IODINE SEED IMPLANTATION AND LYMPHADENECTOMY

1. NURSING DIAGNOSIS: Need for preoperative teaching

Objectives of nursing intervention

If necessary, clarification of reason for hospitalization and type of surgery to be performed

Elimination of any negative or inaccurate notions regarding the forthcoming surgery

Explanation of preoperative tests and procedures

Psychologic preparation for general anesthesia (omit if the patient is to have spinal anesthesia)

Explanation of events expected in the early postoperative period

Explanation of body conditions expected in the early postoperative period

Identification of any known allergies

Expected outcomes

Verbal indication that explanations are understood

Verbal indication of optimistic expectations (within realistic limits) related to forthcoming surgery

Cooperation during preoperative tests and procedures

Verbal or behavioral indication of reduction of anxiety

Absence of postoperative complications

Absence of allergic reactions

Preoperative period

Plan for implementation	Rationale
See master care plan for the patient receiving preoperative teaching.	
In addition to the topics covered in the master care plan, include the following items in the preoperative teaching:	
1. Be aware that, in addition to routine preoperative tests, the following diagnostic studies may have been performed, and answer any questions the patient has regarding them:	
a. Needle biopsy of the prostate	In most cases the definitive diagnosis of carcinoma of the prostate is not made until cytologic examination of the prostatic tissue is performed.
b. Intravenous pyelogram	This is done to detect any associated structural abnormalities such as metastases or obstructive disease.
c. Serum acid phosphatase (prostatic fraction) d. Bone and liver scans e. CT scan of the pelvis for lymph node enlargement f. Lymphangiogram (occasionally done)	These are done to determine the presence of metastatic spread of the disease. If any of the tests are positive, other treatment modalities are usually employed (e.g., radiotherapy or chemotherapy).
2. The preoperative shave is from the umbilicus to mid-thigh.	

522

Plan for implementation	Rationale
3. A light meal may be permitted in the evening after surgery. Otherwise, oral intake will be prohibited until adequate intestinal activity returns (indicated by bowel sounds and passage of flatus). The diet will resume with clear liquids and be advanced as tolerated.	There is sometimes a period of intestinal atony following iliac lymphadenectomy. Within 24 to 48 hours it generally resolves itself, but premature oral intake will cause severe abdominal discomfort, distention, and vomiting.
4. There will be an indwelling urethral catheter in place for approximately 4 days.	
5. The patient will have an incision in his lower abdomen that will be covered by a dressing. The dressing may require frequent changing during the first 24 to 48 hours after surgery.	

2. NURSING DIAGNOSIS: Psychologic distress related to the diagnosis of cancer

Objectives of nursing intervention
{ Provision of an emotionally supportive environment
Achievement of effective communication between patient, family, and staff

Expected outcomes
{ Verbalization by the patient of feelings about the diagnosis
Realistic decision-making
Absence of severe or protracted depression

Plan for implementation	Rationale
See Chapter 20, nursing diagnosis 1.	

Preoperative period

3. NURSING DIAGNOSIS: Anxiety about radiation emitted from radioactive seeds

Objective of nursing intervention	Patient education regarding relative safety of the seeds

Expected outcome	Verbal or behavioral indication of reduction of anxiety

Plan for implementation	Rationale
1. Allow the patient to verablize any concerns he might have regarding radiation dangers.	Any **mis**information must be detected before accurate information can be provided.
2. Provide the following information to dispel the fear that the patient himself might generate radiation that is harmful to others. a. The distance of radiation emitted from these seeds is approximately 2 cm. b. The seeds will slowly disintegrate over a period of 1 year. c. No precautions are necessary for guests, even if they visit frequently.	The half-life of ^{125}I seeds is 60 days. There is no danger to anybody in contact with the patient, including staff members.

4. NURSING DIAGNOSIS: Need for discharge planning

Objectives of nursing intervention	Early commencement of discharge planning Accurate estimate of time required for all discharge teaching

Expected outcome	Smooth transition of care after discharge

Plan for implementation	Rationale
See master care plan for the patient requiring discharge preparations: discharge planning. In addition to the topics covered in the master care plan, the following items should be considered: 1. The duration of hospitalization for this procedure is approximately 10 days. 2. Required teaching includes: a. General postoperative discharge teaching b. Discussion of follow-up care over extended period of time after discharge	

Preoperative period

5. NURSING DIAGNOSIS: Potential for shock

Objective of nursing intervention   Prevention or early detection of shock

Expected outcomes   Vital signs normal, skin dry, color normal
Absence of bright red drainage from wound

Plan for implementation	Rationale
1. Check the patient's vital signs every 4 hours once stable (every 15 minutes if unstable).	Hypovolemic shock is a potential complication after any surgery when there is a risk of considerable blood loss. After removal of lymph nodes, hypovolemic shock might also occur because of excessive loss of lymphatic fluid at the site of the lymphadenectomy.
2. Be alert for increasing pulse and respiratory rates, decreasing blood pressure, diaphoresis, pallor, and feelings of apprehension.	
3. Notify the physician at once if indications of impending shock occur.	

6. NURSING DIAGNOSIS: Potential for wound complications

Objective of nursing intervention   Prevention or early detection of complications arising from the incisional area

Expected outcome   Absence of fever, purulent exudate, erythema, edema, dehiscence, hematoma, and other abnormal wound conditions

Plan for implementation	Rationale
1. Check the dressing every 4 hours during the first 24 to 48 hours and then every shift. Change it when it becomes wet and use sterile technique for the procedure.	These dressings usually require changing at least once a shift in the early postoperative period. The drainage is serosanguineous fluid with a relatively large proportion of lymph.
2. Use caution when removing soiled dressings to prevent the inadvertent removal of the incisional drain(s). Penrose drains, tube drains, or Hemovacs are used. (See pp. 492 and 634 for nursing management of tube drains and Hemovacs.)	Premature removal of a drain may result in prolonged healing.

Early postoperative period

525

Plan for implementation	Rationale
3. Cut and arrange gauze pads around the incisional drain(s).	This prevents the dressings from flattening the drain(s) and possibly obstructing the flow of drainage from the wound.
4. If the dressing requires frequent changing, use Montgomery straps instead of adhesive tape.	This eliminates the need to remove the adhesive tape from the patient's skin each time the dressing is changed. Skin irritation and patient discomfort can be considerably reduced by this method.
5. Note the condition of the suture line. Chart its appearance and the presence of edema, erythema, ecchymosis, hematoma, or other abnormal conditions.	This provides a frame of reference for other staff members caring for the patient.
6. If there is purulent drainage: a. Notify the physician. b. Obtain a wound culture specimen.	This would indicate a wound infection. This will facilitate identification of the infecting organism so that appropriate treatment can be instituted quickly.
7. Check the patient's temperature every 4 hours and notify the physician if there is an elevation above 101°.	Wound infection must always be suspected when the patient runs a fever postoperatively. Other causes include respiratory complications and pharmacologic intervention.

7. NURSING DIAGNOSIS: Need for management of indwelling urethral catheter

Objectives of nursing intervention

Appropriate care of catheter and equipment
Prevention or early detection of infection
Care of tissue surrounding catheter
Maintenance of accurate records of urine output
Appropriate administration of hand-irrigation of catheter
Management of discomfort or pain caused by catheter
Satisfactory collection of urine specimens from catheter

Expected outcomes

Absence of severe bladder spasms
Urine draining freely through system
Absence of fever, chills, and foul-smelling urine
Absence of urethral discharge and tissue inflammation
Minimal discomfort caused by the catheter
Urine specimens in optimum condition for all necessary tests

Early postoperative period

Plan for implementation	Rationale
See master care plan for the patient with an indwelling urethral catheter: care after insertion of the catheter.	
In addition to the topics covered in the master care plan, the following interventions are required: 1. Notify the physician if the urine turns bright red at any time.	The urine is usually lightly blood tinged to clear amber within 24 to 48 hours after surgery.
2. Check drainage bag and tubing for any solid particles. (See p. 529 for interventions regarding displacement of iodine seeds.)	Although it is unlikely, the ^{125}I seeds occasionally become dislodged and are passed in the urine.

8. NURSING DIAGNOSIS: Need for management of intravenous infusion

Objectives of nursing intervention

- Appropriate administration of specific types of intravenous solutions
- Prevention or early detection of local complications
- Prevention or early detection of systemic complications
- Management of discomfort caused by the intravenous infusion
- Maintenance of proper function of intravenous equipment
- Maintenance of accurate records of the patient's hydration status

Expected outcomes

- Normal hydration status
- Normal electrolyte status
- Absence of thrombophlebitis, infiltration, infection, fluid overload, and pulmonary embolism
- Absence of discomfort caused by the intravenous infusion

Plan for implementation	Rationale
See master care plan for the patient receiving intravenous therapy.	These patients usually receive isotonic dextrose and saline solutions, antibiotics, and plasma expanders.

Early postoperative period

527

9. NURSING DIAGNOSIS: Postoperative pain

Objective of nursing intervention   Appropriate management of pain or discomfort

Expected outcome   Behavioral and/or verbal indication that pain is adequately reduced or absent

Plan for implementation	Rationale
Determine the source of the pain. It may be related to the catheter or the surgical wound.	Pain from different sources usually requires different intervention.
1. Question and observe the patient to obtain information about the pain.	
2. Be aware that pain is a unique and individual experience. Although the different sources of pain can usually be determined by their characteristics, there are also many variations.	
3. Be alert for indications (verbal or behavioral) that the patient is experiencing discomfort other than physical pain, and attempt to resolve the problem.	Fear, loneliness, depression, and numerous other conditions may be sources of extreme discomfort for the patient, who may unconsciously translate these feelings into pain.

PERSISTENT, SEVERE, INCREASING PAIN IN SUPRAPUBIC AREA

See Chapter 11, part one, nursing objective 6.	This pain is probably caused by an obstructed catheter.

SPASMODIC, INTERMITTENT PAIN IN SUPRAPUBIC AREA, OR PAIN RADIATING TO URETHRAL AREA

See Chapter 11, part one, nursing objective 6.	This pain is probably caused by the catheter's irritating effect on the bladder.

Early postoperative period

Plan for implementation	Rationale
MODERATE TO SEVERE PAIN AT SURGICAL SITE, USUALLY AGGRAVATED BY PHYSICAL ACTIVITY	
1. Be certain the catheter is not obstructed. Although pain with these characteristics is usually of incisional origin and is expected, it may be difficult to differentiate between incisional pain and pain from an obstructed catheter after this type of surgery.	Catheter obstruction must be ruled out first because it cannot remain untreated. However, after this type of surgery it is unlikely for the catheter to become obstructed because there is rarely enough blood in the drainage for clots to form, and no tissue particles are normally passed in the urine.
2. Administer analgesics as ordered.	Analgesic medication usually provides considerable relief from incisional pain.
3. Plan the patient's activities to coincide with a time when there is a high level of pain medication in the patient's bloodstream.	The patient will cooperate better with coughing exercises, ambulating, bathing, etc. when the pain is well under control.
4. Notify the physician if the patient's requests for pain medication do not decrease within 48 to 72 hours.	Although the intensity of postoperative pain varies enormously between patients, there should be a marked decrease in the apparent severity of the pain within 2 or 3 days. If this does not occur, it may indicate the development of wound complications.

10. NURSING DIAGNOSIS: Potential for displacement of radioactive iodine seeds

Objectives of nursing intervention { Patient education about possibility of seed displacement
Detection and appropriate management of seed displacement

Expected outcomes { Verbal confirmation that information is understood
Detection of seed displacement if it occurs

Plan for implementation	Rationale
1. Be alert for any solid matter passed in the urine.	Although it is unlikely, there is a possibility that one or more of the seeds will become dislodged from the prostate and be excreted in the urine. Unless passed in the immediate postoperative period, these seeds become encrusted with blood and will look like urinary stones or clots.
2. Ask the patient to notify the nurse if he observes any solid particles in his urine.	
3. In the event that a seed is passed: a. Avoid prolonged handling of the seed. b. Send it to the laboratory for analysis. c. Notify the physician.	Usually hospital policy requires that all specimens be sent to the laboratory.

Early postoperative period

529

11. NURSING DIAGNOSIS: Potential for respiratory complications related to surgical intervention

| **Objective of nursing intervention** | Prevention or early detection of atelectasis and/or pneumonia |

Expected outcomes
- Cooperation with therapeutic respiratory regimen
- Absence of fever or audible lung congestion
- Sputum clear or white and easily mobilized

Plan for implementation	**Rationale**
See master care plan for the patient at risk for respiratory complications, nursing objective 3.	

12. NURSING DIAGNOSIS: Potential for deep vein thrombosis

Objectives of nursing intervention
- Explanation and maintenance of precautions against deep vein thrombosis
- Early detection of deep vein thrombosis

Expected outcomes
- Cooperation with regimen to prevent deep vein thrombosis
- Absence of local pain, swelling, and redness of a lower extremity
- Absence of fever

Plan for implementation	**Rationale**
See master care plan for the patient at risk for deep vein thrombosis.	

13. NURSING DIAGNOSIS: Potential for voiding complications following removal of indwelling urethral catheter

| **Objective of nursing intervention** | Prevention or early detection of complications |

Expected outcomes
- Resumption of normal voiding pattern
- Absence of dysuria

Plan for implementation	**Rationale**
See master care plan for the patient with an indwelling urethral catheter: care after removal of the catheter.	

Early postoperative period

Late postoperative period

14. NURSING DIAGNOSIS: Need for discharge teaching

Objectives of nursing intervention

- Explanation of basic information about medications to be taken at home
- Explanation of information regarding follow-up care
- Explanation of residual effects of the condition and/or treatment
- Explanation of instructions concerning postdischarge activities
- Explanation of symptoms that constitute a reason to contact the physician
- Review of admitting diagnosis and mode of treatment

Expected outcomes

- Accurate return verbalization and/or demonstration of all material learned
- Smooth transition of care after discharge
- Absence or early detection of complications arising after discharge
- Ability to provide health care practitioners with important data about health history

Plan for implementation	Rationale
See master care plan for the patient requiring discharge preparations: discharge teaching.	
In addition to the topics covered in the master care plan, include the following items in the discharge teaching: 1. At the initial follow-up office visit, the physician will check the wound for adequate healing and will obtain a urine specimen for culture. The patient will be expected to return for periodic check-ups approximately every 6 months for 2 years and then yearly.	The purpose of these follow-up visits is for the physician to assess the degree of reduction of tumor size and changes in its consistency. It is expected to become smaller and softer as the malignant cells are destroyed.
2. The patient should bring to the physician's office any particles passed in the urine.	These will be examined to determine if any seeds have become displaced.
3. During the next few weeks, expected residual effects of the surgery include incisional discomfort and fatigue.	
4. The patient should notify the physician if any of the following occur: a. Chills, fever, flank pain b. Severe pain or increasing redness at the incisional site c. Blood in the urine d. The passage of any particles in the urine	These might indicate a urinary tract infection. These might indicate a wound infection. This might indicate continued growth of malignant tissue, or it may be caused by a urinary tract infection. These should be examined to determine whether seeds are being excreted or if there is abnormal bleeding resulting in clot formation.

Convalescent period

CHAPTER 46

Management of the patient with acute prostatitis

Acute prostatitis is a urinary tract infection arising in the prostate gland. It is characterized by high fever, chills, urinary frequency, urgency, dysuria, and often suprapubic and low back pain. Although hospitalization is not always necessary, it may be required if the patient is septic or there is any associated urinary retention.

The infecting organism is usually found in the urine, and a specimen for culture and sensitivity tests is obtained at once. However, until the results of the culture are known, the patient may be given trimethoprim and sulfamethoxazole (Septra) because this antimicrobial medication readily diffuses into prostatic tissue.

In the event that edema of the inflamed tissue causes the patient to go into urinary retention, a trocar cystotomy may be performed to provide drainage of urine (Fig. 46-1). This is a bedside procedure for which the patient is given a local anesthetic. A silicone catheter is introduced into the bladder by means of a trocar cannula. The catheter is then secured to the skin with a plastic adhesive and usually left in the bladder for 1 week. Once the patient becomes asymptomatic, the tube is clamped; if the patient voids well for the next 24 hours, the tube is removed. Sometimes an indwelling urethral catheter is used to drain the bladder instead of suprapubic drainage.

Antimicrobial therapy is usually continued for 30 days (despite the relief of symptoms that generally occurs within 2 to 5 days), and follow-up urine specimens are obtained periodically to detect recurrent infection.

Occasionally a fluctuant prostate may be revealed during a rectal examination. This indicates a prostatic abscess for which transurethral drainage is usually performed. (See Chapter 42 for nursing care after transurethral drainage of a prostatic abscess. It is very similar to care after a transurethral prostatectomy.)

ACUTE PROSTATITIS
Outline of Care Plan
ANTICIPATED NURSING DIAGNOSES:

Period of acute symptoms
1. Need for reduction of symptomatic discomfort (urgency, dysuria, pain, urethral discharge, chills, and fever).
2. Potential for urinary retention.
3. Need for management of intravenous infusion.
4. Potential for complications related to bed rest.
5. Need for management of trocar cystostomy.*
6. Need for discharge planning.

Convalescent period
7. Need for discharge teaching.

---

*Used only if the patient goes into urinary retention; may not apply.

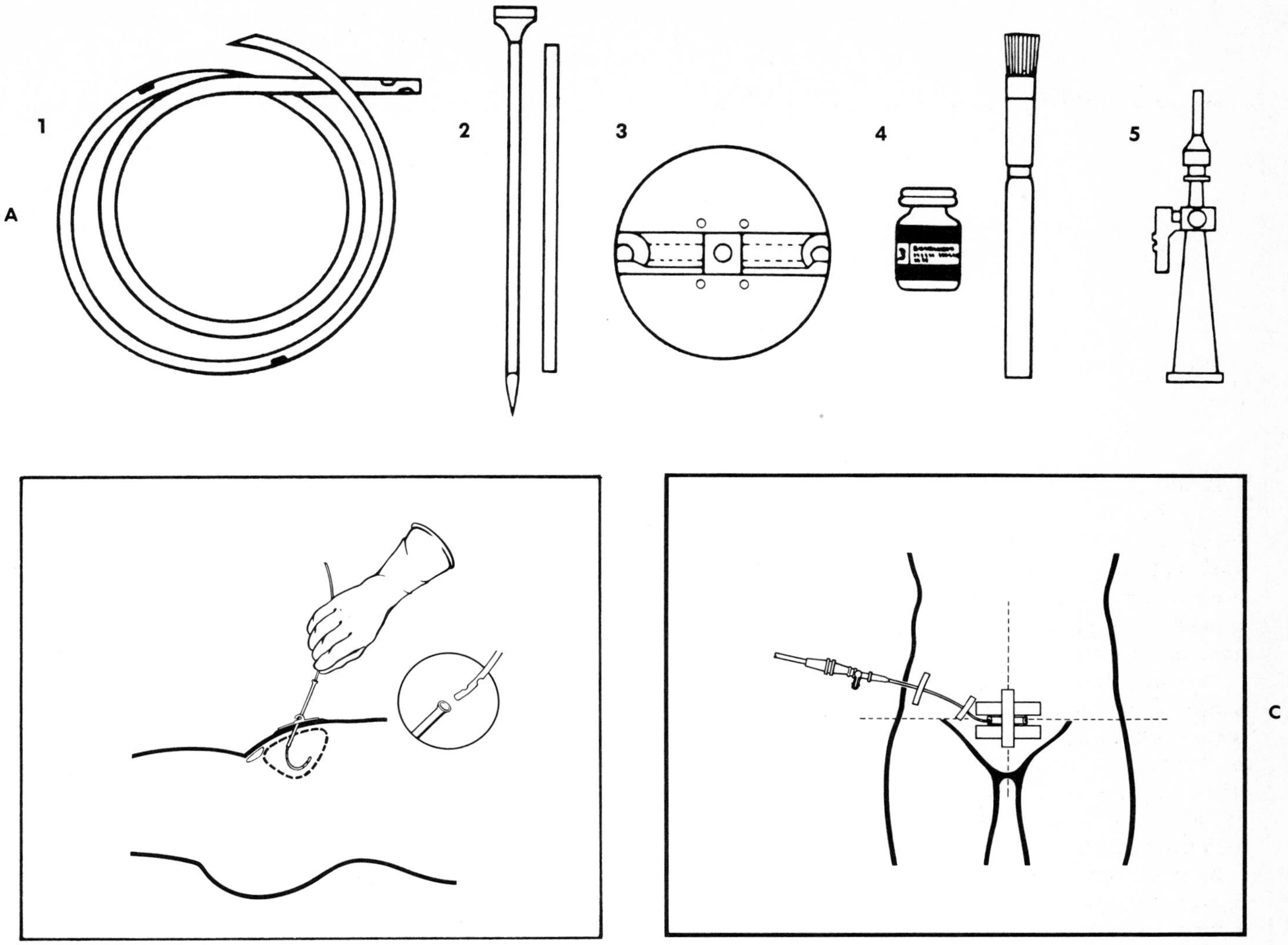

Fig. 46-1. Trocar cystostomy using Silastic brand Cystocath Suprapubic Drainage System (Reif design). **A,** Components of Cystocath System: *1,* Silicone catheter; *2,* trocar and cannula; *3,* body seal; *4,* adhesive; *5,* three-way stopcock. **B,** Catheter is threaded through cannula into bladder. **C,** Cystocath System in place; body seal and catheter taped to abdomen to ensure maximum patient mobility. (Courtesy Dow Corning Corporation, Midland, Mich.)

NURSING CARE PLAN FOR THE PATIENT WITH ACUTE PROSTATITIS

1. NURSING DIAGNOSIS: Need for reduction of symptomatic discomfort (urgency, dysuria, pain, urethral discharge, chills, and fever)

Objective of nursing intervention	Appropriate management of symptoms
Expected outcomes	Verbal or behavioral indication that discomfort is adequately reduced Normal voiding pattern reestablished Absence of urethral discharge, chills, and fever

Period of acute symptoms ↓

533

Plan for implementation	Rationale

URINARY FREQUENCY AND URGENCY

1. Provide antispasmodic medications such as oxybutynin chloride (Ditropan) or propantheline bromide (Pro-Banthine) as ordered (or suggest that these medications be ordered).

    Antispasmodics are effective in reducing the intensity of bladder spasms that cause frequency and urgency. (See Appendix A for contraindications and side effects.)

2. Provide the patient with easy access to urinal or bathroom.

3. Avoid the use of strong sleeping medications.

    If the patient has nocturia, he may fall and become injured while under the effects of a sedative.

DYSURIA

1. Provide the following medications as ordered (or suggest that these medications be ordered).
   a. Urinary tract analgesic such as phenazopyridine HCl (Pyridium)

    Phenazopyridine HCl (Pyridium) may be useful; because it is excreted in the urine, it produces a topical analgesic effect on the urinary tract mucosa.

   b. Antispasmodics

    Antispasmodics are effective in reducing the intensity of bladder spasms that contribute to dysuria.

2. Encourage adequate hydration.

    Dilute urine is less irritating to inflamed tissue. However, fluid intake should be regulated to maintain a urine output of 1 to 1.5 L per day to prevent dilution of antimicrobial medication.

3. Encourage the patient to take slow, deep breaths while voiding if the spasms are very painful.

    Deep breathing promotes general relaxation. Whether or not it has a relaxing effect on the bladder itself has not been proved, but it does seem to relieve some of the discomfort.

SUPRAPUBIC AND BACK PAIN

1. Provide local heat, tub bath, or sitz bath.

    Heat causes vasodilation. This increases the circulation to the area, thus reducing tissue fluid and removing toxins. The process results in the reduction of pressure on nerve endings and reduction of inflammation.

2. Medicate with analgesics as ordered.

URETHRAL DISCHARGE

Provide gauze pads and hydrogen peroxide for cleaning the meatus if discharge is copious.

    This is for esthetic and hygienic purposes.

Period of acute symptoms

Plan for implementation	Rationale

CHILLS AND FEVER

1. Obtain blood and urine specimens for culture as ordered. The urine should be a midstream specimen from a cleansed orifice.

These specimens are obtained to identify the infecting organism and determine its antibiotic sensitivity.

2. Medicate with an antipyretic as ordered.

Measures to reduce fever are usually ordered for temperatures above 101°. However, this is a controversial subject, since the exact role of fever in fighting infection has not yet been determined.

3. Provide alcohol sponge bath, hypothermia blanket, or tepid bath as ordered.

4. Notify the physician at once if there are any indications of septic shock. These include:
   a. Decreasing blood pressure
   b. Mental obtundation
   c. Cool, pale extremities
   d. Increasing pulse and respiratory rates

Although this is an unlikely complication, the possibility of septic shock must be considered if the prostate gland is infected with a gram-negative organism.

2. **NURSING DIAGNOSIS:** Potential for urinary retention

Objective of nursing intervention	Early detection of urinary retention

Expected outcome	Minimal discomfort if urinary retention occurs

Plan for implementation	Rationale

1. Monitor urine output carefully.
   a. Note volume and appearance of urine.
   b. Note frequency of voiding.

2. Be alert for the following indications of urinary retention and notify the physician if any occur:
   a. No urine output for 6 hours despite adequate hydration.
   b. Suprapubic distention and discomfort.
   c. Frequent voiding of small amounts. (The nurse should be aware that this symptom may also be caused by bladder involvement in the infection; it is not necessarily an indication of urinary retention.)

Edema from inflamed prostatic tissue sometimes causes urinary retention. If this occurs, the physician may perform a trocar cystotomy or insert an indwelling urethral catheter.

This is known as retention with overflow. The small amount of urine being voided is that which is in excess of what the bladder can hold. The bladder is not completely emptying itself when this scanty but frequent voiding occurs. Severe bladder spasms usually accompany the voiding.

Period of acute symptoms

535

3. NURSING DIAGNOSIS: Need for management of intravenous infusion

Objectives of nursing intervention

Appropriate administration of specific types of intravenous solutions

Prevention or early detection of local complications

Prevention or early detection of systemic complications

Management of discomfort caused by the intravenous infusion

Maintenance of proper function of intravenous equipment

Maintenance of accurate records of the patient's hydration status

Precautions against adverse effects of nephrotoxic and ototoxic drugs*

Expected outcomes

Normal hydration status

Normal electrolyte status

Absence of thrombophlebitis, infiltration, infection, fluid overload, and pulmonary embolism

Absence of discomfort caused by the intravenous infusion

Normal blood urea nitrogen and creatinine levels*

Normal audiometry test results*

Plan for implementation	Rationale
See master care plan for the patient receiving intravenous therapy.	
In addition to the items mentioned in the master care plan, the following interventions may be required:	
1. If the patient is receiving an aminoglycoside (e.g., gentamicin, kanamycin, tobramycin), be certain laboratory studies are being performed for blood urea nitrogen and serum creatinine levels at least three times per week, and report any irregularities.	These drugs may be nephrotoxic. However, they are highly effective in the treatment of infections caused by gram-negative organisms. They are most commonly given via the intravenous route. If they are given intramuscularly instead, the same precautions apply.
2. If the patient is scheduled for audiometric studies during the period of aminoglycoside administration, explain the purpose.	These drugs are also ototoxic, and the physician may want the patient to have his hearing tested initially for a baseline reading and then periodically throughout aminoglycoside therapy. However, this adverse effect does not commonly occur unless the dosage is unusually high, the duration of treatment is prolonged, or if renal impairment exists.

Period of acute symptoms (side label)

*Applies to patients receiving intravenous nephrotoxic and ototoxic antibiotics.

4. NURSING DIAGNOSIS: Potential for complications related to bed rest*

Objective of nursing intervention	Prevention or early detection of complications associated with bed rest

Expected outcomes
- Absence of adverse psychologic effects of bed rest (e.g., boredom, depression, frustration)
- Normal bowel function and respiratory function
- Good skin integrity
- Absence of deep vein thrombosis and disuse atrophy of muscles

Plan for implementation	Rationale
1. Place all necessary items within easy reach of the patient.	This encourages the patient to remain in bed without causing him to feel overly dependent on others.
2. Provide the patient with diversional activities (e.g., books, television, newspapers).	Boredom and depression are not unusual reactions when a normally active individual is confined to bed.
3. Promote adequate bowel function by encouraging fruit juices and high-residue foods.	Constipation is a common complication of immobility. If the patient is receiving antispasmodic medications, this reaction is even more likely to occur.
4. Keep accurate records of the patient's bowel movements and provide a cathartic or stool softener as needed.	
5. Check the integrity of the patient's skin daily; massage reddened areas over bony prominences and avoid the use of plastic bed shields (e.g., Chux) in direct contact with the patient's skin.	Skin breakdown may occur on areas where there is prolonged pressure. Promoting circulation and keeping the areas as dry as possible will reduce the incidence of pressure necrosis.
6. Encourage periodic abdominal breathing, yawning, and sighing.	These maneuvers are considered to be a deterrent to atelectasis and pneumonia by helping to inflate the alveoli and expand the lungs to total capacity.
7. Encourage frequent changing of position, flexing and relaxing of leg muscles, range of motion exercises, and isometric exercises.	These activities help to prevent venous stasis (a predisposing factor in deep vein thrombosis), disuse atrophy of the muscles, joint contractures, skin breakdown, and respiratory congestion.

Period of acute symptoms

*In most cases these patients will not be required to remain in bed for more than a few days. Therefore many of the hazards resulting from immobility will not be a threat. However, if the patient is elderly or debilitated or if bed rest must be prolonged, related complications are a major nursing consideration.

5. NURSING DIAGNOSIS: Need for management of trocar cystostomy*

Objectives of nursing intervention
Adequate patient preparation for the procedure
Prevention or early detection of complications related to trocar cystostomy

Expected outcomes
Verbal and/or behavioral indication of absence of anxiety before and during procedure
Urine flowing freely through cystostomy tube

Plan for implementation	Rationale
1. Prior to the insertion of the trocar cystostomy tube, explain the procedure. The physician will insert a soft plastic tube into the patient's bladder through a puncture wound in his lower abdomen. Urine will drain through the tube into a collecting container.	
2. Provide assistance with the procedure if requested by the physician.	This is often done at the patient's bedside.
3. Provide encouragement to the patient during the procedure.	When done at the patient's bedside, it is performed with local anesthesia. It should be painless, but the patient may need emotional support.
4. After the procedure, observe the following guidelines:	
a. Keep the tubing taped securely to the side of the patient's abdomen.	This prevents tension on the tubing and inadvertent displacement of it.
b. If it is necessary to disconnect the tubing, close the stopcock prior to disconnection (and **reopen** it after reconnection).	This maintains a column of urine in the catheter, which is necessary for a siphon effect and proper drainage after reconnection.
c. Irrigate the tubing only if ordered and with prescribed irrigating solution. This is a sterile procedure.	Irrigation of the tube is not routinely done because of the risk of introducing microorganisms into the urinary tract. Furthermore, unless there is active bleeding or tissue sloughing, it is unlikely that the tube will become obstructed. However, the relatively narrow lumen of the tubing makes obstruction a potential complication for which the nurse must be alert.
d. Keep the collecting container below the level of the patient's bladder.	Urine flows through the tubing via gravity. Elevation of the container will result in urine flowing back into the bladder from the distal portion of the system, which has the greatest potential for contamination.
e. Keep accurate records of urine output.	
f. Follow the physician's orders for trial closing of the stopcock.	A regimen of periodic closure of the stopcock will be instituted to determine the patient's voiding ability prior to the removal of the tube.
g. Measure residual urine as ordered by the physician by opening the stopcock after the patient voids.	

Period of acute symptoms

*May not apply.

Plan for implementation	**Rationale**

5. After removal of the cystostomy tube:
   a. Periodically check the suprapubic dressing and replace it if it becomes wet.
 	
   b. Allow the patient to shower if he wishes, and change the dressing afterward.
	The physician will place a sterile dressing over the cut-down site after the tube is removed. This will absorb any urine that may continue to seep through the wound for a few days.

6. **NURSING DIAGNOSIS:** Need for discharge planning

Objectives of nursing intervention { Early commencement of discharge planning
Accurate estimate of time required for all discharge teaching

Expected outcome   Smooth transition of care after discharge

Plan for implementation	**Rationale**

See master care plan for the patient requiring discharge preparations: discharge planning.
 	
In addition to the topics covered in the master care plan, the following items should be considered:
1. The duration of hospitalization for treatment of prostatitis varies considerably but may be as long as 1 week.
 	
2. Required teaching includes:
   a. Need for diligent antibiotic administration
   b. Possible diet restrictions
   c. Care of suprapubic wound if trocar cystotomy was performed
	The length of hospitalization depends on the type of treatment required. A patient requiring suprapubic or indwelling urethral catheter drainage will be hospitalized for longer than one who does not go into urinary retention. Generally the patient will remain in the hospital until his fever is down and he is voiding well.

Period of acute symptoms

7. NURSING DIAGNOSIS: Need for discharge teaching

Objectives of nursing intervention

Explanation of basic information about medications to be taken at home

Explanation of information regarding follow-up care

Explanation of residual effects of the condition and/or treatment

Explanation of instructions concerning postdischarge activities

Explanation of symptoms that constitute a reason to contact the physician

Review of admitting diagnosis and mode of treatment

Expected outcomes

Accurate return verbalization and/or demonstration of all material learned

Smooth transition of care after discharge

Absence or early detection of complications arising after discharge

Ability to provide future health care practitioners with important data about health history

Plan for implementation	Rationale
See master care plan for the patient requiring discharge preparations: discharge teaching.	
In addition to the topics covered in the master care plan, include the following items in the discharge teaching:	
1. The patient should understand the importance of continuing the antibiotic medication for the entire length of time prescribed, despite absence of symptoms.	Medication is usually prescribed for 30 days to decrease the risk of resistant microorganisms and the development of chronic prostatitis.
2. At the follow-up office visit the physician will take a urine specimen for culture.	
3. The physician may request that the patient limit his intake of alcohol and highly spiced foods.	Some physicians consider these to be irritating to the prostate.
4. The patient should drink at least 2 L of fluid per day for the next month.	Adequate hydration discourages bacterial multiplication in the urinary tract.
5. The physician may request that the patient refrain from sexual intercourse for 2 weeks or until after the follow-up office visit.	Sexual intercourse stimulates the prostatic secretions. This may aggravate the congestion and inflammation in the gland.
6. The patient should notify the physician at once if there is a recurrence of any of the symptoms (fever, chills, frequency, urgency, or low back or suprapubic pain).	It is not unusual for the infection to recur, and prompt medical intervention is necessary.

Convalescent period

References and bibliography

BIBLIOGRAPHY

Gault, P.: The prostate—coping with dangerous and distressing complications, Nurs. 77 **7:**34-38, April 1977.

Goodman, L.S., and Gilman, A.: The pharmacological basis of therapeutics, ed. 6, New York, 1980, Macmillan Publishing Co., Inc.

Harrison, J.H., et al.: Cambell's urology, vols. 1 and 3, Philadelphia, 1978, W.B. Saunders Co.

Harvey, A.M., et al.: The principles and practice of medicine, ed. 20, New York, 1980, Appleton-Century-Crofts.

Lapides, J.: Fundamentals of urology, Philadelphia, 1976, W.B. Saunders Co.

Luckmann, J., and Sorensen, K.C.: Medical-surgical nursing: a psychophysiologic approach, ed. 2, Philadelphia, 1980, W.B. Saunders Co.

Mitchell, P.H.: Concepts basic to nursing, ed. 2, New York, 1977, McGraw-Hill Book Co., Inc.

Morel, A., and Wise, G.J.: Urologic endoscopic procedures, ed. 2, St. Louis, 1979, The C.V. Mosby Co.

Phipps, W.J., Long, B.C., and Woods, N.F.: Medical-surgical nursing: concepts and clinical practice, St. Louis, 1979, The C.V. Mosby Co.

Physician's desk reference, ed. 35, Oradell, N.J., 1981, Medical Economics Co.

Schumann, D.: Wound healing in your abdominal surgery patient, Nurs. 80 **10:**34-40, April 1980.

Smith, D.R.: General urology, ed. 9, Los Altos, Calif., 1978, Lange Medical Publications.

Thorn, G.W., et al.: Harrison's principles of internal medicine, ed. 8, New York, 1977, McGraw-Hill Book Co., Inc.

Vogel, C.H.: Keeping patients alive in spite of post-obstructive diuresis, Nurs. 79 **9:**50-56, March 1979.

Winter, C.C., and Morel, A.: Nursing care of the patients with urologic diseases, ed. 4, St. Louis, 1977, The C.V. Mosby Co.

UNIT IX

PROCEDURES FOR DISORDERS
OF
THE PENIS

CHAPTER 47

Circumcision

Circumcision (i.e., the removal of the prepuce from the penis) is done for a variety of reasons on a male of any age. It is often performed on the infant for religious reasons, as in the Jewish and Islamic faiths. It may also be done for hygienic purposes or for prophylactic reasons, since penile cancer is very rare in circumcised males. Later on in life it is usually done for medical reasons to correct phimosis and eliminate the infection that frequently occurs as a result of this condition.

The simplest form of the procedure can be done on infants and young children. It involves the use of a bell-shaped plastic device (Plastibell) that is placed onto the tip of the penis under the prepuce. A string is tied tightly around the rim of the bell (over the prepuce), and the bell portion is then disconnected, leaving the glans exposed with the collar of plastic under the foreskin and string remaining around the foreskin. The prepuce distal to the string becomes ischemic and atrophies. Within 1 week the string cuts through the foreskin and the collar falls off, leaving a well-healed line of excision at the base of the glans. There is some evidence to suggest that the incidence of infection is higher with this method than with surgical excision,[1] and a Plastibell cannot be used for religious circumcisions because a small portion of the prepuce remains at the base of the glans.

When circumcision is done surgically, it is performed by either of two methods. The patient is in a supine position for both. In the simpler procedure the prepuce is pulled forward, and a clamp is applied distal to the tip of the glans. The prepuce is then excised and, as the clamp is removed, the skin slides back, exposing the glans. Sutures are applied in the foreskin around the base of the glans to prevent bleeding (Fig. 47-1).

In the other method the outer and inner surfaces of the prepuce are incised and dissected away, without cutting the larger blood vessels within the prepuce. Retraction of these vessels spontaneously occurs, and sutures are applied to approximate the two surfaces of the prepuce. The advantage of this method is that minimal blood loss occurs, so fewer sutures are required, and the incision heals with less induration. A nonadhesive (Telfa or Vaseline) dressing may or may not be applied after either procedure.

CIRCUMCISION
Outline of Care Plan
ANTICIPATED NURSING DIAGNOSES:

Preoperative period
  1. Need for preoperative teaching.
  2. Need for discharge planning.
Postoperative period
  3. Potential for postoperative complications (shock, atelectasis, pneumonia, urinary retention, deep vein thrombosis).
  4. Potential for wound complications.
  5. Postoperative pain.
Convalescent period
  6. Need for discharge teaching.

Fig. 47-1. Surgical procedures for circumcision. **A,** Prepuce is pulled forward and clamped. **B,** Prepuce is excised. **C,** Penile skin is allowed to slide back over shaft of penis. **D,** Area of incision is sutured.

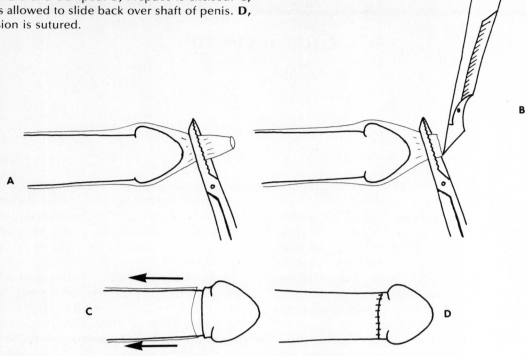

NURSING CARE PLAN FOR THE PATIENT UNDERGOING CIRCUMCISION

1. NURSING DIAGNOSIS: Need for preoperative teaching

Preoperative period

Objectives of nursing intervention

If necessary, clarification of reason for hospitalization and type of surgery to be performed

Elimination of any negative or inaccurate notions regarding the forthcoming surgery

Explanation of preoperative tests and procedures

Psychologic preparation for general anesthesia (omit if the patient is to have spinal or local anesthesia)

Explanation of events expected in the early postoperative period

Explanation of body conditions expected in the early postoperative period

Identification of any known allergies

Expected outcomes

Verbal indication that explanations are understood

Verbal indication of optimistic expectations (within realistic limits) related to forthcoming surgery

Cooperation during preoperative tests and procedures

Verbal or behavioral indication of reduction of anxiety

Absence of postoperative complications

Absence of allergic reactions

Plan for implementation	Rationale
See master care plan for the patient receiving preoperative teaching. In addition to the topics covered in the master care plan, include the following items in the preoperative teaching: 1. If the patient is an adult or an adolescent, the preoperative shave will be of the pubic area. Some surgeons omit the shave altogether.	
2. The patient will be permitted a light meal a few hours after surgery.	These patients can usually tolerate oral intake within a few hours after surgery. For this reason the intravenous infusion used during the surgery is often discontinued in the recovery room or shortly after the patient returns to the urology floor and tolerates fluids.
3. There will be an incision around the corona of the penis, possibly covered by a Vaseline dressing.	

2. NURSING DIAGNOSIS: Need for discharge planning

Objectives of nursing intervention { Early commencement of discharge planning
Accurate estimate of time required for all discharge teaching

Expected outcome Smooth transition of care after discharge

Plan for implementation	Rationale
See master care plan for the patient requiring discharge preparations: discharge planning. In addition to the topics covered in the master care plan, the following items should be considered: 1. The duration of hospitalization for this type of surgery is approximately 24 to 48 hours. Some patients may be discharged in the evening after surgery.	

2. Required teaching includes:
  a. General postoperative discharge teaching
  b. Instructions on removal of dressing on the third postoperative day	

Preoperative period

3. NURSING DIAGNOSIS: Potential for postoperative complications (shock, atelectasis, pneumonia, urinary retention, deep vein thrombosis)

Objective of nursing intervention	Prevention or early detection of postoperative complications

Objective of nursing intervention   Prevention or early detection of postoperative complications

Expected outcomes
  Pulse and blood pressure normal, skin dry, color normal
  Respirations regular and unlabored, absence of pulmonary congestion
  Normal voiding pattern established within 6 hours after surgery
  Early ambulation tolerated well

Plan for implementation	Rationale
1. Check the patient's vital signs every 4 hours and notify the physician of any indications of impending shock. These include: a. Increasing pulse and respiratory rates b. Decreasing blood pressure c. Diaphoresis and pallor d. Feelings of apprehension	Although shock is a potential complication after any kind of surgery, it is a relatively small risk after circumcision because few blood vessels are cut and the duration of surgery is short.
2. Encourage coughing and abdominal breathing if the patient's lungs sound congested, and notify the physician if any of the following conditions are present: a. The patient is unable to cough and his lungs sound congested. b. Sputum volume is copious. c. Sputum color is other than clear or white. d. There is a rise in the patient's temperature. e. Breath sounds are diminished.	Although precautions must be taken, respiratory complications are unlikely after this type of surgery because the period of anesthesia is very short. Furthermore, there is no abdominal incision to inhibit effective coughing. These conditions require additional treatment. The physician may order therapies such as incentive spirometry, nasotracheal suctioning, postural drainage, or intermittent positive pressure breathing, depending on the extent of respiratory embarrassment.
3. Promote resumption of normal voiding pattern by the following actions: a. Be certain the patient is well hydrated. b. Leave urinal at the bedside within reach of the patient. c. Ask the patient to notify the nurse the first time he voids. d. If the patient has not voided within 6 hours after surgery: (1) Assist the patient to a standing position to void. (2) If the patient is still unable to void, notify the physician.	Temporary urinary retention is an occasional result of anesthesia. Assuming the accustomed position for voiding will help the patient to void if the retention is caused by psychologic factors. Catheterization may be required.
4. Use precautions against deep vein thrombosis. (See master care plan for the patient at risk for deep vein thrombosis.) The patient is usually permitted out of bed in the evening after surgery.	Although deep vein thrombosis is a relatively small risk after this type of surgery, it still must be considered, and adequate precautions should be taken.

Postoperative period

4. NURSING DIAGNOSIS: Potential for wound complications

Objective of nursing intervention　　Prevention or early detection of complications arising from the incisional area

Expected outcomes

Absence of fever

Absence of bleeding, edema, erythema, purulent exudate, and other abnormal wound conditions

Suture line intact

Plan for implementation	Rationale
1. Check the dressing (or suture line if no dressing is used) every 4 hours for the first 12 hours after surgery.	Hemorrhage is a potential (though uncommon) complication of circumcision, particularly if the clamp method was employed.
2. If the dressing falls off, do not replace it.	The dressing is not necessary. Many surgeons do not even apply one to the wound in the operating room.
3. If frank bleeding is present, notify the physician.	There should be practically no drainage after circumcision. Any active bleeding is abnormal.
4. Note the condition of the suture line; chart its appearance and the presence of edema, erythema, or other abnormal wound conditions.	This provides a frame of reference for other staff members caring for the patient.
5. If there is purulent drainage: 　a. Notify the physician. 　b. Obtain a wound culture specimen.	This would indicate a wound infection. This will facilitate identification of the infecting organism so that appropriate treatment can be instituted quickly.
6. Check the patient's temperature every 4 hours and notify the physician if there is an elevation above 101°.	Wound infection must be suspected when the patient runs a fever postoperatively.
7. Administer barbiturate sleeping medication as ordered.	If the patient is an adolescent or an adult, some surgeons order a barbiturate to be administered at night for the first few nights after surgery. The purpose of this is to suppress the REM phase of sleep so that the normal sleep pattern erections do not occur. If the sutures are not strong, there is a possibility that they will break if the penis expands. Sleeping medications, other than those in the barbiturate group, do not have this inhibiting effect on the normal erection pattern.

Postoperative period

5. NURSING DIAGNOSIS: Postoperative pain

Objective of nursing intervention   Appropriate management of pain or discomfort

Expected outcome   Behavioral and/or verbal indication that pain is adequately reduced or absent

Plan for implementation	Rationale
1. Determine characteristics of the pain by questioning and observing the patient.	The degree of pain after circumcision varies, but in most cases the pain is minimal.
2. Be alert for indications (verbal or behavioral) that the patient is experiencing discomfort other than physical pain, and attempt to resolve the problem.	Surgery on the sexual organs may give rise to considerable anxiety, which can often be alleviated simply by reassurance from the nurse.
3. If the discomfort is a result of the surgical incision, administer analgesic medication as ordered. A nonnarcotic or a mild narcotic such as codeine is usually adequate.	
4. Note the patient's response to the pain medication.	This provides a frame of reference for evaluation of the patient's condition on subsequent shifts.

6. NURSING DIAGNOSIS: Need for discharge teaching

Objectives of nursing intervention

- Explanation of basic information about medications to be taken at home
- Explanation of information regarding follow-up care
- Explanation of residual effects of the condition and/or treatment
- Explanation of instructions concerning postdischarge activities
- Explanation of symptoms that constitute a reason to contact the physician
- Review of admitting diagnosis and mode of treatment

Expected outcomes

- Accurate return verbalization and/or demonstration of all material learned
- Smooth transition of care after discharge
- Absence or early detection of complications arising after discharge
- Ability to provide future health care practitioners with important data about health history

Postoperative period

Convalescent period

Plan for implementation	**Rationale**
See master care plan for the patient requiring discharge preparations: discharge teaching.	
In addition to the topics covered in the master care plan, include the following items in the discharge teaching:	
1. At the follow-up office visit the physician will check the suture line for adequate healing. The sutures are absorbed and therefore do not need to be removed.	
2. The expected residual effects of this surgery are minimal. The patient should be able to return to his normal activities within a week. Sexual intercourse may be resumed after 1 week.	

3. If the patient has been discharged with a dressing, provide the following instructions:
   a. On the third postoperative day the patient should soak in a warm bath.
   b. The dressing should be allowed to float off.
   c. No medication should be applied to the incision.	

4. If the patient has been given a prescription for barbiturate medication for sleeping: a. Explain the reason (see p. 549).	The patient may not take the medication unless he is aware of its purpose.
b. Inform the patient that after 4 days the sutures are strong enough to withstand erections and the medication is no longer required. (Usually the physician prescribes the medication for 4 days. If it is for a different number of days, make the appropriate changes in the teaching.)	
5. The patient should notify the physician if any of the following occur: a. Swelling at the incisional area	This may indicate an infection or, if the swelling is large, it may be a hematoma.
b. Purulent drainage	This would indicate a wound infection.

Convalescent period

CHAPTER 48

Urethroplasty

The operative repair of a defect in the urethra may be done in numerous ways, depending on the nature of the defect, the age of the patient, and the surgeon's preference. It is indicated in patients with urethral strictures, trauma to the penis, epispadias, hypospadias, and various other conditions. Because the forms of urethroplasty differ considerably, there is no standard nursing care plan that can be applied to all or even a group of these procedures. The duration of hospitalization, the number of operations involved in the correction, the use of catheters and drains, and the type of convalescence vary for each method.

Therefore the most commonly performed procedures are discussed, followed by a description of what the nurse might expect regarding patient care. However, each surgeon has personal preferences in patient management, and the nurse will have to formulate a care plan based on the particular orders given by the surgeon.

Urethroplasty in childhood is most commonly done for hypospadias, a birth defect in which the urethra terminates on the ventral surface of the penis or sometimes at the penoscrotal junction or the perineum. When the degree of hypospadias is not severe, it may be corrected by a single-stage procedure in which an incision is made in the penis to outline a strip of skin extending from the meatus to the corona. The edges of the strip are sutured to form an extension of the urethra, and the remaining skin is sutured together to cover the newly formed urethra (Fig. 48-1).

If the patient has severe hypospadias accompanied by chordee (ventral curvature of the penis), a two-stage repair is used. The first stage consists of excision of the fibrous bands distal to the urethral meatus, which releases the chordee. The skin defect is then covered with foreskin and allowed to heal. Six to 12 months later the second stage is performed, which is similar to the single-stage procedure just described.

If the child had been circumcised prior to correction of hypospadias, multistage, complicated surgery is required.

After these procedures the nurse may expect to find orders regarding a compression dressing around the penis, an indwelling urethral catheter or suprapubic drainage tube, and possibly daily enemas to prevent straining and rectal distention.

One of the more common forms of urethroplasty performed on the adult is the patch urethroplasty, which is used for strictures of the pendulous urethra. The procedure involves a longitudinal incision along the ventral aspect of the penis to expose the strictured portion of the urethra. This area of the urethra is then incised, and the lumen is laid open. A full-thickness graft is taken from a hairless area (the prepuce) and trimmed to the appropriate size. The edges of the graft are then sutured to the edges of the urethra (Fig. 48-2). The skin incision is closed without drainage, and a dressing is applied. A urethral catheter may or may not be left indwelling, depending on the surgeon's preference. Sometimes a suprapubic tube is used.

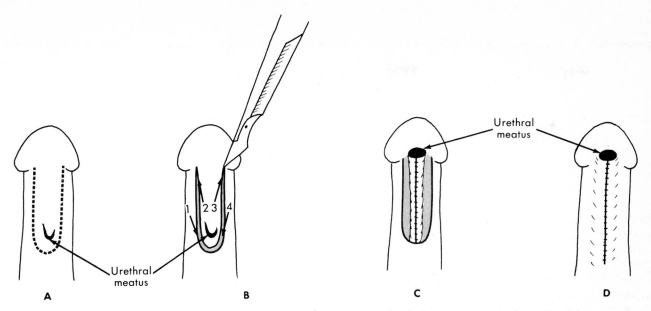

Fig. 48-1. Single-stage urethroplasty for hypospadias. **A,** Location of incision is outlined. **B,** Incision is made, producing four edges of skin (*1, 2, 3* and *4*). **C,** Skin edges *2* and *3* are sutured together in a tubelike fashion to form the new urethra. **D,** Skin edges *1* and *4* are sutured together to cover the new urethra. NOTE: The new meatus is now located in a functional position for voiding, sexual intercourse, and insemination. If desired, additional surgery may be done to bring the meatus to the tip of the glans for cosmetic purposes.

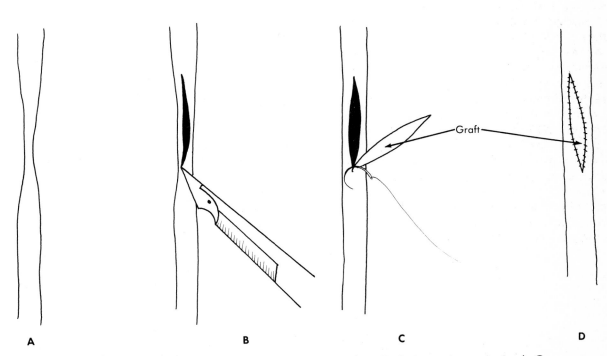

Fig. 48-2. "Patch" urethroplasty. **A,** Strictured urethra. **B,** Strictured area incised. **C,** Graft is sutured into incision to augment urethra. **D,** Completed urethroplasty.

CHAPTER 49

Partial or total penectomy

Penectomy is a procedure done primarily for carcinoma of the penis when the lesion cannot be successfully treated by radiotherapy. The amputation may be partial or total, depending on the extent of the lesion.

When the lesion is limited only to the glans, a partial penectomy is performed. For the procedure the patient is placed in a lithotomy position, and a tourniquet is applied around the penis. Skin flaps are marked, and an incision is made to amputate a portion of the corpora cavernosa and corpus spongiosum. Hemostasis is achieved by ligating arterial branches in the corpora. The urethra is anastomosed to the skin, and a dressing is applied.

Total penectomy is required when the lesion has penetrated the shaft of the penis or when the tumor has recurred after radiation treatment and conservation of an adequate stump is impossible.

For total penectomy the patient is placed in a lithotomy position and an incision is made, starting at the pubic bone. The incision encircles the penis and extends into the perineum. The roots of both corpora cavernosa are exposed and excised, and the penis is amputated. Hemostasis is achieved by ligation of bleeding vessels. A perineal urethrotomy is then performed by anastomosing the bulbar urethra to the skin. An indwelling urethral catheter is inserted, an incisional drain is placed in the wound, and the incision is then closed (Fig. 49-1). A compression dressing is applied to prevent scrotal edema.

Fig. 49-1. Location for drains and incision after total penectomy.

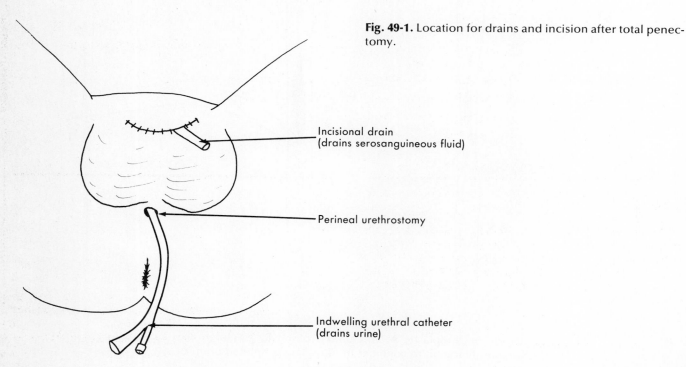

Incisional drain
(drains serosanguineous fluid)

Perineal urethrostomy

Indwelling urethral catheter
(drains urine)

PARTIAL OR TOTAL PENECTOMY
Outline of Care Plan
ANTICIPATED NURSING DIAGNOSES:

Preoperative period
1. Need for preoperative teaching.
2. Need for discharge planning.
3. Psychologic distress related to forthcoming changes in body image.

Early postoperative period
4. Potential for shock.
5. Potential for wound complications.
6. Need for management of indwelling urethral catheter.*

7. Need for management of intravenous infusion.
8. Postoperative pain.
9. Potential for respiratory complications related to surgical intervention.
10. Potential for deep vein thrombosis.
11. Continued need for psychologic assistance in coping with partial or total loss of the penis.

Late postoperative period
12. Potential for voiding complications following removal of indwelling urethral catheter.*

Convalescent period
13. Need for discharge teaching.

*May not apply.

*May not apply.

NURSING CARE PLAN FOR THE PATIENT UNDERGOING PARTIAL OR TOTAL PENECTOMY

1. NURSING DIAGNOSIS: Need for preoperative teaching

Objectives of nursing intervention

If necessary, clarification of reason for hospitalization and type of surgery to be performed

Elimination of any negative or inaccurate notions regarding the forthcoming surgery

Explanation of preoperative tests and procedures

Psychologic preparation for general anesthesia (omit if the patient is to have spinal anesthesia)

Explanation of events expected in the early postoperative period

Explanation of body conditions expected in the early postoperative period

Identification of any known allergies

Expected outcomes

Verbal indication that explanations are understood

Verbal indication of optimistic expectations (within realistic limits) related to forthcoming surgery

Cooperation during preoperative tests and procedures

Verbal or behavioral indication of reduction of anxiety

Absence of postoperative complications

Absence of allergic reactions

Plan for implementation	Rationale

See master care plan for the patient receiving preoperative teaching.
 	
In addition to the topics covered in the master care plan, include the following items in the preoperative teaching:
1. Be aware that, in addition to routine preoperative tests, the following diagnostic studies may have been performed, and answer any questions the patient has regarding them:
  a. Biopsy of penile lesion
 	
  b. Chest x-ray examination and tomogram
	
	This is frequently done before admission. It establishes the diagnosis of carcinoma of the penis.
	These are done to determine the presence of distal metastasis.

Preoperative period

555

Plan for implementation	Rationale
c. Bone and liver scans	Same as preceding rationale.
d. Computerized tomography (CT scan) of the pelvis	Same as preceding rationale.
e. Bilateral pedal lymphangiogram	This is sometimes done to determine the presence of malignant tissue in the lymph nodes (particularly the inguinal and subinguinal nodes).

2. The preoperative shave will be from umbilicus to mid-thigh.

3. The patient will probably be permitted fluids a few hours after surgery and a light meal in the evening.

4. If the patient is to have a total penectomy:
   a. There will be an indwelling urethral catheter in place for 24 to 48 hours.
   b. There will be a dressing over the incisional area that will be held tightly in place against the perineum.

5. If the patient is to have a partial penectomy:
   a. There will be a dressing around his penis.
   b. The patient may have an indwelling urethral catheter for 24 to 48 hours after surgery.

Preoperative period

2. NURSING DIAGNOSIS: Need for discharge teaching

Objectives of nursing intervention { Early commencement of discharge planning
Accurate estimate of time required for all discharge teaching

Expected outcome Smooth transition of care after discharge

Plan for implementation	Rationale
See master care plan for the patient requiring discharge preparations: discharge planning.	
In addition to the topics covered in the master care plan, the following items should be considered: 1. Hospitalization for partial penectomy is approximately 1 week; for a total penectomy it is approximately 10 days.	

2. Required teaching includes:
  a. General postoperative discharge teaching
  b. Discussion of the need for frequent follow-up examinations	

3. Available community resources for psychiatric and sexual counseling should be sought out and identified.	If the nurse is aware of the types of services available in the community, he or she will be more capable of making appropriate referrals.

Preoperative period

3. NURSING DIAGNOSIS: Psychologic distress related to forthcoming changes in body image

Objective of nursing intervention Provision of a supportive environment in which the patient can begin to adjust to the forthcoming changes in his body image

Expected outcomes
- Ability to express feelings concerning his condition
- Absence of severe or protracted depression

Preoperative period

Plan for implementation	Rationale
1. Be aware that, no matter how accepting the patient may appear, the forthcoming surgery will create severe emotional difficulties.	After partial penectomy the patient will have to adjust to considerable changes in his body image. After total penectomy those changes will be far greater, and he will also have to adjust to major changes in body functions. He will no longer be able to have penile-vaginal intercourse, and he will no longer be able to void in a standing position.
2. Encourage the patient (and wife) to verbalize any feelings he (they) might have regarding the forthcoming surgery.	
3. Convey willingness to listen.	
4. Provide emotional support and encouragement.	
5. Without negating the patient's feelings, present alternative points of view. For example:	
a. If the patient is to have a partial penectomy, it sometimes helps to emphasize the fact that at least the patient will avoid the radical changes associated with a total penectomy. b. If the patient is to have a total penectomy, he is sometimes helped by the reminder that the alternative to the surgery would mean continued spread of a disease that would eventually be fatal.*	The patient is usually so preoccupied with the sense of impending loss of manhood that he is unable to see his situation from any other point of view. However, mentioning the alternatives may help. It will also help the patient indirectly if the **nurse** remembers the alternatives and is therefore able to maintain a positive attitude. This is very disturbing surgery for anybody to confront, even caregivers; but **pity** on the part of the nurse can have no beneficial value.
6. Suggest psychiatric counseling for the patient (and/or wife) if deemed appropriate.	Usually it is the attending physician who makes the official request that the patient be seen by a psychiatrist during his hospitalization. However, since nurses are with the patient on a more continual basis, they may be the first to detect the need for psychiatric assistance.
7. Provide information regarding sexual counseling services available in the community.	

*For most patients the possibility that death will eventually result from this "small" lesion on the penis (if it is not treated) seems remote. They are rarely suffering from any severe systemic symptoms and, except for the discomfort caused by the lesion, they usually feel quite well. Therefore the impending loss of the penis is frequently their consuming thought, not the potential loss of their life. For this reason, a section on the psychologic difficulties in adjusting to the diagnosis of cancer has been omitted from this chapter. However, the immediate problem (i.e., the changes brought on by the surgery) can sometimes be dealt with in a more realistic way once the patient **fully** recognizes what the long-range ramifications of his illness actually are.

4. NURSING DIAGNOSIS: Potential for shock

Objective of nursing intervention   Prevention or early detection of shock

Expected outcomes { Vital signs normal, skin dry, color normal
Absence of bright red drainage

Plan for implementation	Rationale
1. Check the patient's vital signs every 4 hours once stable (every 15 minutes if unstable).	Although there is relatively little blood loss during the surgery, if any of the internal sutures slip, considerable bleeding may occur, and hemorrhagic shock is a definite possibility.
2. Be alert for increasing pulse and respiratory rates, decreasing blood pressure, diaphoresis, pallor, and feelings of apprehension.	
3. Notify the physician at once if indications of impending shock occur.	

5. NURSING DIAGNOSIS: Potential for wound complications

Objective of nursing intervention   Prevention or early detection of complications arising from the incisional area

Expected outcome   Absence of dehiscence, hemorrhage, fever, purulent exudate, erythema, edema, hematoma, and other abnormal wound conditions

Plan for implementation	Rationale
1. Check the dressing frequently (every 2 to 4 hours) during the first 24 to 48 hours after surgery.	There may be a moderate amount of drainage after total penectomy because one or two incisional drains are usually used.
2. Notify the physician if there is any unusual bleeding.	Drainage from the incision is usually serosanguineous. Frank bleeding is abnormal.
3. Change the dressing if necessary, using sterile technique.	

Early postoperative period

Plan for implementation	Rationale
4. After total penectomy, maintain a dressing with mild compression for at least 12 to 24 hours postoperatively. This type of dressing can be constructed by applying a scrotal support over a few gauze pads tightly packed against the perineum.	

5. If there is purulent drainage:
  a. Notify the physician.
  b. Obtain a wound culture specimen.
	This would indicate a wound infection.
	
	This will facilitate identification of the infecting organism so that appropriate treatment can be instituted quickly.

6. Check the patient's temperature every 4 hours and notify the physician if there is an elevation above 101°.	Wound infection must always be suspected when a patient runs a fever postoperatively. Other causes include respiratory complications and pharmacologic intervention.
7. Administer barbiturate sleeping medication as ordered (only applies to the patient who has undergone a partial penectomy).	Some surgeons order a barbiturate to be administered at night for the first few nights after surgery. The purpose is to suppress the REM phase of sleep so that normal sleep pattern erections do not occur. Such erections might disrupt the surgical site. Sleeping medications, other than those in the barbiturate group, do not have this inhibiting effect on the normal erection pattern.

Early postoperative period

6. NURSING DIAGNOSIS: Need for management of indwelling urethral catheter*

Objectives of nursing intervention
- Appropriate care of catheter and equipment
- Prevention or early detection of infection
- Care of tissue surrounding catheter
- Maintenance of accurate records of urine output
- Appropriate administration of hand-irrigation of catheter
- Management of discomfort or pain caused by catheter
- Satisfactory collection of urine specimens from catheter

Expected outcomes
- Absence of severe bladder spasms and suprapubic distention
- Urine draining freely through system
- Absence of fever, chills, and foul-smelling urine
- Absence of urethral discharge and tissue inflammation
- Minimal discomfort caused by the catheter
- Urine specimens in optimum condition for all necessary tests

Plan for implementation	Rationale
See master care plan for the patient with an indwelling urethral catheter: care after insertion of the catheter.	
In addition to the topics covered in the master care plan, the following interventions are required:	
1. Use caution when performing catheter care to prevent disruption of the surgical site.	
2. Notify the physician if there is any blood in the urine.	Catheter drainage after this surgery should be clear amber.

Early postoperative period

*May not apply.

561

Early postoperative period

7. NURSING DIAGNOSIS: Need for management of intravenous infusion

Objectives of nursing intervention
- Appropriate administration of specific types of intravenous solutions
- Prevention or early detection of local complications
- Prevention or early detection of systemic complications
- Management of discomfort caused by the intravenous infusion
- Maintenance of proper function of intravenous equipment
- Maintenance of accurate records of the patient's hydration status

Expected outcomes
- Normal hydration status
- Normal electrolyte status
- Absence of thrombophlebitis, infiltration, infection, fluid overload, and pulmonary embolism
- Absence of discomfort caused by the intravenous infusion

Plan for implementation	Rationale
See master care plan for the patient receiving intravenous therapy.	Although the patient can usually tolerate fluids shortly after surgery, an intravenous line may be left in place until the following morning, when the risk of hemorrhage has passed.

8. NURSING DIAGNOSIS: Postoperative pain

Objective of nursing intervention
Appropriate management of pain or discomfort

Expected outcome
Behavioral and/or verbal indication that pain is adequately reduced or absent

Plan for implementation	Rationale
Determine the source of the pain. It may be related to the catheter (if used) or the surgical wound.	Pain from different sources usually requires different intervention.
1. Question and observe the patient to obtain information about the pain.	
2. Be aware that pain is a unique and individual experience. Although the different sources of pain can usually be determined by their characteristics, there are also many variations.	

Plan for implementation	**Rationale**
3. Be alert for indications (verbal or behavioral) that the patient is experiencing discomfort other than physical pain, and attempt to resolve the problem.	Fear, loneliness, depression, and numerous other conditions may be sources of extreme discomfort for the patient, who may unconsciously translate these feelings into pain.

PERSISTENT, SEVERE, INCREASING PAIN IN SUPRAPUBIC AREA*

See Chapter 11, part one, nursing objective 6.	This pain is probably caused by an obstructed catheter.

SPASMODIC, INTERMITTENT PAIN IN SUPRAPUBIC AREA, OR PAIN RADIATING TO URETHRAL AREA*

See Chapter 11, part one, nursing objective 6.	This pain is probably caused by the catheter's irritating effect on the bladder.

MODERATE TO SEVERE PAIN AT SURGICAL SITE, USUALLY AGGRAVATED BY PHYSICAL ACTIVITY

1. Be certain the catheter is not obstructed.* Although pain with these characteristics is usually of incisional origin and is expected, the patient may not be able to identify accurately the precise location of the pain.	Catheter obstruction must be ruled out first because it cannot remain untreated. However, after this type of surgery it is unlikely for the catheter to become obstructed because there is no blood in the drainage for clots to form, and no tissue particles are normally passed in the urine.
2. Administer analgesics as ordered.	Analgesic medication usually provides considerable relief from incisional pain.
3. Plan the patient's activities to coincide with a time when there is a high level of pain medication in the patient's bloodstream.	The patient will cooperate better with ambulating, bathing, etc. when the pain is well under control.
4. Notify the physician if the patient's requests for pain medication do not decrease within 48 to 72 hours.	Although the intensity of postoperative pain varies enormously between patients, there should be a marked decrease in the apparent severity of the pain within 2 or 3 days. If this does not occur, it may indicate the development of wound complications.

Early postoperative period

*Only applies to the patient with an indwelling urethral catheter.

9. NURSING DIAGNOSIS: Potential for respiratory complications related to surgical intervention

Objective of nursing intervention	Prevention or early detection of atelectasis and/or pneumonia

Expected outcomes	Cooperation with therapeutic respiratory regimen Absence of fever or audible lung congestion Sputum clear or white and easily mobilized

Plan for implementation	Rationale
See master care plan for the patient at risk for respiratory complications, nursing objective 1.	

10. NURSING DIAGNOSIS: Potential for deep vein thrombosis

Objectives of nursing intervention	Explanation and maintenance of precautions against deep vein thrombosis Early detection of deep vein thrombosis

Expected outcomes	Cooperation with regimen to prevent deep vein thrombosis Absence of local pain, swelling, and redness of a lower extremity Absence of fever

Plan for implementation	Rationale
See master care plan for the patient at risk for deep vein thrombosis.	

Early postoperative period

11. NURSING DIAGNOSIS: Continued need for psychologic assistance in coping with partial or total loss of penis

Objectives of nursing intervention { Careful surveillance of the patient's psychologic status
Maintenance of a supportive environment

Expected outcomes { Ability to look at the operative site
Ability to verbalize feelings
Absence of severe or protracted depression

Plan for implementation	Rationale
1. Maintain accurate records of the patient's psychologic status throughout the postoperative and convalescent periods.	This provides a frame of reference for other staff members caring for the patient.
2. Report any sudden mood changes or prolonged depression.	The possibility of suicide attempts should never be entirely ruled out after this type of surgery. The symbolic meaning a man attaches to his penis may appear more important to him than his life. He may feel completely unable to cope with the radical changes in his body image, especially after a total penectomy.
3. Provide adequate privacy for the patient whenever dressing changes or examinations are required.	
4. Be aware that the initial sight of the surgical area may be extremely upsetting for the patient.	
5. Be careful not to communicate one's **own** feelings when viewing the surgical site; be particularly aware of facial expressions.	Although urology nurses eventually become accustomed to the sight of a penectomy incision, there are few who can look at it without some emotional reaction to the change in the patient's body. These feelings can be easily transmitted by minute facial movements and can hinder the patient's adjustment. On the other hand, if nurses convey to the patient that they still see him as a whole person, his concept of himself may become less identified with his physical being, and he may begin to view himself as still a complete man.
6. Provide continued emotional support of the patient (and his wife).	
7. If the patient (and/or his wife) has previously rejected the possibility of psychiatric or sexual counseling, be alert for any indications that the attitude might be changing, and take appropriate actions if this is the case.	Professional assistance in dealing with the massive psychologic and sexual adjustments can make a tremendous difference in the patient's future psychologic well-being.

Early postoperative period

12. NURSING DIAGNOSIS: Potential for voiding complications following removal of indwelling urethral catheter (if used)

Objective of nursing intervention	Prevention or early detection of complications

Expected outcomes { Resumption of normal voiding pattern
Absence of dysuria

Plan for implementation	**Rationale**
See master care plan for the patient with an indwelling urethral catheter: care after removal of the catheter.	
In addition to the items covered in the master care plan, if total penectomy was performed, the psychologic aspects of having to void in a sitting position must be considered.	
1. Provide the patient with privacy at all times.	
2. Mention that some patients initially feel uneasy voiding in a sitting position. With time, however, they adjust.	This indirectly reminds the patient that he is not the only one who has had this kind of surgery. It also lets him know that his feelings are normal and probably temporary.

Late postoperative period

13. NURSING DIAGNOSIS: Need for discharge teaching

Objectives of nursing intervention

Explanation of basic information about medications to be taken at home
Explanation of information regarding follow-up care
Explanation of residual effects of the condition and/or treatment
Explanation of instructions concerning postdischarge activities
Explanation of symptoms that constitute a reason to contact the physician
Review of admitting diagnosis and mode of treatment

Expected outcomes

Accurate return verbalization and/or demonstration of all material learned
Smooth transition of care after discharge
Absence or early detection of complications arising after discharge
Ability to provide future health care practitioners with important data about health history

Plan for implementation	Rationale
See master care plan for the patient requiring discharge preparations: discharge teaching.	
In addition to the topics covered in the master care plan, include the following items in the discharge teaching:	
1. At the follow-up office visit the physician will check the wound for adequate healing. The patient will then be scheduled for follow-up examinations approximately every 6 months, during which the physician will palpate the local skin area to check for recurrence of the lesion. Chest x-ray examinations and bone scans may be done on a yearly basis.	Careful follow-up management is necessary because of the possibility of local recurrence or metastatic spread of the disease.
2. During the next few weeks the expected residual effects of the surgery include incisional discomfort and fatigue.	
3. The patient should notify the physician if any of the following occur:	
a. Severe pain, swelling, or increasing redness at the incisional site.	This may indicate an infection.
b. Any exudate or changes in the integrity of the skin at or near the incisional area.	This may indicate recurrence of the lesion.
4. Give the patient written information regarding where he can turn for psychologic assistance if he is not being seen by a psychiatrist at the time of discharge.	Sometimes the most difficult period of psychologic adjustment occurs after the patient leaves the hospital. He should know that there are places to which he can turn for help if needed.

Convalescent period

CHAPTER 50

Implantation of penile prosthesis

The implantation of a penile prosthesis is a relatively new surgical procedure. It enables a man whose erection is inadequate for genital intercourse to have satisfactory coitus.* It is usually only performed after other methods to correct sexual impotence have failed. Many patients who are candidates for a penile prosthesis suffer from impotence secondary to diabetes.

There are two kinds of devices—the inflatable and the noninflatable or semirigid types (Figs. 50-1 to

*Occasionally a prosthesis is used for patients with severe incontinence where phallus size or configuration makes fitting of an external catheter difficult or impossible.

50-3). Although there may be some variations in the surgical approach, in general, for implantation of the inflatable type the patient is placed in a supine position. A vertical or transverse suprapubic incision is made, and the spherical reservoir is placed in the prevesical space. The corpora cavernosa are then exposed at the base of the penis, and they are dilated distally and proximally. After determining the appropriate size, the surgeon inserts the rods into the corpora. The pump is then positioned in the most dependent portion of the scrotum. Once the three components are connected (rods, reservoir, and pump), the device is checked for proper inflation and deflation. It is then left in the partially

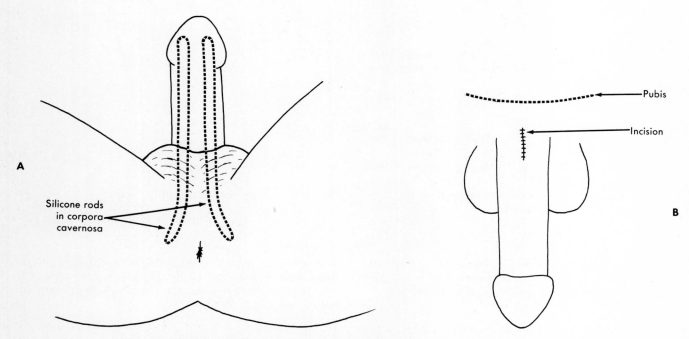

Fig. 50-1. Noninflatable penile prosthesis. **A,** Location of silicone rods. **B,** Location of incision.

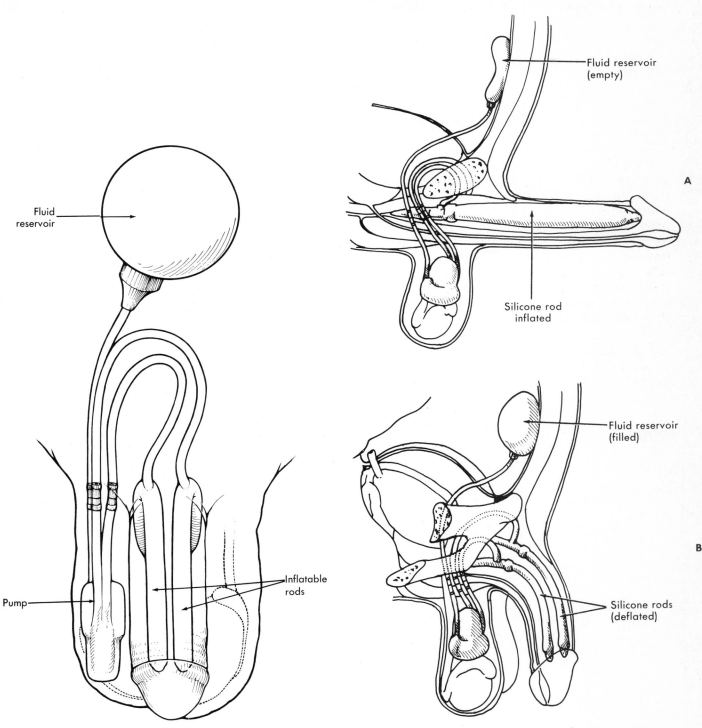

Fig. 50-2. Inflatable penile prosthesis, frontal view. (Courtesy American Medical Systems, Inc., Minneapolis, Minn.)

Fig. 50-3. Inflatable penile prosthesis, sagittal view. **A,** Penis in erect position. **B,** Penis in flaccid position. (Courtesy American Medical Systems, Inc., Minneapolis, Minn.)

inflated position to promote proper healing and reduce bleeding. The incision is then closed, and a dressing is applied. An indwelling urethral catheter may be inserted to prevent urinary retention due to edema.

For implantation of the noninflatable semirigid type the patient is placed in a supine position. A vertical incision is made at the base of the dorsal surface of the penis. Each corpus cavernosum is incised and dilated distally and proximally, and the rods are inserted. The main incision is then closed. A mild compression dressing may be applied, and an indwelling urethral catheter may be inserted to prevent urinary retention from edema.

The psychologic aspects of this surgery are far more complicated than the actual physical procedure. Although this is certainly elective surgery, the patient may still have ambiguous feelings about having a mechanical device implanted in his penis. The primary concern is usually related to his partner's response to the prosthesis. If he is married, his wife is encouraged to be present in the preliminary discussions with the physician. If, however, there is no sex partner at the time of surgery, the uncertainty about the acceptance of his prosthesis by some future sex partner may be a source of considerable anxiety for the patient.

IMPLANTATION OF PENILE PROSTHESIS
Outline of Care Plan
ANTICIPATED NURSING DIAGNOSES:

Preoperative period
1. Embarrassment about the nature of the surgery.*
2. Need for preoperative teaching.
3. Potential for disturbances in diabetes control.*
4. Need for discharge planning.

Early postoperative period
5. Potential for postoperative complications (shock, atelectasis, pneumonia, urinary retention, deep vein thrombosis).
6. Potential for wound complications.
7. Postoperative pain.
8. Continued potential for disturbance in diabetes control.*
9. Need for management of indwelling urethral catheter.*
10. Need for management of intravenous infusion.

Late postoperative period
11. Potential complications after removal of indwelling urethral catheter.*
12. Need for instruction on inflation and deflation procedure.†
13. Need for assistance in adjusting to change in body image.‡

Convalescent period
14. Need for discharge teaching.

---

*May not apply.
†Only applies to the patient with an inflatable prosthesis.
‡Only applies to the patient with a noninflatable prosthesis.

NURSING CARE PLAN FOR THE PATIENT UNDERGOING SURGICAL IMPLANTATION OF A PENILE PROSTHESIS

1. NURSING DIAGNOSIS: Embarrassment about the nature of the surgery*

Objective of nursing intervention	Provision of an accepting environment in which the patient feels comfortable expressing his feelings
Expected outcome	Ability to discuss forthcoming surgery without indications of anxiety

Preoperative period

Plan for implementation	Rationale
1. Convey acceptance of the nature of the surgery, and express willingness to discuss it with the patient.	In spite of his decision to have the surgery, the patient may be somewhat apprehensive about it. If the nurse is a female, the patient may be particularly self-conscious. A positive attitude toward the surgery on the part of a female nurse may help the patient in the following ways: 1. If the patient is unmarried, the nurse may be the first woman with whom he is discussing the surgery. Unconsciously the patient may regard her reactions as

---

*This may not apply; some patients are quite comfortable with their decision to have an implant.

Plan for implentation	Rationale
	indicative of a woman's reaction **in general.** If her reaction is one of acceptance, the patient may develop a more optimistic expectation about a future sex partner's reactions.
	2. If the patient is married, the nurse's positive attitude may help the wife's psychologic adjustment.
2. Convey having had prior experience in caring for patients undergoing the same type of surgery.	This will help the patient realize that there are many others like him who have had this surgery (i.e., he is not a "freak"). It will also increase his confidence in the nurse, and he will be more willing to ask questions.
3. Use a scientific, impersonal approach when discussing the surgery.	An objective approach is less threatening to the patient. It will also help to decrease any anxiety the nurse may have about the discussion of intimate sexual matters, if the patient chooses to discuss them.
4. Respect the patient's desire for privacy by using drapes and curtains whenever needed, and avoid unnecessary discussion whenever other patients are within hearing distance.	If the patient is aware that the nurse is sensitive to his feelings, it will increase his sense of trust and his willingness to communicate any problems.

2. **NURSING DIAGNOSIS:** Need for preoperative teaching

Objectives of nursing intervention

- Elimination of any negative or inaccurate notions regarding the forthcoming surgery
- Explanation of preoperative tests and procedures
- Psychologic preparation for general anesthesia (omit if the patient is to have spinal or local anesthesia)
- Explanation of events expected in the early postoperative period
- Explanation of body conditions expected in the early postoperative period
- Identification of any known allergies

Expected outcomes

- Verbal indication that explanations are understood
- Verbal indication of optimistic expectations (within realistic limits) related to forthcoming surgery
- Cooperation with preoperative tests and procedures
- Verbal or behavioral indication of reduction of anxiety
- Absence of postoperative complications
- Absence of allergic reactions

Plan for implementation	Rationale

See master care plan for the patient receiving preoperative teaching.

In addition to the topics covered in the master care plan, include the following items in the preoperative teaching:

Preoperative period

Plan for implementation	Rationale
1. The preoperative shave will be from umbilicus to mid-thigh. Sometimes Betadine scrubs to the abdomen and genitalia will also be prescribed for the day before surgery.	Since infection is the major complication associated with this type of surgery, additional cleansing measures are sometimes employed to promote as clean a skin surface as possible.
2. The patient will probably be permitted fluids a few hours after surgery and a light meal that evening.	
3. There will be an incision covered by a dressing either in the suprapubic area or on the dorsal side of the patient's penis, depending on the type of prosthesis to be implanted.	
4. There may be an indwelling urethral catheter in place for 1 or 2 days.	The use of a catheter is at the physician's discretion. The risk of urinary retention from edema must be weighed against the risk of infection associated with catheter drainage.
5. The patient will receive parenteral antibiotics preoperatively as well as for a few days after surgery.	Infection is the major complication of all prosthetic surgery. Prophylactic use of antibiotics is therefore an important aspect of patient management. The parenteral (IV or IM) route is used, despite the patient's ability to have oral intake shortly after surgery because some of the antibiotics that may be given (e.g., gentamicin) are not effective when taken orally.

Preoperative period

3. NURSING DIAGNOSIS: Potential for disturbances in diabetes control*

Objective of nursing intervention	Prevention or early detection of hypoglycemia or severe hyperglycemia

Expected outcomes

{
- Serum glucose levels close to baseline readings
- Glycosuria absent or within acceptable range
- Absence of ketonuria
- Absence of diaphoresis, tremor, tachycardia, hunger, irritability, headache, and other symptoms of hypoglycemia
}

Plan for implementation	Rationale
1. Carefully monitor the patient's urine for sugar and acetone. a. Keep accurate records of all measurements. b. Administer insulin according to levels of glycosuria as ordered.	The stress of hospitalization and change in routine may affect insulin requirements in an otherwise stable diabetic.
2. Check laboratory values for serum glucose and report any values differing considerably from the baseline levels when the patient was admitted.	
3. Check with the physician before administering any insulin to a patient who is fasting.	Administration of insulin to a fasting patient could result in severe hypoglycemia. However, frequently the stress of anesthesia and surgery more than compensates for lack of dietary carbohydrate, and insulin may still be required.
4. If glycosuria is absent, observe the patient for indications of hypoglycemia. These include diaphoresis, tremor, tachycardia, hunger, irritability, pallor, headache, blurred vision, confusion, and loss of consciousness.	
5. If any of the conditions in no. 4 are observed, notify the physician at once, and do the following: a. If the patient is able to have oral intake, administer 2 teaspoons of sugar in an 8-ounce glass of orange juice at once. b. If the patient is unable to have oral intake, administer intravenous dextrose in water (D/50/W) and possibly glucagon as ordered by the physician.	A rapid intake of sugar will reverse hypoglycemia within 10 to 20 minutes. Rapid administration of dextrose will reverse the patient's condition within a few minutes. Administration of glucagon will have similar effects.
6. In general, ensure that patients who are diabetic are scheduled for surgery early in the day.	This minimizes the effects of fasting on ketosis.

Preoperative period

*May not apply. However, since many of these patients suffer from impotence secondary to diabetes, this section has been included. For detailed nursing management of a diabetic surgical patient, consult a medical-surgical nursing textbook.

4. NURSING DIAGNOSIS: Need for discharge planning

Objectives of nursing intervention { Early commencement of discharge planning
Accurate estimate of time required for all discharge teaching

Expected outcome   Smooth transition of care after discharge

Plan for implementation	Rationale

Preoperative period

See master care plan for the patient requiring discharge preparations: discharge planning.

In addition to the topics covered in the master care plan, the following items should be considered:
1. The duration of hospitalization for this surgery is approximately 5 to 10 days, depending on the type of prosthesis implanted. The inflatable kind requires longer hospitalization.

2. Required teaching includes:
   a. General postoperative discharge teaching
   b. Instruction on manipulation of inflatable type of prosthesis

---

5. NURSING DIAGNOSIS: Potential for postoperative complications (shock, atelectasis, pneumonia, urinary retention, deep vein thrombosis)

Objective of nursing intervention   Prevention or early detection of postoperative complications

Expected outcomes { Pulse and blood pressure normal, skin dry, color normal

Respirations regular and unlabored, absence of pulmonary congestion

Normal voiding pattern established within 6 hours after surgery (if no catheter is present)

Early ambulation tolerated well

Plan for implementation	Rationale

Early postoperative period

1. Check the patient's vital signs every 4 hours, and notify the physician of any indications of impending shock. These include:
   a. Increasing pulse and respiratory rates
   b. Decreasing blood pressure
   c. Diaphoresis and pallor
   d. Feelings of apprehension

Although shock is a potential complication after any kind of surgery, it is a relatively small risk after implantation of a penile prosthesis because few blood vessels are cut and the duration of surgery is short.

Plan for implementation	**Rationale**
2. Encourage coughing and abdominal breathing if the patient's lungs sound congested, and notify the physician if any of the following conditions are present:	Although precautions must be taken, respiratory complications are unlikely after this type of surgery because the period of anesthesia is short and effective coughing is usually not hindered by pain from the incision.

a. The patient is unable to cough and his lungs sound congested.
  b. Sputum volume is copious.
  c. Sputum color is other than clear or white.
  d. There is a rise in the patient's temperature.
  e. Breath sounds are diminished.
	These conditions require additional treatment. The physician may order therapies such as incentive spirometry, nasotracheal suctioning, postural drainage, or intermittent positive pressure breathing, depending on the extent of respiratory embarrassment.

3. Promote resumption of normal voiding pattern by the following actions*:
  a. Be certain the patient is well hydrated.
  b. Leave a urinal at the bedside within reach of the patient.
  c. Ask the patient to notify the nurse the first time he voids.
  d. If the patient has not voided within 6 hours after surgery:
    (1) Assist the patient to a standing position to void.
 	
    (2) If the patient is still unable to void, notify the physician.
	Temporary urinary retention is occasionally a result of anesthesia and/or edema near the urethra.
	
	Assuming the accustomed position for voiding will help the patient to void if the retention is due to psychologic factors.
	Catheterization may be required.

4. Use precautions against deep vein thrombosis. (See master care plan for the patient at risk for deep vein thrombosis.) These patients are sometimes permitted out of bed in the evening after surgery.	Although deep vein thrombosis is a relatively small risk after this type of surgery, it still must be considered, and adequate precautions should be taken.

Early postoperative period →

---

*Only applies to the patient who does not have an indwelling urethral catheter after surgery.

Early postoperative period

6. NURSING DIAGNOSIS: Potential for wound complications

Objective of nursing intervention	Prevention or early detection of complications arising from the incisional area
Expected outcome	Absence of fever, purulent exudate, erythema, edema, hematoma, and other abnormal wound conditions

Plan for implementation	Rationale
1. Check the dressing every shift. If it requires changing:	Drainage is very slight or absent after this type of surgery, since no incisional drains are used. However, if the patient has a penile dressing (i.e., for the noninflatable type of prosthesis), it may slip and/or become saturated with urine. In either case it should be changed to prevent irritation of the incision.
a. Use sterile technique for the procedure.	
b. Note the condition of the suture line; chart its appearance and the presence of edema, erythema, or other abnormal wound conditions.	This provides a frame of reference for other staff members caring for the patient.
c. If there is any purulent drainage:	This would indicate a wound infection.
(1) Notify the physician.	
(2) Obtain a wound culture specimen.	This will facilitate identification of the infecting organism so that appropriate treatment can be instituted quickly.
2. Check the patient's temperature every 4 hours, and notify the physician if there is an elevation above 101°.	Infection is a frequent complication after this type of surgery, and the incidence is even higher if the patient is diabetic. If infection appears to be present, the physician will order blood and urine specimens to be taken to determine the type and sensitivity of the offending organism, and the antibiotic currently being given may be changed accordingly.
3. If the patient has an inflatable type of prosthesis, be certain that it remains in the semirigid position for at least 4 days postoperatively.	The first time the prosthesis is to be inflated, the patient's physician will probably do it. This is usually done between the fourth and sixth postoperative day to prevent wound disruption, which might occur in the early postoperative period.

7. NURSING DIAGNOSIS: Postoperative pain

Objective of nursing intervention	Appropriate management of pain or discomfort
Expected outcome	Behavioral and/or verbal indications that pain is adequately reduced or absent

Plan for implementation	Rationale
1. Determine characteristics of the pain by questioning and observing the patient.	Patients will vary considerably in the degree of pain they experience after this type of surgery. Moderate incisional pain is expected for approximately 24 to 48 hours after surgery.
2. Be alert for indications (verbal or behavioral) that the patient is experiencing discomfort other than physical pain, and attempt to resolve the problem.	The patient may still have some psychologic conflicts with regard to the nature of the surgery.
3. If the discomfort is from surgical manipulation, administer analgesic medication and provide ice packs to scrotum and penis as ordered.	
4. Note the patient's response to the pain medication.	This provides a frame of reference for evaluation of the patient's condition on subsequent shifts.
5. Notify the physician if the patient's requests for pain medication do not decrease within 24 to 48 hours.	There should be a marked decrease in the apparent severity of pain within 1 or 2 days. If this does not occur, it may indicate the development of wound complications.

Early postoperative period

8. NURSING DIAGNOSIS: Continued potential for disturbances in diabetes control*

| Objective of nursing intervention | Prevention or early detection of hypoglycemia or severe hyperglycemia |

Expected outcomes
- Serum glucose levels close to baseline readings
- Glycosuria absent or within acceptable range
- Absence of ketonuria
- Absence of diaphoresis, tremor, tachycardia, hunger, irritability, pallor, headache, and other symptoms of hypoglycemia

Plan for implementation	Rationale
1. Carefully monitor the patient's urine for sugar and acetone. a. Keep accurate records of all measurements. b. Administer insulin according to levels of glycosuria as ordered.	The stress of anesthesia and surgery may aggravate hyperglycemia because of the increased secretion of epinephrine and glucocorticoids. The patient may require larger than usual doses of insulin, despite recent preoperative fasting.
2. If glycosuria is absent, observe the patient for indications of hypoglycemia. These include diaphoresis, tremor, tachycardia, hunger, irritability, pallor, headache, blurred vision, confusion, and loss of consciousness.	Glycosuria does not usually occur until the serum glucose levels exceeds the renal threshold, which is approximately 150 to 180 mg glucose per 100 ml blood. Absence of sugar in the urine could indicate very mild hyperglycemia, as well as normal serum glucose levels. However, it could also indicate hypoglycemia, which is a less likely situation but one that presents a more immediate threat to the patient than does hyperglycemia. It is more likely to occur in patients receiving parenteral insulin than in those taking oral hypoglycemics.
3. If any of the conditions in no. 2 are observed, notify the physician at once and do the following:	Severe hypoglycemia can be an emergency situation. If there is any doubt about whether the patient is actually in a state of hypoglycemia, some form of sugar should still be given because progressive hypoglycemia is more hazardous than a temporarily induced hyperglycemia.
a. If the patient is able to have oral intake, administer 2 teaspoons of sugar in an 8-ounce glass of orange juice at once.	A rapid intake of sugar will reverse hypoglycemia within 10 to 20 minutes.
b. If the patient is unable to have oral intake, administer intravenous dextrose in water (D/50/W) and possibly glucagon as ordered by the physician.	Rapid administration of dextrose will reverse the patient's condition within a few minutes. Administration of glucagon will have similar effects.
4. Check intravenous orders carefully regarding the type of solution. This includes piggyback solutions as well.	Isotonic dextrose solutions are a hidden source of sugar. Piggyback bottles (which are usually dextrose solutions) are a frequently overlooked hazard for diabetic patients.
5. If hypotension is noted postoperatively, notify the physician and make arrangements for the patient's serum glucose level to be checked.	Hypoglycemia should be ruled out as a possible cause of postoperative hypotension.

Early postoperative period

---

*Only applies to the diabetic patient.

Plan for implementation	Rationale
6. If the patient develops an infection, be particularly alert for a rise in serum glucose levels and consequent increase in insulin requirements.	Infection usually exacerbates hyperglycemia.
7. In general, be certain the patient's serum glucose is being monitored on a regular basis. Usually daily blood specimens are obtained during the early postoperative period.	

9. NURSING DIAGNOSIS: Need for management of indwelling urethral catheter*

Objectives of nursing intervention
Appropriate care of catheter and equipment
Prevention or early detection of infection
Care of tissue surrounding catheter
Maintenance of accurate records of urine output
Appropriate administration of hand-irrigation of catheter
Management of discomfort or pain caused by catheter
Satisfactory collection of urine specimens from catheter

Expected outcomes
Absence of severe bladder spasms and suprapubic distention
Urine draining freely through system
Absence of fever, chills, and foul-smelling urine
Absence of urethral discharge and tissue inflammation
Minimal discomfort caused by the catheter
Urine specimens in optimum condition for all necessary tests

Plan for implementation	Rationale
See master care plan for the patient with an indwelling urethral catheter: care after insertion of the catheter.	
In addition to the topics covered in the master care plan, the following interventions are required: 1. Provide catheter care gently to prevent discomfort.	
2. Notify the physician if the urine is cloudy, blood tinged, or foul smelling. It should be clear amber.	Although there is no communication between the location of the prosthesis and the urinary tract, the urethra may occasionally become perforated during surgery. Even minimal trauma to the urethra may give rise to a urinary tract infection, which should be treated as soon as possible.

*May not apply; an indwelling urethral catheter is used at the surgeon's discretion after this type of surgery.

Early postoperative period

10. NURSING DIAGNOSIS: Need for management of intravenous infusion

Objectives of nursing intervention

{
Appropriate administration of specific types of intravenous solutions

Prevention or early detection of local complications

Prevention or early detection of systemic complications

Management of discomfort caused by the intravenous infusion

Maintenance of proper function of intravenous equipment

Maintenance of accurate records of the patient's hydration status

Precautions against adverse effects of nephrotoxic antibiotics*
}

Expected outcomes

{
Normal hydration status

Normal electrolyte status

Absence of thrombophlebitis, infiltration, infection, fluid overload, and pulmonary embolism

Absence of discomfort caused by the intravenous infusion

Normal blood urea nitrogen and creatinine levels*
}

Plan for implementation	Rationale
See master care plan for the patient receiving intravenous therapy.	Although these patients can usually tolerate oral intake within a few hours after surgery, the intravenous infusion may be left in place for a few days to provide a route for antibiotics.
In addition to the items covered in the master care plan, the following interventions may be required:	
1. Be certain the antibiotics are administered in the prescribed dosage and only for the prescribed length of time.	Because the risk of infection is relatively high after this type of surgery, more than one antibiotic may be prescribed. Antibiotics with serious toxic effects may be ordered only for a predetermined number of doses while the patient continues to receive another antibiotic for a longer time. This may give rise to some confusion if orders are not carefully transcribed and carried out.
2. If the patient is receiving an aminoglycoside (e.g., gentamicin, tobramycin, kanamycin), be certain laboratory studies are being performed for blood urea nitrogen and serum creatinine levels, and report any irregularities.	These drugs may be nephrotoxic. However, they are highly effective in the treatment of infections caused by gram-negative organisms. They are most commonly given via the intravenous route. If they are given intramuscularly instead, the same precautions apply.

Early postoperative period

*Applies to patients receiving potentially nephrotoxic antibiotics.

11. NURSING DIAGNOSIS: Potential for voiding complications following removal of indwelling urethral catheter*

Objective of nursing intervention Prevention or early detection of complications

Expected outcomes Resumption of normal voiding pattern
Absence of dysuria

Plan for implementation	Rationale
See master care plan for the patient with an indwelling urethral catheter: care after removal of the catheter.	

*May not apply.

12. NURSING DIAGNOSIS: Need for instruction on inflation and deflation procedures*

Objective of nursing intervention Appropriate explanation and supervision of procedures

Expected outcomes Ability to manipulate prosthesis with ease
Absence of severe pain on inflation

Plan for implementation	Rationale
1. Describe the procedures to the patient and supervise his ability to perform them. (Frequently the patient's physician will do the initial teaching and inflation.)	
2. Inflate and deflate the prosthesis according to the prescribed schedule. It is usually started between the fourth and the sixth postoperative day and done twice a day. Sometimes analgesics are given prior to the first inflation.	
3. Notify the physician if the patient has severe pain during the procedure.	Although the initial inflation may be uncomfortable, severe pain should not occur. If it does, it may be an indication of an infection or improper fit of the appliance.
4. Do not permit the prosthesis to remain in the inflated position for prolonged periods of time.	This can cause tissue necrosis.

Late postoperative period

*Only applies to the patient with an inflatable prosthesis.

13. NURSING DIAGNOSIS: Need for assistance in adjusting to change in body image*

Objective of nursing intervention	Suggestion of methods to facilitate adjustment to the prosthesis
Expected outcome	Absence of verbal or behavioral indication of psychologic discomfort with regard to the prosthesis

Late postoperative period

Plan for implementation	Rationale
1. Provide the patient with pajama bottoms in addition to his hospital gown as soon as his catheter is removed.	This facilitates the patient's adjustment to wearing regular clothing.
2. If the patient expresses concern that the implant is protruding unnaturally under his clothing: a. Suggest that he wear snug-fitting jockey shorts and place the penis upward against the abdomen. b. Provide reassurance that there is no unnatural prominence visible under his clothing.	

*Only applies to the patient with a noninflatable type of prosthesis.

14. NURSING DIAGNOSIS: Need for discharge teaching

Objectives of nursing intervention	Explanation of basic information about medications to be taken at home Explanation of information regarding follow-up care Explanation of residual effects of the condition and/or treatment Explanation of instructions concerning postdischarge activities Explanation of symptoms that constitute a reason to contact the physician
Expected outcomes	Accurate return verbalization and/or demonstration of all material learned Smooth transition of care after discharge Absence or early detection of complications arising after discharge

Convalescent period

Plan for implementation	Rationale

See master care plan for the patient requiring discharge preparations: discharge teaching.

In addition to the topics covered in the master care plan, include the following items in the discharge teaching:

Plan for implementation	Rationale
1. Have the patient demonstrate his ability to inflate and deflate the prosthesis, and provide instruction if necessary.* Use a mechanical teaching model and printed materials whenever possible.	
2. At the follow-up office visit the physician will check the wound for adequate healing and determine whether the patient is having any problems with operating the prosthesis (if he has the inflatable type).	
3. The expected residual effects of this surgery are minimal except for some tenderness around the surgical area. This should decrease over the next 3 or 4 weeks. The patient can resume most of his usual activities within 1 week after surgery. However, he should not have sexual intercourse until his physician gives him permismision to do so.	If the patient has an inflatable prosthesis, he is usually told to refrain from sexual intercourse for approximately 4 to 6 weeks. If he has the noninflatable type, usually 3 weeks is sufficient for adequate healing to take place. In either case the importance of lubrication is emphasized to minimize trauma to penile tissue.
4. The patient should notify the physician if any of the following occur:	
a. Severe pain and/or increasing discomfort at the incisional site	This may indicate an infection.
b. Chills and/or fever	This also may indicate an infection.
c. Failure of the device to inflate or deflate*	This indicates either a mechanical failure within the device or the patient's inability to manipulate it properly.
d. Protrusion of the device through the skin or urethra	These may indicate improper fit of the device, and additional surgery will be required to replace the device with one of appropriate size.
e. Buckling of the glans during intercourse	

*Applies only to the patient with an inflatable prosthesis.

Convalescent period

References and bibliography

REFERENCES
Chapter 47
1. Gee, W.F., and Ansell, J.S.: Neonatal circumcision: a ten-year overview: with comparison of the Gomco clamp and the Plasti-bell device, Pediatrics **58:**824, 1976.

BIBLIOGRAPHY
Furlow, W.L.: Current status of the inflatable penile prosthesis in the management of impotence: Mayo Clinic experience updated, J. Urol. **119:**363, 1978.

Gee, W.F., and Ansell, J.S.: Neonatal circumcision: a ten-year overview: with comparison of the Gomco clamp and the Plasti-bell device, Pediatrics **58:**824, 1976.

Golgi, H.: Experience with penile prosthesis in spinal cord injury patients, J. Urol. **121:**288, 1979.

Goodman, L.S., and Gilman, A.G.: The pharmacological basis of therapeutics, ed. 5, New York, 1975, Macmillan Publishing Co., Inc.

Horton, C.E., editor: Plastic and reconstructive surgery of the genital area, Boston, 1973, Little, Brown & Co.

Karminsky-Binkhorst, M.D.: Female partner perception of Small-Carrion implant, Urology **12:**545, 1978.

Renshaw, D.C.: Inflatable penile prosthesis (editorial), J.A.M.A. **241:**2637, 1979.

Schwartz, S.I., et al.: Principles of surgery, ed. 3, New York, 1979, McGraw-Hill Book Co., Inc.

Scott, F.B., et al.: Erectile impotence treated with an implantable, inflatable prosthesis. Five years of clinical experience, J.A.M.A. **241:**2609, 1979.

Small, M.P.: Small-Carrion penile prosthesis: a report on 160 cases and review of the literature, J. Urol. **119:**365, 1978.

Smith, A.D., Lange, P.H., and Fraley, E.E.: A comparison of the Small-Carrion and Scott-Bradley penile prostheses, J. Urol. **121:**609, 1979.

Winter, C.C., and Morel, A.: Nursing care of patients with urologic disease, ed. 4, St. Louis, 1977, The C.V. Mosby Co.

Wood, R.Y., and Rose, K.: Penile implants for impotence, Am. J. Nurs. Feb. 1978, p. 234.

UNIT X

**PROCEDURES FOR DISORDERS
WITHIN
THE SCROTUM**

CHAPTER 51

Hydrocelectomy

A hydrocele is a cystic mass filled with straw-colored fluid that forms around the testicle. Unless it remains small, it should be surgically removed. In a young child this may be done simply by aspiration of the fluid from the scrotum. However, in an adult this method is rarely satisfactory, and hydrocelectomy is usually performed.

For the procedure the patient is placed in a supine position, and a horizontal incision is made between the visible blood vessels in the scrotum. The hydrocele sac is defined and removed from the scrotal sac and is then incised close to the testicle. Hemostasis is carried out by ligation and fulguration. A dependent incisional drain is inserted, the wound is closed (Fig. 51-1), and a dressing and scrotal support or suspensory are applied.

Some surgeons use a slightly different technique in which the hydrocele sac is plicated instead of excised (Lord's procedure). This method eliminates the possibility of redevelopment of the hydrocele by permanently collapsing its wall. After this form of the procedure no incisional drain is used.

HYDROCELECTOMY
Outline of Care Plan
ANTICIPATED NURSING DIAGNOSES:

Preoperative period
1. Need for preoperative teaching.
2. Need for discharge planning.
Postoperative period
3. Potential for postoperative complications (shock, atelectasis, pneumonia, urinary retention, deep vein thrombosis).
4. Potential for wound complications.
5. Postoperative pain.
Convalescent period
6. Need for discharge teaching.

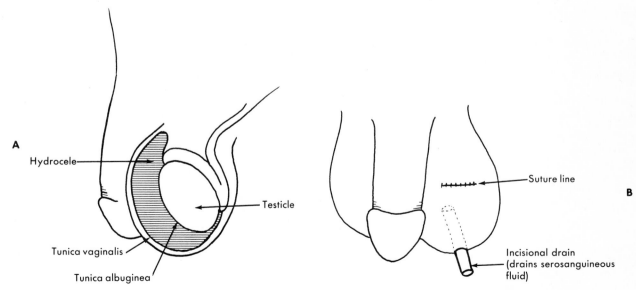

Fig. 51-1. Surgical correction of hydrocele. **A,** Hydrocele. **B,** Hydrocelectomy. Note asymmetry of scrotum caused by edema in the early postoperative period.

NURSING CARE FOR THE PATIENT UNDERGOING HYDROCELECTOMY

1. NURSING DIAGNOSIS: Need for preoperative teaching

Objectives of nursing intervention

If necessary, clarification of reason for hospitalization and type of surgery to be performed

Elimination of any negative or inaccurate notions regarding the forthcoming surgery

Explanation of preoperative tests and procedures

Psychologic preparation for general anesthesia (omit if the patient is to have spinal anesthesia)

Explanation of events expected in the early postoperative period

Explanation of body conditions expected in the early postoperative period

Identification of any known allergies

Expected outcomes

Verbal indication that explanations are understood

Verbal indication of optimistic expectations (within realistic limits) related to forthcoming surgery

Cooperation during preoperative tests and procedures

Verbal or behavioral indication of reduction of anxiety

Absence of postoperative complications

Absence of allergic reactions

Plan for implementation	Rationale
See master care plan for the patient receiving preoperative teaching.	
In addition to the topics covered in the master care plan, include the following items in the preoperative teaching:	
1. Be aware that, in addition to routine preoperative tests, the following diagnostic studies may have been performed, and answer any questions the patient has regarding them:	
a. Manual palpation of the scrotum	
b. Transillumination of the scrotum	A rounded, cystic, nontender intrascrotal mass that transilluminates (permits light to show through when a flashlight is held against it) is pathognomonic of a hydrocele and a spermatocele. In the former case the mass appears to surround the testicle.
c. Tests to rule out testicular tumor (see p. 621)	These additional tests **may** be performed in certain cases, since hydrocele sometimes develops secondarily to a testicular tumor.
2. The preoperative shave will be from umbilicus to midthigh.	

Preoperative period

Plan for implementation	Rationale
3. The patient will be permitted a light meal a few hours after surgery.	These patients can usually tolerate oral intake a few hours after surgery. For this reason the intravenous infusion used during surgery is often discontinued in the recovery room or shortly after the patient returns to the urology floor and tolerates fluids.
4. There will be an incision in the patient's scrotum covered by a dressing and a scrotal support or suspensory. The dressing may require frequent changing for the first 24 to 48 hours.	If the hydrocele is excised, an incisional drain will be in place, which will drain a moderate amount of fluid. If the hydrocele is plicated (Lord's procedure), there will be no drain and relatively little drainage. The nurse should know which method the particular surgeon prefers and provide the appropriate information.

2. NURSING DIAGNOSIS: Need for discharge planning

Objectives of nursing intervention
{ Early commencement of discharge planning
Accurate estimate of time required for all discharge teaching

Expected outcome   Smooth transition of care after discharge

Plan for implementation	Rationale
See master care plan for the patient requiring discharge preparations: discharge planning.	
In addition to the topics covered in the master care plan, the following items should be considered:	
1. The duration of hospitalization for this procedure is approximately 3 or 4 days.	
2. Required teaching includes only general postoperative discharge teaching.	

Preoperative period

3. NURSING DIAGNOSIS: Potential for postoperative complications (shock, atelectasis, pneumonia, urinary retention, deep vein thrombosis)

Objectives of nursing intervention	Prevention or early detection of postoperative complications

Expected outcomes
- Pulse and blood pressure normal, skin dry, color normal
- Respirations regular and unlabored, absence of pulmonary congestion
- Normal voiding pattern established within 6 hours after surgery
- Early ambulation tolerated well

Plan for implementation	Rationale
1. Check the patient's vital signs every 4 hours, and notify the physician of any indications of impending shock. These include: a. Increasing pulse and respiratory rates b. Decreasing blood pressure c. Diaphoresis and pallor d. Feelings of apprehension	Although shock is a potential complication after any kind of surgery, it is a relatively small risk after this procedure because few blood vessels are cut and the duration of surgery is short.
2. Encourage coughing and abdominal breathing if the patient's lungs sound congested, and notify the physician if any of the following conditions are present: a. The patient is unable to cough and his lungs sound congested. b. Sputum volume is copious. c. Sputum color is other than clear or white. d. There is a rise in the patient's temperature. e. Breath sounds are diminished.	Although precautions must be taken, respiratory complications are unlikely after this type of surgery because the period of anesthesia is very short. Furthermore, there is no abdominal incision to inhibit effective coughing. These conditions require additional treatment. The physician may order therapies such as incentive spirometry, nasotracheal suctioning, postural drainage, or intermittent positive pressure breathing, depending on the extent of respiratory embarrassment.
3. Promote resumption of normal voiding pattern by the following actions: a. Be certain the patient is well hydrated. b. Leave a urinal at the bedside within reach of the patient. c. Ask the patient to notify the nurse the first time he voids. d. If the patient has not voided within 6 hours after surgery: (1) Assist the patient to a standing position to void. (2) If the patient is still unable to void, notify the physician.	Temporary urinary retention is occasionally a result of anesthesia. Assuming the accustomed position for voiding will help the patient to void if the retention is caused by psychologic factors. Catheterization may be required.
4. Use precautions against deep vein thrombosis. (See master care plan for the patient at risk for deep vein thrombosis.) These patients are sometimes permitted out of bed in the evening after surgery.	Although deep vein thrombosis is a relatively small risk after this type of surgery, it still must be considered, and adequate precautions should be taken.

Postoperative period

4. NURSING DIAGNOSIS: Potential for wound complications

Objective of nursing intervention Prevention or early detection of complications arising from the incisional area

Expected outcome Absence of fever, purulent exudate, erythema, edema, hematoma, or other abnormal wound conditions

Plan for implementation	Rationale
1. Check the dressing every 2 to 4 hours for the first 24 hours.	There is usually moderate to heavy serosanguineous drainage for the first 24 to 48 hours after surgery if an incisional drain is present. However, if Lord's procedure is used, there will be no drain and thus minimal drainage.
a. Change the dressing if it becomes wet, and use sterile technique for the procedure.	
b. Make any adjustments in the scrotal support or suspensory that increase patient comfort.	The scrotal support serves two purposes. It keeps the scrotal dressing in place, and it elevates the scrotum, which helps to prevent edema from developing. If the patient is ambulatory, the support tends to slip out of place and may need periodic tightening.
2. If the dressing requires changing:	
a. Use caution when removing soiled dressing to prevent inadvertent removal of an incisional drain (if used).	The drain should remain in place for 24 to 48 hours to prevent an excessive accumulation of fluid in the scrotum.
b. Note the condition of the suture line. Chart its appearance and the presence of edema, erythema, or other abnormal wound conditions.	This provides a frame of reference for other staff members caring for the patient.
c. If there is purulent drainage:	This would indicate a wound infection.
(1) Notify the physician.	
(2) Obtain a wound culture specimen.	This will facilitate identification of the infecting organism so that appropriate treatment can be instituted quickly.
3. Check the patient's temperature every 4 hours, and notify the physician if there is an elevation above 101°.	Wound infection must always be suspected when the patient runs a fever postoperatively. It is the most common complication following this type of surgery.
4. Have the soiled scrotal supports laundered, and order extra ones so that there will always be a clean, dry one available.	If there is heavy drainage from the incision, the scrotal support, as well as the dressing, often gets saturated. Whenever a new dressing is applied, a soiled scrotal support also should be replaced to maintain maximum cleanliness in the area.

Postoperative period

5. NURSING DIAGNOSIS: Postoperative pain

Objective of nursing intervention   Appropriate management of pain or discomfort

Expected outcome   Behavioral and/or verbal indication that pain is adequately reduced or absent

Plan for implementation	Rationale
1. Determine characteristics of the pain by questioning and observing the patient.	Patients will vary considerably in the degree of pain they experience after this type of surgery. Moderate incisional pain is expected for approximately 24 hours after surgery.
2. Be alert for indications (verbal or behavioral) that the patient is experiencing discomfort other than physical pain, and attempt to resolve the problem.	Fear, loneliness, depression, and numerous other conditions may be sources of extreme discomfort for the patient, who may unconsciously translate these feelings into pain. Also, surgery involving the sexual organs may give rise to considerable anxiety, which often can be alleviated simply by reassurance from the nurse.
3. If the discomfort is a result of surgical manipulation: a. Be certain the scrotal support is positioned properly. b. Provide analgesic medication as ordered.	The scrotal support elevates the scrotum, thereby enhancing drainage from the area. This reduces discomfort caused by edema.
4. Note the patient's response to the pain medication.	This provides a frame of reference for evaluation of the patient's condition on subsequent shifts.
5. Notify the physician if the patient's requests for pain medication do not decrease within 24 to 48 hours.	There should be a marked decrease in the apparent severity of pain within 1 or 2 days. If this does not occur, it may indicate the development of wound complications.

Postoperative period

6. NURSING DIAGNOSIS: Need for discharge teaching

Objectives of nursing intervention
- Explanation of basic information about medications to be taken at home
- Explanation of information regarding follow-up care
- Explanation of residual effects of the condition and/or treatment
- Explanation of instructions concerning postdischarge activities
- Explanation of symptoms that constitute a reason to contact the physician
- Review of admitting diagnosis and mode of treatment

Expected outcomes
- Accurate return verbalization and/or demonstration of all material learned
- Smooth transition of care after discharge
- Absence or early detection of complications arising after discharge
- Ability to provide future health care practitioners with important data about health history

Plan for implementation	Rationale
See master care plan for the patient requiring discharge preparations: discharge teaching.	
In addition to the topics covered in the master care plan, include the following items in the discharge teaching: 1. At the follow-up office visit the physician will check the wound for adequate healing and will palpate the scrotum for any evidence of infection, such as extreme tenderness or bogginess.	
2. The expected residual effects of this surgery are minimal. However, after hydrocelectomy the scrotum may remain swollen from residual inflammation for as long as 1 month. The patient should be reassured that this is normal and that the edema will eventually subside.	
3. The patient should notify the physician if any of the following symptoms occur: a. Chills and/or fever b. Increasing scrotal tenderness c. Increasing pain and redness around the incision d. Persistent scrotal enlargement that lasts longer than 1 month	These are symptoms of infection, which is the most common postoperative complication. It should be treated as soon as possible to prevent epididymoorchitis and other serious complications. Reevaluation of the testicular mass may be required.

CHAPTER 52

Spermatocelectomy

A spermatocele is a cystic mass that occasionally develops at the upper pole of the testicle and is filled with milky-white fluid. Usually it is relatively small and asymptomatic. However, if it becomes large enough to be disturbing to the patient, spermatocelectomy may be required.

For the procedure the patient is placed in a supine position, and a horizontal incision is made between the visible blood vessels in the scrotum. The scrotal sac is opened, the affected testicle is exteriorized, and the spermatocele is excised. Hemostasis is achieved by fulguration. The incision is then closed without drainage (Fig. 52-1), and a dressing and scrotal support are applied.

In the event that additional small cysts are found, the patient may later be advised by his physician of the possibility of recurrence, since multiple small cysts are usually inoperable.

SPERMATOCELECTOMY
Outline of Care Plan
ANTICIPATED NURSING DIAGNOSES:

Preoperative period
1. Need for preoperative teaching. (See p. 588.)*
2. Need for discharge planning. (See p. 589.)*

Postoperative period
3. Potential for postoperative complications (shock, atelectasis pneumonia, urinary retention, deep vein thrombosis). (See p. 590.)*
4. Potential for wound complications. (See p. 591. No incisional drain is used; therefore only slight drainage is expected. The dressing will not require frequent changing.)*
5. Postoperative pain. (See p. 592.)*

Convalescent period
6. Need for discharge teaching. (See p. 593. Revise no. 2; residual swelling will be minimal.)*

*Nursing care is the same as for the patient undergoing hydrocelectomy.

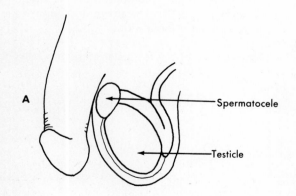
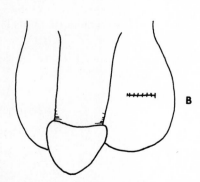

Fig. 52-1. Surgical correction of spermatocele. **A,** Spermatocele. **B,** Spermatocelectomy.

CHAPTER 53

Varicocelectomy

A varicocele is a cluster of dilated veins posterior to and above the testicle (Fig. 53-1, *A*). It can be identified on scrotal palpation, particularly during a Valsalva maneuver and can be either unilateral or bilateral. In many cases it is asymptomatic and requires no treatment. However, in some individuals it causes pain and is associated with infertility because of the increased scrotal temperature from venous stasis near the testicle. In these cases varicocelectomy is often performed. The sudden appearance of a varicocele in an older man may be a late sign of a renal tumor that has invaded the renal vein and interfered with venous drainage from the testicle. This requires a complete diagnostic investigation of the underlying cause of the condition.

A varicocelectomy can be performed by two different approaches. The patient is in a supine position for either.

For a low-ligation varicocelectomy an inguinal incision is made, and the contents of the inguinal canal are exposed. Trunks of the spermatic vein are identified and ligated at the level of the inguinal ring (Fig. 53-1, *B*). The incision is then closed without a drain, and a dressing is applied.

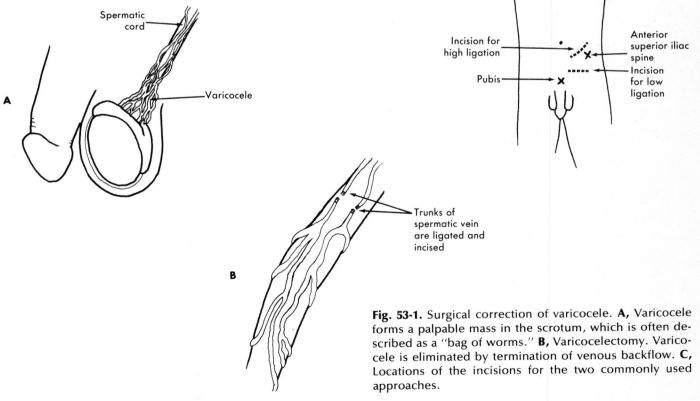

Fig. 53-1. Surgical correction of varicocele. **A,** Varicocele forms a palpable mass in the scrotum, which is often described as a "bag of worms." **B,** Varicocelectomy. Varicocele is eliminated by termination of venous backflow. **C,** Locations of the incisions for the two commonly used approaches.

595

For a high-ligation varicocelectomy the incision is made adjacent to the anterior superior iliac spine (Fig. 53-1, *C*). Trunks of the spermatic vein are approached and ligated in the retroperitoneal space. The incision is then closed without a drain, and a dressing is applied.

After either procedure, venous drainage from the testicle is accomplished by other venous channels. The high-ligation technique is preferred by some surgeons because it provides better access to the main trunks of the spermatic veins and reduces the risk of recurrence.

VARICOCELECTOMY
Outline of Care Plan
ANTICIPATED NURSING DIAGNOSES:

Preoperative period
1. Need for preoperative teaching.
2. Need for preliminary discharge planning.

Postoperative period
3. Potential for postoperative complications (shock, atelectasis, pneumonia, urinary retention, deep vein thrombosis).
4. Potential for wound complications.
5. Potential for alterations in gastrointestinal function.*
6. Postoperative pain.
7. Need for management of intravenous infusion.*

Convalescent period
8. Need for discharge teaching.

---

*May not apply.

NURSING CARE PLAN FOR THE PATIENT UNDERGOING VARICOCELECTOMY

1. NURSING DIAGNOSIS: Need for preoperative teaching

Preoperative period

Objectives of nursing intervention

- If necessary, clarification of reason for hospitalization and type of surgery to be performed
- Elimination of any negative or inaccurate notions regarding the forthcoming surgery
- Explanation of preoperative tests and procedures
- Psychologic preparation for general anesthesia (omit if the patient is to have spinal anesthesia)
- Explanation of events expected in the early postoperative period
- Explanation of body conditions expected in the early postoperative period
- Identification of any known allergies

Expected outcomes

- Verbal indication that explanations are understood
- Verbal indication of optimistic expectations (within realistic limits) related to forthcoming surgery
- Cooperation during preoperative tests and procedures
- Verbal or behavioral indication of reduction of anxiety
- Absence of postoperative complications
- Absence of allergic reactions

Plan for implementation	**Rationale**
See master care plan for the patient receiving preoperative teaching. In addition to the topics covered in the master care plan, include the following items in the preoperative teaching: 1. Be aware that, in addition to routine preoperative tests, the following diagnostic studies may have been per-	

Plan for implementation	Rationale
formed, and answer any questions the patient has regarding them:	
a. Manual palpation of the scrotum	A mass of dilated veins lying posterior to and above the testis is pathognomonic of a varicocele. This dilatation can be increased by the Valsalva maneuver.
b. Semen analysis	This test would be done only if the varicocele is suspected of being the cause of infertility. The test provides information about the concentration, morphology, and motility of the patient's sperm.
2. The preoperative shave will be from umbilicus to mid-thigh.	
3. Resumption of oral intake will depend on the surgical approach used. a. Inguinal approach: the patient will probably be permitted a light meal a few hours after surgery. b. Retroperitoneal approach: oral intake may be prohibited for 24 hours or until bowel sounds are heard.	If the retroperitoneal approach is used, the patient may experience a period of intestinal atony from the manipulation in the area. The nurse should know which approach the particular surgeon prefers and provide the appropriate information.
4. There will be a small incision in the inguinal area or a few inches higher if the retroperitoneal approach is used. The incision will be covered with a dressing.	

Preoperative period

2. NURSING DIAGNOSIS: Need for discharge planning

Objectives of nursing intervention { Early commencement of discharge planning
Accurate estimate of time required for all discharge teaching

Expected outcome   Smooth transition of care after discharge

Plan for implementation	Rationale
See master care plan for the patient requiring discharge preparations: discharge planning.	
In addition to the topics covered in the master care plan, the following items should be considered: 1. The duration of hospitalization for this procedure is approximately 2 to 4 days, depending on the surgical approach.	
2. Required teaching includes only general postoperative discharge teaching.	

3. NURSING DIAGNOSIS: Potential for postoperative complications (shock, atelectasis, pneumonia, urinary retention, deep vein thrombosis)

Objective of nursing intervention	Prevention or early detection of postoperative complications

Expected outcomes
- Pulse and blood pressure normal, skin dry, color normal
- Respirations regular and unlabored, absence of pulmonary congestion
- Normal voiding pattern established within 6 hours after surgery
- Early ambulation tolerated well

Plan for implementation	Rationale
1. Check the patient's vital signs every 4 hours, and notify the physician of any indications of impending shock. These include: a. Increasing pulse and respiratory rates b. Decreasing blood pressure c. Diaphoresis and pallor d. Feelings of apprehension	Although shock is a potential complication after any kind of surgery, it is a relatively small risk after varicocelectomy because few blood vessels are cut and the duration of surgery is short.
2. Encourage coughing and abdominal breathing if the patient's lungs sound congested, and notify the physician if any of the following conditions are present: a. The patient is unable to cough and his lungs sound congested. b. Sputum volume is copious. c. Sputum color is other than clear or white. d. There is a rise in the patient's temperature. e. Breath sounds are diminished.	Although precautions must be taken, respiratory complications are unlikely after this type of surgery because the period of anesthesia is short and the incision is not high enough to inhibit effective coughing. These conditions require additional treatment. The physician may order therapies such as incentive spirometry, nasotracheal suctioning, postural drainage, or intermittent positive pressure breathing, depending on the extent of respiratory embarrassment.
3. Promote resumption of normal voiding pattern by the following actions: a. Be certain the patient is well hydrated. b. Leave a urinal at the bedside within reach of the patient. c. Ask the patient to notify the nurse the first time he voids. d. If the patient has not voided within 6 hours after surgery: (1) Assist the patient to a standing position to void. (2) If the patient is still unable to void, notify the physician.	Temporary urinary retention is occasionally a result of anesthesia. Assuming the accustomed position for voiding will help the patient to void if the retention is caused by psychologic factors. Catheterization may be required.

Plan for implementation	Rationale
4. Use precautions against deep vein thrombosis. (See master care plan for the patient at risk for deep vein thrombosis.) These patients are sometimes permitted out of bed in the evening after surgery.	Although deep vein thrombosis is a relatively small risk after this type of surgery, it still must be considered, and adequate precautions should be taken.

4. NURSING DIAGNOSIS: Potential for wound complications

Objective of nursing intervention   Prevention or early detection of complications arising from the incisional area

Expected outcome   Absence of fever, purulent exudate, erythema, edema, hematoma, and other abnormal wound conditions

Plan for implementation	Rationale
1. Check the dressing every shift. If it requires changing:	Drainage is very slight or absent after this type of surgery, since no incisional drains are used.
a. Use sterile technique for the procedure.	
b. Note the condition of the suture line; chart its appearance and the presence of edema, erythema, or other abnormal wound conditions.	This provides a frame of reference for other staff members caring for the patient.
c. If there is purulent drainage:	This would indicate a wound infection.
(1) Notify the physician.	
(2) Obtain a wound culture specimen.	This will facilitate identification of the infecting organism so that appropriate treatment can be instituted quickly.
2. Check the patient's temperature every 4 hours, and notify the physician if there is elevation above 101°.	Wound infection must always be suspected when a patient runs a fever postoperatively.

Postoperative period

5. NURSING DIAGNOSIS: Potential for alterations in gastrointestinal function*

Objective of nursing intervention   Prevention and/or early detection of gastrointestinal complications

Expected outcomes { Compliance with orders prohibiting oral intake
Absence of abdominal distention, tympany, nausea, or vomiting
Presence of bowel sounds and passage of flatus within 12 to 24 hours after surgery

Plan for implementation	Rationale
1. If oral intake is prohibited by the patient's physician: a. Inform the patient that he is not to eat or drink anything. b. Notify the auxiliary staff of the orders. c. Provide mouth care as needed. d. Check periodically for bowel sounds and passage of flatus, and notify the physician when they occur.	When the retroperitoneal approach is used, there is sometimes a period of intestinal atony postoperatively from manipulation of the peritoneal contents during surgery. Premature oral intake could cause abdominal pain, distention, and vomiting. Lack of salivary stimulation often causes dryness and an unpleasant taste in the mouth. These are indications that the intestines are regaining their function.
2. When oral intake is permitted: a. Begin the patient's dietary intake with clear fluids. b. Note the presence of distention, tympany, nausea, or vomiting. c. Advance the diet as tolerated.	

*This only applies if the retroperitoneal approach was used for the surgery.

6. NURSING DIAGNOSIS: Postoperative pain

Objective of nursing intervention   Appropriate management of pain or discomfort

Expected outcome   Behavioral and/or verbal indication that pain is adequately reduced or absent

Plan for implementation	Rationale
1. Determine the characteristics of the pain by questioning and observing the patient. It may be related to the surgical wound, scrotal engorgement, or gastrointestinal manipulation. 2. Be alert for indications (verbal or behavioral) that the patient is experiencing discomfort other than physical pain, and attempt to resolve the problem.	Patients will vary considerably in the degree of pain they experience after this type of surgery. Mild to moderate incisional pain is expected for approximately 24 hours after surgery. Scrotal pain may be more severe and last longer. Surgery involving the sexual organs may give rise to considerable anxiety, which often can be alleviated simply by reassurance from the nurse.

Postoperative period

600

Plan for implementation	Rationale
3. Notify the physician if the patient's apparent need for pain medication does not decrease within 24 to 48 hours.	There should be a marked decrease in the severity of the pain within 1 or 2 days. If this does not occur, it may indicate the development of wound complications.

INCISIONAL PAIN

1. Provide analgesic medication as ordered.	Incisional pain is usually well controlled with analgesics.
2. Note the patient's response to the medication.	This provides a frame of reference for evaluation of the patient's condition on subsequent shifts.

SCROTAL PAIN

1. Elevate the scrotum while the patient is in bed. This can be done by placing a rolled towel or an adhesive strip under the scrotum (see Fig. 59-1).	Engorgement of the scrotum is common after this type of surgery because of the changed circulation in the area. The pressure from the excessive fluid may cause pain. Any process that enhances drainage from the area (e.g., elevation of the scrotum) will bring considerable relief.
2. While the patient is ambulating, have him use a scrotal support.	
3. Provide analgesic medication as ordered.	
4. Apply ice to the scrotum if ordered.	
5. Note the patient's response to whichever interventions are used.	This enables continuity of the most successful means of managing the scrotal pain.

COLICKY, INTERMITTENT VISCERAL PAIN, USUALLY ACCOMPANIED BY ABDOMINAL DISTENTION*

1. Check the patient's abdomen for the presence and extent of distention. 2. Encourage ambulation as soon as possible.	Because some areas of the intestines regain function before others, abdominal distention and "gas" pains may occur. General activity often helps to relieve the discomfort.
3. Administer neostigmine methylsulfate (Prostigmin) as ordered for relief of distention.	Neostigmine is a cholinergic drug that occasionally relieves postoperative abdominal distention.
4. Suggest that a rectal tube be ordered for insertion two to four times per day for approximately 30 minutes.	This may provide some relief from flatus.

*Abdominal pain is very unlikely unless a high-ligation (retroperitoneal approach) varicocelectomy is performed.

Postoperative period

Plan for implementation	**Rationale**

5. Check laboratory values for the patient's serum potassium level, and if it is lower than normal:
  a. Notify the physician.
  b. Monitor the patient's pulse and cardiac status.
	Hypokalemia may contribute to distention and decreased intestinal motility. However, there are more important reasons for correction of deficient serum potassium levels as soon as possible (e.g., cardiac arrhythmias).

7. NURSING DIAGNOSIS: Need for management of intravenous infusion*

Objectives of nursing intervention
- Appropriate administration of specific types of intravenous solutions
- Prevention or early detection of local complications
- Prevention or early detection of systemic complications
- Management of discomfort caused by the intravenous infusion
- Maintenance of proper function of intravenous equipment
- Maintenance of accurate records of the patient's hydration status

Expected outcomes
- Normal hydration status
- Normal electrolyte status
- Absence of thrombophlebitis, infiltration, infection, fluid overload, and pulmonary embolism
- Absence of discomfort caused by the intravenous infusion

Plan for implementation	**Rationale**
See master care plan for the patient receiving intravenous therapy.	These patients usually receive intravenous dextrose and saline solutions until they are able to tolerate oral intake.

*Only applies if the retroperitoneal approach was used and oral intake is withheld.

Postoperative period

8. NURSING DIAGNOSIS: Need for discharge teaching

Objectives of nursing intervention

- Explanation of basic information about medications to be taken at home
- Explanation of information regarding follow-up care
- Explanation of residual effects of the condition and/or treatment
- Explanation of instructions concerning postdischarge activities
- Explanation of symptoms that constitute a reason to contact the physician
- Review of admitting diagnosis and mode of treatment

Expected outcomes

- Accurate return verbalization and/or demonstration of all material learned
- Smooth transition of care after discharge
- Absence or early detection of complications arising after discharge
- Ability to provide future health care practitioners with important data about health history

Plan for implementation	Rationale
See master care plan for the patient requiring discharge preparations: discharge teaching.	
In addition to the topics covered in the master care plan, include the following items in the discharge teaching:	
1. At the follow-up office visit the physician will remove the sutures and check the wound for adequate healing. It is usually done on the sixth postoperative day.	
2. The expected residual effects of this surgery are minimal. The patient can usually resume most of his usual activities 1 week after discharge.	
3. The patient should notify the physician if any of the following occur:	
a. Severe pain and/or increasing discomfort at the incisional site	This may indicate a wound infection.
b. Increasing discomfort in the scrotal area	This may indicate that the circulation to the testicle has been impaired. Testicular atrophy is a rare complication of this surgery if the blood supply to the testicle is insufficient.

Convalescent period

CHAPTER 54

Orchidopexy

Orchidopexy is most commonly done on young children who are born with undescended testicles. The surgery is generally performed prior to school age so that the child does not suffer psychologic distress by feeling different from other male children. If it is not done before puberty, spermatogenesis in the affected testicle will be permanently impaired. The testicle will, however, produce normal amounts of testosterone.

Occasionally an orchidopexy will be performed on an adult whose condition was not diagnosed in childhood. In this case it is done for prophylactic reasons, based on the evidence that there is a significantly higher incidence of testicular cancer in cryptorchid testicles, whether or not they have been surgically corrected.[1,2] Therefore bringing them into the scrotum allows periodic manual examination of the testicles to detect early pathologic changes. Usually orchidopexy is done only if the condition is bilateral, since testosterone production must be maintained. If the condition is unilateral, many surgeons prefer to do an orchiectomy of the undescended testicle, since testosterone production will be carried on by the normal testicle.

For the procedure the patient is placed in a supine position, and an inguinal incision is made to free the spermatic cord from the surrounding fascia and to obtain maximum length. Care is taken not to injure the blood supply to the cord or to the vas deferens. Once sufficient length has been achieved, the scrotal sac is dilated to accommodate the testicle. The testicle is then placed in the scrotal sac and held in position by a suture into the tunica albuginea of the testicle and the dartus muscle of the scrotum. Some surgeons transpose the testicle into the opposite scrotal sac so the interscrotal septum maintains its position (Fig. 54-1). The incision is then closed and a dressing is applied.

ORCHIDOPEXY
Outline of Care Plan
ANTICIPATED NURSING DIAGNOSES:

Preoperative period
1. Need for preoperative teaching.
2. Need for discharge planning.

Postoperative period
3. Potential for postoperative complications (shock, atelectasis, pneumonia, urinary retention, deep vein thrombosis).
4. Potential for wound complications.
5. Postoperative pain.

Convalescent period
6. Need for discharge teaching.

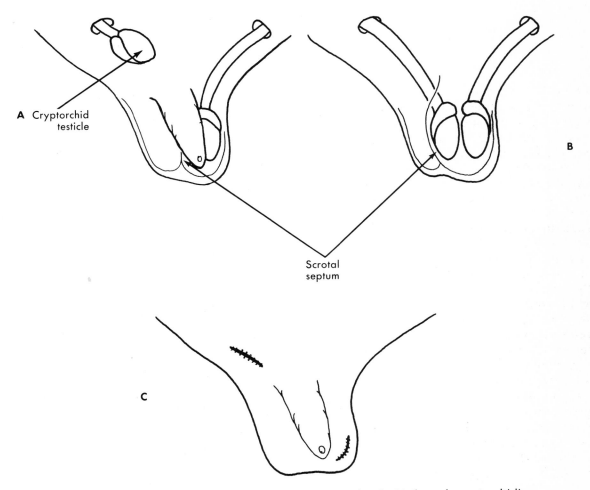

A Cryptorchid
testicle

Scrotal
septum

B

C

Fig. 54-1. Surgical correction of undescended testicle. **A,** Unilateral cryptorchidism.
B, Orchidopexy. The testicle is manually placed into the opposite scrotal sac to maintain its position. **C,** Result of orchidopexy after a few months. Testicles lie symmetrically
in the scrotum.

NURSING CARE PLAN FOR THE PATIENT UNDERGOING ORCHIDOPEXY

1. NURSING DIAGNOSIS: Need for preoperative teaching

Objectives of nursing intervention

- If necessary, clarification of reason for hospitalization and type of surgery to be performed
- Elimination of any negative or inaccurate notions regarding the forthcoming surgery
- Explanation of preoperative tests and procedures
- Psychologic preparation for general anesthesia
- Explanation of events expected in the early postoperative period
- Explanation of body conditions expected in the early postoperative period
- Identification of any known allergies

Expected outcomes

- Verbal indication that explanations are understood
- Verbal indication of optimistic expectations (within realistic limits) related to forthcoming surgery
- Cooperation during preoperative tests and procedures
- Verbal or behavioral indication of reduction of anxiety
- Absence of postoperative complications
- Absence of allergic reactions

Preoperative period

Plan for implementation	Rationale
See master care plan for the patient receiving preoperative teaching.	
In addition to the topics covered in the master care plan, include the following items in the preoperative teaching:	
1. Be aware that, in addition to routine preoperative tests, a thorough manual examination of the scrotum will be performed, and answer any questions the patient may have regarding it.	The visual appearance of the scrotum is not adequate for diagnosing cryptorchidism. A retractile testicle (a normally located testicle that is temporarily retracted out of the scrotum by the cremasteric reflex) requires no treatment and therefore must be ruled out by careful palpation. The manual examination also enables the physician to determine the location of the undescended testicle, since it may be in the inguinal canal, perineal area, or the abdomen.
2. If the patient is an adult or an adolescent, the preoperative shave will be from umbilicus to midthigh.	
3. The patient will be permitted a light meal a few hours after surgery.	These patients can usually tolerate oral intake within a few hours after surgery. For this reason the intravenous infusion used during surgery is often discontinued in the recovery room or shortly after the patient returns to the floor and tolerates fluids.
4. There will be a small incision in the inguinal area of the affected side(s) that will be covered by a dressing. There may also be a suture(s) in the scrotum that will be covered by a dressing and a scrotal support.	

2. NURSING DIAGNOSIS: Need for discharge planning

Objectives of nursing intervention
{ Early commencement of discharge planning
Accurate estimate of time required for all discharge teaching

Expected outcome Smooth transition of care after discharge

Plan for implementation	Rationale
See master care plan for the patient requiring discharge preparations: discharge planning. In addition to the topics covered in the master care plan, the following items should be considered: 1. The duration of hospitalization for this procedure is approximately 4 or 5 days. 2. Required teaching includes: a. General discharge teaching b. If the patient is an adult, discussion of the need for periodic testicular examination c. If the patient is a child, discussion with the parents of the need for periodic testicular examination	There is a higher incidence of testicular cancer in individuals who have, **or had,** undescended testicles.[1,2]

3. NURSING DIAGNOSIS: Potential for postoperative complications (shock, atelectasis, pneumonia, urinary retention, deep vein thrombosis)

Objective of nursing intervention Prevention or early detection of postoperative complications

Expected outcomes
{ Pulse and blood pressure normal, skin dry, color normal
Respirations regular and unlabored, absence of pulmonary congestion
Normal voiding pattern established within 6 hours after surgery
Early ambulation tolerated well

Plan for implementation	Rationale
1. Check the patient's vital signs every 4 hours and notify the physician of any indications of impending shock. These include: a. Increasing pulse and respiratory rates b. Decreasing blood pressure c. Diaphoresis and pallor d. Feelings of apprehension	Although shock is a potential complication after any kind of surgery, it is a relatively small risk after orchidopexy because few blood vessels are cut and the duration of surgery is short.

Preoperative period

Postoperative period

Plan for implementation	Rationale

2. Encourage coughing and abdominal breathing if the patient's lungs sound congested, and notify the physician if any of the following conditions are present:
 	
  a. The patient is unable to cough and his lungs sound congested.
  b. Sputum volume is copious.
  c. Sputum color is other than clear or white.
  d. There is a rise in the patient's temperature.
  e. Breath sounds are diminished.
	Although precautions must be taken, respiratory complications are unlikely after this type of surgery because the period of anesthesia is short and the incision is not high enough to inhibit effective coughing.
	These conditions require additional treatment. The physician may order therapies such as incentive spirometry, nasotracheal suctioning, postural drainage, or intermittent positive pressure breathing, depending on the extent of respiratory embarrassment.

3. Promote resumption of normal voiding pattern by the following actions:
  a. Be certain the patient is well hydrated.
  b. Leave a urinal at the bedside within reach of the patient.
  c. Ask the patient to notify the nurse the first time he voids.
  d. If the patient has not voided within 6 hours after surgery:
    (1) Assist the patient to a standing position to void.
 	
    (2) If the patient is still unable to void, notify the physician.
	Temporary urinary retention is occasionally a result of anesthesia.
	
	Assuming the accustomed position for voiding will help the patient to void if the retention is caused by psychologic factors.
	Catheterization may be required.

4. Use precautions against deep vein thrombosis. (See master care plan for the patient at risk for deep vein thrombosis.) These patients are sometimes permitted out of bed in the evening after surgery.	Although deep vein thrombosis is a relatively small risk after this type of surgery, it still must be considered, and adequate precautions should be taken.

Postoperative period

4. NURSING DIAGNOSIS: Potential for wound complications

Objective of nursing intervention Prevention or early detection of complications arising from the incisional area

Expected outcome Absence of fever, purulent exudate, erythema, edema, hematoma, and other abnormal wound conditions

Plan for implementation	Rationale
1. Check the inguinal and scrotal dressings every shift. If they require changing: a. Use sterile technique for the procedure.	Drainage is very slight or absent after this type of surgery, since no incisional drains are used.

Plan for implementation	Rationale
b. Note the condition of the suture line; chart its appearance and the presence of edema, erythema, or other abnormal wound conditions.	This provides a frame of reference for other staff members caring for the patient.
c. If there is purulent drainage:	This would indicate a wound infection.
(1) Notify the physician.	
(2) Obtain a wound culture specimen.	This will facilitate identification of the infecting organism so that appropriate treatment can be instituted quickly.
2. Check the patient's temperature every 4 hours, and notify the physician if there is an elevation above 101°.	Wound infection must always be suspected when a patient runs a fever postoperatively.

5. NURSING DIAGNOSIS: Postoperative pain

Objective of nursing intervention	Appropriate management of pain or discomfort
Expected outcome	Behavioral and/or verbal indication that pain is adequately reduced or absent

Plan for implementation	Rationale
1. Determine characteristics of the pain by questioning and observing the patient.	Patients will vary considerably in the degree of pain they experience after this type of surgery. Moderate incisional pain is expected for approximately 24 hours.
2. Be alert for indications (verbal or behavioral) that the patient is experiencing discomfort other than physical pain, and attempt to resolve the problem.	Surgery on the sexual organs may give rise to considerable anxiety, which often can be alleviated simply by reassurance from the nurse.
3. If the discomfort is from surgical manipulation:	
a. Be certain the scrotal support is positioned properly.	The scrotal support elevates the scrotum, thereby enhancing drainage from the area. This reduces discomfort caused by edema.
b. Provide analgesic medication as ordered.	
4. Note the patient's response to the pain medication.	This provides a frame of reference for the evaluation of the patient's condition on subsequent shifts.
5. Notify the physician if the patient's requests for pain medication do not decrease within 24 to 48 hours.	There should be a marked decrease in the apparent severity of pain within 1 or 2 days. If this does not occur, it may indicate the development of wound complications.

Postoperative period

6. NURSING DIAGNOSIS: Need for discharge teaching

Objectives of nursing intervention
- Explanation of basic information about medications to be taken at home
- Explanation of information regarding follow-up care
- Explanation of residual effects of the condition and/or treatment
- Explanation of instructions concerning postdischarge activities
- Explanation of symptoms that constitute a reason to contact the physician
- Review of admitting diagnosis and mode of treatment

Expected outcomes
- Accurate return verbalization and/or demonstration of all material learned
- Smooth transition of care after discharge
- Absence or early detection of complications arising after discharge
- Ability to provide future health care practitioners with important data about health history

Plan for implementation	Rationale
See master care plan for the patient requiring discharge preparations: discharge teaching.	
In addition to the topics covered in the master care plan, include the following items in the discharge teaching:	
1. At the follow-up office visit the physician will check the incision for adequate healing and will palpate the testicles.	
2. The expected residual effects after this type of surgery are minimal. The patient can usually resume most of his normal activities 1 week after discharge.	
3. The patient will be expected to return to the physician's office for periodic testicular examinations and/or will be taught how to examine his own testicles for pathologic changes. Testicular self-examination includes the following guidelines: a. It should be done approximately every month. b. It should be done after a warm bath or shower.	Warmth causes relaxation of the cremaster muscle. This facilitates palpation.
c. Each testicle should be explored with the thumb and forefingers, one at a time, with slow, gentle palpation. d. The patient should become thoroughly familiar with normal consistency of the testicle and its adjacent structures (epididymis and spermatic cord).	

Convalescent period

610

Plan for implementation	Rationale
4. The patient should notify the physician if any of the following occur:	
a. Severe pain and/or increased swelling at the incisional site	This may indicate a wound infection.
b. Scrotal pain or swelling	In the period shortly after surgery, this may indicate an infection or ischemia of the testicle.
c. Any changes in the consistency or shape of the testicle or its adjacent structures	The early sign of a testicular tumor is usually a smooth, nontender, hard, freely movable mass that does not transilluminate.

Convalescent period

CHAPTER 55

Orchiectomy

An orchiectomy may be performed for a variety of reasons, but it is most commonly done for patients with advanced prostatic cancer and for patients with testicular cancer. The surgical approach varies depending on the patient's diagnosis, so the nursing care also differs for each procedure. The first part of the chapter concerns advanced prostatic cancer, and the second part concerns testicular cancer.

Orchiectomy for the patient with advanced prostatic cancer

Some prostatic tumors have been found to be testosterone dependent, and their growth is retarded when the amount of circulating testosterone decreases. The nonsurgical method of reducing testosterone levels is by oral administration of estrogen in the form of diethylstilbestrol. Surgically, testosterone production can be reduced by bilateral orchiectomy. In some cases both methods are used together.

For the procedure the patient is placed in a supine position, and a horizontal incision is made between visible blood vessels on the anterolateral aspect of the scrotum. The scrotal sac is opened and the testicle is exteriorized. A clamp is applied to the testicular pedicle, the vas and blood vessels are ligated separately, and the testicle is excised. The incision is closed without drainage. The same procedure is then repeated on the other side. (Occasionally both testicles are removed through the same scrotal incision.) A dressing and scrotal support are then applied.

ORCHIECTOMY FOR THE PATIENT WITH ADVANCED PROSTATIC CANCER
Outline of Care Plan
ANTICIPATED NURSING DIAGNOSES:

Preoperative period
1. Need for preoperative teaching.
2. Psychologic distress about forthcoming changes in body image.
3. Need for discharge planning

Postoperative period
4. Potential for postoperative complications (shock, atelectasis, pneumonia, urinary retention, deep vein thrombosis).
5. Potential for wound complications.
6. Postoperative pain.

Convalescent period
7. Need for discharge teaching.

NURSING CARE PLAN FOR THE PATIENT UNDERGOING ORCHIECTOMY FOR ADVANCED PROSTATIC CANCER

1. NURSING DIAGNOSIS: Need for preoperative teaching

Objectives of nursing intervention

If necessary, clarification of reason for hospitalization and type of surgery to be performed

Elimination of any negative or inaccurate notions regarding the forthcoming surgery

Explanation of preoperative tests and procedures

Psychologic preparation for general anesthesia (omit if the patient is to have spinal or local anesthesia)

Explanation of events expected in the early postoperative period

Explanation of body conditions expected in the early postoperative period

Identification of any known allergies

Expected outcomes

Verbal indication that explanations are understood

Verbal indication of optimistic expectations (within realistic limits) related to forthcoming surgery

Cooperation during preoperative tests and procedures

Verbal or behavioral indication of reduction of anxiety

Absence of postoperative complications

Absence of allergic reactions

Plan for implementation	Rationale
See master care plan for the patient receiving preoperative teaching.	
In addition to the topics covered in the master care plan, include the following items in the preoperative teaching:	
1. Be aware that, in addition to routine preoperative tests, the following diagnostic studies may have been performed, and answer any questions the patient has regarding them:	
a. Blood specimen for acid and alkaline phosphatase	There is an elevation of these products in the blood when prostatic cancer has metastasized to the bone.
b. Blood specimen for complete blood count	Although this is a routine test for all preoperative patients, it is particularly important for patients with prostatic cancer because, when tumor cells invade the bone, severe anemia can occur.
c. Bone and liver scans	These are done to determine the presence and location of metastases to these organs.
d. Chest x-ray examination	This will determine the presence of metastatic lesions in the lungs, hilar nodes, and ribs.
2. The preoperative shave will be from umbilicus to mid-thigh.	
3. The patient will be permitted a light meal a few hours after surgery.	These patients can usually tolerate oral intake within a few hours after surgery. For this reason the intravenous infusion used during surgery is often discontinued in the

Preoperative period

613

Plan for implementation	Rationale
	recovery room or shortly after the patient returns to the floor and tolerates fluids.
4. There will be one or two incisions in the patient's scrotum that will be covered by a dressing and scrotal support.	
5. If the patient has been taking oral medication for bone pain prior to admission, he will be given the equivalent medication via injection during the period when he is to have no oral intake.	Many of these patients suffer from severe pain in their lower back, thighs, and other bony areas. They may be taking narcotic analgesics regularly and need reassurance that control of this pain will be continued.

2. NURSING DIAGNOSIS: Psychologic distress about forthcoming changes in body image

Objective of nursing intervention   Provision of a supportive environment

Expected outcomes
- Willingness and ability to express feelings about forthcoming changes
- Absence of severe or protracted depression
- Optimistic outlook on the benefits of the surgery

Plan for implementation	Rationale
1. Encourage the patient to verbalize his feelings. His primary concerns about his body image will probably include:	
a. A sense of loss of manhood	The symbolic meaning a man attaches to his testicles usually involves his sense of virility, strength, and power.
b. Loss of sexual potency	The reduction of testosterone will reduce the patient's sexual desire and his ability to have an erection and orgasm. Sterility will, of course, also occur. However, these patients are generally over the age of 60, and sterility is not a major concern to them.
c. Feminization (redistribution of fat, breast enlargement, loss of facial hair)	These changes may occur because of the reduction of testosterone. Sometimes small doses of radiation to the areolar area may be given to reduce the possibility of gynecomastia (breast enlargement).
2. Provide emotional support.	Although the patient may be quite elderly, do not assume that he is sexually inactive or that he is disinterested in being attractive in a "manly" way. This is traumatic surgery for a man of any age.
3. Emphasize the positive results that are expected from the surgery (i.e., the patient will probably have considerable pain reduction).	

Preoperative period

3. NURSING DIAGNOSIS: Need for discharge planning

Objectives of nursing intervention
{ Early commencement of discharge planning
Accurate estimate of time required for all discharge teaching

Expected outcome   Smooth transition of care after discharge

Plan for implementation	Rationale
See master care plan for the patient requiring discharge preparations: discharge planning. In addition to the topics covered in the master care plan, the following items should be considered: 1. The duration of hospitalization for this procedure is approximately 4 days. 2. Required teaching includes: a. General postoperative discharge teaching b. Explanation of the need for reevaluation of analgesic requirements after a few weeks	

4. NURSING DIAGNOSIS: Potential for postoperative complications (shock, atelectasis, pneumonia, urinary retention, deep vein thrombosis)

Objective of nursing intervention   Prevention or early detection of postoperative complications

Expected outcomes
{ Pulse and blood pressure normal, skin dry, color normal
Respirations regular and unlabored, absence of pulmonary congestion
Normal voiding pattern established within 6 hours after surgery
Early ambulation tolerated well

Plan for implementation	Rationale
1. Check the patient's vital signs every 4 hours, and notify the physician of any indications of impending shock. These include: a. Increasing pulse and respiratory rates b. Decreasing blood pressure c. Diaphoresis and pallor d. Feelings of apprehension	Although shock is a potential complication after any kind of surgery, it is a relatively small risk after orchiectomy because few blood vessels are cut and the duration of surgery is short.

Plan for implementation	Rationale
2. Encourage coughing and abdominal breathing if the patient's lungs sound congested, and notify the physician if any of the following conditions are present:	Although precautions must be taken, respiratory complications are unlikely after this type of surgery because the period of anesthesia is very short. Furthermore, there is no abdominal incision to inhibit effective coughing.
a. The patient is unable to cough and his lungs sound congested. b. Sputum volume is copious. c. Sputum color is other than clear or white. d. There is a rise in the patient's temperature. e. Breath sounds are diminished.	These conditions require additional treatment. The physician may order therapies such as incentive spirometry, nasotracheal suctioning, postural drainage, or intermittent positive pressure breathing, depending on the extent of respiratory embarrassment.
3. Promote resumption of normal voiding pattern by the following actions: a. Be certain the patient is well hydrated. b. Leave a urinal at the bedside within reach of the patient. c. Ask the patient to notify the nurse the first time he voids. d. If the patient has not voided within 6 hours after surgery:	Temporary urinary retention is occasionally a result of anesthesia.
(1) Assist the patient to a standing position to void.	Assuming the accustomed position for voiding will help the patient to void if the retention is caused by psychologic factors.
(2) If the patient is still unable to void, notify the physician.	Catheterization may be required.
4. Use precautions against deep vein thrombosis. (See master care plan for the patient at risk for deep vein thrombosis.)	Although deep vein thrombosis is a relatively small risk after this type of surgery, it still must be considered, and adequate precautions should be taken.

Postoperative period

5. NURSING DIAGNOSIS: Potential for wound complications

Objective of nursing intervention	Prevention or early detection of complications arising from the incisional area
Expected outcome	Absence of fever, purulent exudate, erythema, edema, hematoma, and other abnormal wound conditions

Plan for implementation	Rationale
1. Check the dressing every shift. a. Change the dressing if it becomes wet, and use sterile technique for the procedure.	Drainage is very light or absent after this type of surgery, since no incisional drains are used.
b. Make any adjustments in the scrotal support that increase patient comfort.	The scrotal support serves two purposes. It keeps the scrotal dressing in place, and it elevates the scrotum, which helps to prevent edema from developing. If the patient is ambulatory, the support tends to slip out of place and may need periodic tightening.
2. If dressing requires changing: a. Note the condition of the suture line. Chart its appearance and the presence of edema, erythema, or other abnormal wound conditions.	This provides a frame of reference for other staff members caring for the patient.
b. If there is purulent drainage: (1) Notify the physician.	This would indicate that the patient has a wound infection.
(2) Obtain a wound culture specimen.	This will facilitate identification of the infecting organism so that appropriate treatment can be instituted quickly.
3. Check the patient's temperature every 4 hours, and notify the physician if there is an elevation above 101°.	Wound infection must always be suspected when the patient runs a fever postoperatively.
4. Have the soiled scrotal supports laundered, and order extra ones so that there will always be a clean dry one available.	

Postoperative period

6. NURSING DIAGNOSIS: Postoperative pain

Objective of nursing intervention   Appropriate management of pain or discomfort

Expected outcome   Behavioral and/or verbal indication that pain is adequately reduced or absent

Plan for implementation	Rationale
1. Determine characteristics of the pain by questioning and observing the patient.	Patients will vary considerably in the degree of pain they experience after this type of surgery. Moderate incisional pain is expected for approximately 24 hours postoperatively. However, many patients with advanced prostatic cancer have severe chronic pelvic and thigh pain from metastatic infiltration into adjacent bones. They may need relatively high doses of pain medication postoperatively, since many of them have been taking narcotic analgesics for a long time and have developed a degree of tolerance to these drugs. On the other hand, there are patients who hardly complain of any incisional pain because the bone pain has been so severe that any other pain appears mild by comparison.
2. Be alert for indications (verbal or behavioral) that the patient is experiencing discomfort other than physical pain, and attempt to resolve the problem.	Fear, loneliness, depression, and numerous other conditions may be sources of extreme discomfort for the patient, who may unconsciously translate these feelings into pain.
3. If the discomfort is from surgical manipulation: a. Be certain the scrotal support is positioned properly. b. Provide analgesic medication as ordered.	The scrotal support elevates the scrotum, thereby enhancing drainage from the area. This reduces the discomfort caused by edema.
4. If the discomfort is chronic bone pain, provide medication as ordered.	The bone pain will not be reduced at once after surgery, although the response is usually dramatic after a few weeks.
5. Note the patient's response to the pain medication.	This provides a frame of reference for evaluation of the patient's condition on subsequent shifts.
6. Notify the physician if the patient continues to complain of incisional pain for more than 24 to 48 hours after surgery.	There should be a marked decrease in the apparent severity of the incisional pain within 1 or 2 days. If this does not occur, it may indicate the development of wound complications.

Postoperative period

7. NURSING DIAGNOSIS: Need for discharge teaching

Objectives of nursing intervention

Explanation of basic information about medications to be taken at home

Explanation of information regarding follow-up care

Explanation of residual effects of the condition and/or treatment

Explanation of instructions concerning postdischarge activities

Explanation of symptoms that constitute a reason to contact the physician

Review of admitting diagnosis and mode of treatment

Expected outcomes

Accurate return verbalization and/or demonstration of all material learned

Smooth transition of care after discharge

Absence or early detection of complications arising after discharge

Ability to provide future health care practitioners with important data about health history

Plan for implementation	Rationale
See master care plan for the patient requiring discharge preparations: discharge teaching.	
In addition to the topics covered in the master care plan, include the following items in the discharge teaching:	
1. At the follow-up office visit the physician will check the wound for adequate healing. At subsequent follow-up examinations, the patient's favorable response to the surgery will be assessed by the amount of pain reduction he experiences.	
2. The expected residual effects of this surgery are minimal. The patient should be able to resume his usual activities 1 week after discharge.	
3. The patient should notify the physician if any of the following symptoms occur: a. Chills and/or fever b. Increasing scrotal tenderness c. Increasing pain and tenderness around the incision	These symptoms probably indicate the presence of infection, which is the most common complication after this type of surgery and should be treated as soon as possible.

Convalescent period

ORCHIECTOMY FOR THE PATIENT WITH TESTICULAR CANCER

The patient who is suspected of having testicular cancer will undergo surgical exploration of the scrotum and, if malignant tissue is found, unilateral orchiectomy. Needle or transscrotal biopsies are not done for suspected neoplasms, since there is considerable risk of spreading malignant cells into healthy tissue with these procedures.

For the procedure the patient is placed in a supine position, and an inguinal incision is made on the affected side. The spermatic cord is approached, and a noncrushing clamp is applied. The testicle is mobilized and examined, and a frozen section may be taken. If the mass proves to be malignant, the cord is ligated at the base where the clamp was placed, and the testicle and cord are excised. The wound is then closed without incisional drains, and a dressing and scrotal support are applied. If the mass is nonmalignant (e.g., it may be a hematoma or an organized abscess), only the mass is removed, and the testicle and spermatic cord are left intact.

Since most testicular tumors are highly prone to metastasis, additional treatment may be employed, depending on the type of tumor. If it is a pure semi-noma, radiation therapy may be administered. If it is an embryonal cell carcinoma, teratoma, or teratocarcinoma, chemotherapy may be given (see pp. 640 to 645) with or without retroperitoneal lymphadenectomy (see p. 628). If it is a choriocarcinoma, chemotherapy alone is usually employed, since these tumors metastasize so early that surgery would not be of value.

ORCHIECTOMY FOR THE PATIENT WITH TESTICULAR CANCER
Outline of Care Plan
ANTICIPATED NURSING DIAGNOSES:

Preoperative period
1. Need for preoperative teaching.
2. Psychologic distress related to forthcoming changes in body image.
3. Need for discharge planning.

Postoperative period
4. Potential for postoperative complications (shock, atelectasis, pneumonia, urinary retention, deep vein thrombosis).
5. Potential for wound complications.
6. Postoperative pain.

Convalescent period
7. Need for discharge teaching.

NURSING CARE PLAN FOR THE PATIENT UNDERGOING ORCHIECTOMY FOR TESTICULAR CANCER

1. NURSING DIAGNOSIS: Need for preoperative teaching

Preoperative period

Objectives of nursing intervention

If necessary, clarification of reason for hospitalization and type of surgery to be performed

Elimination of any negative or inaccurate notions regarding the forthcoming surgery

Explanation of preoperative tests and procedures

Psychologic preparation for general anesthesia (omit if the patient is to have spinal anesthesia)

Explanation of events expected in the early postoperative period

Explanation of body conditions expected in the early postoperative period

Identification of any known allergies

Expected outcomes

Verbal indication that explanations are understood

Verbal indication of optimistic expectations (within realistic limits) related to forthcoming surgery

Cooperation during preoperative tests and procedures

Verbal or behavioral indication of reduction of anxiety

Absence of postoperative complications

Absence of allergic reactions

Plan for implementation	Rationale
See master care plan for the patient receiving preoperative teaching. In addition to the topics covered in the master care plan, include the following items in the preoperative teaching: 1. Be aware that, in addition to the routine preoperative tests, the following diagnostic studies may have been performed, and answer any questions the patient has regarding them: a. Blood specimens for alpha-fetoprotein (AFP) and human chorionic gonadotropin (HCG) b. Bilateral pedal lymphangiogram c. Intravenous pyelogram d. Chest x-ray examination and tomogram e. Bone, liver, and brain scans f. Abdominal and pelvic CT scan (computerized tomography) 2. The preoperative shave will be from umbilicus to mid-thigh. 3. The patient will be permitted a light meal a few hours after surgery. 4. There will be a small incision in the inguinal area on the affected side that will be covered with a dressing.	It is especially important to give these patients as comprehensive an explanation as they can understand. They are usually extremely anxious about these tests, since the results will affect the rest of their lives. Knowing when they can expect the results and what the results might mean gives them a chance to deal with their anxiety in a concrete way. Serum levels of these substances (known as tumor markers) are elevated in testicular tumors. The tests are also important in determination of tumor metastasis; after orchiectomy, elevated tumor markers will return to normal if the tumor has not metastasized. This may be done to determine retroperitoneal lymph node involvement. This is done to determine renal and/or ureteral involvement. These are done to determine the presence of metastatic lesions in the lung. These are done to determine metastatic involvement of these organs. This is done to further determine the presence of metastatic lesions in the abdomen and/or pelvis. These patients can usually tolerate oral intake within a few hours after surgery. For this reason the intravenous infusion used during surgery is often discontinued in the recovery room or shortly after the patient returns to the floor and tolerates fluids. The scrotal approach is not used for orchiectomy when the patient has testicular cancer. The inguinal approach permits high ligation of the cord at the internal ring.

Preoperative period

2. NURSING DIAGNOSIS: Psychologic distress related to forthcoming changes in body image

Objectives of nursing intervention { Provision of a supportive environment
Correction of any inaccurate notions

Expected outcomes { Willingness and ability to express feelings about forthcoming changes
Absence of prolonged or protracted depression

Plan for implementation	Rationale
1. Encourage the patient to verbalize his feelings. His primary concerns about his body image will probably be: a. Loss of sexual attractiveness b. Feared infertility and impotence	The idea of having only one testicle and therefore looking different from a "normal" man may be very threatening for the patient. The patient's physician has probably told him that (provided his other testicle is normal) he will not become sterile (although his sperm count may be lowered), nor will his ability to have an erection and orgasm be affected. However, the nurse cannot be certain how much the patient has actually **heard,** since usually the patient's anxiety level is very high when discussing his diagnosis and treatment.
2. Provide emotional support.	
3. Provide information that may alleviate some of the patient's distress. a. Surgical implantation of a gel-filled silicone prosthesis can usually be performed at a later date if the patient so desires. b. The surgery will not impair fertility or sexual functioning. NOTE: The nurse should use caution when reassuring the patient about his fertility because, in the event that he requires radiotherapy or chemotherapy, his fertility will probably be impaired for approximately 2 years. Both chemotherapy and radiotherapy have an adverse effect on spermatogenesis during the period of treatment, which is usually approximately 2 years. Furthermore, if lymphadenectomy is required, the patient might suffer from ejaculatory failure, depending on the extent of the node dissection. If bilateral dissection is required of the nodes below the renal vessels, L1 sympathetic ganglia will be interrupted, resulting in the inability to ejaculate. (See p. 630 for discussion of bilateral versus unilateral dissection.)	

Preoperative period

3. NURSING DIAGNOSIS: Need for discharge planning

Objectives of nursing { Early commencement of discharge planning
intervention { Accurate estimate of time required for all discharge teaching

Expected outcome   Smooth transition of care after discharge

Plan for implementation	Rationale

See master care plan for the patient requiring discharge preparations: discharge planning.

In addition to the topics covered in the master care plan, the following items should be considered:
1. Hospitalization for orchiectomy (when performed for testicular cancer) is approximately 1 week. However, it may need to be extended if the patient is to receive chemotherapy and/or additional surgery. Since additional treatment will depend on the type of tumor, and this is frequently not known until after the orchiectomy has been performed, discharge planning may need to be deferred until the postoperative period.

2. Discharge teaching will vary according to the type of tumor. It will include:
   a. General postoperative discharge teaching
   b. Possible radiation treatment regimen
   c. Possible chemotherapy regimen
   d. Discussion of the need for frequent follow-up examinations

Preoperative period

4. NURSING DIAGNOSIS: Potential for postoperative complications (shock, atelectasis, pneumonia, urinary retention, deep vein thrombosis)

Objective of nursing intervention	Prevention or early detection of postoperative complications

Expected outcomes

- Pulse and blood pressure normal, skin dry, color normal
- Respirations regular and unlabored, absence of pulmonary congestion
- Normal voiding pattern established within 6 hours after surgery
- Early ambulation tolerated well

Plan for implementation	Rationale
1. Check the patient's vital signs every 4 hours, and notify the physician of any indications of impending shock. These include: a. Increasing pulse and respiratory rates b. Decreasing blood pressure c. Diaphoresis and pallor d. Feelings of apprehension	Although shock is a potential complication after any kind of surgery, it is a relatively small risk after orchiectomy because few blood vessels are cut and the duration of surgery is short.
2. Encourage coughing and abdominal breathing if the patient's lungs sound congested, and notify the physician if any of the following conditions are present: a. The patient is unable to cough and his lungs sound congested. b. Sputum volume is copious. c. Sputum color is other than clear or white. d. There is a rise in the patient's temperature. e. Breath sounds are diminished.	Although precautions must be taken, respiratory complications are unlikely after this type of surgery because the period of anesthesia is short and the incision is not high enough to prevent effective coughing. These conditions require additional treatment. The physician may order therapies such as incentive spirometry, nasotracheal suctioning, postural drainage, or intermittent positive pressure breathing, depending on the extent of respiratory embarrassment.
3. Promote resumption of normal voiding pattern by the following actions: a. Be certain the patient is well hydrated. b. Leave a urinal at the bedside within reach of the patient. c. Ask the patient to notify the nurse the first time he voids. d. If the patient has not voided within 6 hours after surgery: (1) Assist the patient to a standing position to void. (2) If the patient is still unable to void, notify the physician.	Temporary urinary retention is occasionally a result of anesthesia. Assuming the accustomed position for voiding will help the patient to void if the retention is caused by psychologic factors. Catheterization may be required.
4. Use precautions against deep vein thrombosis. (See master care plan for the patient at risk for deep vein thrombosis.)	Although deep vein thrombosis is a relatively small risk after this type of surgery, it still must be considered, and adequate precautions should be taken.

Postoperative period

5. NURSING DIAGNOSIS: Potential for wound complications

Objective of nursing intervention   Prevention or early detection of complications arising from the incisional area

Expected outcome   Absence of fever, purulent exudate, erythema, edema, hematoma, and other abnormal wound conditions

Plan for implementation	Rationale

1. Check the dressing every shift.
  a. Change the dressing if it becomes wet, and use sterile technique for the procedure.
  b. Make any adjustments in the scrotal support that increase patient comfort.
	Drainage should be very slight or absent after this type of surgery, since no incisional drain is used.
	The scrotal support elevates the scrotum and thus prevents edema from developing. If the patient is ambulatory, the support tends to slip out of place and may need tightening.

2. If the dressing requires changing:
  a. Note the condition of the suture line. Chart its appearance and the presence of edema, erythema, or other abnormal wound conditions.
  b. If there is purulent drainage:
    (1) Notify the physician.
    (2) Obtain a wound culture specimen.
	This provides a frame of reference for other staff members caring for the patient.
	
	This would indicate a wound infection.
	
	This will facilitate identification of the infecting organism so that appropriate treatment can be instituted quickly.

3. Check the patient's temperature every 4 hours, and notify the physician if there is an elevation above 101°.	Wound infection must always be suspected when the patient runs a fever postoperatively.

Postoperative period

Postoperative period

6. NURSING DIAGNOSIS: Postoperative pain

Objective of nursing intervention Appropriate management of pain or discomfort

Expected outcome Behavioral and/or verbal indication that pain is adequately reduced or absent

Plan for implementation	Rationale
1. Determine characteristics of the pain by questioning and observing the patient.	Patients will vary considerably in the degree of pain they experience after this type of surgery. Moderate incisional pain is expected for approximately 24 hours after surgery.
2. Be alert for indications (verbal or behavioral) that the patient is experiencing discomfort other than physical pain, and attempt to resolve the problem.	Fear, loneliness, depression, and numerous other conditions may be sources of extreme discomfort for the patient, who may unconsciously translate these feelings into pain.
3. If the discomfort is from surgical manipulation:	
a. Be certain the scrotal support is positioned properly.	The scrotal support elevates the scrotum, thereby enhancing drainage from the area. This reduces discomfort caused by edema.
b. Provide analgesic medication as ordered.	
4. Note the patient's response to the pain medication.	This provides a frame of reference for evaluation of the patient's condition on subsequent shifts.
5. Notify the physician if the patient's requests for pain medication do not decrease within 24 to 48 hours.	There should be a marked decrease in the apparent severity of pain within 1 or 2 days. If this does not occur, it may indicate the development of wound complications.

Convalescent period

7. NURSING DIAGNOSIS: Need for discharge teaching*

Objectives of nursing intervention
- Explanation of basic information about medications to be taken at home
- Explanation of information regarding follow-up care
- Explanation of residual effects of the conditon and/or treatment
- Explanation of instructions concerning postdischarge activities
- Explanation of symptoms that constitute a reason to contact the physician
- Review of admitting diagnosis and mode of treatment

*May not apply here; many of these patients will need further surgery (see p. 628) and/or chemotherapy (see p. 640) for which they will require continued hospitalization. Only the patient whose diagnosis is a pure seminoma (or a nonmalignant mass) will be discharged at this time.

Expected outcomes
{
Accurate return verablization and/or demonstration of all material learned

Smooth transition of care after discharge

Absence or early detection of complications arising after discharge

Ability to provide future health care practitioners with important data about health history
}

Plan for implementation	Rationale

See master care plan for the patient requiring discharge preparations: discharge teaching.

In addition to the topics covered in the master care plan, include the following items in the discharge teaching:

1. At the follow-up office visit the physician will check the wound for adequate healing. If the tumor was a seminoma, he may also schedule the patient for a series of radiotherapy treatments.

The physician will usually wait until the wound is considerably healed before beginning radiation treatments.

2. Additional follow-up examinations will be scheduled at least every 6 months for the next 2 years, during which the physician will examine the patient's abdomen and other testicle and take blood specimens. The patient may also be scheduled for periodic chest x-ray examinations.

The physician will palpate for any evidence of metastatic tumor growth and the presence of a tumor in the other testicle. He will also check the patient's blood for elevations of AFP and HCG. Chest x-ray examinations will be done periodically to identify any metastatic lesions in the patient's lungs.

3. Expected residual effects of the surgery are minimal. The patient may resume most of his normal activities 1 week after discharge. He might experience the following as a result of the radiation treatments:
   a. Sterility during the period he is undergoing radiation therapy (usually for approximately 2 years)
   b. Nausea and vomiting

4. The patient should notify the physician if any of the following occur:
   a. Severe pain or increasing discomfort at the incisional site
   b. Appearance of a mass in the neck, inguinal area, or opposite testicle (see p. 610 for testicular self-examination)

This may indicate a wound infection.

This may indicate metastatic spread of the tumor.

Convalescent period

CHAPTER 56

Additional surgery for testicular cancer: retroperitoneal lymphadenectomy

Retroperitoneal lymphadenectomy is frequently employed as adjuvant therapy in the treatment of certain types of testicular tumors after orchiectomy is performed (see Chapter 55). These tumors fall into five main categories: seminoma, teratocarcinoma, embryonal carcinoma, teratoma, and choriocarcinoma. A pure seminoma will usually respond to radiation therapy, which is therefore considered the treatment of choice to eradicate any metastases following orchiectomy. The other tumors usually respond to chemotherapy, which may be employed with or without a lymphadenectomy. This additional surgery is performed a few days after orchiectomy if there is lymph node infiltration (identified on the lymphangiogram or CT scan) but no further evidence of metastases.

The surgery involves the retroperitoneal nodes in the iliac and lumbar regions. A wide excision is necessary, since the blood supply and the lymphatic vessels of the testicles and the kidneys are directly related. This occurs because, in the embryo, the testicles develop adjacent to the kidneys. Although the testicles later descend and the kidneys ascend from their original positions in the abdomen, the circulatory vessels of these organs remain closely connected.

For the procedure the patient is placed either in a supine or a side-lying position (see Fig. 22-1), and a midline incision, a transthoracic incision, or a combination of the two incisions is made. The adjacent section of the colon is mobilized medially, thereby exposing the perinephric area. The perinephric fat and nodes are removed on the affected side, along with the nodes near the aorta and both renal hila. The node dissection continues along the iliac vessels to the inguinal area of the affected side (Fig. 56-1). Incisional drains are inserted at the lateral end

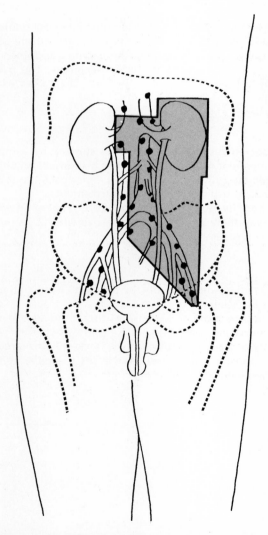

Fig. 56-1. Area of lymph node dissection in lymphadenectomy for testicular cancer, left side.

of the transthoracic incision (or via a stab wound if it is a midline incision). The incision is then closed, and a dressing is applied.

RETROPERITONEAL LYMPHADENECTOMY
Outline of Care Plan
ANTICIPATED NURSING DIAGNOSES:

Preoperative period
1. Psychologic distress related to the diagnosis of cancer.
2. Need for preoperative teaching.
3. Need for discharge planning.

Early postoperative period
4. Potential for shock.
5. Postoperative pain.
6. Potential for wound complications.
7. Need for management of intravenous infusion.
8. Alterations in gastrointestinal function.
9. Potential for respiratory complications related to surgical intervention.
10. Potential for urinary retention.
11. Potential for deep vein thrombosis.

Late postoperative period
12. Continued potential for circulatory and respiratory complications.
13. Potential for gastrointestinal complications related to resumption of oral intake.

Convalescent period
14. Potential for side effects and complications resulting from chemotherapy.*
15. Need for discharge teaching.

---

*May not apply.

NURSING CARE PLAN FOR THE PATIENT UNDERGOING RETROPERITONEAL LYMPHADENECTOMY

---

1. NURSING DIAGNOSIS: Psychologic distress related to the diagnosis of cancer

Objectives of nursing intervention
{ Provision of an emotionally supportive environment
Achievement of effective communication between patient, family, and staff

Expected outcomes
{ Verbalization by the patient of feelings about the diagnosis
Realistic decision-making
Absence of severe or protracted depression

Plan for implementation	Rationale
See Chapter 20, nursing objective 1.	
In addition to the interventions mentioned in Chapter 20, do the following:	
Avoid identification with the patient, which is a common problem in nurse-patient relationships when the nurse and patient are roughly the same age. Since many of these patients are under 30, this situation frequently occurs, often without the nurse even being aware of it.	If nurses permit themselves to identify too strongly with a patient, they may become caught up in their **own** feelings and fears about how **they** would cope with the condition if it were to happen to them. Personal feelings such as these can, if not recognized, interfere with direct communication and understanding of what the **patient** is feeling.

Preoperative period

2. NURSING DIAGNOSIS: Need for preoperative teaching

Objectives of nursing intervention

- If necessary, clarification of type of surgery to be performed
- Elimination of any negative or inaccurate notions regarding the forthcoming surgery
- Explanation of preoperative tests and procedures
- Explanation of events expected in the early postoperative period
- Explanation of body conditions expected in the early postoperative period

Expected outcomes

- Verbal indication that explanations are understood
- Verbal indication of optimistic expectations (within realistic limits) related to forthcoming surgery
- Cooperation during preoperative tests and procedures
- Verbal or behavioral indication of reduction of anxiety
- Absence of postoperative complications

Plan for implementation	Rationale
1. Briefly review with the patient the items mentioned prior to his orchiectomy.	Retroperitoneal lymphadenectomy is usually performed a few days after an orchiectomy (after the pathology reports on the type of tumor have been completed).
2. In addition to the topics already covered in the initial preoperative teaching explain the following: a. The preoperative shave will be from nipple line to midthigh. b. Oral intake will be prohibited for at least 24 to 48 hours after surgery. During this time the patient will have a nasogastric tube connected to a suction machine by his bedside to remove gastric secretions and gas. c. Once the patient passes flatus and bowel sounds are heard, he will be given a clear fluid diet. If this is tolerated, the diet will be advanced to the patient's normal diet. d. The patient will have an incision on his abdomen that will be covered by a dressing. There is usually drainage from the incision, so the dressing will require frequent changing for the first few days after surgery.	Oral intake, as well as gastric secretions and gas, would cause severe discomfort during the period of intestinal atony, which almost always occurs after this type of surgery.
3. Determine from the physician if he anticipates that the patient will be sterile after surgery and, if so, whether he has thoroughly discussed this with the patient and explored the option of using a sperm bank prior to surgery.*	Usually complete sexual function can be preserved if the surgeon avoids dissecting the aortic lymph nodes on the **unaffected** side below the renal vessels. The purpose is to avoid interrupting the sympathetic ganglia at L1. Otherwise, ejaculatory failure will occur. (The patient will still be able to experience erection and orgasm.) In some cases, however, bilateral dissection cannot be avoided, and the patient will have to face the prospect of perma-

Preoperative period

*Although sperm banking does not guarantee fertility, in many cases sperm that have been frozen and stored for a period of time are still capable of fertilizing an egg (via artificial insemination). Generally three semen specimens are required, and these should be collected 48 hours apart to ensure adequate sperm concentration.

Plan for implementation	Rationale
	nent sterility as well as all the other potentially devastating consequences of testicular cancer.

4. If sterility is anticipated and **after** the physician has discussed it with the patient:
   a. Encourage the patient to express his feelings.
   b. Provide emotional support (see Chapter 19).
   c. Reassure the patient that, although he may become infertile, he will still be capable of having sexual intercourse.

3. NURSING DIAGNOSIS: Need for discharge planning

Objectives of nursing intervention
Early commencement of discharge planning
Accurate estimate of time required for all discharge teaching

Expected outcome Smooth transition of care after discharge

Plan for implementation	Rationale

See master care plan for the patient requiring discharge preparations: discharge planning.

In addition to the topics covered in the master care plan, the following items should be considered:
1. The duration of hospitalization for the combined orchiectomy and lymphadenectomy is approximately 2 to 3 weeks, unless it is prolonged for chemotherapy.

2. The required teaching includes:
   a. General postoperative discharge teaching
   b. Discussion of the need for frequent follow-up examinations
   c. Possible instructions on chemotherapeutic regimen, if one is required

4. NURSING DIAGNOSIS: Potential for shock

Objective of nursing intervention   Prevention or early detection of shock

Expected outcomes   { Vital signs normal, skin dry, color normal
                          Absence of bright red drainage

Plan for implementation	Rationale
1. Check the patient's vital signs every 4 hours once stable (every 15 minutes if unstable).	Hypovolemic shock is a potential complication after this type of surgery because of the possibility of excessive loss of lymphatic fluid at the site of the lymphadenectomy. Furthermore, the painstaking removal of numerous lymph nodes makes the duration of this surgery relatively long, predisposing the patient to neurogenic shock from prolonged anesthesia.
2. Be alert for increasing pulse and respiratory rates, decreasing blood pressure, diaphoresis, pallor, and feelings of apprehension.	
3. Notify the physician at once if indications of impending shock occur.	

5. NURSING DIAGNOSIS: Postoperative pain

Objective of nursing intervention   Appropriate management of pain or discomfort

Expected outcome   Behavioral and/or verbal indication that pain is adequately reduced or absent

Plan for implementation	Rationale
Determine the source of the pain. It may be related to the surgical wound, musculoskeletal manipulation, or pharyngeal irritation.	Pain from different sources usually requires different intervention.
1. Question and observe the patient to obtain information about the pain.	
2. Be aware that pain is a unique and individual experience. Although the different sources of pain can usually be determined by their characteristics, there are also many variations.	
3. Be alert for indications (verbal or behavioral) that the patient is experiencing discomfort other than physical pain, and attempt to resolve the problem.	Numerous conditions, including fear of unknown factors in the future course of his disease, may be sources of extreme discomfort for the patient, who may unconsciously translate these feelings into pain. However, in the early postoperative period the pain after this type of surgery is very real.

Early postoperative period

Additional surgery for testicular cancer: retroperitoneal lymphadenectomy

Plan for implementation	Rationale

MODERATE TO SEVERE PAIN AT SURGICAL SITE, USUALLY AGGRAVATED BY PHYSICAL ACTIVITY

1. Administer analgesics as ordered.

Pain with these characteristics is usually incisional in origin, which is expected and often quite severe after this type of surgery.

2. Plan the patient's activities to coincide with a time when there is a high level of pain medication in the patient's bloodstream.

The patient will cooperate better with coughing exercises, ambulating, bathing, etc. when the pain is well under control.

3. Notify the physician if the patient's requests for pain medication do not begin to decrease within 48 to 72 hours.

Although the intensity of postoperative pain varies enormously between patients, there should be some decrease in the apparent severity of the pain within 2 or 3 days. If this does not occur, the possibility of wound complications should be considered. However, the extensive nature of this surgery, combined with the emotional stress most patients experience in relation to their diagnosis, may result in the patient expressing a need for analgesia for considerably longer than the average surgical patient.

MUSCULAR DISCOMFORT IN NECK, SHOULDERS, EXTREMITIES, ETC.

1. Provide the patient with an explanation for the pain and reassurance that it is transient.

Because of the relatively long duration of this operation and the side-lying position sometimes used for the surgery, the patient may feel stiffness or soreness in various parts of his body. For the first few days after surgery the administration of narcotic analgesics and the presence of severe incisional pain may mask this discomfort. Generally, reassurance that it does not indicate complications is sufficient to take the patient's mind off it.

2. Apply warm compresses to affected area.

3. Provide back rubs as needed.

SORE THROAT

1. Explain the reason for the discomfort.

The nasogastric tube and possible trauma caused by the endotracheal tube may cause this discomfort. Explanation and reassurance reduces patient anxiety and therefore may provide some relief.

2. Provide reassurance that, after the removal of the nasogastric tube, the discomfort will be considerably reduced and should disappear within a day or two.

3. Suggest that 2% lidocaine mouthwash (Xylocaine 2% Viscous) be ordered for gargling as needed.

This topical anesthetic may provide some temporary relief from the discomfort.

Early postoperative period

6. NURSING DIAGNOSIS: Potential for wound complications

**Objective of nursing
intervention**   Prevention or early detection of complications arising from the incisional area

Expected outcome   Absence of fever, purulent exudate, erythema, edema, hematoma, dehiscence,
and other abnormal wound conditions

Plan for implementation	Rationale
1. Check the dressing frequently (every 4 hours during the first 24 to 48 hours after surgery). Change it when it becomes wet, and use sterile technique for the procedure.	There is usually a moderate amount of drainage on the dressing for the first 1 or 2 days after the surgery. If a Hemovac drain is used, the dressing will not require changing as frequently as it would with a Penrose drain because most of the drainage will be drawn into the Hemovac vacuum bottle.
2. If a Hemovac drain is used, employ the following guidelines*: a. Avoid contamination of the spout and inner portion of the cap while emptying the vacuum bottle.	Because the drain communicates with the interior of the wound, care must be taken to prevent the possibility of organisms ascending from any point in the system.
b. Keep accurate records of the amount and character of the drainage. c. Notify the physician when the drainage ceases.	Usually the termination of drainage indicates that the Hemovac can be removed. However, if drainage stops within 24 hours after surgery, this may also indicate an obstruction in the lumen or a malfunctioning vacuum. The physician may want to irrigate the tube or change the vacuum bottle.
d. Reapply pressure to the vacuum bottle before closing it.	The negative pressure in the drain facilitates drainage from the wound.
e. Keep the vacuum bottle tied loosely around the patient's waist, hanging from his shoulder, or pinned to his gown.	This prevents inadvertent removal of the drain by accidental pulling on the vacuum bottle.
3. Use caution when removing soiled dressings to prevent inadvertent removal of the incisional drain.	Premature removal of a drain may result in prolonged wound healing.
4. Cut and arrange gauze pads around the incisional drain.	This prevents the dressings from flattening the drain and possibly obstructing the flow of drainage from the wound.
5. Note the condition of the suture line. (Usually retention and skin sutures are used.) Chart its appearance and the presence of edema, erythema, ecchymosis, or other abnormal conditions.	This provides a frame of reference for other staff members caring for the patient.

*These guidelines can also be applied to Jackson-Pratt suction devices, which are used in some hospitals instead of Hemovacs.

Early postoperative period

Plan for implementation	Rationale
6. Notify the physician if there is any evidence of dehiscence.	

7. If there is purulent drainage:
  a. Notify the physician.
  b. Obtain a wound culture specimen.
	This would indicate a wound infection.
	
	This will facilitate identification of the infecting organism so that appropriate treatment can be instituted quickly.

8. Check the patient's temperature every 4 hours, and notify the physician if there is an elevation above 101°.	Wound infection must always be suspected when a patient runs a fever postoperatively. Other causes include respiratory complications and pharmacologic intervention.

7. NURSING DIAGNOSIS: Need for management of intravenous infusion

Objectives of nursing intervention
- Appropriate administration of specific types of intravenous solutions
- Prevention or early detection of local complications
- Prevention or early detection of systemic complications
- Management of discomfort caused by the intravenous infusion
- Maintenance of proper function of intravenous equipment
- Maintenance of accurate records of the patient's hydration status

Expected outcomes
- Normal hydration status
- Normal electrolyte status
- Absence of thrombophlebitis, infiltration, infection, fluid overload, and pulmonary embolism
- Absence of discomfort caused by the intravenous infusion

Plan for implementation	Rationale
See master care plan for the patient receiving intravenous therapy.	These patients usually receive isotonic dextrose and saline solutions until they are able to tolerate oral intake. Potassium supplements are frequently given to compensate for losses in nasotracheal and wound drainage. Sometimes plasma expanders are also given.

Early postoperative period

8. NURSING DIAGNOSIS: Alterations in gastrointestinal function

Objectives of nursing intervention
{ Appropriate management of nasogastric suction
Prevention or early detection of complications heralded by changes in nasogastric drainage

Expected outcomes
{ Moderate amount of greenish brown drainage through suction apparatus
Absence of pain, abdominal distention, nausea, and vomiting

Plan for implementation	Rationale
1. Keep nasogastric tube securely taped to the patient's nose and pinned to the patient's gown.	This prevents inadvertent traction on the tube, which would cause discomfort.
2. Maintain suction through the tube as ordered, and irrigate it with normal saline at regular intervals (usually every 2 hours).	
3. Record volume and characteristics of drainage each shift. (Drainage is usually greenish.)	Records of the volume of drainage are extremely important. Frequently the physician will order intravenous replacement of fluid and electrolytes to compensate for what was lost in the gastrointestinal secretions.
4. Be alert for sudden changes in color or volume of the drainage.	
a. If drainage ceases, irrigate with normal saline; if no results, check the suction device and replace it if necessary.	Sudden reduction of output may indicate obstruction of tubing or faulty suction equipment.
b. If there appears to be blood in the drainage: (1) Notify the physician at once. (2) Obtain a specimen for a test for occult blood.	Drainage that is bright red or has brownish particles in it indicates bleeding somewhere in the gastrointestinal tract.
5. Prohibit oral intake as ordered.	
6. Provide mouth care as needed.	The mouth often becomes uncomfortably dry when nasogastric suction is in use.
7. Lubricate the nares with petroleum jelly as needed.	This reduces some of the irritation caused by the nasogastric tube.
8. Check periodically for bowel sounds and passage of flatus.	These indicate that the intestines are regaining function.

Early postoperative period

9. NURSING DIAGNOSIS: Potential for respiratory complications related to surgical intervention

Objectives of nursing intervention
- Early detection of pneumothorax
- Prevention or early detection of atelectasis and/or pneumonia

Expected outcomes
- Cooperation with therapeutic respiratory regimen
- Absence of dyspnea and other symptoms of pneumothorax
- Absence of fever or audible lung congestion
- Sputum clear or white and easily mobilized

Plan for implementation	Rationale
See master care plan for the patient at risk for respiratory complications, nursing objectives 4 and 5.	This surgery involves the removal of perinephric fat and lymph nodes adjacent to the lung under the diaphragm. Therefore, as with any renal surgery, the risk of pneumothorax must be considered along with the more common respiratory complications.

10. NURSING DIAGNOSIS: Potential for urinary retention

Objectives of nursing intervention
- Maintenance of accurate records of urinary output
- Early detection of retention

Expected outcome   Normal voiding pattern resumed within 6 hours after surgery

Plan for implementation	Rationale
1. Instruct the patient to notify the nurse when he needs to void for the first time after surgery, and leave a urinal by the bedside.	The effects of the anesthesia may cause temporary urinary retention. If this occurs, it should be corrected as soon as possible to prevent discomfort and possible renal damage. However, this is an infrequent complication in patients who are relatively young.
2. Keep accurate records of the volume, frequency, and character of each voiding for at least 72 hours (or as long as the patient has an intravenous infusion).	

3. If the patient has not voided within 6 hours after surgery:
  a. Be certain he is receiving adequate fluids.
  b. Palpate suprapubic area for distention. (This may be difficult if the incision and dressing are very low on the abdomen.)
  c. Depending on the condition of the patient, assist the patient to a standing position with the urinal. Permission from the physician may be required because bed rest is ordered in the immediate postoperative period.
	Occasionally dehydration may be the cause of anuria.
	If the patient is in severe retention, the suprapubic area will be hard and distended.
	
	Assuming the accustomed position for voiding will help the patient to void if the retention is caused by psychologic factors.

Early postoperative period

Plan for implementation	Rationale
d. Provide the patient with adequate privacy.	
e. Notify the physician if the patient has not voided despite these measures.	Catheterization may be necessary.

11. NURSING DIAGNOSIS: Potential for deep vein thrombosis

Objectives of nursing intervention
Explanation and maintenance of precautions against deep vein thrombosis
Early detection of deep vein thrombosis

Expected outcomes
Cooperation with regimen to prevent deep vein thrombosis
Absence of local pain, swelling, and redness of a lower extremity
Absence of fever

Plan for implementation	Rationale
See master care plan for the patient at risk for deep vein thrombosis.	These patients are at risk for deep vein thrombosis because of the manipulation of the retroperitoneal and iliac blood vessels during removal of the adjacent lymph nodes.

12. NURSING DIAGNOSIS: Continued potential for circulatory and respiratory complications

Objective of nursing intervention
Prevention or early detection of deep vein thrombosis, atelectasis, and pneumonia

Expected outcomes
Cooperation with regimen to promote adequate circulation
Absence of lung congestion
or
Cooperation with regimen to improve respiratory function

Plan for implementation	Rationale
1. Encourage the patient to sit in a chair at least twice daily and to ambulate (with assistance if necessary).	Because of the extensive nature of this surgery, the patient may be reluctant to move around, and adequate circulation and lung expansion may be compromised.
2. Do not permanently remove antiembolic stockings or Ace bandages until the patient is ambulating well.	Until the patient is out of bed most of the day, elastic support of the legs is considered useful in preventing venous stasis.

Early postoperative period

Late postoperative period

638

Plan for implementation	Rationale
3. Auscultate for lung congestion and continue coughing and abdominal breathing exercises as needed.	The patient may be reluctant to breathe deeply because of the proximity of the incision to the lung.
4. Note changes in characteristics of cough, and notify the physician if the sputum becomes yellow, green, or brown and/or is foul smelling.	Any indications of pneumonia must be reported to the physician so appropriate treatment can be started as soon as possible.

13. NURSING DIAGNOSIS: Potential for gastrointestinal complications related to resumption of oral intake

Objective of nursing intervention   Early detection of gastrointestinal complications

Expected outcome   { Absence of abdominal distention, tympany, nausea, and vomiting
             Return to normal bowel function

Plan for implementation	Rationale
1. Disconnect the nasogastric tube as ordered.	Once bowel sounds are heard and the patient passes flatus, nasogastric suction is no longer required. The patient will usually be permitted sips of water with the nasogastric tube clamped. If this is tolerated, the tube will be removed.
2. If a long (intestinal) tube is used, assist the physician with its removal.	A tube that extends into the intestines must be removed gradually over a period of a few hours to prevent damage to the gastrointestinal tract.
3. Notify the physician if nausea and vomiting occur.	
4. Note the patient's response to the diet, which usually begins with clear fluids and is then advanced as tolerated. The development of distention, tympany, nausea, or vomiting indicates that the patient is not yet able to tolerate oral intake.	

Late postoperative period

Convalescent period

14. NURSING DIAGNOSIS: Potential for side effects and complications resulting from chemotherapy

Objectives of nursing intervention

Reduction of the patient's fears and negative expectations regarding chemotherapy

Prevention or limitation of stomatitis

Maintenance of adequate gastrointestinal and nutritional status

Reduction of alopecia and related psychologic discomfort

Prevention and/or early detection of toxicity

Safe administration of specific chemotherapeutic medications

Expected outcomes

Expression of realistic expectations regarding chemotherapy

Compliance with regimen to prevent or limit stomatitis

Compliance with feasible nutritional regimen

Absence of embarrassment regarding alopecia

Normal blood urea nitrogen and creatinine levels, absence of tinnitus or hearing deficits, white blood cell, red blood cell, and platelet counts within acceptable range

Chemotherapeutic agents may be used as adjuvant therapy for testicular tumors (except seminomas) when there is evidence of metastasis. The three most commonly used medications are bleomycin sulfate, vinblastine sulfate, and cisplatin. The specific combination of these or other drugs and the commencement, frequency, or duration of treatment vary considerably, depending on the extent of the disease and the particular protocol being followed by the physician. Occasionally these drugs are used preoperatively to shrink an inoperable lesion to an operable size. In most cases considerable nursing intervention is required to prevent or minimize the untoward effects of the medications. Furthermore, there is a fine line between the expected side effects and dangerous toxic effects. The nurse must be aware of what side effects to look for in relation to a particular drug and be able to identify toxic effects that may indicate the need for termination of that drug.

Plan for implementation	Rationale
PSYCHOLOGIC ATTITUDE TOWARD CHEMOTHERAPY	
1. Ask the patient what he has heard about chemotherapy and how he thinks it will affect him.	There has been a considerable amount of negative publicity regarding the side effects of chemotherapy. Much of it is inaccurate or only partially accurate.
2. Provide accurate information regarding the effects of chemotherapy.	The patient should be aware that some aspects of his treatment will be unpleasant, although inaccurate or distorted information should be corrected. The nurse should emphasize that chemotherapy is considered a highly successful means of treating certain kinds of testicular cancer.[3] This reduces the possibility of the patient's expectations affecting his responses to the medication. This is particularly important with regard to nausea and vomiting, which may be somewhat influenced by the patient's mental state.
3. When discussing the side effects, avoid definitive statements. Instead, say that **some** patients **may** have a particular response.	
4. Throughout the period of treatment, help the patient maintain a sense of autonomy by conveying the importance of **his** reports on what he is experiencing in relation to the chemotherapy.	Although objective data (e.g., blood tests, x-rays, etc.) provide an important basis for the continuation or modification of the chemotherapeutic protocol, the patient's subjective response is also extremely important. He should be made to feel that he is taking an active role in

Plan for implementation	Rationale
	his treatment. Too often, the debilitating effects of the chemotherapy increase the patient's sense of being a victim, not only of a life-threatening disease but also of the health care team that is trying to help him.
5. When possible, include the patient in the decision-making process regarding possible modifications in his treatment. This is particularly important once the patient is discharged and is receiving chemotherapy on an outpatient basis. He should be helped to maintain as much of a normal life-style as possible.	

STOMATITIS

Plan for implementation	Rationale
1. Examine the patient's mouth before commencement of treatment; report any abnormal findings.	Any urgent dental work may have to be completed before the treatment to prevent the risk of life-threatening hemorrhage or infection. The patient will be more prone to these complications because of the decreased platelet count and the immunosuppression resulting from the chemotherapy.
2. Chart the appearance of the patient's mouth (i.e., color of gums, bleeding, ulceration).	This provides a baseline for an accurate evaluation of the patient's mouth during treatment.
3. Maintain good oral hygiene during treatment and for at least 2 to 3 weeks afterward (or until all signs of inflammation disappear). This includes: a. Brushing with a soft toothbrush b. Using hydrogen peroxide mouthwash solution every 4 hours; hydrogen peroxide can be diluted with equal parts water and a nonirritating flavored mouthwash if desired c. Discontinuation of brushing (and the use of dental floss if used before treatment) if the platelet count drops below 10,000 to 15,000/mm^3 d. Avoiding the use of lemon and glycerine swabs at all times	Vinblastine and other chemotherapeutic agents cause disturbances of the buccal mucosa. Ulceration, bleeding, and infection are common. This minimizes irritation of the buccal mucosa. This provides mild antiseptic action and should be done regularly. Any irritation of the gums should be avoided when bleeding tendencies are severe. Although these swabs may be refreshing for the normal mouth, they should not be used when the mucosa is deteriorated because they have a drying effect and they also change the pH of the mouth.
4. Encourage appropriate nutritional habits, such as: a. Eating soft, nonabrasive foods b. Eating bland, nonacid foods	This reduces mechanical irritation of the buccal mucosa. This prevents chemical irritation of the buccal mucosa.
5. If eating becomes painful, suggest that the physician order a topical anesthetic such as 2% lidocaine mouthwash (Xylocaine 2% Viscous) to precede meals or every 4 hours.	This reduces mouth pain, which in some cases can be severe.
6. Obtain a culture specimen from any new mouth lesions.	This enables appropriate antimicrobial treatment to be determined.

Convalescent period

Convalescent period

Plan for implementation	Rationale
ANOREXIA, NAUSEA, VOMITING	
1. Before commencement of chemotherapy, weigh the patient (for a baseline) and then continue to weigh him periodically throughout the duration of the treatment and during follow-up care.	This provides a general indicator of the patient's nutritional status.
2. During the period of treatment, keep the emesis basin within reach **but out of sight of the patient.**	This reduces the psychologic component of nausea and vomiting during chemotherapy.
3. Suggest that the physician order antiemetics to be administered as needed or prophylactically during treatment. Although not always effective, the following drugs may provide some relief: a. Prochlorperazine (Compazine) b. Chlorpromazine (Thorazine) c. Trimethobenzamide (Tigan) d. THC (tetrahydrocannabinol)*	The majority of chemotherapeutic agents cause nausea and vomiting to some degree. Cisplatin almost always causes vomiting beginning approximately 1 hour after administration and lasting for 24 to 36 hours or more after the treatment ends. Nausea may persist even longer.
4. Keep accurate records of the volume of vomitus.	Fluids lost during vomiting should be replaced by an increase in the volume of intravenous infusion fluids. These patients must be kept well hydrated to prevent renal damage, another common complication from chemotherapy, especially with cisplatin. If vomiting is copious, additional electrolytes will probably be ordered, since sodium, potassium, chloride, and hydrogen ions are lost.
5. Determine the patient's food preferences and provide him with the most appetizing meals, if he is able to tolerate oral intake.	Anorexia is very common during treatment. The patient should be encouraged to eat as much as possible whenever he is capable of doing so to avoid nutritional deficiencies.
6. Determine whether there is a particular time during the day when the nausea is least disturbing, and encourage high food intake at that time.	Sometimes a patient will tolerate food better in the morning than at other times during the day. Therefore breakfast (or whichever meal is served at the particular time when he feels best) should be as nutritionally complete as possible.
LOWER GASTROINTESTINAL TRACT DISTURBANCES	
1. If the patient develops cramps and/or diarrhea: a. Record volume of liquid stool and frequency of episodes of diarrhea. b. Encourage the patient to follow a bland, low-residue diet. c. Suggest that the physician order an antidiarrhetic such as diphenoxylate (Lomotil).	These symptoms often result from hypermotility of the gastrointestinal tract due to cellular damage.

*This derivative of marijuana is being used experimentally in some cancer centers.

Plan for implementation	**Rationale**
2. If the patient develops anal tenderness, apply A & D ointment or petroleum jelly.	This may result from excoriation of the anal mucosa after frequent bowel movements.
3. If the patient develops constipation:	This is a side effect of vinblastine and a few other chemotherapeutic agents.
a. Encourage the patient to follow a high-residue diet (unless stomatitis is present and the texture of the food is irritating to his gums).	
b. Encourage the patient to drink fruit juices.	
c. Suggest that the physician order a stool softener or cathartic to be administered as needed.	

ALOPECIA

1. Explain ahead of time that hair loss might occur but that the hair usually regrows within about 8 weeks after termination of treatment. However, the hair may be a different color and texture when it grows in.	Hair loss is a possible side effect of bleomycin, vinblastine, and certain other chemotherapeutic agents.
2. Attempt to reduce the severity of hair loss in one of the following ways:	These measures limit the circulation to the hair follicles during the period when there is a relatively high concentration of the medication in the patient's bloodstream.
a. Apply a scalp tourniquet during intravenous administration of the particular drug, and keep it in place for 10 to 15 minutes after the infusion has ended.[2]	
b. Apply ice packs to the scalp area during the period of drug administration and for 10 to 15 minutes after the infusion has ended.	
3. If alopecia occurs and the patient is very distressed about it, suggest the use of a cap or a bandanna worn around the head.	

DANGEROUS, TOXIC EFFECTS

1. Reduce or limit the incidence of renal toxicity by the following actions:	Cisplatin and certain other chemotherapeutic agents are highly nephrotoxic.
a. Keep the patient well hydrated during treatment. The precise amount of intravenous fluid will be prescribed by the patient's physician.	
b. Maintain accurate records of intake and output.	
c. Be certain blood urea nitrogen and creatinine levels are being measured daily.	
d. Report any abnormal laboratory values for renal function tests.	
e. Verify with the physician any concomitant use of aminoglycoside medications.	Antibiotics in this group (e.g., gentamicin, kanamycin, and tobramycin) are nephrotoxic. This added insult to the kidneys should certainly be avoided.

Convalescent period

Plan for implementation	Rationale
2. Reduce or limit the incidence of ototoxicity by the following actions: 　a. Check that a baseline audiogram has been obtained for the patient before treatment. 　b. Be certain the patient continues to have periodic audiometry during the treatment. 　c. Notify the physician if the patient complains of tinnitus or if he appears to be having hearing difficulty.	Cisplatin and certain other chemotherapeutic agents are highly ototoxic.
3. Reduce or limit the incidence of liver toxicity by the following actions: 　a. Be certain blood specimens are being drawn for liver function tests on a regular basis. 　b. Notify the physician if there are any abnormal values on liver function tests.	Bleomycin and certain other chemotherapeutic agents are hepatotoxic. The physician will order these tests to be done at a frequency based on the patient's general condition and the specific drug being used.
4. Reduce or limit the effects of bone marrow depression by the following actions: 　a. Be certain specimens for complete blood counts are being obtained on a regular basis. 　b. If the patient's white blood cell count falls below normal: 　　(1) Wash hands before any contact with the patient. 　　(2) Avoid having the patient in contact with anybody who has an infection. This includes other patients, visitors, and staff members who have colds. 　　(3) Carefully monitor the patient's temperature, and notify the physician at once if there is any elevation. It may be an indication of an infection, although the possibility that it may be a side effect of a particular medication (e.g., bleomycin) should also be considered. 　c. If the patient's red blood cell count falls below normal: 　　(1) Explain to the patient the reason for his decreased tolerance to activity. 　　(2) Plan the patient's activities to include frequent rest periods. 　　(3) Encourage activities that do not require a great expenditure of energy (e.g., television and reading). 　d. If the patient's platelet level falls below normal:	Almost all chemotherapeutic agents have an adverse effect on the bone marrow; they reduce the rate of production of white blood cells, red blood cells, and platelets. These are usually taken daily unless the patient's platelet count is so low that the process of withdrawing blood could result in an episode of bleeding. A depressed white blood cell count increases the patient's susceptibility to infection. Because an infection can be life threatening when the patient's immune system is compromised, early detection and treatment are essential. Blood and urine culture specimens will probably be obtained, and the patient may be given a broad-spectrum antibiotic until results of the cultures are known. A depressed red blood cell count will cause the patient to tire easily. The decrease in the number of red blood cells reduces the oxygen-carrying capacity of the blood. This is usually a temporary effect of the chemotherapy and should reverse itself once treatment is terminated. A depressed platelet count will cause an increased bleeding tendency, manifested by delayed clotting, ecchymosis, and bleeding from the gastrointestinal and urinary tracts.

Convalescent period

644

Plan for implementation	Rationale
(1) Minimize the number of injections the patient must receive by having as many medications as possible reordered for intravenous or oral routes.	
(2) Maintain pressure over puncture sites after injections and blood specimen withdrawals until bleeding has completely stopped.	
(3) Warn the patient that he might bruise more easily. Explain the reason and that it is a temporary effect of the chemotherapy.	
(4) Pad any bony prominences if ecchymosis is occurring.	
(5) Be certain the patient is using a soft toothbrush.	
(6) Observe urine, vomitus, and stool for indications of gastrointestinal and urinary tract bleeding, and report any abnormal findings.	

SPECIAL PROBLEMS CONCERNING ONLY BLEOMYCIN, VINBLASTINE, AND CISPLATIN

1. If the patient is receiving bleomycin:
   a. Be alert for changes in the patient's respiratory status.
   b. Notify the physician if dyspnea occurs or if rales are noted on auscultation.
   c. Be certain the patient is receiving chest x-ray examinations at regular intervals.

Pneumonitis, developing into pulmonary fibrosis, is a serious side effect of bleomycin.
These are early symptoms of pneumonitis.

Chest x-ray examinations should be scheduled approximately every 1 or 2 weeks during treatment to detect any irregularities in the lungs.

2. If the patient is receiving vinblastine:
   a. Take special precautions to avoid splashing medication into the patient's or your own eyes.
   b. If accidental contact with the eye occurs, irrigate the affected eye thoroughly with water.

Vinblastine will cause severe irritation of the eye and possibly corneal ulceration.

3. If the patient is receiving cisplatin:
   a. Keep unreconstituted drug in the refrigerator, but keep reconstituted drug at room temperature until ready for use.
   b. Do not use intravenous sets, catheters, or needles that contain aluminum when administering cisplatin.

If reconstituted solution is refrigerated, it will precipitate.[1]

Cisplatin may react with the aluminum to form a black precipitate.[4]

Convalescent period

15. NURSING DIAGNOSIS: Need for discharge teaching

Objectives of nursing intervention

Explanation of basic information about medications to be taken at home

Explanation of information regarding follow-up care

Explanation of residual effects of the condition and/or treatment

Explanation of instructions concerning postdischarge activities

Explanation of symptoms that constitute a reason to contact the physician

Review of admitting diagnosis and mode of treatment

Expected outcomes

Accurate return verbalization and/or demonstration of all material learned

Smooth transition of care after discharge

Absence or early detection of complications arising after discharge

Ability to provide future health care practitioners with important data about health history

Plan for implementation	Rationale
See master care plan for the patient requiring discharge preparations: discharge teaching.	
In addition to the topics covered in the master care plan, include the following items in the discharge teaching:	
1. At the initial follow-up visit the physician will check the wound for adequate healing, take blood specimens, and examine the patient's abdomen. If a chemotherapy regimen is to be started (or continued), plans for this will be discussed. Chemotherapy may be continued intermittently for up to 2 years.	
2. Additional check-ups and chest x-ray examinations will be scheduled periodically throughout the next 2 years.	
3. The patient may experience some fatigue for the next few weeks as a residual effect of the surgery. Any reactions encountered during treatment with chemotherapeutic agents (see pp. 640 to 645) should gradually subside once medication is terminated.	
4. The patient should notify the physician if any of the following occur:	
a. Fever	This may be caused by an infection or a reaction to the chemotherapeutic regimen.
b. Unusual bleeding or bruising	This is probably a reaction to the chemotherapy and warrants reevaluation of the patient's red blood cell, white blood cell, and platelet counts.
c. Appearance of a mass in the neck, inguinal area, or opposite testicle (see p. 610 for testicular self-examination)	This may indicate metastatic spread of the tumor.
d. Severe pain or increasing redness at the incisional site	This may indicate a wound infection.

Convalescent period

CHAPTER 57

Vasectomy and vasovasotomy

Vasectomy and vasovasotomy are presented together because one procedure is virtually the reverse of the other. Vasectomy is an elective procedure for a man who wants a permanent and totally reliable method of contraception. Vasovasotomy is done in instances where a vasectomized man has changed his mind and wants to attempt conception. The success rate of vasovasotomy in restoring fertility is approximately 20%.[3]

For a vasectomy the patient is in a supine position.

The vas deferens is palpated near the upper part of the scrotum, and an incision is made into the scrotal skin. The vas is identified, approximately 1 cm of it is resected, and the edges are ligated (Fig. 57-1). The scrotal skin is closed, without drainage, and the procedure is repeated on the opposite side. A dressing and scrotal support are then applied.

The patient is informed that he must continue to use another means of contraception until after the follow-up semen analysis is performed (usually 1

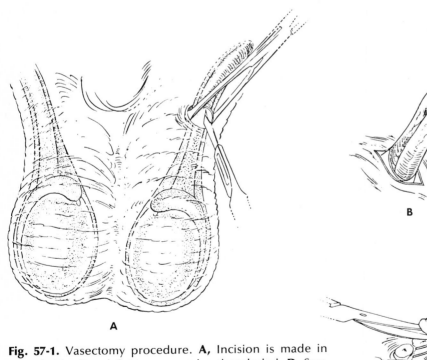

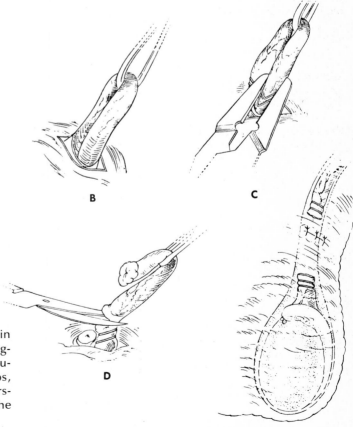

Fig. 57-1. Vasectomy procedure. **A,** Incision is made in scrotal skin. **B** and **C,** Vas exposed and occluded. **D,** Segment is excised. **E,** Vas is replaced in sheath and skin sutured. Procedure is repeated on other side. (From Phipps, W.J., Long, B.C., and Woods, N.F.: Medical-surgical nursing: concepts and clniical practice, St. Louis, 1979, The C.V. Mosby Co.)

month after surgery) and aspermia is confirmed. Prior to this time infertility cannot be ensured because any sperm present in the seminal vessicles will be released during the next few ejaculations.

Vasovasotomy is performed under an operating microscope with 16 to 25× magnification. For the procedure the patient is placed in a supine position, and an incision is made into the scrotal skin at the location of the vasectomy. The strictured part of the vas is excised, and anastomosis is performed. This is usually done in two layers, with the mucosa anastomosed in one layer and the muscular tissue joined in a second layer. The scrotal incision is closed without drainage, the procedure is repeated on the opposite side, and a scrotal support and dressing are applied. Sperm analyses are done at 3-month intervals to assess the extent of improvement of semen quality.

Usually the hospital nurse will see only patients who are undergoing vasovasotomy because most vasectomies are performed in the physician's office under local anesthesia. When vasectomy is done on an inpatient basis with general anesthesia, the nursing care is almost identical to that for the vasovasotomy patient. For this reason the nursing care plans for both procedures are combined.

VASECTOMY OR VASOVASOTOMY
Outline of Care Plan
ANTICIPATED NURSING DIAGNOSES:

Preoperative period
1. Need for preoperative teaching.
2. Need for discharge planning.

Postoperative period
3. Potential for postoperative complications (shock, atelectasis, pneumonia, urinary retention, deep vein thrombosis).
4. Potential for wound complications.
5. Postoperative pain.

Convalescent period
6. Need for discharge teaching.

NURSING CARE PLAN FOR THE PATIENT UNDERGOING VASECTOMY OR VASOVASOTOMY

1. NURSING DIAGNOSIS: Need for preoperative teaching

Objectives of nursing intervention	Elimination of any negative or inaccurate notions regarding the forthcoming surgery
	Explanation of preoperative tests and procedures
	Psychologic preparation for general anesthesia (omit if the patient is to have spinal or local anesthesia)
	Explanation of events expected in the early postoperative period
	Explanation of body conditions expected in the early postoperative period
	Identification of any known allergies
Expected outcomes	Verbal indication that explanations are understood
	Verbal indication of optimistic expectations (within realistic limits) related to forthcoming surgery
	Cooperation during preoperative tests and procedures
	Verbal or behavioral indication of reduction of anxiety
	Absence of postoperative complications
	Absence of allergic reactions

Plan for implementation	Rationale
See master care plan for the patient receiving preoperative teaching.	

Preoperative period

Plan for implementation	Rationale
In addition to the topics covered in the master care plan, include the following items in the preoperative teaching: 1. The preoperative shave will be of the pubic area.	
2. The patient will be permitted a light meal in the evening after surgery.	These patients can usually tolerate oral intake within a few hours after surgery. For this reason the intravenous infusion used during surgery is often discontinued in the recovery room or shortly after the patient returns to the floor and tolerates fluids.
3. There will be two small incisions in the patient's scrotum that will be covered with a dressing and a scrotal support.	

2. NURSING DIAGNOSIS: Need for discharge planning

Objectives of nursing intervention
Early commencement of discharge planning
Accurate estimate of time required for all discharge teaching

Expected outcome   Smooth transition of care after discharge

Plan for implementation	Rationale
See master care plan for the patient requiring discharge preparations: discharge planning. In addition to the topics covered in the master care plan, the following items should be considered: 1. The duration of hospitalization for either of these procedures is approximately 2 or 3 days. 2. Required teaching includes: a. General postoperative discharge teaching b. Discussion of the need for follow-up semen analyses to determine the effectiveness of the surgery	

Preoperative period

649

3. NURSING DIAGNOSIS: Potential for postoperative complications (shock, atelectasis, pneumonia, urinary retention, deep vein thrombosis)

Objective of nursing intervention	Prevention or early detection of postoperative complications

Expected outcomes

Pulse and blood pressure normal, skin dry, color normal

Respirations regular and unlabored, absence of pulmonary congestion

Normal voiding pattern established within 6 hours after surgery

Early ambulation tolerated well

<table>
<tr><th>Plan for implementation</th><th>Rationale</th></tr>
<tr>
<td>

1. Check the patient's vital signs every 4 hours, and notify the physician of any indications of impending shock. These include:
   a. Increasing pulse and respiratory rates
   b. Decreasing blood pressure
   c. Diaphoresis and pallor
   d. Feelings of apprehension

</td>
<td>

Although shock is a potential complication after any kind of surgery, it is a relatively small risk after vasectomy or vasovasotomy because few blood vessels are cut and the duration of surgery is short.

</td>
</tr>
<tr>
<td>

2. Encourage coughing and abdominal breathing if the patient's lungs sound congested, and notify the physician if any of the following conditions are present:

   a. The patient is unable to cough and his lungs sound congested.
   b. Sputum volume is copious.
   c. Sputum color is other than clear or white.
   d. There is a rise in the patient's temperature.
   e. Breath sounds are diminished.

</td>
<td>

Although precautions must be taken, respiratory complications are unlikely after this type of surgery because the period of anesthesia is very short. Furthermore, there is no abdominal incision to inhibit effective coughing.
These conditions require additional treatment. The physician may order therapies such as incentive spirometry, nasotracheal suctioning, postural drainage, or intermittent positive pressure breathing, depending on the extent of respiratory embarrassment.

</td>
</tr>
<tr>
<td>

3. Promote resumption of normal voiding pattern by the following actions:
   a. Be certain the patient is well hydrated.
   b. Leave a urinal at the bedside within reach of the patient.
   c. Ask the patient to notify the nurse the first time he voids.
   d. If the patient has not voided within 6 hours after surgery:
      (1) Assist the patient to a standing position to void.

      (2) If the patient is still unable to void, notify the physician.

</td>
<td>

Temporary urinary retention is occasionally a result of anesthesia.

Assuming the accustomed position for voiding will help the patient to void if the retention is caused by psychologic factors.
Catheterization may be required.

</td>
</tr>
</table>

Postoperative period

Plan for implementation	Rationale
4. Use precautions against deep vein thrombosis. (See master care plan for the patient at risk for deep vein thrombosis.) These patients are usually permitted out of bed in the evening after surgery.	Although deep vein thrombosis is a relatively small risk after this type of surgery, it still must be considered, and adequate precautions should be taken.

4. NURSING DIAGNOSIS: Potential for wound complications

Objective of nursing intervention   Prevention or early detection of complications arising from the incisional area

Expected outcome   Absence of fever, purulent exudate, erythema, edema, and other abnormal wound conditions

Plan for implementation	Rationale
1. Check the dressing every shift. If it requires changing:	Drainage is very slight or absent after this type of surgery, since no incisional drains are used.
a. Use sterile technique for the procedure.	
b. Note the condition of the suture lines; chart their appearances and the presence of edema, erythema, or other abnormal wound conditions.	This provides a frame of reference for other staff members caring for the patient.
c. If there is purulent drainage:	This would indicate a wound infection.
(1) Notify the physician.	
(2) Obtain a wound culture specimen.	This will facilitate identification of the infecting organism so that appropriate treatment can be instituted quickly.
2. Check the patient's temperature every 4 hours, and notify the physician if there is an elevation above 101°.	Wound infection must always be suspected when the patient runs a fever postoperatively.

Postoperative period

5. NURSING DIAGNOSIS: Postoperative pain

Objective of nursing intervention   Appropriate management of pain or discomfort

Expected outcome   Behavioral and/or verbal indication that pain is adequately reduced or absent

Plan for implementation	Rationale
1. Determine characteristics of the pain by questioning and observing the patient.	The degree of pain patients experience after this type of surgery varies, but in most cases mild pain may be expected for the first 24 hours.
2. Be alert for indications (verbal or behavioral) that the patient is experiencing discomfort other than physical pain, and attempt to resolve the problem.	Surgery involving the sexual organs may give rise to considerable anxiety, which often can be alleviated simply by reassurance from the nurse.

3. If the discomfort is from surgical manipulation:
  a. Be certain the scrotal support is positioned properly.
 	
  b. Provide analgesic medication as ordered.
	The scrotal support elevates the scrotum, thereby enhancing drainage from the area. This reduces discomfort caused by edema.

4. Note the patient's response to the pain medication.	This provides a frame of reference for evaluation of the patient's condition on subsequent shifts.

Postoperative period

6. NURSING DIAGNOSIS: Need for discharge teaching

Objectives of nursing intervention
{ Explanation of basic information about medications to be taken at home
Explanation of information regarding follow-up care
Explanation of residual effects of the condition and/or treatment
Explanation of instructions concerning postdischarge activities
Explanation of symptoms that constitute a reason to contact the physician

Expected outcomes
{ Accurate return verbalization and/or demonstration of all material learned
Smooth transition of care after discharge
Absence or early detection of complications arising after discharge

Plan for implementation	Rationale
See master care plan for the patient requiring discharge preparations: discharge teaching.	
In addition to the topics covered in the master care plan, include the following items in the discharge teaching:	
1. At the follow-up office visit the physician will check the incisions for adequate healing. The sutures are absorbed and do not require removal.	

2. If the patient had a vasectomy:
  a. He should use additional contraception until after the follow-up semen analysis.
 	
  b. He should have the follow-up semen analysis approximately 1 month after the surgery.
	The vasectomy is not effective until all sperm remaining in the seminal vesicles are depleted. This takes approximately four or five ejaculations.

3. If the patient had a vasovasotomy:
  a. He should have follow-up semen analyses at 3-month intervals to determine the presence of sperm in the semen and their morphology, motility, and concentration.
  b. If semen quality has not improved considerably, he may require further investigation and possible treatment for the presence of sperm antibodies.
	There is a higher incidence of sperm antibodies in vasectomized men than in men who have not undergone this surgery.[1,2] There is some evidence to suggest that these antibodies can sometimes be eradicated with corticosteroid administration.[4]

4. The patient should notify the physician if any of the following occur:
  a. Severe pain or increased swelling at the surgical site
  b. Chills or fever
	This may indicate a wound infection.
	
	This may also indicate an infection.

Convalescent period

CHAPTER 58

Testicular biopsy for infertility

A testicular biopsy is performed for patients with aspermia to determine if the problem is at the level of the testicles (i.e., no sperm is being produced) or if the defect is in the sperm transport system.

For the procedure the patient is placed in a supine position, and the testicle is held so that the skin around it is tense. An incision is made into the scrotal skin to reach the surface of the testicle, and then a separate incision is made into the testicle. A small portion of the testicle is excised, and the specimen is immediately placed into a special solution that will not change cellular morphology. The specimen must **not** be placed in formalin. The scrotal skin is then closed without drainage, and the procedure is repeated on the other side. A dressing and scrotal support are applied when the biopsies are completed.

TESTICULAR BIOPSY FOR INFERTILITY
Outline of Care Plan
ANTICIPATED NURSING DIAGNOSES:

Preoperative period
1. Need for preoperative teaching.
2. Need for discharge planning.

Postoperative period
3. Potential for postoperative complications (shock, atelectasis, pneumonia, urinary retention, deep vein thrombosis).
4. Potential for wound complications.
5. Postoperative pain.

Convalescent period
6. Need for discharge teaching.

NURSING CARE PLAN FOR THE PATIENT UNDERGOING TESTICULAR BIOPSY FOR INFERTILITY

Preoperative period

1. NURSING DIAGNOSIS: Need for preoperative teaching

Objectives of nursing intervention

Elimination of any negative or inaccurate notions regarding the forthcoming surgery

Explanation of preoperative tests and procedures

Psychologic preparation for general anesthesia (omit if the patient is to have spinal or local anesthesia)

Explanation of events expected in the early postoperative period

Explanation of body conditions expected in the early postoperative period

Identification of any known allergies

Expected outcomes
- Verbal indication that explanations are understood
- Verbal indication of optimistic expectations (within realistic limits) related to forthcoming surgery
- Cooperation during preoperative tests and procedures
- Verbal or behavioral indication of reduction of anxiety
- Absence of postoperative complications
- Absence of allergic reactions

Plan for implementation	Rationale
See master care plan for the patient receiving preoperative teaching.	
In addition to the topics covered in the master care plan, include the following items in the preoperative teaching: 1. Be aware that, in addition to the routine preoperative tests, the following diagnostic studies may have been performed, and answer any questions the patient has regarding them:	
a. Complete physical examination	Endocrine or genital abnormalities associated with infertility are sought. These include hypogonadism, Kleinfelter's syndrome, cryptorchidism, absence of vasa deferentia and varicocele.
b. Complete health and sexual history	Illnesses that may cause infertility include mumps orchitis and untreated gonorrhea. Infection with T-mycoplasma has also been implicated in certain cases of infertility.[1] Prolonged fever and the ingestion of certain drugs may temporarily suppress spermatogenesis. Impotence may also be the underlying factor in the condition.
c. Semen analysis	This is done to determine the morphology, motility, and concentration of the sperm, fructose content of the semen, and the presence of sperm antibodies.
d. Blood tests for gonadotropic hormones and testosterone	Pituitary and hypothalamic hormones control spermatogenesis and testosterone production. Abnormal levels may result in infertility.
e. Urine test for 17-ketosteroids	These substances are metabolites of hormones controlling sexual function. Abnormal levels may indicate diseases such as hypogonadism or other conditions associated with infertility.
2. The preoperative shave will be of the pubic area.	
3. The patient will be permitted a light meal in the evening after surgery.	These patients can usually tolerate oral intake a few hours after surgery. For this reason the intravenous infusion used during surgery is often discontinued in the recovery room or shortly after the patient returns to the floor and tolerates fluids.
4. There will be an incision on both sides of the patient's scrotum that will be covered by a dressing and a scrotal support.	

Preoperative period

Preoperative period

2. NURSING DIAGNOSIS: Need for discharge planning

Objectives of nursing intervention
{ Early commencement of discharge planning
Accurate estimate of time required for all discharge teaching

Expected outcome Smooth transition of care after discharge

Plan for implementation	Rationale
See master care plan for the patient requiring discharge preparations: discharge planning. In addition to the topics covered in the master care plan, the following items should be considered: 1. The duration of hospitalization for this procedure is approximately 24 to 48 hours. 2. Required teaching includes general postoperative discharge teaching.	

Postoperative period

3. NURSING DIAGNOSIS: Potential for postoperative complications (shock, atelectasis, pneumonia, urinary retention, deep vein thrombosis)

Objective of nursing intervention Prevention or early detection of postoperative complications

Expected outcomes
{ Pulse and blood pressure normal, skin dry, color normal
Respirations regular and unlabored, absence of pulmonary congestion
Normal voiding pattern established within 6 hours after surgery
Early ambulation tolerated well

Plan for implementation	Rationale
1. Check the patient's vital signs every 4 hours, and notify the physician of any indications of impending shock. These include: a. Increasing pulse and respiratory rates b. Decreasing blood pressure c. Diaphoresis and pallor d. Feelings of apprehension	Although shock is a potential complication after any kind of surgery, it is a relatively small risk after testicular biopsy because few blood vessels are cut and the duration of surgery is short.

656

Plan for implementation	**Rationale**
2. Encourage coughing and abdominal breathing if the patient's lungs sound congested, and notify the physician if any of the following conditions are present:	Although precautions must be taken, respiratory complications are unlikely after this type of surgery because the period of anesthesia is very short. Futhermore, there is no abdominal incision to inhibit effective coughing.
a. The patient is unable to cough and his lungs sound congested. b. Sputum volume is copious. c. Sputum color is other than clear or white. d. There is a rise in the patient's temperature. e. Breath sounds are diminished.	These conditions require additional treatment. The physician may order therapies such as incentive spirometry, nasotracheal suctioning, postural drainage, or intermittent positive pressure breathing, depending on the extent of respiratory embarrassment.
3. Promote resumption of normal voiding pattern by the following actions: a. Be certain the patient is well hydrated. b. Leave a urinal at the bedside within reach of the patient. c. Ask the patient to notify the nurse the first time he voids. d. If the patient has not voided within 6 hours after surgery:	Temporary urinary retention is occasionally a result of anesthesia.
(1) Assist the patient to a standing position to void.	Assuming the accustomed position for voiding will help the patient to void if the retention is caused by psychologic factors.
(2) If the patient is still unable to void, notify the physician.	Catheterization may be required.
4. Use precautions against deep vein thrombosis. (See master care plan for the patient at risk for deep vein thrombosis.) These patients are sometimes permitted out of bed in the evening after surgery.	Although deep vein thrombosis is a relatively small risk after this type of surgery, it still must be considered, and adequate precautions should be taken.

Postoperative period

4. NURSING DIAGNOSIS: Potential for wound complications

Objective of nursing intervention   Prevention or early detection of complications arising from the incisional area

Expected outcome   Absence of fever, purulent exudate, erythema, edema, and other abnormal wound conditions

Plan for implementation	Rationale
1. Check the dressing every shift. If it requires changing:	Drainage is very slight or absent after this type of surgery, since no incisional drains are used.
a. Use sterile technique for the procedure.	
b. Note the condition of the suture lines; chart their appearance and the presence of edema, erythema, or other abnormal wound conditions.	This provides a frame of reference for other staff members caring for the patient.
c. If there is purulent drainage:	This would indicate a wound infection.
(1) Notify the physician.	
(2) Obtain a wound culture specimen.	This will facilitate identification of the infecting organism so that appropriate treatment can be instituted quickly.
2. Check the patient's temperature every 4 hours, and notify the physician if there is an elevation above 101°.	Wound infection must always be suspected when the patient runs a fever postoperatively.

5. NURSING DIAGNOSIS: Postoperative pain

Objective of nursing intervention   Appropriate management of pain or discomfort

Expected outcome   Behavioral and/or verbal indication that pain is adequately reduced or absent

Plan for implementation	Rationale
1. Determine characteristics of the pain by questioning and observing the patient.	The degree of pain patients experience after this type of surgery varies, but in most cases mild pain may be expected for the first 24 hours.
2. Be alert for indications (verbal or behavioral) that the patient is experiencing discomfort other than physical pain, and attempt to resolve the problem.	Fear of the outcome of the biopsy, depression, and numerous other conditions may be sources of extreme discomfort for the patient, who may unconsciously translate these feelings into pain. Also, surgery involving the sexual organs may give rise to considerable anxiety which often can be alleviated simply by reassurance from the nurse.
3. If the discomfort is from surgical manipulation:	
a. Be certain the scrotal support is positioned properly.	The scrotal support elevates the scrotum, thereby enhancing drainage from the area. This reduces discomfort caused by edema.

Postoperative period

658

Plan for implementation	Rationale
b. Provide analgesic medication as ordered.	
4. Note the patient's response to the pain medication.	This provides a frame of reference for evaluation of the patient's condition on subsequent shifts.

6. NURSING DIAGNOSIS: Need for discharge teaching

Objectives of nursing intervention

Explanation of basic information about medications to be taken at home

Explanation of information regarding follow-up care

Explanation of residual effects of the condition and/or treatment

Explanation of instructions concerning postdischarge activities

Explanation of symptoms that constitute a reason to contact the physician

Expected outcomes

Accurate return verbalization and/or demonstration of all material learned

Smooth transition of care after discharge

Absence or early detection of complications arising after discharge

Plan for implementation	Rationale
See master care plan for the patient requiring discharge preparations: discharge teaching.	
In addition to the topics covered in the master care plan, include the following items in the discharge teaching:	
1. At the follow-up office visit the physician will check the incisions and discuss plans for further treatment on the basis of the histology reports.	
2. The expected residual effects of this surgery are minimal. The patient can usually resume most of his normal activities within 1 week after discharge.	
3. The patient should notify the physician if any of the following occur:	
a. Severe pain or increased swelling at the incisional site	This may indicate a wound infection.
b. Chills and fever	This may also indicate an infection.

Postoperative period

Convalescent period

CHAPTER 59

Management of the patient with epididymoorchitis

Epididymoorchitis is an inflammation of the testicle and epididymis. Although orchitis and epididymitis may occur separately, they are discussed here as a single condition because infection of one of these organs can quickly spread to the other, and it is often difficult to distinguish whether the inflammation is limited to only one of the organs. Furthermore, the treatment is very similar for both disorders.

Epididymoorchitis occurs most commonly from a urinary tract infection that descends via the vas to the epididymis and testicle. Previous prostatectomy, urethral instrumentation, and chronic prostatitis are frequently associated factors. The condition may also occur as a result of metastasis via the blood and/or lymphatic vessels from localized foci of the infection elsewhere in the body, or from systemic disease, most notably mumps (parotitis).

The infecting organisms include staphylococci, streptococci, colon bacilli, gonococci, and mumps virus.

Symptoms vary from mild testicular pain and low-grade fever to those which usually require hospitalization, i.e., high fever, sudden, severe testicular pain that might radiate to the groin and flank, nausea, vomiting, and urethral discharge. The involved testicle is usually swollen and exquisitely tender. The scrotum may be reddened and edematous, and an associated hydrocele may be present.

Treatment includes aggressive antibiotic therapy, bed rest, and symptomatic relief, including support of the scrotum and hot or cold compresses. If a testicular abscess occurs, orchiectomy may be required.

It may take 1 or 2 weeks before all the pain is gone, and it is not uncommon for subacute chronic epididymitis to recur, especially if chronic prostatitis is present. Long-term effects may include testicular atrophy and sterility from fibrosis and destruction of the tubules.

The incidence of postoperative epididymoorchitis has decreased considerably as a result of prophylactic vasectomy, which is often performed before surgical instrumentation when there is evidence of a urinary tract infection. Gonococcal epididymoorchitis has also become relatively infrequent because of the early use of antibiotics in the treatment of gonorrhea.

EPIDIDYMOORCHITIS
Outline of Care Plan
ANTICIPATED NURSING DIAGNOSES:

Period of acute symptoms
1. Dependence on reduction of symptomatic discomfort (scrotal pain, nausea and vomiting, urethral discharge, and chills and fever).
2. Potential for septic shock.
3. Need for management of intravenous infusion.
4. Potential for complications related to bed rest.
5. Need for precautions if the infection is associated with gonorrhea.*
6. Need for precautions if the infection is associated with mumps.*
7. Need for discharge planning.

Convalescent period
8. Need for discharge teaching.

---

*May not apply.

NURSING CARE PLAN FOR THE PATIENT WITH EPIDIDYMOORCHITIS

1. NURSING DIAGNOSIS: Dependence on reduction of symptomatic discomfort (scrotal pain, nausea and vomiting, urethral discharge, and chills and fever)

Objective of nursing intervention Appropriate management of symptoms

Expected outcomes
{ Verbal and/or behavioral indication of reduction of pain
Absence of nausea and vomiting
Reduction and eventual absence of fever

Plan for implementation	Rationale
SCROTAL PAIN THAT MAY RADIATE TO GROIN AND FLANK AREA	
1. Provide the most comfortable type of support for the scrotum. a. Apply scrotal support or suspensory if the swelling is not so severe that it creates pressure against the scrotum. **or** b. Elevate the scrotum on a rolled towel placed under the scrotum with the patient in a supine position. **or** c. Apply a Bellevue bridge (Fig. 59-1).	Elevation of the scrotum promotes drainage from the area, thus decreasing the pain and pressure of edema. The degree of swelling varies considerably, and the patient's comfort is the best indicator of the most advantageous method of scrotal support.

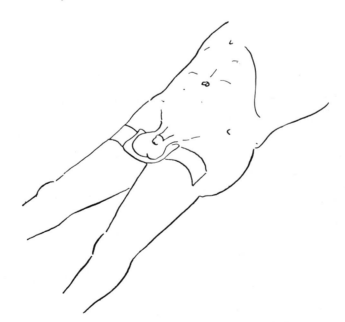

Fig. 59-1. Bellevue bridge: elevation of scrotum on adhesive strip in patient confined to bed. (From Winter, C., and Morel, A.: Nursing care of patients with urologic diseases, ed. 4, St. Louis, 1977, The C.V. Mosby Co.)

Period of acute symptoms

Plan for implementation	Rationale
2. Medicate with analgesics as ordered.	The pain may be severe. Narcotic analgesia is often required.
3. Provide local heat, tub bath, or sitz bath, **if ordered.**	Heat causes vasodilatation. This increases circulation to the area, thus reducing tissue fluid and removing toxins. The process results in alleviation of pressure on nerve endings and reduction of inflammation. But the value of heat applied directly to the scrotum must be weighed against the possible temporary harm to spermatogenesis. (For spermatogenesis to occur, the temperature of the testicle must be a few degrees lower than the normal body temperature.) However, massive inflammation can also impair fertility. Therefore the decision to apply heat to the scrotum should be left to the patient's physician.
4. If ordered, provide ice packs intermittently to the scrotum (20 minutes on and 20 minutes off).	Ice may also reduce swelling by causing vasoconstriction and reduction of the fluid accumulating in the area.

NAUSEA AND VOMITING

1. Administer an antiemetic such as trimethobenzamide (Tigan) or prochlorperazine (Compazine) as ordered (or suggest that such medication be ordered) **before** the symptoms become severe.	Since nausea and vomiting frequently accompany epididymoorchitis, anticipation and early treatment may spare the patient considerable discomfort.
2. Encourage slow deep breathing if nausea is severe.	Concentration on slow abdominal breathing promotes general relaxation and may provide distraction from the nausea.
3. If the patient is vomiting: a. Prohibit oral intake. b. Keep the patient lying on his side or sitting up. c. Provide frequent mouth care. d. Maintain accurate records of volume and character of vomitus.	This prevents aspiration of vomitus. If vomiting is severe, the patient may become dehydrated and develop electrolyte imbalances, since sodium, chloride, potassium, and hydrogen ions are lost in the gastric juices. Fluid and electrolyte replacements may be ordered to correct losses before they become severe.

Period of acute symptoms

Plan for implementation	Rationale

URETHRAL DISCHARGE

1. Provide gauze pads and hydrogen peroxide to clean the meatus if discharge is copious.

   This is for esthetic and hygienic purposes.

2. If the infection is associated with gonorrhea or mumps, observe the precautions listed on pp. 667 and 668.

   Certain isolation precautions should be observed to protect other patients and staff.

CHILLS AND FEVER

1. Explain why blood and urine specimens are necessary and assist with procedures.

   These specimens are obtained to identify the infecting organism and determine its antibiotic sensitivity. The urine should be a midstream specimen from a cleansed orifice.

2. Medicate with an antipyretic as ordered.

   Measures to reduce fever are usually ordered for patients with temperatures above 101°. However, this is a controversial subject, since the exact role of fever in fighting infection has not yet been determined.

3. Provide an alcohol sponge bath or hypothermia blanket as ordered.

4. Be alert for symptoms of septic shock (see nursing diagnosis 2).

Period of acute symptoms

2. NURSING DIAGNOSIS: Potential for septic shock

Objective of nursing intervention	Prevention or early detection and treatment of septic shock

Expected outcomes
- Vital signs normal, extremities warm, color normal
- Patient alert and oriented
- Urinary output approximately 60 ml per hour

Plan for implementation	Rationale
1. Check the patient's vital signs every 4 hours (or more often if unstable).	Septic shock, as with other forms of shock, occurs as a result of inadequate tissue perfusion. However, unlike hypovolemic shock, which has been discussed in relation to most surgical procedures, septic shock is a result of abnormalities in the vascular bed rather than in the volume of circulating blood, and it occurs in the setting of a preexisting infection. Endotoxins released from gram-negative bacteria are implicated in the pathogenesis of the syndrome, sometimes referred to as endotoxic shock. The condition progresses rapidly, resulting in severe tissue anoxia, coagulation defects, and respiratory, renal, and cardiac failure. **Prompt recognition and treatment are essential, or the condition is irreversible.** The patient is usually given aggressive antibiotic and steroid therapy. The administration of massive doses of corticosteroids is controversial but appears to be effective. Changes in the type of antibiotic may be made after the results of the culture are known, but broad-spectrum antibiotics, effective against gram-negative bacteria, are given initially.
2. Be alert for the following symptoms of septic shock (keeping in mind that there may be other causes for some of these symptoms): a. Decreasing blood pressure b. Cool, pale extremities, often with peripheral cyanosis c. Increasing pulse and respiratory rates d. Chills and fever (not always present) e. Mental obtundation f. Oliguria	
3. Be aware that in an elderly or debilitated patient septic shock may not be readily detectable, and the only clues may be the following signs: a. Unexplained hypotension b. Increasing confusion and disorientation c. Hyperventilation	
4. Notify the physician **at once** it septic shock is suspected.	
5. Obtain blood and urine specimens for cultures.	

Period of acute symptoms

3. NURSING DIAGNOSIS: Need for management of intravenous infusion

Objectives of nursing intervention

Appropriate administration of specific types of intravenous solutions
Prevention or early detection of local complications
Prevention or early detection of systemic complications
Management of discomfort caused by the intravenous infusion
Maintenance of proper function of intravenous equipment
Maintenance of accurate records of the patient's hydration status
Precautions against adverse effects of nephrotoxic and ototoxic antibiotics*

Expected outcomes

Normal hydration status
Normal electrolyte status
Absence of thrombophlebitis, infiltration, infection, fluid overload, and pulmonary embolism
Absence of discomfort caused by the intravenous infusion
Normal blood urea nitrogen and creatinine levels*
Normal audiometry tests*

Plan for implementation	Rationale
See master care plan for the patient receiving intravenous therapy.	
In addition to the items mentioned in the master care plan, the following interventions may be required*: 1. If the patient is receiving an aminoglycoside (e.g., gentamicin, kanamycin, tobramycin), be certain laboratory studies are being performed for blood urea nitrogen and serum creatinine levels at least three times per week.	These drugs may be nephrotoxic. However, they are highly effective in the treatment of infections caused by gram-negative organisms. They are most commonly given via the intravenous route. If they are given intramuscularly, instead, the same precautions apply.
2. If the patient is scheduled for audiometric studies during the period of aminoglycoside administration, explain the purpose.	These drugs are also ototoxic, and the patient's physician may want the patient to have his hearing tested initially for a baseline reading and then periodically throughout the period in which he is receiving aminoglycoside therapy. However, this adverse effect does not commonly occur unless the dosage is unusually high, the duration of treatment is prolonged, or if renal impairment exists.

Period of acute symptoms

*Applies to patients receiving nephrotoxic and ototoxic antibiotics.

4. NURSING DIAGNOSIS: Potential for complications related to bed rest*

Objective of nursing intervention	Prevention or early detection of complications associated with bed rest

Expected outcomes
- Absence of adverse psychologic effects of bed rest (boredom, depression, frustration, etc.)
- Normal bowel function and respiratory function
- Good skin integrity
- Absence of deep vein thrombosis and disuse atrophy of the muscles

Plan for implementation	Rationale
1. Place all necessary items within easy reach of the patient.	This encourages the patient to remain in bed (as ordered) without causing him to feel overly dependent on others.
2. Provide the patient with diversional activities (e.g., books, television, newspapers).	Boredom and depression are not unusual reactions when a normally active individual is confined to bed.
3. Promote adequate bowel function by encouraging fruit juices and high-residue foods.	Constipation is a common complication of immobility. If the patient is taking narcotic analgesics, such as codeine, it is even more likely to occur.
4. Keep accurate records of the patient's bowel movements and provide a cathartic or stool softener as needed.	
5. Check the integrity of the patient's skin daily; massage reddened areas over bony prominences and avoid the use of plastic bed shields (e.g., Chux) in direct contact with the patient's skin.	Skin breakdown may occur on areas where there is prolonged pressure. Promoting circulation and keeping the areas as dry as possible will reduce the incidence of pressure necrosis.
6. Encourage periodic abdominal breathing, yawning, and sighing.	These maneuvers are considered a deterrent to atelectasis and pneumonia by helping to inflate the alveoli and expand the lungs to total capacity.
7. Encourage frequent changing of position, flexing and relaxing of leg muscles, range of motion exercises, and isometric exercises.	These activities help to prevent venous stasis (a predisposing factor in deep vein thrombosis), disuse atrophy of the muscles, joint contractures, skin breakdown, and respiratory congestion.

Period of acute symptoms

---

*In most cases these patients will not be required to remain in bed for more than a week. Therefore many of the hazards resulting from immobility will not be a threat. However, if the patient is elderly or debilitated or if for some reason bed rest must be prolonged, related complications are a major nursing consideration.

5. NURSING DIAGNOSIS: Need for precautions if the infection is associated with gonorrhea*

Objectives of nursing intervention
{ Maintenance of a nonjudgmental attitude regarding the nature of the infection
Enforcement of regimen to prevent spread of the infection to others

Expected outcomes
{ Absence of embarrassment about having a venereal disease
Absence of spread of the infection to others

Plan for implementation	Rationale
1. Convey attitude of acceptance by approaching the condition like any other infectious disease.	Venereal disease is often a social stigma, and the patient may feel embarrassed about his diagnosis.
2. Maintain the following precautions to prevent cross-contamination of others and self:	Although gonorrhea is almost always transmitted through sexual contact, certain routine hospital activities may promote spread of the disease.
a. When emptying the patient's urinal, take particular care not to splash urine in the eyes.	The urethra may be heavily contaminated with the infecting organism, and the conjunctivae are susceptible to this particular organism.
b. Use double-bagging technique when disposing of any material in contact with contaminated secretions.	These are general precautions for **any** infected drainage. Their value in preventing the spread of venereal disease has not been established, but common sense and good nursing habits dictate that they be observed.
c. If there is any broken skin on the hands of the caregiver, wear gloves during perineal care or any treatments that require contact with the urethral secretions.	
3. See Chapter 18 for additional nursing considerations for the patient with a venereal disease.	

Period of acute symptoms

*May not apply.

6. NURSING DIAGNOSIS: Need for precautions if the infection is associated with mumps*

Objective of nursing intervention	Enforcement of a regimen to prevent the spread of the infection to others

Expected outcome	Absence of additional cases of mumps among staff and other patients

Plan for implementation	**Rationale**

1. Keep the patient in respiratory isolation.
  a. The patient must be in a private room.
  b. Masks must be worn by all susceptible persons who enter the room.
  c. Masks must be worn when disposing of urine.
	The mumps virus is spread by the respiratory route.
	
	Mumps virus is excreted in the urine. Inhalation of airborne droplets during disposal is a potential source of infection.

2. If possible, eliminate all contact between the patient and any male staff member who has not had the disease and is therefore susceptible to it.	Although it is not considered a serious disease in a child, mumps can cause considerable discomfort in an adult and may result in sterility in a man.

*May not apply.

7. NURSING DIAGNOSIS: Need for discharge planning

Objectives of nursing intervention	{ Early commencement of discharge planning { Accurate estimate of time required for all discharge teaching

Expected outcome	Smooth transition of care after discharge

Plan for implementation	**Rationale**
See master care plan for the patient requiring discharge preparations: discharge planning. In addition to the topics covered in the master care plan, the following items should be considered: 1. The duration of hospitalization for the treatment of epididymoorchitis varies considerably but may be as long as 1 week to 10 days, particularly if it is bilateral. 2. Required teaching includes discussion of the need for diligent antibiotic administration after discharge.	

Period of acute symptoms

8. NURSING DIAGNOSIS: Need for discharge teaching

Objectives of nursing intervention
Explanation of basic information about medications to be taken at home
Explanation of information regarding follow-up care
Explanation of residual effects of the condition and/or treatment
Explanation of instructions concerning postdischarge activities
Explanation of symptoms that constitute a reason to contact the physician
Review of admitting diagnosis and mode of treatment

Expected outcomes
Accurate return verbalization and/or demonstration of all material learned
Smooth transition of care after discharge
Absence or early detection of complications arising after discharge
Ability to provide future health care practitioners with important data about health history

Plan for implementation	Rationale
See master care plan for the patient requiring discharge preparations: discharge teaching.	
In addition to the topics covered in the master care plan, include the following items in the discharge teaching:	
1. It is extremely important that the patient continue the antibiotic medication for the entire length of time prescribed, despite absence of symptoms.	Medication is usually prescribed for approximately 10 days to decrease the risk of resistant microorganisms.
2. At the follow-up office visit the physician will take a urine specimen for culture and will examine the scrotum to assess the degree of healing.	
3. The patient should notify the physician at once if there is a recurrence of any of the symptoms (fever, chills, or scrotal tenderness and/or swelling).	

Convalescent period

UNIT X

References and bibliography

REFERENCES
Chapter 54

1. Altman, B.L., and Malament, M.: Carcinoma of the testis following orchiopexy, J. Urol. **97:**498, 1967.
2. Batata, M.A., et al.: Cancer of the undescended or maldescended testis, Am. J. Roentgenol. **126:**302, Feb. 1976.

Chapter 56

1. Bristol Laboratories: Platinol-Cisplatin Product Monograph, Syracuse, N.Y., 1979, Brystol-Meyers Co.
2. Burns, N.: Cancer chemotherapy: a systemic approach, Nurs. 78 **8:**56, 1978.
3. Fraley, E.E., editor: The Urologic Clinics of North America, vol. 4, Philadelphia, 1977, W.B. Saunders Co.
4. Gever, L.N.: Cisplatin—a breakthrough for the cancer patient; a nursing challenge for you, Nurs. 80 **10:**53, Dec. 1980.

Chapter 57

1. Ansbacher, R., Keung-Yeung, K., and Wurster, J.C.: Sperm antibodies in vasectomized men, Fertil. Steril. **23:**640, 1972.
2. Cochran, J.S.: Immunobiology of reproductive processes in men, Urology **4:**367, Oct. 1974.
3. Dorsey, J.W.: Surgical correction of post-vasectomy sterility, J. Urol. **110:**554, 1973.
4. Shulman, S., Harlin, B., and Davis, P.: New method of treatment for immune infertility, Urology **12:**582, 1978.

Chapter 58

1. Khatamee, M.A., and Decker, W.H.: Recovery of genital mycoplasma from infertile couples using New York City Medium, Infertility **1**(2):155, 1978.

BIBLIOGRAPHY

Altman, B.L., and Malament, M.: Carcinoma of the testis following orchiopexy, J. Urol. **97:**498, 1967.
Amelar, R.D., Dubin, L., and Walsh, P.C.: Male infertility, Philadelphia, 1977, W.B. Saunders Co.
Andrysiak, T., Carroll, R., and Ungerleider, J.T.: Marijuana for the oncology patient, Am. J. Nurs. Aug. 1979, p. 1396.

Batata, M.A., et al.: Cancer of the undescended or maldescended testis, Am. J. Roentgenol. **126:**302, Feb. 1976.
Bristol Laboratories: Platinol-Cisplatin Product Monograph, Syracuse, N.Y., 1979, Brystol-Meyers Co.
Burns, N.: Chemotherapy: a systemic approach, Nurs. 78 **8:**56, 1978.
Cochran, J.S.: Immunobiology of reproductive processes in men, Urology **4:**367, 1974.
Conklin, M., et al.: Should health teaching include self-examination of the testes? Am. J. Nurs. **78:**2073, 1978.
Cox, C.E., editor: The Urologic Clinics of North America, vol. 2, Philadelphia, 1975, W.B. Saunders Co.
Culp, D.A., Boatman, D.L., and Wilson, V.B.: Testicular tumors: 40 years' experience, J. Urol. **110:**548, 1973.
Dorsey, J.W.: Surgical correction of post-vasectomy sterility, J. Urol. **110:**554, 1973.
Fraley, E.E., editor: The Urologic Clinics of North America, vol. 4, Philadelphia, 1977, W.B. Saunders Co.
Gault, P.L.: Taking your part in the fight against testicular cancer, Nurs. 81 **11:**47, May 1981.
Gever, L.N.: Cisplatin—a breakthrough for the cancer patient; a nursing challenge for you, Nurs. 80 **10:**53, Dec. 1980.
Howards, S.S., and Lipshutz, L.I., editors: The Urologic Clinics of North America, vol. 5, Philadelphia, 1978, W.B. Saunders Co.
Lum, J.L.J., et al.: Nursing care of oncology patients receiving chemotherapy, Nurs. Res. **27:**340, Nov.-Dec. 1978.
Murray, B.L.S., and Wilcox, L.J.: Testicular self-examination, Am. J. Nurs. Dec. 1978, p. 2074.
Ostchega, C.Y.: Preventing and treating cancer chemotherapy's oral complications, Nurs. 80 **10:**47, Aug. 1980.
Scogna, D.M., and Smalley, R.V.: Chemotherapy-induced nausea and vomiting, Am. J. Nurs. **79:**1562, 1979.
Shulman, S., Harlin, B., and Davis, P.: New method of treatment for immune infertility, Urology **12:**582, 1978.
Todres, R., Wojtiuk, R.: The cancer patient's view of chemotherapy, Cancer Nurs. **2:**283, Aug. 1979.
Van Scoy-Mosher, M.B.: Chemotherapy: a manual for patients and their families, Cancer Nurs. **1:**234, June 1978.

UNIT XI

PROCEDURES FOR DISORDERS
WITHIN
THE URETHRA

CHAPTER 60

Fulguration of urethral warts

Condylomata acuminata (urethral warts) is a sexually transmitted disease of viral origin. The lesions occur on the external genitalia, perianal area, and within the urethra. Initially they are usually treated with podophyllum (applied daily for 2 weeks). If they do not respond to this treatment, surgery is performed.

For the procedure the patient is placed in a lithotomy position, and the superficial lesions are treated with a needle electrode and low-coagulation current. For the lesions within the urethra, cystoscopy is performed to assess the extent of the growths, and then they are treated with a fulguration electrode. Care is taken not to produce excessive burning, since this may cause scarring and the development of stricture formation. An indwelling urethral catheter is inserted at the end of the procedure.

FULGURATION OF URETHRAL WARTS
Outline of Care Plan
ANTICIPATED NURSING DIAGNOSES:

Preoperative period
1. Need for preoperative teaching.
2. Need for discharge planning.

Postoperative period
3. Potential for postoperative complications (shock, atelectasis, pneumonia, deep vein thrombosis, infection).
4. Need for management of indwelling urethral catheter.
5. Postoperative pain.

Convalescent period
6. Potential for voiding complications following removal of indwelling urethral catheter.
7. Need for discharge teaching.

NURSING CARE PLAN FOR THE PATIENT UNDERGOING FULGURATION OF URETHRAL WARTS

1. NURSING DIAGNOSIS: Need for preoperative teaching

Objectives of nursing intervention	If necessary, clarification of reason for hospitalization and type of surgery to be performed
	Elimination of any negative or inaccurate notions regarding the forthcoming surgery
	Explanation of preoperative tests and procedures
	Psychologic preparation for general anesthesia (omit if the patient is to have spinal anesthesia)
	Explanation of events expected in the early postoperative period
	Explanation of body conditions expected in the early postoperative period
	Identification of any known allergies

Preoperative period

Expected outcomes

Verbal indication that explanations are understood

Verbal indication of optimistic expectations (within realistic limits) related to forth-coming surgery

Cooperation during preoperative tests and procedures

Verbal or behavioral indication of reduction of anxiety

Absence of postoperative complications

Absence of allergic reactions

Plan for implementation	Rationale
See master care plan for the patient receiving preoperative teaching.	
In addition to the topics covered in the master care plan, include the following items in the preoperative teaching: 1. The preoperative shave (if ordered) will be of the pubic area.	The shave is ordered at the surgeon's discretion.
2. The patient will be permitted a light meal in the evening after surgery.	These patients can usually tolerate oral intake a few hours after surgery. For this reason the intravenous infusion used during surgery is often discontinued in the recovery room or shortly after the patient returns to the floor and tolerates fluids.
3. There will be an indwelling urethral catheter in place for approximately 24 to 48 hours.	

2. NURSING DIAGNOSIS: Need for discharge planning

Objectives of nursing intervention

Early commencement of discharge planning

Accurate estimate of time required for all discharge teaching

Expected outcome   Smooth transition of care after discharge

Plan for implementation	Rationale
See master care plan for the patient requiring discharge preparations: discharge planning.	
In addition to the topics covered in the master care plan, the following items should be considered: 1. The duration of hospitalization for this procedure is approximately 3 or 4 days.	
2. Required teaching includes general postoperative discharge teaching.	

Preoperative period

3. NURSING DIAGNOSIS: Potential for postoperative complications (shock, atelectasis, pneumonia, deep vein thrombosis, infection)

Objective of nursing intervention	Prevention or early detection of postoperative complications

Expected outcomes
- Pulse and blood pressure normal, skin dry, color normal
- Respirations regular and unlabored, absence of pulmonary congestion
- Early ambulation tolerated well
- Absence of chills or fever

Plan for implementation	**Rationale**
1. Check the patient's vital signs every 4 hours, and notify the physician of any indications of impending shock. These include: a. Increasing pulse and respiratory rates b. Decreasing blood pressure c. Diaphoresis and pallor d. Feelings of apprehension	Although shock is a potential complication after any kind of surgery, it is a relatively small risk after this kind of procedure because few blood vessels are cut and the duration of surgery is short.
2. Encourage coughing and abdominal breathing if the patient's lungs sound congested, and notify the physician if any of the following conditions are present: a. The patient is unable to cough and his lungs sound congested. b. Sputum volume is copious. c. Sputum color is other than clear or white. d. There is a rise in the patient's temperature. e. Breath sounds are diminished.	Although precautions must be taken, respiratory complications are unlikely after this type of surgery because the period of anesthesia is very short. Furthermore, there is no abdominal incision to inhibit effective coughing. These conditions require additional treatment. The physician may order therapies such as incentive spirometry, nasotracheal suctioning, postural drainage, or intermittent positive pressure breathing, depending on the extent of respiratory embarrassment.
3. Use precautions against deep vein thrombosis. (See master care plan for the patient at risk for deep vein thrombosis.) These patients are sometimes permitted out of bed in the evening after surgery.	Although deep vein thrombosis is a relatively small risk after this type of surgery, it still must be considered, and adequate precautions should be taken.
4. Notify the physician if the patient shows any indications of infection: a. Chills b. Fever c. Flushed skin	Bacteremia can occur after any instrumentation of the urinary tract. This happens as a result of absorption of bacteria through the walls of the urethral mucosa. Blood and urine specimens are often ordered to determine the type and sensitivity of the offending organism, and the patient is usually given antibiotic therapy.

Postoperative period

4. NURSING DIAGNOSIS: Need for management of indwelling urethral catheter

Objectives of nursing intervention

Appropriate care of catheter and equipment

Prevention or early detection of infection

Care of tissue surrounding catheter

Maintenance of accurate records of urine output

Appropriate administration of hand-irrigation of catheter

Management of discomfort or pain caused by catheter

Satisfactory collection of urine specimens from catheter

Expected outcomes

Absence of severe bladder spasms and suprapubic distention

Urine draining freely through system

Absence of fever, chills, and foul-smelling urine

Absence of urethral discharge and tissue inflammation

Minimal discomfort caused by the catheter

Urine specimens in optimum condition for all necessary tests

Plan for implementation	Rationale
See master care plan for the patient with an indwelling urethral catheter: care after insertion of the catheter.	
In addition to the topics covered in the master care plan, the following interventions are required:	
1. Notify the physician if there is a considerable amount of blood in the urine.	The urine should be clear amber or only slightly blood tinged after this type of procedure. Some bleeding, however, is expected **around** the catheter (i.e., a bloody urethral discharge).
2. Use caution when giving catheter care, to avoid irritation of healing tissue.	

Postoperative period

5. NURSING DIAGNOSIS: Postoperative pain

Objective of nursing intervention	Appropriate management of pain or discomfort
Expected outcome	Behavioral and/or verbal indications that pain is adequately reduced or absent

Plan for implementation	Rationale
Determine the source of the pain. It may be related to the catheter or surgical manipulation.	Pain from different sources usually requires different intervention.
1. Question and observe the patient to obtain information about the pain.	
2. Be aware that pain is a unique and individual experience. Although the different sources of pain can usually be determined by their characteristics, there are also many variations.	
3. Be alert for indications (verbal or behavioral) that the patient is experiencing discomfort other than physical pain, and attempt to resolve the problem.	The patient may be anxious about having a venereal disease (see Chapter 18) or about having surgery on his genitalia. The nurse's attitude and reassurance may be sufficient to alleviate these sources of discomfort, which the patient may unconsciously translate into feelings of pain.

PERSISTENT, SEVERE, INCREASING PAIN IN SUPRAPUBIC AREA

See Chapter 11, part one, nursing objective 6.	This pain is probably caused by an obstructed catheter.

SPASMODIC, INTERMITTENT PAIN IN SUPRAPUBIC AREA, OR PAIN RADIATING TO URETHRAL AREA

See Chapter 11, part one, nursing objective 6.	This pain is probably caused by the catheter's irritating effect on the bladder or by urethral manipulation during surgery. In either case analgesic medication should provide adequate relief.

Postoperative period

6. NURSING DIAGNOSIS: Potential for voiding complications following removal of indwelling urethral catheter

| **Objective of nursing intervention** | Prevention or early detection of complications |

Expected outcomes { Resumption of normal voiding pattern
Absence of dysuria

Plan for implementation	**Rationale**
See master care plan for the patient with an indwelling urethral catheter: care after removal of the catheter.	

7. NURSING DIAGNOSIS: Need for discharge teaching

Objectives of nursing intervention {
Explanation of basic information about medications to be taken at home
Explanation of information regarding follow-up care
Explanation of residual effects of the condition and/or treatment
Explanation of instructions concerning postdischarge activities
Explanation of symptoms that constitute a reason to contact the physician
Review of admitting diagnosis and mode of treatment

Expected outcomes {
Accurate return verbalization and/or demonstration of all material learned
Smooth transition of care after discharge
Absence or early detection of complications arising after discharge
Ability to provide future health care practitioners with important data about health history

Plan for implementation	**Rationale**
See master care plan for the patient requiring discharge preparations: discharge teaching.	

In addition to the topics covered in the master care plan, include the following items in the discharge teaching:
1. At the follow-up office visit the physician will check any visible areas from which warts were removed.

2. The expected residual effects of this surgery are minimal. The patient can usually resume most of his activities within 1 week. Sexual intercourse should be avoided for at least 4 days after discharge.

Convalescent period

678

Plan for implementation	Rationale
3. The patient should encourage any sexual partners suspected of having urethral warts to seek medical attention.	
4. The patient should notify the physician if any of the following are present:	
a. Hematuria	Tissue sloughing and bleeding occasionally occur. If it is severe or persistent, treatment will be required.
b. Urinary retention or poor urinary stream	Occasionally edema of the urethra will result in occlusion of the lumen and inability to void. Recatheterization will be necessary until the edema subsides.

Convalescent period

CHAPTER 61

Excision of urethral caruncle

A caruncle is a fleshy, vascular tumor that occasionally forms at the external urethral meatus in postmenopausal women. It often becomes irritated and may bleed and cause pain. If the condition is asymptomatic, no treatment is required, although biopsy may be necessary to rule out urethral carcinoma.

For excision of urethral caruncle the patient is placed in a lithotomy position, and an indwelling urethral catheter is inserted. The mass and protruding urethral mucosa are excised in a circumferential manner. Sutures are applied for hemostasis, and a Vaseline dressing is placed around the catheter to maintain lubrication between the catheter and surgical site.

EXCISION OF URETHRAL CARUNCLE
Outline of Care Plan
ANTICIPATED NURSING DIAGNOSES:

Preoperative period
1. Need for preoperative teaching. (See p. 673.)*
2. Need for discharge planning. (See p. 674.)*

Postoperative period
3. Potential for postoperative complications (shock, atelectasis, pneumonia, deep vein thrombosis, infection). (See p. 675.)*
4. Need for management of indwelling urethral catheter. (See p. 676.)* A Vaseline dressing should be kept on the surgical site until the catheter is removed.
5. Postoperative pain. (See p. 677. The mention of a venereal disease in rationale 3 does not apply. A urethral caruncle is not a venereal disease.)*

Convalescent period
6. Potential voiding complications following removal of indwelling urethral catheter. (See p. 678.)*
7. Need for discharge teaching. (See p. 681.)†

---

*Nursing care is the same as for the patient undergoing fulguration of urethral warts.
†Nursing care is described on the following page.

7. NURSING DIAGNOSIS: Need for discharge teaching

Objectives of nursing intervention
- Explanation of basic information about medications to be taken at home
- Explanation of information regarding follow-up care
- Explanation of residual effects of the condition and/or treatment
- Explanation of instructions concerning postdischarge activities
- Explanation of symptoms that constitute a reason to contact the physician
- Review of admitting diagnosis and mode of treatment

Expected outcomes
- Accurate return verbalization and/or demonstration of all material learned
- Smooth transition of care after discharge
- Absence or early detection of complications arising after discharge
- Ability to provide future health care practitioners with important data about health history

Plan for implementation	Rationale
See master care plan for the patient requiring discharge preparations: discharge teaching.	
In addition to the topics covered in the master care plan, include the following items in the discharge teaching:	
1. At the follow-up office visit the physician will check the urethral meatus for adequate healing.	
2. The expected residual effects of this surgery are minimal. The patient can usually resume most of her activities within 1 week. Sexual intercourse, however, should be postponed for at least 2 weeks after discharge, and liberal amounts of water-soluble lubricant should be used.	
3. During the next week the patient should take daily sitz baths or warm tub baths (without bath oils or soaps, which may be irritating to healing tissue).	These baths will remove sloughed tissue and mucus and will soothe healing tissue.
4. The patient should notify the physician if significant meatal bleeding occurs.	Tissue sloughing and therefore bleeding occasionally occur. If it is severe, additional treatment may be required. However, light spotting is expected during the first week after discharge.

Convalescent period

References and bibliography

BIBLIOGRAPHY

Lapides, J.: Fundamentals of urology, Philadelphia, 1976, W.B. Saunders Co.

Smith, D.R.: General urology, ed. 8, Los Altos, Calif., 1975, Lange Medical Publications.

Winter, C.C., and Morel, A.: Nursing care of patients with urologic diseases, ed. 4, St. Louis, 1977, The C.V. Mosby Co.

APPENDIX A

Medications commonly used for the urology patient

ANTIMICROBIAL DRUGS

Drug group	Drug	Urologic indications	Usual adult dosage*	Adverse reactions and contraindications	Nursing considerations
Penicillin	Penicillin G procaine (Crysticillin, Wycillin, others)	Treatment of syphilis and gonorrhea	Syphilis (primary, secondary, and latent): Intramuscular, 600,000 units for 8 days. Syphilis (tertiary): intramuscular, 600,000 units daily for 10-15 days. Gonorrhea (uncomplicated): intramuscular, 4.8 million units divided into at least 2 doses and administered in 2 different sites. This is preceded by oral administration of 1 g probenecid at least 30 minutes before the injections.	ADVERSE REACTIONS: Dermatologic reactions, fever, serum sickness, blood dyscrasias, polyarthritis, superinfection by resistant organisms. CONTRAINDICATIONS: Hypersensitivity to penicllins, procaine, and possibly to cephalosporins.	1. Question the patient about previous allergic reactions to penicillin. This drug can cause potentially fatal anaphylactic reactions in susceptible people. 2. If any indications of hypersensitivity occur after administration of the drug (e.g., red flare or wheal at injection site, flushing, wheezing, itching, dyspnea), notify the physician at once and be prepared to administer epinephrine, antihistamines, and corticosteroids. Have a fully equipped emergency tray and oxygen readily available. 3. Advise any patient who manifests an allergic reaction to wear a Medic-Alert tag or to inform future health care providers of this reaction. Place a note on a conspicuous part of the patient's chart as well.
	Oxacillin sodium (Prostaphlin, Bactocill)	Treatment of penicillin-resistant staphylococcal infections such as septicemia of urologic origin (e.g., renal abscess or renal carbuncle).	Oral, intramuscular, intravenous: 250 mg to 1 g every 4-6 hours.	ADVERSE REACTIONS: Dermatologic reactions, gastrointestinal disturbances, superinfections, blood dyscrasias, fever, and elevated serum aspartate aminotransferase (SGOT) CONTRAINDICATIONS: See penicillin G.	1. See penicillin G. 2. Administer oral preparation 1 hour before or at least 2 hours after meals. 3. If intravenous medication is to be administered directly, give slowly (over a 10-minute period).

*For pediatric dosages consult *Physician's Desk Reference.*

ANTIMICROBIAL DRUGS—cont'd

Drug group	Drug	Urologic indications	Usual adult dosage	Adverse reactions and contraindications	Nursing considerations
	Ampicillin (Omnipen, Polycillin, others)	Treatment of urinary tract infections such as acute pyelonephritis.	Oral, intramuscular, intravenous: 500 mg every 6 hours.	ADVERSE REACTIONS: Diarrhea, skin rash; see also penicillin G. CONTRAINDICATIONS: See penicillin G.	1. See penicillin G. 2. Administer oral preparation 1 hour before or at least 2 hours after meals. 3. Administer parenteral preparations within 1 hour after reconstitution. 4. High urine concentration of this drug may cause false positive tests for glycosuria using Clinitest, Benedict's or Fehling's solution, but not with Clinistix or Tes-Tape.
	Carbenicillin disodium (Geopen, Pyopen)	Treatment of severe systemic or genitourinary infections, particularly those caused by *Pseudomonas* organisms.	Dosage varies according to the type and severity of the infection. Serious urinary tract infections: intravenous, 200/mg/kg/day. Uncomplicated urinary tract infections: intramuscular or intravenous, 1-2 g every 6 hours.	ADVERSE REACTIONS: Dermatologic reactions, nausea, blood dyscrasias, elevated serum aspartate aminotransferase (SGOT), hemorrhagic manifestations in patients with uremia, convulsions in patients with renal failure (if given in high doses). CONTRAINDICATIONS: See penicillin G.	1. See penicillin G. 2. Do not give more than 2 g in an intramuscular injection, per site. 3. If gentamicin is used concurrently with this medication, do not mix them in the same infusion fluid. 4. The patient may complain of an unpleasant taste in the mouth after rapid intravenous administration. 5. Use with caution in patients on sodium restriction (1 g of carbenicillin disodium contains 4.7 mEq sodium).

Continued.

Appendix

ANTIMICROBIAL DRUGS—cont'd

Drug group	Drug	Urologic indications	Usual adult dosage	Adverse reactions and contraindications	Nursing considerations
Cephalosporin	Cephalothin sodium (Keflin)	Initial treatment of urinary tract infections because of its wide spectrum of bactericidal activity. Once the results from the culture and sensitivity tests are known, another drug may be substituted or added to the regimen.	Intravenous or (rarely) intramuscular: 500 mg to 2 g every 4-6 hours.	ADVERSE REACTIONS: Dermatologic reactions, superinfections, blood dyscrasias, fever, phlebitis, elevated serum aspartate aminotransferase (SGOT), possibly nephrotoxicity. CONTRAINDICATIONS: Hypersensitivity to cephalosporins and possibly to penicillin.	1. This medication may cause a false positive reaction in tests for glycosuria with Fehling's or Benedict's solutions or with Clinitest, but not with Tes-Tape. 2. Repeated intramuscular injections may cause increasing pain and induration at the site. 3. Slight darkening of the concentrated solution at room temperature is permissible.
	Cefazolin sodium (Ancef, Kefzol)	See cephalothin.	Intramuscular or intravenous: 250 mg to 1 g every 6-12 hours.	ADVERSE REACTIONS: Same as cephalothin; also gastrointestinal disturbances. CONTRAINDICATIONS: See cephalothin.	1. See cephalothin, nursing consideration 1. 2. Intramuscular injections are better tolerated with this drug than with cephalothin.
	Cephalexin (Keflex)	See cephalothin.	Oral: 250-500 mg every 6 hours.	ADVERSE REACTIONS: Diarrhea and other gastrointestinal disturbances, superinfections, vaginitis, dizziness, headache. CONTRAINDICATIONS: See cephalothin.	1. See cephalothin, nursing consideration 1.
Tetracycline	Tetracycline and tetracycline hydrochloride (Achromycin, Panmycin, others)	Treatment of nonspecific urethritis and prostatitis; may also be used in place of penicillin if the patient is allergic to penicillin.	Oral: 1-2 g/24 hours divided into 2 to 4 equal doses. Intramuscular: 250 mg/24 hours or 300 mg every 8-12 hours. Intravenous: 250-500 mg every 12 hours.	ADVERSE REACTIONS: Dermatologic reactions, gastrointestinal disturbances, superinfections, photosensitivity, hepatotoxicity. CONTRAINDICATIONS: Hypersensitivity to tetracyclines, pregnancy, and period of breast feeding.	1. Check expiration date prior to administration. Tetracyclines decompose with age, exposure to light, and extreme humidity, and may become toxic. 2. Give oral preparation 1 hour before meals or at least 2 hours after meals. 3. Do not give oral tetracycline with milk products, antacids containing aluminum, magnesium, calcium, or zinc, or with oral iron preparations. 4. Advise the patient to avoid exposure to sunlight because of the risk of a photosensitive reaction.

686

ANTIMICROBIAL DRUGS—cont'd

Drug group	Drug	Urologic indications	Usual adult dosage	Adverse reactions and contraindications	Nursing considerations
	Doxycycline hyclate or doxy-cycline monohy-drate (Vibramy-cin)	See tetracycline.	Oral: 50-100 mg every 12 hours. Intravenous: 100-200 mg/day in a single dose or 2 infusions.	ADVERSE REACTIONS: See tetracycline. CONTRAINDICATIONS: See tetracycline.	1. See tetracycline, nursing considerations 1 and 4. 2. If gastrointestinal disturbances occur, this drug may be given with milk or food. 3. Do not give oral preparation at the same time as antacid administration. 4. Intravenous infusions must be completed within 12 hours and should be protected from direct light by silver foil or other light-resistant material. 5. Check dosage and administration schedule carefully. Lower and less frequent doses characterize this drug, and inadvertent overmedication may result in an increase of side effects.
Aminoglycoside	Gentamicin sulfate (Garamycin)	Treatment of septicemia when other, less toxic, drugs cannot be used because of resistant organisms; combined treatment with other drugs in severe septicemia; prophylaxis for a very limited period for patients at high risk for infection (e.g., prosthetic surgery).	Intramuscular or intravenous: 3-5 mg/kg/day in three equally divided doses. Dosage may be adjusted according to serum levels. Lower doses are recommended for patients with impaired renal function.	ADVERSE REACTIONS: Nephrotoxicity, ototoxicity, superinfections, dermatologic reactions, fever, joint pain, laryngeal edema, blood dyscrasias, nausea, vomiting, headache, alopecia, pulmonary fibrosis, respiratory depression, mental changes. CONTRAINDICATIONS: Hypersensitivity to gentamicin or other aminoglycosides.	1. Obtain specimens for blood urea nitrogen and serum creatinine levels at least every other day during treatment. 2. Audiometry may be ordered if the therapy is prolonged. 3. Advise the patient to report tinnitus, roaring in the ears, decreased hearing ability, or dizziness. If these symptoms occur, consult with the physician before giving the next dose because they are indications of toxicity. 4. Do not mix in a syringe or solution with any other medication. 5. Keep the patient well hydrated.

Continued.

ANTIMICROBIAL DRUGS—cont'd

Drug group	Drug	Urologic indications	Usual adult dosage	Adverse reactions and contraindications	Nursing considerations
	Tobramycin sulfate (Nebcin)	See gentamicin.	Intramuscular or intravenous: 3 mg/kg/day in 3 equal doses, every 8 hours.	ADVERSE REACTIONS: Nephrotoxicity, ototoxicity, blood dyscrasias, dermatologic reactions, gastrointestinal disturbances. CONTRAINDICATIONS: Hypersensitivity to tobramycin or other aminoglycosides.	See gentamicin.
	Neomycin sulfate (Mycifradin, Neobiotic, others)	Preoperative disinfection of the bowel.	Oral: 1 g every hour for 4 doses, and then 1 g every 4 hours for the next 24 hours.	ADVERSE REACTIONS: Diarrhea, nausea, vomiting. CONTRAINDICATIONS: Hypersensitivity to neomycin or other aminoglycosides, intestinal obstruction.	If surgery is postponed, check with the physician before continuing administration of this drug. Preoperative treatment rarely extends beyond 72 hours because the toxicity of this drug increases with duration of therapy.
Sulfonamide	Sulfisoxazole (Gantrisin, SK-Soxazole)	Treatment of uncomplicated urinary tract infection.	Oral: 4-8 g/24 hours divided into 4 to 6 doses. Intravenous: 100 mg/kg/24 hours divided into 4 doses. Subcutaneous: same as above divided into 3 doses. Intramuscular: same as above divided into 2 to 3 doses.	ADVERSE REACTIONS: Dermatologic reactions, photosensitivity, gastrointestinal disturbances, blood dyscrasias, central nervous system abnormalities, headache, fever, chills joint pain, crystalluria, hematuria, proteinuria, reduced sperm count, nephrotoxicity, hepatotoxicity. CONTRAINDICATIONS: Hypersensitivity to sulfonamides, pregnancy, period of breast feeding.	1. Maintain the patient on a high fluid intake to ensure solubility of the drug. Urine output should be at least 1500 ml/24 hours. 2. Notify the physician if skin rash or oral ulcerations occur. Either may indicate toxicity. 3. Advise the patient to avoid exposure to direct sunlight. 4. Warn the patient that para-aminobenzoic acid (an ingredient in many suntan lotions) is contraindicated during sulfonamide therapy. 5. Monitor serum glucose levels in patients taking oral hypoglycemics because sulfonamides may cause hypoglycemia. 7. Advise the patient not to take aspirin, which may increase the nephrotoxicity and tendency for crystalluria.

ANTIMICROBIAL DRUGS—cont'd

Drug group	Drug	Urologic indications	Usual adult dosage	Adverse reactions and contraindications	Nursing considerations
	Trimethoprim and sulfamethoxazole (Septra, Septra DS, Bactrim, Bactrim DS)	Treatment of uncomplicated urinary tract infection; prostatitis (this drug has a greater concentration in prostatic tissue than other antimicrobials); long-term prophylaxis against urinary tract infections.	Oral: 1 Septra DS (or Bactrim DS) every 12 hours; or 2 Septra (or Bactrim) every 12 hours.	ADVERSE REACTIONS: See sulfisoxazole. CONTRAINDICATIONS: See sulfisoxazole.	See sulfisoxazole.
Urinary tract antiseptics	Methenamine mandelate (Mandelamine)	Treatment of uncomplicated urinary tract infections, particularly in patients allergic to sulfonamides and penicillins. This drug releases formaldehyde in urine when the pH is below 5.5 and has a bacteriostatic effect on most urinary tract pathogens.	Oral: 500 mg to 1 g every 6 hours (usually given with 500 mg ascorbic acid to ensure urinary acidification).	ADVERSE REACTIONS: Gastrointestinal disturbances, generalized skin rash, dysuria. CONTRAINDICATIONS: Hypersensitivity to methenamine mandelate, hepatic insufficiency.	1. Give after meals or with a full glass of water to minimize gastric irritation. 2. Check urine pH frequently and report readings above 5.5. 3. Do not encourage high fluid intake because the antiseptic effect is dependent on a relatively high concentration of formaldehyde in the urine.
	Nitrofurantoin macrocrystals (Macrodantin)	Treatment of uncomplicated urinary tract infections, particularly in patients allergic to sulfonamides and penicillins.	Oral: 50-100 mg every 6 hours.	ADVERSE REACTIONS: Pulmonary reactions, hemolytic anemia, peripheral neuropathy, gastrointestinal disturbances, hepatitis, dermatologic reactions, blood dyscrasias, superinfection with resistant organisms within the genitourinary tract. CONTRAINDICATIONS: Hypersensitivity to nitrofurantoin preparations, renal failure, pregnancy at term.	1. Give with food or milk to minimize gastric irritation. 2. Maintain urine output of at least 1500 ml/ 24 hours. 3. Warn the patient that the drug may turn his urine brownish. 4. Consult with the physician before giving next dose if the patient complains of numbness or tingling of the extremities.

ANALGESICS

Drug group	Drug	Urologic indications	Usual adult dosage	Adverse reactions and contraindications	Nursing considerations
Narcotic	Morphine sulfate	Severe pain.	Subcutaneous: 5-15 mg every 3-4 hours as needed.	ADVERSE REACTIONS: Respiratory depression, decreased cough reflex, bradycardia, postural hypotension, nausea, vomiting, constipation, urinary retention, pruritus, diaphoresis. CONTRAINDICATIONS: Hypersensitivity to opiates, respiratory depression, increased intracranial pressure, head injuries, convulsive disorders, acute bronchial asthma, undiagnosed acute abdominal conditions.	1. Consult with the physician prior to administering this medication if the respiratory rate is below 12/minute or if the pupils are constricted or dilated. 2. Encourage the postoperative patient to turn, cough, and breathe deeply to prevent atelectasis. 3. Monitor urinary output. Encourage the patient to void every 4 hours, and notify the physician if the output decreases, despite adequate fluid intake. 4. Caution the ambulatory patient about severe postural hypotension. 5. Ambulatory patients experiencing nausea and vomiting may obtain relief of these symptoms by lying down. 6. Encourage a high-residue diet to counteract the constipating effects of the drug. 7. Tolerance, as well as physiologic and psychic dependence, may occur with repeated use. Therefore evaluate the pain carefully and suggest that the physician order a milder narcotic or nonnarcotic analgesic when deemed appropriate.
	Meperidine hydrochloride (Demerol)	Preoperative sedation; moderate to severe pain.	Oral, subcutaneous, intramuscular: 50-150 mg every 3-4 hours as needed.	ADVERSE REACTIONS: Similar to morphine in equianalgesic doses but less constipating and less likely to cause urinary retention. CONTRAINDICATIONS: Similar to morphine; use of MAO inhibitors within 14 days.	1. See morphine, nursing considerations 1, 2, 4, 5, and 7. 2. Do not mix this drug in the same syringe with barbiturates.

ANALGESICS—cont'd

Drug group	Drug	Urologic indications	Usual adult dosage	Adverse reactions and contraindications	Nursing considerations
	Codeine	Mild to moderate pain.	Oral, subcutaneous, intramuscular: 15-60 mg 4 times a day as needed.	ADVERSE REACTIONS: Depression of cough reflex, constipation, light-headedness, dizziness, sedation, nausea, vomiting, dermatologic reactions, euphoria, dysphoria. CONTRAINDICATIONS: Hypersensitivity to codeine.	1. See morphine, nursing considerations 1, 2, 6, and 7. 2. Concomitant administration of acetaminophen or aspirin enhances analgesic effect.
	Pentazocine hydrochloride (Talwin)	Moderate to severe pain.	Oral: 50-100 mg every 3-4 hours, not to exceed 600 mg/day. Intramuscular, intravenous, subcutaneous: 30 mg every 3-4 hours.	ADVERSE REACTIONS: Sedation, respiratory depression, hallucinations, sweating, dizziness, nausea, hypertension. CONTRAINDICATION: Hypersensitivity to pentazocine.	1. This drug is a mild narcotic antagonist and therefore may precipitate withdrawal symptoms in a patient who has been receiving opiates regularly. 2. Rotate injection sites and be alert for sloughing, induration, or nodule formation. 3. Tolerance to analgesic effect may occur, but psychic or physical dependence is unlikely unless the patient has a history of drug abuse.
Nonnarcotic	Propoxyphene hydrochloride (Darvon, Dolene, others)	Mild to moderate pain.	Oral: 65 mg every 4 hours as needed.	ADVERSE REACTIONS: Dizziness, sedation, nausea. CONTRAINDICATIONS: Hypersensitivity to propoxyphene; patients who are suicidal or addiction prone.	1. Concomitant administration of aspirin enhances the analgesic effect. 2. Caution the ambulatory patient about dizziness. 3. Caution the patient to limit his intake of alcohol while taking this drug. 4. Tolerance, as well as physical and psychic dependence, may occur after excessive use.

Continued.

ANALGESICS—cont'd

Drug group	Drug	Urologic indications	Usual adult dosage	Adverse reactions and contraindications	Nursing considerations
Urinary tract analgesic	Phenazopyridine hydrochloride (Pyridium)	Pain associated with irritation of the urinary tract mucosa.	Oral: 200 mg 3 times a day.	ADVERSE REACTIONS: Mild gastrointestinal disturbances, headache, vertigo, blood dyscrasias, jaundice, renal stones. CONTRAINDICATIONS: Hypersensitivity to phenazopyridine, impaired renal function.	1. Administer this drug after meals. 2. Warn the patient that his urine will be reddish orange. 3. Check skin and sclerae periodically for a yellowish tinge. If this occurs, consult with the physician before giving the next dose. It may indicate drug accumulation due to renal impairment. 4. Maintain adequate hydration. 5. Urine tests that rely on color reactions may be invalidated.

DRUGS ACTING ON THE AUTONOMIC NERVOUS SYSTEM

Drug group	Drug	Urologic indications	Usual adult dosage	Adverse reactions and contraindications	Nursing considerations
Anticholinergics (parasympatholytics)	Belladonna and opium suppository (B & O Supprette no. 15A and no. 16A)	Reduction of bladder spasms and ureteral colic, most commonly caused by catheters and suprapubic tubes. This drug has antispasmodic as well as analgesic actions.	One Supprette per rectum once or twice a day, as needed.	ADVERSE REACTIONS: Drowsiness, dry mouth, urinary retention, photophobia, rapid pulse, dizziness, blurred vision, nausea, vomiting, constipation, dermatologic reactions. CONTRAINDICATIONS: Glaucoma, severe cardiac, renal, or hepatic disease, bronchial asthma, narcotic idiosyncrasies, respiratory depression, convulsive disorders, acute alcoholism, within 72 hours of most types of prostatic surgery.	1. Explain to the patient that the medication is to relieve pain and is not for catharsis, as many assume when they see a suppository. 2. Moisten Supprette with water or water-soluble lubricant before inserting. 3. Notify the physician if there is a considerable rise in the patient's pulse rate. 4. Repeated use of this drug may result in tolerance as well as physiologic and psychic dependence.
	Propantheline bromide (Pro-Banthine)	Reduction of bladder spasms and ureteral colic, most commonly caused by catheters and suprapubic tubes; also used in urodynamic evaluation and in the treatment of certain types of hyperreflexive neurogenic bladder.	Oral: 15 mg 4 times a day (dosage is adjusted according to individual response).	ADVERSE REACTIONS: Tachycardia, drowsiness, dizziness, dry mouth, decreased sweating, blurred vision, constipation. CONTRAINDICATIONS: Glaucoma, severe cardiovascular disease, gastrointestinal obstruction, ulcerative colitis, intestinal atony, hiatal hernia associated with reflux esophagitis, myasthenia gravis, patients with prostatic hyperplasia (unless they have an indwelling urethral catheter).	1. Give after meals to avoid the effects of decreased salivary secretion (difficulty swallowing due to dry mouth). 2. Warn the patient that the drug may cause blurred vision. 3. Encourage a high-residue diet to counteract the constipating effects of the drug. 4. Suggest chewing gum or hard candy if the patient has a dry mouth. 5. Administration of this drug in high environmental temperature may result in heat prostration due to decreased sweating. 6. This drug may delay the absorption of other oral medications given concomitantly.

Continued.

DRUGS ACTING ON THE AUTONOMIC NERVOUS SYSTEM—cont'd

Drug group	Drug	Urologic indications	Usual adult dosage	Adverse reactions and contraindications	Nursing considerations
	Oxybutynin chloride (Ditropan)	Management of certain types of hyper-reflexive neurogenic bladder conditions. (It causes an increase in bladder capacity and a delay in the initial desire to void.)	Oral: 5 mg twice or three times a day.	ADVERSE REACTIONS: See propantheline bromide. CONTRAINDICATIONS: See propantheline bromide.	See propantheline bromide.
Cholinergic (parasympatho-mimetic)	Bethanechol chloride (Urecholine, Myotonachol, others)	Reduction of nonobstructive urinary retention and management of certain types of atonic neurogenic bladder conditions (it increases bladder contractility).	Oral or subcutaneous: 10-50 mg 3 or 4 times a day (dosage and route of administration are individualized).	ADVERSE REACTIONS: Abdominal discomfort, salivation, sweating, flushed skin. Larger doses are more likely to result in symptoms related to parasympathetic stimulation: headache, colicky pain, diarrhea, nausea, vomiting, asthma, decrease in blood pressure. CONTRAINDICATIONS: Hypersensitivity to bethanechol chloride, peptic ulcer, bronchial asthma, severe bradycardia or hypotension, following recent bladder surgery or gastrointestinal resection and anastomosis, bladder neck obstruction, others (consult *Physician's Desk Reference*).	1. Observe the patient closely for untoward effects, particularly at the commencement of treatment. 2. Monitor pulse and blood pressure. 3. When administering the drug subcutaneously, aspirate before injecting to avoid inadvertent administration directly into the bloodstream, and have a subcutaneous syringe of atropine (0.6 mg) on hand to counteract severe side effects if they occur. 4. Give oral preparation at a time when the stomach is relatively empty to prevent nausea and vomiting.

DRUGS ACTING ON THE AUTONOMIC NERVOUS SYSTEM—cont'd

Drug group	Drug	Urologic indications	Usual adult dosage	Adverse reactions and contraindications	Nursing considerations
Antiadrenergic (sympatholytic)	Phenoxybenz-amine hydro-chloride (Diben-zyline)	Autonomic hyperre-flexia due to neuro-genic bladder. Moderate outflow obstruction (e.g., prostatism).	Route and dosage are individualized. Oral: 10 mg 1 to 3 times a day.	ADVERSE REACTIONS: Nasal congestion, miosis, postural hypotension, tachycardia, gastrointestinal irritation, ejaculatory inhibition. CONTRAINDICATIONS: Hypersensitivity to phenoxybenzamine hydrochloride, conditions where a fall in blood pressure would be undesirable.	1. Administer with food or milk to decrease gastric irritation. 2. Monitor blood pressure and report significant decreases. 3. Caution the patient about possible dizziness. 4. Explain to the patient about the possibility of ejaculatory failure and that it is a temporary condition that will subside if the medication is discontinued.
	Phentolamine hydrochloride (Regitine)	Diagnostic test for pheochromocytoma; urodynamic evaluation of internal sphincter resistance.	Intravenous: 1 mg/minute infusion.	ADVERSE REACTIONS: Acute and prolonged hypotension, cardiac arrhythmias, dizziness, flushing, orthostatic hypotension, gastrointesinal disturbances. CONTRAINDICATIONS: Hypersensitivity to phentolamine, history of myocardial infarction, coronary artery disease.	1. Check the patient's blood pressure after urodynamic test. 2. Have the patient sit and dangle his legs before standing up, to reduce orthostatic hypotension.
Adrenergic (sympathomimetic)	Ephedrine sulfate	Correction of mild stress incontinence (it increases bladder neck and urethral resistance); management of certain types of enuresis.	Oral: 15-50 mg every 3-4 hours (dosage is individualized).	ADVERSE REACTIONS: Insomnia, tachycardia, nervousness, nausea, headache. CONTRAINDICATIONS: Severe cardiac disease, hypertension.	1. If possible, avoid administering this drug at bedtime (unless used for enuresis) to reduce the risk of insomnia. 2. Monitor blood pressure 30 minutes after administration and report significant elevations.

Continued.

MISCELLANEOUS DRUGS FREQUENTLY USED IN UROLOGY

Drug group	Drug	Urologic considerations	Usual adult dosage	Adverse reactions and contraindications	Nursing considerations
	Ascorbic acid (Vitamin C)	Concomitant use with methenamine mandelate to ensure low urinary pH; prevention of formation of urinary calculi such as calcium phosphate; reduction of skin breakdown due to alkaline urine in patients with urostomies.	Oral: 2 g or more daily in divided dosage (usually 4 times a day).	ADVERSE REACTIONS: Diarrhea (rare), precipitation of cystine or uric acid stones.	1. High doses of ascorbic acid may cause invalid results in tests for glycosuria (e.g., false positive results with Benedict's solution and Clinitest; false negative results with Clinistix and Tes-Tape). 2. Caution the patient with conduit diversion or ureterosigmoidostomy not to take ascorbic acid without the physician's knowledge and not to exceed the prescribed dosage.
	Castor oil	Elimination of fecal matter from the bowel prior to diagnostic x-ray examination.	Oral: 15 mg.	ADVERSE REACTIONS: Nausea, severe diarrhea, abdominal cramps, dehydration, hypokalemia, acidosis, alkalosis. CONTRAINDICATIONS: Symptoms of appendicitis (e.g., nausea, vomiting, abdominal pain).	1. Administer on an empty stomach. 2. Mix with cold fruit juice or soft drink to disguise unpleasant taste. 3. Provide the patient with a bedpan or easy access to bathroom. 4. Elderly patients may be incontinent of stool. 5. Reassure the patient that it is not abnormal to be unable to move the bowels for 1 or 2 days after catharsis.

MISCELLANEOUS DRUGS FREQUENTLY USED IN UROLOGY—cont'd

Drug group	Drug	Urologic indications	Usual adult dosage	Adverse reactions and contraindications	Nursing considerations
	Diethylstilbestrol	Palliative therapy in advanced prostatic cancer.	Oral: 1-3 mg daily.	ADVERSE REACTIONS: Sodium retention, hypertension, thromboembolic and cardiovascular disorders, gynecomastia, testicular atrophy, loss of libido, impotence. CONTRAINDICATIONS: Active thromboembolic disorders, history of angina.	1. Monitor the patient's weight and blood pressure and report significant increases. 2. Advise the patient to report any leg pain or soreness so that deep vein thrombosis can be detected and treated as soon as possible. 3. Provide emotional support to help the patient cope with changes in his body image.
	Methionine (Pedameth)	Reduction of urinary odor in incontinent patients or those with urostomies who are self-conscious about urinary odor; reduction of dermatitis and ulceration caused by ammoniacal urine in the incontinent patient.	Oral: one capsule 3-4 times a day.	CONTRAINDICATION: Liver disease.	1. Correct other causes of urinary odor (e.g., infection, poor hygiene) before using as a deodorant. 2. Give with food or milk.
	Methylene blue (Urolene Blue)	Detection of urinary drainage in surgical wounds.	Intravenous: one 10-ml ampule of 1% solution.	CONTRAINDICATION: Hypersensitivity to methylene blue.	1. Warn the patient that his urine may have a blue-green color. 2. Hypochlorite solution can be used to remove methylene blue stains.
	Aminocaproic acid (Amicar)	Treatment of bleeding due to fibrinolysis following prostatic surgery or neoplastic disease.	Intravenous, oral: 4-5 gm in the first hour followed by 1 gm every hour for 8 hours.	ADVERSE REACTIONS: Gastrointestinal disturbances, tinnitus, dizziness, conjunctival suffusion, nasal stuffiness, headache, skin rash. CONTRAINDICATIONS: Evidence of active intravascular clotting process.	1. When giving intravenous preparation, observe all precautions against thrombophlebitis. 2. Avoid rapid intravenous administration because it may produce hypotension, bradycardia, and arrhythmias.

Goodman, L.S., and Gilman, A.: The pharmacological basis of therapeutics, ed. 5, New York, 1975, Macmillan Publishing Co., Inc.
Govoni, L.E., and Hayes, J.E.: Drugs and nursing implications, ed. 3, New York, 1978, Appleton-Century-Crofts.
Meyers, F.H., Jawetz, E., and Goldfein, A.: Review of medical pharmacology, ed. 5, Los Altos, Calif., 1976, Lange Medical Publications.
Physician's desk reference, ed. 35, Oradell, N.J., 1980, Medical Economics Co.

APPENDIX B

Urologic glossary

androgen Masculinizing hormone (e.g., testosterone).

anuria Absence of urinary output.

azospermia Absence of sperm in the seminal fluid.

azotemia Excess of urea or other nitrogenous bodies in the blood.

bacteriuria Bacteria in the urine.

catheter A hollow tube used for drainage of urine.

chordee Ventral curvature of the penis.

cryptorchidism Failure of the testes to descend into the scrotum.

cystitis Inflammation of the bladder.

dyspareunia Painful intercourse.

dysuria Painful or difficult urination.

enuresis Bed-wetting due to involuntary nocturnal micturition.

epispadias A congenital defect in which the urethra opens onto the dorsum of the penis.

glycosuria The presence of glucose in the urine.

hematuria The presence of blood in the urine.

Hemovac Incisional drainage device using negative pressure produced by a portable suction receptacle.

hesitancy Difficulty initiating urination.

hypospadias A congenital defect in which the urethra opens on the ventral aspect of the penis or on the perineum in the male and in the vagina in the female.

incontinence Involuntary urination.

  overflow (paradoxical) incontinence Leakage of urine from a distended bladder in the absence of effective contractions.

  stress incontinence Loss of urine associated with sudden increase of intraabdominal pressure.

  urgency (irritative) incontinence The urge to void occurring simultaneously with bladder contraction, so urine is expressed before the individual is prepared to void.

Jackson-Pratt drain Incisional drainage device using negative pressure produced by a portable suction receptacle.

lithotomy position Supine position with hips and knees abducted and flexed.

micturition Urination.

nocturia Urinary frequency occurring at night.

oligospermia Subnormal sperm count.

oliguria Diminished urinary output in relation to fluid intake.

paraphimosis Contraction of the foreskin in the retracted position so that it cannot be replaced to its normal position.

Penrose drain Incisional drainage device composed of a flexible rubber tube that acts as a conduit for drainage from a wound onto a dressing.

Pfannenstiel incision A curved transverse suprapubic incision used for many types of urologic and gynecologic surgery.

phimosis Contraction of the foreskin (in its normal position) preventing it from being retracted back over the glans.

priapism Persistent, abnormal, sustained erection, usually without sexual desire.

prostatism Obstruction of the urethra secondary to prostatic enlargement, resulting in varying degrees of urinary retention.

pyocystis Accumulation of pus in the bladder.

resectoscope Urologic endoscopic instrument used for removal of tissue via a cutting electrode.

residual urine Urine that remains in the bladder after voiding.

staghorn calculus A type of renal stone characterized by irregular branches of calculus material.

stenosis Any narrowing of a tubelike structure that conveys substances.

stent A device (often a thin catheter) used to support and maintain the patency of a tubelike structure (e.g., ureter).

strangury Painful urination.

tenesmus Painful bladder spasms.

trabeculation Honeycomb appearance of the bladder wall resulting from hypertrophy of the bladder muscles.

tube drain A semirigid plastic incisional drain that acts as a conduit for drainage from a wound into a bag connected to the distal end of the drain and strapped to the patient's thigh.

undiversion Surgical procedure that reestablishes the normal route of urine after prior surgery, such as ileal conduit diversion.

uremia The retention of excessive by-products of protein metabolism (urea) in the blood and the toxicity resulting from it.

urgency An intense desire to void.

urinary calculus A "stone"; a solid concretion of substances precipitated from urine.

urinary cast A mold of a renal tubule composed of blood cells or other abnormal constituents in the urine; one of the microscopic findings in a urinalysis.

urinoma An abnormal collection of urine anywhere near the urinary tract resulting from previous extravasation.

uroncus *See* Urinoma.

urolithiasis The formation of urinary calculi.

uropathy Urinary tract disease.

urosanguineous Fluid composed of urine and serosanguineous drainage from a surgical wound.

urostomy A stoma surgically created from the ileum, colon, or ureter through which **urine** flows.

urothelium Transitional cell epithelium that lines the entire urinary tract.

vesical Pertaining to the bladder.

APPENDIX C

Catheterization procedures

INDWELLING URETHRAL CATHETERIZATION: FEMALE

EQUIPMENT: Nos. 16 to 22 F Foley catheter
                Sterile drapes
                Sterile forceps
                Sterile sponges
                Povidone-iodine solution
                Sterile lubricant
                Basin to collect urine
                Sterile field
                Syringe with 5 to 30 ml sterile water
                Drainage bag and tubing
                (See step 2 for optional equipment)

Procedure steps	Rationale
1. Explain the procedure to the patient.	Understanding a procedure reduces patient anxiety.
2. Assemble all equipment on a tray to the right of the nurse performing the catheterization.* In addition to the equipment listed above, an extra catheter and a pair of sterile gloves of an appropriate size to fit the nurse are often included. These gloves are particularly important if a disposable catheter tray is being used. Such prepackaged kits include a pair of one-size-fits-all gloves which are usually big and cumbersome for female nurses.	Having the extra catheter at the bedside saves time if the original one is contaminated during the procedure. The nurse is also more likely to change a contaminated catheter if a replacement is readily available. The fitted gloves enable the nurse to perform the procedure with better dexterity. Some nurses put the one-size-fits-all glove **over** the fitted glove on the right hand and wear it for steps 9 through 13. It is then shaken off, leaving a completely uncontaminated, well-fitting glove on the hand that inserts the catheter.
3. Place waste receptacle at a convenient location near the patient's bed.	
4. Place the patient in either a dorsal recumbent position with lower limbs flexed and rotated outward or the Sims position (i.e., the patient is on her side with the inferior arm behind her back and the superior thigh and knee flexed as much as possible).	The Sims position is useful if the patient has hip contractures.

*Instructions referring to right and left hand concern right-handed individuals. Those who are left-handed should reverse all such references.

Procedure steps	Rationale
5. Place a moisture-proof pad under the patient's hips.	
6. Direct a light onto the perineal area.	
7. Open the prepackaged catheter tray (or arrange a sterile field if a disposable kit is not used).	
8. Drape the patient with sterile drapes, taking care to handle them only by the corners.	Draping is necessary to prevent contamination of the catheter if it should inadvertently touch the area around the perineum.
9. Apply sterile gloves of appropriate size.	
10. Lubricate the tip of the catheter and leave it on the sterile field.*	
11. Pour povidone-iodine onto the sterile sponges.*	
12. With the left thumb and forefinger, separate the labia minora so that the urethral meatus is exposed. (If the patient is in the Sims position, lift the superior labium to expose the urethral meatus.)	
13. Clean the meatus with forceps and sponges soaked in povidine-iodine, wiping from the urethral meatus toward the rectum. Discard each sponge after each wipe. If the meatus is not immediately identifiable, take advantage of the wiping maneuvers to find it between the folds of mucosa.	Cleaning in this manner prevents contamination of the urethral meatus by rectal flora.
14. Insert a well-lubricated catheter 2 or 3 inches into the urethra, keeping distal end over the basin. Insert it an additional inch after urine begins to flow.	This ensures that the balloon portion of the catheter is in the bladder and not the urethra.
If urine does not flow through the catheter after inserting it 3 or 4 inches, the catheter is in the vagina and not the urethra. In such an instance, leave the catheter in place and insert the extra catheter into the urethra. Be certain to reglove after opening the second catheter package, and clean the meatal area again prior to inserting the catheter.	The urethral meatus is not always easy to find in older, multiparous women. Leaving the first catheter in place usually prevents a repeat of the first mistake. Under no circumstances should the same catheter be withdrawn and reinserted because it is highly contaminated with vaginal flora.
15. Inflate the balloon with sterile water via the syringe, and connect the catheter to the tubing and drainage bag.	**Sterile** water is used because, in the unlikely event that the balloon breaks, the bladder will not be contaminated.
If the patient has any pain during inflation, deflate the balloon at once, insert the catheter farther up into the bladder, and reinflate the balloon.	Pain during inflation of the balloon indicates that the balloon is in the urethra instead of the bladder. This could be hazardous to the patient.
16. Gently apply traction to the catheter until resistance is felt (i.e., the catheter is resting at the base of the bladder).	
17. Tape the tubing (not the catheter) to the patient's thigh.	

*It is assumed that a disposable kit is being used and that the packages of lubricant and antiseptic are sterile and therefore will not contaminate the sterile gloves. Otherwise, steps 10 and 11 must be done **before** donning gloves.

INDWELLING URETHRAL CATHETERIZATION: MALE

EQUIPMENT: Nos. 16 to 18 F Foley catheter
Sterile drapes
Sterile forceps
Sterile sponges
Povidone-iodine solution
Sterile lubricant
Basin to collect urine
Sterile field
Syringe with 5 to 30 ml sterile water
Drainage bag and tubing
(See step 2 for optional equipment)

Procedure steps	Rationale
1. Explain the procedure to the patient.	Understanding a procedure reduces patient anxiety.
2. Assemble all equipment on a tray to the right of the nurse performing the catheterization.* In addition to the equipment listed above, an extra catheter and a pair of sterile gloves of an appropriate size to fit the nurse are often included. These gloves are particularly important if a disposable catheter tray is being used. Such prepackaged kits include a pair of one-size-fits-all gloves, which are usually big and cumbersome for female nurses.	Having the extra catheter at the bedside saves time if the original one is contaminated during the procedure. The nurse is also more likely to change a contaminated catheter if a replacement is readily available. The fitted gloves enable the nurse to perform the procedure with better dexterity. Some nurses put the one-size-fits-all glove **over** the fitted glove on the right hand and wear it for steps 9 through 12. It is then shaken off, leaving a completely uncontaminated, well-fitting glove on the hand that inserts the catheter.
3. Place a waste receptacle at a convenient location near the bed.	
4. Place the patient in a dorsal recumbent position with legs extended.	
5. Place a moisture-proof pad under the patient's hips.	
6. Direct a light onto the perineal area.	
7. Open the prepackaged catheter tray (or arrange sterile field if disposable kit is not being used).	
8. Drape the patient with the sterile drapes, handling them only by the corners.	Draping is necessary to prevent contamination of the catheter if it inadvertently touches the area around the penis.

*Instructions referring to right and left hand concern right-handed individuals. Those who are left-handed should reverse all such references.

Procedure steps	Rationale

9. Apply sterile gloves.

10. Apply lubricant to approximately 7 inches of the catheter, starting at the tip.*

11. Pour antiseptic solution onto sterile sponges.*

12. Grasp the shaft of the penis with the left hand and clean the glans and meatus with sterile forceps and sponges soaked in povidone-iodine. Maintain the position of the left hand through step 15.

13. Hold the catheter with the right hand so that the distal portion of it is folded in the palm of the hand and the tip is controlled by the thumb and forefinger.

    Keeping the distal portion of the catheter within the hand prevents inadvertent contamination of it during insertion. In the male patient this is particularly important because almost the entire length of the catheter is passed into the urethra.

14. While holding the penis almost perpendicular to the body, insert the catheter into the urethra, keeping distal end over the basin. If resistance is encountered, increase traction on the penis while applying gentle pressure to the catheter. If the catheter still cannot be advanced, do not attempt to force it; notify the urologist.

    Frequently there is some resistance at the bladder neck. Patients with enlarged prostates may be extremely difficult to catheterize, and a nurse should not attempt it. A Coudé-tip catheter is sometimes used in these instances because the curve at the tip of the catheter facilitates passage through the obstructed area.

15. Continue to insert the catheter beyond the point where urine begins to flow, almost to its bifurcation.

    This ensures that the balloon portion is well within the bladder and not in the prostatic urethra.

16. Inflate the balloon with sterile water via the syringe, and connect the catheter to the drainage bag.

    If the patient has pain during inflation of the balloon, deflate it and advance the catheter farther into the bladder before reinflating.

    Pain during inflation of the balloon indicates that the balloon is in the urethra instead of the bladder. This could be hazardous to the patient.

17. After inflation, gently apply traction to the catheter until resistance is felt (i.e., the balloon is resting at the base of the bladder).

18. Tape the tubing (not the catheter) to the patient's thigh or abdomen.

*It is assumed that a disposable kit is being used and that the packages of lubricant and antiseptic are sterile and therefore will not contaminate sterile gloves. Otherwise steps 10 and 11 must be done **before** donning gloves.

STRAIGHT CATHETERIZATION
Sterile straight catheterization

Sterile straight catheterization is used when a "clean catch" urine specimen for culture is inappropriate or unobtainable. It is also used to empty the bladder when the underlying disorder is not known. The procedure is similar to insertion of an indwelling urethral catheter, except that a nonretention catheter is used. (See steps 1 to 14 of catheterization with an indwelling urethral catheter.) The equipment must include a sterile specimen container as well as a basin if a urine specimen is to be collected, and care must be taken not to contaminate the distal end of the catheter. When the bladder is empty, the catheter is withdrawn. The volume of urine output should be recorded.

PROCEDURE FOR CLEAN INTERMITTENT SELF-CATHETERIZATION

EQUIPMENT: No. 14 F clear plastic catheter; regular length for a male, cut to a shorter, more convenient size for a female (a Coudé-tip catheter may be required for a male)
Lubricant (optional for a female)
Basin for urine
Soap and water

Clean intermittent self-catheterization

Clean intermittent catheterization is used to manage urinary retention when the cause of the bladder dysfunction has been established (e.g., atonic neurogenic bladder). It must be done on a regular basis to be safe and effective. It is usually taught to the patient (or significant other) so that the procedure can be performed anywhere the patient happens to be.

The importance of performing this procedure regularly cannot be emphasized enough. Overdistention of the bladder between catheterizations predisposes the patient to infection. Introduction of a few bacteria into the urethra is not considered hazardous, provided that the bladder is not permitted to become distended beyond a volume of 500 ml.

Procedure steps	Rationale
Female	
1. Position the patient on the examination table with her feet on the table, her lower extremities flexed, and her knees apart. Place a mirror in front of her, and adjust the light so that her perineum is easily visualized. Later the mirror will be unnecessary, and the patient will do the procedure either standing in front of or sitting on the toilet.	
2. Explain to the patient how to palpate the meatus. With her left hand* she should hold the labia apart with her index and ring fingers and palpate the urethra with the middle finger.	Eventually, most patients can perform the procedure entirely by touch. This should be encouraged because reliance on lighting and a mirror will limit the patient's ability to catheterize herself under less than optimum conditions.
3. Instruct the patient to hold the catheter in her right hand between thumb and forefinger and insert it into the meatus. (In the initial period, while the patient is becoming accustomed to performing the procedure, a water-soluble sterile lubricant is sometimes used on the tip of the catheter.) Be certain the distal end of the catheter is held over the basin.	Although it is unnecessary to lubricate this catheter for the female, it facilitates insertion of the catheter the first few times the patient attempts to catheterize herself, when inexperience with the procedure may result in trauma to urethral tissue.

*Instructions referring to right and left hand concern right-handed individuals. Those who are left-handed should reverse all such references.

Procedure steps	**Rationale**

4. Have the patient advance the catheter until urine flows and leave it in place until the flow ceases. If possible, the patient should bear down with her abdominal muscles to facilitate complete emptying of the bladder.

5. Instruct the patient to remove the catheter and to wash her hands and the catheter in soap and water. The catheter should be rinsed thoroughly on the inside and outside with clear water.

6. Emphasize to the patient the importance of regular catheterization. The physician will determine the frequency in accordance with the particular patient's bladder capacity and volume of fluid intake. It is usually prescribed every 4 to 6 hours.

Male

1. Position the patient either standing or sitting.

2. Have him apply a liberal amount of sterile, water-soluble lubricant to the catheter.

3. Instruct him to grasp his penis with his left hand* and insert the catheter into the meatus until urine begins to flow (approximately 6 inches). He may have to apply a small amount of traction to his penis and move it perpendicular to his body to maneuver the catheter past the bladder neck. Be certain the distal end of the catheter is held over the basin.

4. Have the patient leave the catheter in place until urine ceases to flow. If possible, he should bear down with his abdominal muscles to facilitate complete emptying of his bladder.

5. Instruct the patient to remove the catheter and wash his hands and the catheter in soap and water. The catheter should be rinsed thoroughly on the inside and outside with clear water.

6. Emphasize to the patient the importance of regular catheterization. The physician will determine the frequency in accordance with the particular patient's bladder capacity and volume of fluid intake. It is usually prescribed every 4 to 6 hours.

*Instructions referring to right and left hand concern right-handed individuals. Those who are left-handed should reverse all such references.

DOUBLE-LUMEN CATHETERIZATION OF ILEAL OR COLON CONDUIT STOMA

Although a urostomy patient can be catheterized by inserting a standard urethral catheter (nos. 12 to 16 F) into the stoma, the use of a double-lumen catheter has become popular because it decreases the risk of a contaminated specimen and may limit the retrograde ascent of bacteria from the distal portion of the stoma (Fig. C-1).

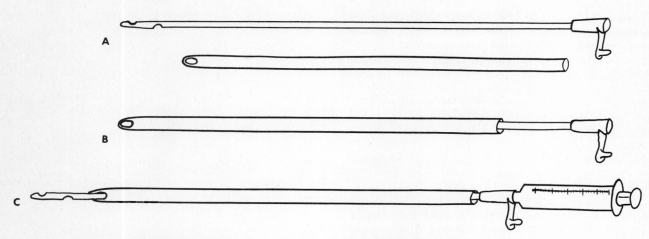

Fig. C-1. Formation of double-lumen catheter for catheterization of ileal or colon conduit stoma. **A,** Infant feeding tube and whistle-tip catheter prior to formation of double-lumen catheter. **B,** Infant feeding tube within the catheter, ready for insertion into stoma. **C,** After insertion, syringe is attached to distal end and feeding tube is advanced through catheter hole to withdraw urine specimen.

EQUIPMENT: Sterile no. 16 F whistle-tip catheter
Sterile no. 8 F polyethylene infant feeding tube
Sterile scissors
Sterile drapes
Sterile sponges
Sterile forceps
Sterile gloves
Sterile water-soluble lubricant
Sterile 10-ml syringe
Povidone-iodine
Sterile culture container
Soap, water, and 4 × 4-inch gauze pads

Procedure steps	Rationale
1. Explain the procedure to the patient.	Understanding a procedure reduces patient anxiety.
2. Place a waterproof pad under the patient's body and have the patient in a comfortable supine or semi-Fowler's position.	Some urine may drain from the stoma during the period when the ostomy pouch is removed.
3. Remove the ostomy pouch and clean the stoma and peristomal area with soap and water. Rinse well.	

Procedure steps	Rationale
4. Arrange sterile field on a tray to the right* of the nurse, with all sterile equipment readily available.	
5. Pour povidone-iodine onto sterile sponges.	These steps are done before sterile gloves are donned because the containers are often not sterile. If, however, the lubricant and antiseptic are in sterile packages, these steps can be done later.
6. Pour a liberal amount of lubricant onto a small area of the sterile field so that the catheter tip can be dipped into it immediately prior to insertion.	
7. Remove the catheter and feeding tube from their wrappers and drop them onto the sterile field (without touching them).	
8. Don sterile gloves.	
9. Using the sterile scissors, cut the end of the catheter so that it is 1 inch shorter than the feeding tube. Insert the feeding tube into the catheter, keeping the tip retracted within the lumen of the catheter (Fig. C-1, B). Leave it on the sterile field.	
10. Place sterile drapes around the stoma.	This prevents contamination of the catheter if it touches anything around the stoma.
11. Clean the stoma with the sponges saturated with povidone-iodine, holding the sponges with the sterile forceps and working from the center of the stoma outward.	
12. Lubricate the catheter tip and insert the catheter (and feeding tube within it) into the stoma, approximately 2 inches. Do not force it; insert it gently and gradually. It is sometimes necessary to wait until the stoma and conduit relax before the catheter can be inserted the full 2 inches.	
13. After the catheter is in place, attach the syringe to the feeding tube and then advance the feeding tube into the catheter as far as it will go (Fig. C-1, C). it may be necessary to rotate the inner tube to manipulate it through the opening of the catheter.	
14. Gently withdraw 2 to 5 ml of urine into the syringe. If the urine is difficult to aspirate, having the patient cough, sit up, or turn onto the stoma side may help express the urine.	
15. Retract the feeding tube so that the tip is within the catheter, and remove the catheter from the stoma.	
16. Transfer the urine from the syringe into a sterile container.	
17. Apply the ostomy pouch.	

*Instructions referring to right and left hand concern right-handed individuals. Those who are left-handed should reverse all such references.

Index